Lecture Notes in
Medical Informatics

Edited by D. A. B. Lindberg and P. L. Reichertz

W0043429

1

Medical Informatics Europe 78

First Congress of the European Federation
for Medical Informatics

Proceedings, Cambridge, England
September 4 – 8, 1978

Edited by J. Anderson

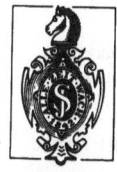

Springer-Verlag
Berlin Heidelberg New York 1978

Editor

John Anderson
Department of Medicine
King's College Hospital
Medical School
Denmark Hill
London SE5 9RS/GB

Congress of the European Federation for Medical Infor-
    matics, 1st, Cambridge, Eng., 1978.
    Medical informatics Europe 78.

    (Lecture notes in medical informatics ; 1)
    Bibliography: p.
    Includes index.
    1. Medicine--Data processing--Congresses.
I. Anderson, John, 1921-   II. Title. III. Se-
ries.
R858.A1C66 1978   610'.28'54   78-15019

ISBN-13:978-3-540-08916-2   e-ISBN-13:978-3-642-93095-9
DOI: 10.1007/978-3-642-93095-9

2145/3140-543210

INTRODUCTION

These proceedings reflect the major scientific contribution by the First
International Congress of the European Federation for Medical Informatics. The
European Federation for Medical Informatics is a co-operative venture between the
National Informatics Societies of Europe. It is sponsoring this first inter-
national meeting organised by the Medical Specialist Groups of the British
Society under the guidance of a European Scientific Programme Committee.

The challenge of medical informatics has been well taken and the scientific papers
by its members cover a wide range of topics dealing with medical records,
laboratory investigation, indexing and administrative systems, nursing records,
planning and administration modelling, data bases, text processing, transferability,
user education, privacy, etc. Not published in this volume are presentations by
industry about hardware and software. Also at the meeting there will be teaching
sessions for doctors, nurses, scientists and administrators who are just entering
this field which are also not published.

Medical informatics has established itself as an important area of medical activity
and its growing application, as this conference illustrates, suggests a very rich
potential for the future. Aids to medical decision making and modelling are newer
areas of activity, where significant progress has been made.

Sociological changes have taken place to meet this challenge and developments in
the issues of privacy and confidentiality are important, as also are user education,
and the teaching of medical informatics to medical students and to doctors.
Inevitably these changes illustrate that medical informatics has already had a
significant impact on medical teaching and training as well as in the relationship
of medicine to society.

I should like to thank the Programme Committee for their hard work in selecting
papers for the congress and the authors for their contributions. I have had a
great deal of help from Mrs E Mills and Miss M O'Hara and thank them for their
valuable support. Mrs Paula Stockham of Online Conferences has also rendered
invaluable assistance and smoothed out any difficulties.

I leave it to the reader to decide if our objectives in bringing readers up-to-date in this important area of medical informatics have been attained.

Professor J Anderson
Editor and
Chairman of the Programme Committee

CONTENTS

CORONARY CARE INFORMATION SYSTEM :
ITS USE IN THE ASSESSMENT OF PROGNOSIS
IN ACUTE MYOCARDIAL INFARCTION

Jos L. Willems, J. Pardaens
L. De Wolf, H. Ector and H. De Geest
Divisions of Medical Informatics
and Cardiology,
University of Leuven, Belgium

INTRODUCTION

As of October 1, 1973 data are collected in a standardized and prospective way from all patients admitted to the coronary care unit (CCU) in our institution. Information is gathered in a similar way from all patients admitted to the emergency department and the medical intensive care unit, whenever suspicion of acute myocardial infarction (MI) exists.

The primary objectives of these efforts are a study of the short and long term prognostic determinants in patients with acute MI and an assessment of critical factors in the management of these patients.

The collection and storage of the various data items in a coronary care information system and the use of these data in the off- and on-line determination of prognosis in patients suffering from acute myocardial infarction are described in this paper.

DATA BASE CONTENT

A total of over 250 different fixed items are coded and collected. The data collection primarily concerns non-invasive parameters, routinely gathered in a CCU.

Punch card oriented coding documents are filled in by physicians in the CCU and on the wards. Administrative data are collected from the patient admission subsystem of the hospital information system.

The data can be divided into 5 parts, as listed below.

1. Patient identification and historical data :

1.1 Patient identification and registration data :
  - patient name, address, sex, date of birth
  - source of admission, referring physician

1.2 Information with regard to the early stages of the acute episode :
  - date, time and place of onset of symptoms
  - reason and mode of admission, type of transportation
  - state of the patient at the time of registration
  - time of arrival in the hospital and CCU
  - ventricular fibrillation or standstill and anti-antiarrhythmic treatment given prior to admission

1.3 Symptoms in the 28 days preceding the onset of the present acute episode are coded according the WHO recommendations for the registration of ischaemic heart disease (1) with respect to their presence or absence, or are coded "unknown" in the absence of information.

1.4 Previous medical history with regard to cardiovascular diseases :
  - previous myocardial infarction, confirmation data available yes or no, number of "confirmed" infarctions, date of last attack
  - angina pectoris present before the 28-day period preceding the onset of the acute attack
  - intermittent claudication, history of cerebro-vascular accident, arterial hypertension, diabetes mellitus, atrioventricular conduction disturbances, congestive cardiac failure in the past, valvular heart disease
  - up to two other cardiovascular abnormalities.

1.5 Smoking habits:
  - consumption of cigarettes, cigars, pipes.

2. <u>Medical examination at admission</u> :

2.1 Physical examination :
  - body weight and height
  - overall hemodynamic status : absence or presence of signs of heart failure, pulmonary oedema, shock
  - heart rate, arterial blood pressure, respiratory rate
  - presence or absence of basal rales, 3rd and 4th heart sound, abnormal precordial pulsations, cardiomegaly, elevated systemic venous pressure, heart murmurs

2.2 ECG at admission :
- presence of unequivocal signs of acute myocardial infarction
- location and depth of infarction

2.3 Estimation of heart size and of presence of pulmonary conges-
tion or oedema, based on RX chest.

3. Data obtained during the stay and at discharge of the CCU :

3.1 Complications during stay in the CCU :

3.1.1 Presence or absence of various arrhythmias : sinus bra-
dycardia, sinus or atrial tachycardia, supraventricular
and ventricular extrasystoles, atrial flutter and fibrillation, ventricular tachycardia, idioventricular
rhythm, 2nd or 3rd degree AV-block, ventricular conduction disturbances, ventricular fibrillation or asystole.

3.1.2 Pumpfailure : congestive cardiac failure, hypotension,
pulmonary oedema, cardiogenic shock.

3.1.3 Thrombo-embolic complications.

3.1.4 Other complications : pericardial rub, papillary dys-
function, volume deficit, acute psychiatric disturbances, rupture of the septum or myocardial wall.

3.2 Laboratory results :
peak serum enzymes (SGOT, SGPT, LDH, CPK), peak leucocytosis,
cholesterol level, ABO and Rhesus blood group.

3.3 Indications wether special investigations have been performed
e.g. coronary arteriography, invasive hemodynamic monitoring,
His bundle recordings ....

3.4 Therapy :
- a check is made whether the patient received any of the following medications : digitalis, diuretics, atropine, lido-
caïne, quinidine, procaïnamide, aprindine, beta-block agents,
anticoagulant or fibrinolytic drugs, pressor-amines, corti-
coïds or one other drug not listed above.
- the reason and timing of eventual cardiac pacing and the
number of synchronous or asynchronous electrical cardiover-
sions are noted, as well as the application of artificial
ventilation and counter pulsation.

3.5 Clinical state and time of discharge.

3.6 CCU discharge diagnosis :
Allocation to categories of "definite", "possible" or "no"
acute myocardial infarction is made according the WHO defini-

tions and the criteria for the diagnosis are registered.

4. Hospital discharge information :

- clinical state at discharge (alive or dead)
- date and time of hospital discharge
- summary diagnosis and registration of complications if any since discharge out of the CCU.

5. Middle- and long-term survival information :

The dead or alive status of the patient is gathered from local community population registers at 2 year intervals.

DATA ANALYSIS

The data are checked for errors before and after entry into the information system. A plausibility program has been developed to test for inconsistencies and missing information. This program also stores the data in a sequential data file on disc and on magnetic tape.

Factors determining CCU, hospital and long-term survival have been studied using uni- and multivariate statistical analysis techniques with the help of the SPSS package (2) on an IBM 370/158 computer.

Cross tabulation of the data was carried out first for various data items in different subgroups. Differences in frequency distribution were tested using chi-square and t-tests. Discriminant analysis techniques were applied next in an attempt to detect the prognostic determinants in acute myocardial infarction. Multidimensional analysis is indeed needed in order to detect the independent contribution of each of the variables in the evolution of the disease.

Results of the univariate analysis and prior clinical knowledge served as basis for the preselection of a total of 38 variables. In a first run only clinical data obtained at admission were used. In the second run data gathered during the CCU stay were added. The 5 variables used in the Norris index (3), namely age, systolic blood pressure, ECG localisation of infarction, presence of pulmonary oedema and cardiomegaly based on chest X-ray findings, served as a third set of variables. In addition to the linear component the squared age, respiratory rate, heart rate and systolic blood pressure

were used, in the first two sets of variables, in order to take into
account the non-linear influence of these variables on mortality after acute myocardial infarction. Coding of the overall hemodynamic
clinical assessment was weighted accordingly. Multivariate discriminant analysis based on the stepwise addition of the variable that
contributed the largest increase in Rao V value, as computed by the
SPSS program, was applied.

Results of the off-line analysis (4) as well as a selection of the
data have been transferred, in a second phase, to an HP 2100 data management system and are on-line accessible in the CCU. For each new
patient survival scores can be derived in the CCU based on discriminant analysis functions, using data obtained at admission or during
the CCU stay. The scores are based on the data from the learning
population i.e. patients admitted between October 1, 1973 and September 30, 1976. The performance in survival prediction is being
tested on a new independent sample of patients admitted since October
1, 1976.

RESULTS
‾‾‾‾‾‾‾

Basic information on the learning population.

The learning population was drawn out of 2206 patients admitted
to the data base during the first 3 years of the project. Only patients who were still alive when they entered the hospital are included in the study.

1091 patients (818 male, 273 female) of the total population proved to have a documented acute MI, using WHO criteria. The mean age
of this group was 63.3 (SD 12) years. The difference in age between
men (61.3 $\pm$ 11) and women (69.5 $\pm$ 10) was highly significant.

The total hospital mortality was 20.2 % (N = 225). 23 (2.1 %)
patients died in the emergency department before they could be admitted to the CCU. 155 (14.2 %) patients did not survive the CCU
stay and 47 (4.3 %) died on the wards after the discharge of the CCU.

The median CCU and hospital stay for the total group with acute
MI was 3 1/2 and 12 days.

Prognostic determinants of short term mortality in acute MI.

Parameters which proved to have a significant independent influence on either CCU or hospital mortality were the following : hemodynamic state of the patient, presence of signs of heart failure, shock, pulmonary oedema (based on clinical or RX findings), cardiomegaly, age, sex, presence or absence of diabetes mellitus, systolic blood pressure, heart rate and respiratory rate at admission, ECG localisation of infarction, presence or absence of different arrhythmias : primary ventricular fibrillation, ventricular-, AV- or persistent (> 2 hr) sinus-tachycardia, AV-block, conduction disturbances and high risk PVC's.

Clinical assessment of the overall hemodynamic status of the patient proved to be by far, the most important predicting factor. Sex came out as a significant factor only once. A combination of the 16 parameters mentioned in the preceding paragraph resulted in correct prediction of CCU and hospital survival in 92 to 95 % of survivors and in 73 to 79 % of non-survivors in the training set (Tables 1 and 2). The highest accuracy figures apply to the prediction of CCU survival.

CONCLUSION

The discriminant analysis functions proved to have a high ability in predicting short-term survival after acute myocardial infarction. The performance in the prediction of mortality was significantly less. Figures between 73 and 79 % are nevertheless still high. The overall accuracy rate varied between 85 and 92.5 % in the training set. The formulas are presently being tested in a new independent group. Preliminary results obtained in the group of patients admitted between October 1, 1976 and December 31, 1977 will be presented at the conference. Long-term survival is similarly being analyzed.

Results obtained in this study, based on non-invasive measurements, made through careful bedside examination, compare favorably with the 72 % accuracy figure obtained in a recent study using a discriminant function based on invasive measurement of pulmonary capillary wedge pressure and heart rate. Addition of other clinical or hemodynamic variables did not improve significantly the discrimination. The pre-

Table 1 : Results in predicting CCU survival, based on data from the learning set (N = 1091)

		Survivors predicted		Non-Survivors predicted		Accuracy of prediction		
		Alive	Dead	Alive	Dead	Morta-lity	Survi-val	Total
I	N	872	41	68	110			
	%	95.5	4.5	38.2	61.8	72.8	92.8	90.0
II	N	876	37	45	133			
	%	95.9	4.1	25.3	74.7	78.2	95.1	92.5

I : using data obtained at admission.
II : using data gathered during the CCU stay.

Table 2 : Results in predicting hospital survival and mortality (learning set data N = 1091).

		Survivors predicted		Non-Survivors predicted		Accuracy of prediction		
		Alive	Dead	Alive	Dead	Morta-lity	Survi-val	Total
I	N	835	36	88	132			
	%	95.9	4.1	40.0	60.0	78.5	90.5	88.6
II	N	831	40	72	148			
	%	95.4	4.6	32.7	67.3	78.7	92.1	89.7
III	N	840	31	131	89			
	%	96.4	3.6	59.5	40.5	74.1	86.6	85.2

I : using data obtained at admission.
II : using data gathered during the CCU stay.
III : using the so-called Norris variables.

sent study proves that analysis of variables available at the bedside and at an early stage has good predictive ability, apparently at least as good as that obtained with laboratory data.

Linear discriminant analysis has been described as a method that closely approximates the formation of judgments by clinicians. In the evaluation of multiple factors it allows for consistent quantitation of the significance of each factor. In complex diagnostic problem situations it may well serve clinical medicine.

In summary : The coronary care information system which we implemented, has so far been primarily research oriented. The system has inherent advantages for teaching purposes. The system allows for on-line prediction of survival after acute myocardial infarction which may be useful for routine patient care. High risk patients can be identified and compared to patients treated previously in the CCU.

ACKNOWLEDGMENT

This study has been supported by grants from the Ministry of Science and the NFWO foundation (Project N° 20332).

REFERENCES

1. Report EURO 5010 (4) of the WHO Regional office for Europe on "Ischaemic Heart Disease Registers", Copenhagen, 1970.

2. NIE, N.H., HULL, C.H., JENKINS, J.G., STEINBRENNER, K. and BENT, D.H. : Statistical Package for the Social Sciences. Mc Graw-Hill, New York, 2nd Edition, 1975.

3. NORRIS, R.M., BRANDT, P.W.T., CAUGHEY, D.E., LEE, A.J. and SCOTT, P.J. : A new coronary prognostic index. The Lancet, Febr. 8, 1969, p. 274-278.

4. WILLEMS, J.L., PARDAENS, J., ECTOR, H. en DE GEEST, H. : Determinerende factoren voor de prognose na een acuut myocardinfarct. In "Aanwinsten in de Interne Geneeskunde" Vol. V. European Press, Ghent, 1978, in press.

5. WEBER, K.T., JANICKI, J.S., RUSSELL, R.O. and RACKLEY, C.E. : Identification of high risk subsets of acute myocardial infarction. Derived from the myocardial Infarction Research Units Cooperative Study Data Bank. Amer. J. Cardiol. 41 : 197-203, 1978.

ACIS

A CLINICAL INFORMATION SYSTEM

Michael A. Fox, Departments of Biomathematics
City of Hope National Medical Center, California
University of California at Los Angeles 90024

ABSTRACT

ACIS is a file generating system in which a compiler, using a simple data definition and schema language, accepts a description of the data and structures that are to be applied to this data and generates a series of PL/1 programs. These programs are immediately available for use or can be user modified. This is far more powerful than providing the user with the conventional subroutine links.

Central to this system is a series of string manipulation programs including a file and core management program which offers and accepts variable length strings to and from routines and moves these strings between buffers and a variety of protected disc files.

A string of data is a member of a variable group and consists of one or more keys together with descriptors or modifiers to these keys. Two main structural forms apply to the data, internal and external. The former relates items, which are themselves members of strings, hierarchically or relationally. The latter associates independently maintained files of pointers to the data base, thus creating inverted files.

Incorporated into ACIS as an option is the Systematized Nomenclature of Medicine (SNOMED). This and other translation modalities translate coded variables into English. Also available are routines which interface hyper-rectangular retrievals to statistical packages which accept case-wise data.

I. INTRODUCTION

ACIS evolved from a data base system, designed by the author, which currently maintains information on approximately 30,000 patients at the City of Hope Medical Center. Subsequent development of the system has been motivated by its use in clinical trials and other areas of biomedical research.

The system is a compiler designed to generate custom programs for a data base using a file description language composed of very simple elements provided by the user. The first generated program actually builds the data base and the second is used for retrieval.

The data may be viewed and manipulated either hierarchically, relationally or both, depending on the options invoked during compilations.

All the programming for this system has been written in PL/1, with much use being made of the pre-processor features of the language to write the expanding compiler sections. Care has been exercised in the design of the system to allow current development in enquiry languages to be acceptable adjuncts to the system.

During the compilation phase ACIS operates on user supplied clauses and generates viable PL/1 programs which incorporate variable group names and variable names chosen by the user. The program produced is then link-edited to the nucleus system and is ready to use.

To the readable PL/1 code the user may add lines of code to those sections which operate on the data to incorporate features not supported by the Data and Schema Definition Language. For example, the values of the context-dependent variables can be evaluated.

The building of a data-base consists of adding new cases, adding to established cases, and modifying existing cases. During an ACIS run an audit is maintained of the data and rejected data is reproduced together with error messages. The retrieval program is created using the same Data Definition Language as that used to build the data base.

II. STRUCTURING THE DATA BASE

Although many of the procedures performed in a hospital eventually find expression in the patient's charts, these recorded sagas in many cases serve to entomb information rather than preserve it. It was with the conviction that a data base should be evolutionary rather than historical that a design was produced and implemented that not only would have a diverse appearance to different users but would permit growth and allow restructuring.

A physician is concerned with individual patients while a chemist is making measurements on a series of bloods and an admission clerk is concerned with bed occupancy. The data pertinent for all of these facets of hospital activity can each be described independently in a rectangular or tabular manner. Such tableaux or relations constitute relational files. Lines from different tableaux are, however, related when one considers the individual patient. The essential rectangular nature of the data is, though obscured, not lost. This follows from the axiom that all data can be written in a series of rectangular arrays with repeated groups as seperate subrectangles. Existing rectangles may be manipulated to produce new rectangles or relations by the 'cut and paste' functions of 'projection' and 'join' of relational algebra. Fig. 1 depicts a series of such arrays covering some of the recordings that are ubiquitous to hospitals. Each row of these arrays or sets is a variable group or relation, and elements within a row are the variables or tuples. Describing some of these sets, there is the general index of patients or the set P, which contains the chart number, name and certain demographic information. The set L shows the location of the patients within the hospital. The set B produced by the technician drawing blood contains the patient chart numbers, acquisition numbers applied to the blood samples, together with the dates and times the bloods were drawn. The clinical chemist reports the results of his analysis as the set R while the surgery performed on a patient appears as an element in set O.

Although each of these sets has utility in isolation, for example, the occupancy can be obtained from the location set alone, such use is generally of transient value. It is when the relations that are inherent in the data are brought together that the power of the data becomes evident.

Consider the members of each of these sets that are attributed to a particular patient, γ. Since the patient is unique there will be one member or row from the set P, i.e. $P(\gamma)$. There may be several different hospital stays for this patient $L(\gamma_1)$, $L(\gamma_2)$... and during each of these stays several bloods may be drawn $B(\gamma_{11})$, $B(\gamma_{12})$...$B(\gamma_{21})$, $B(\gamma_{22})$... Further, for each of these bloods a variety of tests may be performed producing results $R(\gamma_{111})$, $R(\gamma_{112})$...$R(\gamma_{221})$, $R(\gamma_{212})$... The notation is to add a suffix for each additional level of data viewed in a hierarchical sense. This illustrates the need for a linking variable or key which picks out a specific variable group in a hierarchical schema. For example, the blood acquisition number will link a set of results to a specific sample of blood drawn.

The representation of a patient by a hierarchical tree of strings is shown in Fig. 2. This figure also shows links to operations, diagnoses and so forth. Additional primary sets, for example, services, can immediately be incorporated into this schema.

When the data base is naturally hierarchical, as is normally the case with clinical information then the structural form implied by Fig. 2 using embedded pointers is preferred rather than re-creating the structure implied by Fig. 2, from Fig. 1 each time these structures are required. The choice to build a relational or hierarchical file is a compiler option. There is, of course, no reason why part of Fig. 1 may not be maintained independently of Fig. 2 if storage is cheap with respect to processing. The various sets from which Fig. 2 is obtained do not necessarily come from the same physical file, neither are the lines or elements of these sets of the same length. A means of storing and retrieving variable length strings from different physical files is thus essential. This task is provided by a core management sub-system which will be described later.

An inverted file is an additional structure applied to the data, which allows complex logical operations to be performed without reference to actual data. For each category of interest a membership file is created; for example, there may be cases with a particular pathological condition (hepatocellular changes determined by biopsy), with a specific diagnosis recorded (cirrhosis), but no evidence of a specific microorganism (klebsiella, determined by culture). References to these cases can be found by operations on the inverted structure rather than multiple passes through a diminishing number of cases. Such a partial forward pass is only necessary to extract the required variables on that subset of patients with the requested attributes.

Three distinct types of data are being considered: the actual data itself, as shown in Fig. 1; those internal linkages of the data as implied in Fig. 2, which can, if pointers or reference numbers are used, be internally maintained as part of the data structure, and thirdly a structure which is external to the main body of information and can be maintained as a separate entity.

There are many instances where the information maintained on a patient exists, by design, in different types of files. He may be recorded as an inpatient, as an outpatient, as a patient who is part of a particular drug study protocol, or he may exist only as a blood or tissue sample sent to the institution for study. By creating a master file which upon reference gives the particulars of the files in which this person is to be found, an effective method for linking totally new types of files is available. Further, files of limited use can be maintained and deleted with no effect on the other files. This is essential in a research environment where many unusual tests may be performed on a select group of people, and the files holding this information, though linked to other information on the patient, have to be segregated from the main body of information.

III. STORAGE AND RETRIEVAL OF DATA

Examination of Fig. 2 reveals the enactment of three main operations, obtaining a free record from an appropriate file of free records to hold the data items. Linking this record to a chain of like records (to add to a repeating group for one patient or if the data base were relational add this relation to the appropriate set of relations). In some cases a pointer has to be provided to link a chain lower in the hierarchy. Each of these functions is highly generalized and the specific coding and call sequences required for them are generated by the compiler when the system is generated. The specific programming code to call the appropriate routines is generated by providing the compiler with the following information: the types of files that the input forms imply, whether forward or direct, inpatient or outpatient, a description of the data elements and the associated structures (forward and inverted files).

Although there is a fundamental dichotomy between the data elements, which are stored, and the structures applied to them, which are also stored, the mechanism of storing and retrieving is universal to these two distinct quantities. It is useful to introduce the notion of internal and external structures to distinguish them. Thus the implied structure in Figures 1 and 2 can be thought of as internal, whilst structures which reference the data in special ways, say inverted files, are defined as external structures. These external files are in general constructed to satisfy specific uses for the data. By manipulating external structures which reference data rather than retrieving the actual data, logical relations can be generated, which may be of temporary or permanent interest. Such relations will themselves be subject to an external storage class. Particular external files then provide candidates for analysis. For example, the extraction of patients to provide statistically matched sets for drug protocol testing is not only facilitated by storing inverted files, but by maintaining counts within them, the existence of comparable patients can be ascertained without lengthy file searches.

The core management sub-system accepts or provides variable length character strings and either writes these to or takes them from particular locations within blocks of records. Such a block is moved to and from a variable number of buffers within the core and the appropriate direct access devices. During a run, blocks of records are transferred to these in-core buffers as required. Hash tables provide the particular buffer and location in it of the string of interest. When all the buffers are filled an algorithm is used to determine the buffer which contains the records that are least expected to be used, and if any of these records have been updated, they are written to an external auxiliary file instead of their home files to prevent destruction of dynamic pointers in the case of machine failure. After a predetermined number of transactions have been made, a fail safe condition is invoked, in which a reference matrix that maps from the auxiliary or working files to the main files is transferred to another peripheral device. Using this mapping matrix the main or permanent files can then be updated. Should machine malfunction occur during this period of transformation, the information being transferred and the mapping matrix are protected as they reside on peripheral devices. At the end of the fail safe period when all transfers have been made, processing can continue.

IV. EXPERIENCE WITH THE SYSTEM

Apart from maintaining information on current patients and being a pool of knowledge for research purposes, the data base has a further important role. Increasing requirements are placed by both insurance and governmental agencies on hospitals for information that describes the activities within a hospital and to document variances from expected standards of care. Specific external structures have, therefore, been included to facilitate the production of such reports as summary statistics of length of stay by diagnosis and operation with detailed percentiles for specific age groups. Although the methodology of retrieval is uniform, specialized application programs for certain reports have been found to be more economical to use than to rely on a single more generalized report generator.

An interactive retrieval program may also be generated for the data base. This program is particularly attractive to researchers. This program presents the user with information on the state of the file, consisting of such things as the names of the inverted variables and the amount of information contained in each. Code book information can be directed to a hard copy device. Various browsing facilities are provided to give an overview of the data base as a whole. Commands are solicited from the investigator together with the choice to limit the amount of data viewed on the interactive device and then to direct either this subset or the complete set to either a hard copy medium or a pre-assigned data set. Thus the viewer is not subjected to a lengthy list of extractions he may not wish to examine but rather a brief selection of cases to decide if the complete set is worthy of further analysis. This has been found useful for research purposes to ascertain whether enough patients are available with specific qualities, and if not, relatively close groups can then be combined to provide adequate numbers for comparable analysis. Since the generated retrieval program is written in PL/1, code can be added to provide calculations to be performed by command on interactively retrieved groups of data.

An interactive system is only acceptable when the user is able to obtain enough information at a session without being subjected to a surfeit of irrelevant information thus default print options may be overridden for the duration of a session.

V. AUTOMATIC DECODING

Medical data bases are often partially encoded. As an adjunct to ACIS the approximately 40,000 terms of SNOMED (Systematized Nomenclature of Medicine) are available to all data bases created by ACIS. During a retrieval session variables encoded into SNOMED can be automatically translated into English.

In addition any inverted list of variables (for example, diagnosis) may be browsed. This produces a list sorted by code and translated into English. Codes present in SNOMED but not present in the data base are also available for decoding.

Although SNOMED is featured in this description the decode facility may be applied to any coding scheme.

VI. OUTPUT TO STATISTICAL PACKAGES

Data held within an information system may differ in important ways from data presented to statistical packages. The latter often requires categorized information to be numerical, the variable sex, for example, may be categorized as Male = 1, Female = 2. Recoding from the English of the data base values, to the numeric values required by the statistical packages is then required.

Statistical packages are often oriented to accept case-wise information but because of the nature of some data a case can consist of a block of unrelated repeating groups. For example, several diagnosis and many laboratory findings.

Understanding the implications of both repeating groups and unrelated groups will enable the investigator to construct sensible rectangles by only asking for those variables in which analysis will have meaning within the context of the generated case.

The program allows selection of variable groups and particular variables for these groups to be displayed and/or passed to an output medium. The user has total control, therefore, over this output with respect to its subsequent disposition.

VII. INTERFACING ACIS TO STATISTICAL PACKAGES

A semi-customized approach where the user supplies a sub-routine is often used. In a study of a few hundred cases of non-Hodgkins lymphomas, the statistical analysis was performed on the survivorship of the patients. Although much information was stored with respect to treatments, classification of lymphomas, and so forth, this was only used to select the cases and was passed to the statistical program as descriptors or classifying variables. The variables used for survivorship were either numeric, or for "alive", "dead", etc. converted to numeric. A routine was constructed to generate the control language for the BMDP statistical program, and for this particular study survivorship was obtained from a two-step job. Thus for a particular study the problem of interfacing may be straight forward, but specialized.

For a more generalized approach there are two options; both of these depend upon rectangularizing the output. The first method relies on a direct interface to BMDQ5S, a generalized rectangularizing program which functionally collapses repetitive values by taking their means, maximum values, etc., and produces a single row consisting of the concatenation of collapsed variable groups composed of the selected variables. The cases so produced are then written out as a BMD Save File. The second method is to expand or pad a case on the left with repetitions of variable groups in their entirety each time a group or level in the hierarchy is retrieved. This together with the recoding from alpha to numeric is the technique used in providing an interface to PSTAT.

VIII. THE LANGUAGE

The language has the following syntactic form.

VARIABLE_GROUP_NAME: COMMAND ( ): COMMAND ( ):.........:

There are commands which operate between variable groups (giving the group-by-group relational dependency), commands which apply to the data base as a whole, and commands which supply information with respect to particular variables within a variable group... For example,

PROFILE: CONTAINS (MEASURES, PROBLEMS...):
           CONSISTS_OF (FILE_NO(1,4,N3)...DATE(5,D)...RACE(85,1,I)..):
           KEY(FILE_NO)::

PROFILE is the name of the variable group (relation). CONTAINS is the command which builds directive links to the variable groups (or sub-relations) Measures, Problems. CONSISTS_OF is the command which specifies variables (tuples) which constitute the variable group (relation). Following each variable are a series of parenthesized parameters which provide information both about the external form of the variable and for its internal packing (e.g. D directs a date to be transformed from the conventional mm dd yy to a two byte Julian representation). Other parameters are used when the variable is to be inverted, to allow choices with respect to blanks and similar purposes. For instance, RACE(85,1,I) informs the compiler that the value of the variable called RACE is in column 85 and is to be treated as a simple inverted variable. The command KEY identifies the variable FILE_NO as the prime access key to the profile, and that all first level hierarchies are to have this as an implied domain in hierarchical data bases and as the prime entity KEY in relational data bases. Similarly the command MATCH identifies the variable used to link variable groups in a hierarchy deeper than the first level. It is an implied domain in a hierarchical representation and an actual domain in a relation and its sub-relations. If one elects to use the relational structure, the data can be operated without reference to implied hierarchies.

The following example is abstracted from an interactive retrieval session, the annotations are printed in *italics*. For the PROBLEMS, which were encoded in SNOMED, a comparison was made between the original English and that obtained from decoding SNOMED. This study showed SNOMED to be an extremely viable lexicon.

THIS DATA BASE CONTAINS THE FOLLOWING VARIABLE GROUPS

PROFILE	D	*demography 'D' is synonymous with PROFILE*
MEASURES	M	
PROBLEMS	P	
PROB_TEXT	T	

A particular patient in this data base has the hierarchical structure

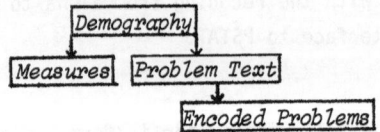

Instructions follow

DO YOU WISH TO BROWSE INVERTED VARIABLES? (PRINTS SORTED MEMBER CODES AND NO. OF REFS.) Y/N
>y
THE FOLLOWING INVERTED VARIABLES ARE AVAILABLE:
1. MEASURES_B_P_ARM
2. MEASURES_SMOKER
    ⋮
8. PROBLEMS_T_FIELD

We select the inverted variable T-field or Topography from the variable group PROBLEMS.

```
TXX000 (2)   XX EYE AND EYE APPENDAGES, EYE NOS, EYEBALL
TXX200 (1)   CORNEA NOS
   .
   .
   .
IF YOU WISH TO TAKE PRINT DEFAULTS ENTER Y?
>n
```
*Using the prompt mode decisions on how much to print are being made. These to-
gether with the selection made under will for this run become the default.*

```
LINES OF PRINT CORRESPONDING TO THE FOLLOWING ACRONYM ARE AVAILABLE
D M P T ENTER WORD CONSTRUCTED FROM THESE LETTERS.
>dt
```
*For the variable groups known to this user demography and text are to be dis-
played.*

```
FROM "PROFILE" IF YOU WANT THE VARIABLE PRINTED THEN ANSWER Y/N/P/ALL
FILE_NO
>p
DATE
>n
NAME
>y
   .
   .
   .
```
*p - in addition to displaying the variable FILE_NO on the screen write
this in an appropriate format to an output data set suitable for
post-retrieval analysis*
n - no
y - only display this on the screen

```
REQUESTED VARIABLES FOR DEMOGRAPHY    1. FILE_NO   3. NAME   12. AGE   13. SEX...
   .
   .
   .
```
variables are then selected from other variable groups e.g. PROBLEMS
```
THE FOLLOWING GROUP OF RETRIEVALS ARE AVAILABLE
A) INDIVIDUAL PATIENTS
B) INDIVIDUAL CODES OR BOOLEAN EXPRESSIONS
C) CATEGORIES OF AN INVERTED VARIABLE
Z) QUIT.    PLEASE ENTER YOUR CHOICE OF RETRIEVAL WITH A/B/C/A
>b
```
We are ready to retrieve using boolean (logical) expressions
```
WHEN REQUESTED SUPPLY EITHER RETRIEVAL CODES OR "LOGICAL COMMANDS".  WHEN YOU
HAVE FINISHED ENTER "ALL".  ENTER FIRST OF CODES TO BE "ANDED".
>bp1
```
This is the code for normal blood pressure
```
         CODE REQUESTED IS BP1

ENTER NEXT CODE OR COMMAND "OR/NOT/ALL"
>f7170
```
This is the SNOMED code for hypertension
```
         CODE REQUESTED IS f7170
   .
   .
   .
ENTER NEXT CODE OR COMMAND "AND/NOT/ALL"
>not
ENTER CODE
>d2350
```
This is the SNOMED code for diabetes mellitus
```
         CODE REQUESTED IS d2350

ENTER NEXT CODE OR COMMAND "ALL"
>all

PROFILE           1712      ANN            29  F  C  M
PROB_TEXT      01 OBESITY
PROB_TEXT      06 ANEMIA (PROBABLE IRON DEFICIENCY)
PROB_TEXT      05 HYPERTENSION
PROB_TEXT      04 VARICOSE VEINS
PROB_TEXT      03 BACKACHES
PROB_TEXT      02 CHOLECYSTECTOMY
                          .
                          .
                          .
```
*This patient is a 29 year old Caucasian
married female and these are her medical
problems*

There were 5 patients retrieved which constitute the set

$$BPl \cap \left[F \ 7170 \cup F \ 7460 \right] \cap \overline{D \ 2350}$$

*that is non diabetics who suffer from hypertension or heart murmur but manifest
normal blood pressure (on medication)*

⋮

Retrieval Continues

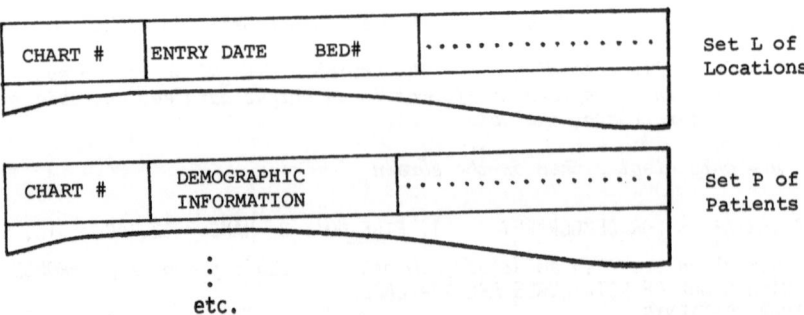

Figure (1)   RELATIONAL TABLEAUX

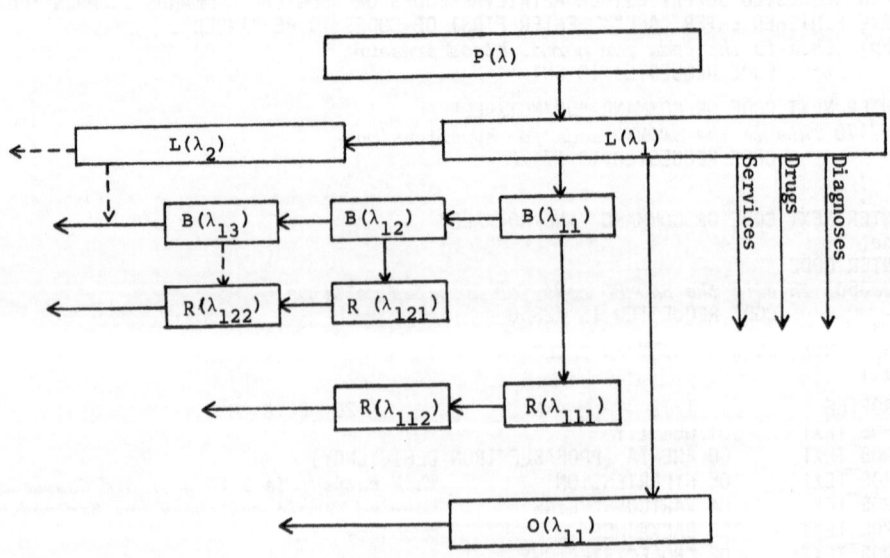

Figure (2)   HIERARCHICAL ARRANGEMENT

AN ANALYSIS OF 3 YEARS EXPERIENCE WITH THE RE-DESIGNED SYSTEM FOR BASIC MEDICAL DOCUMENTATION WITHIN THE MSH

G. von Gaertner-Holthoff, P.R. Pocklington

Department of Biometrics and Medical Informatics
Medical School Hannover

Introduction

At the end of 1975 a system for the acquisition of basic medical documentation within the Medical System Hannover (MSH) was introduced as a replacement for the inital system that had been in use since 1969. The reasons behind the re-design and the underlying principles thereof have been described in detail (1,3,5), and may be summarized as follows:

- switching data acquisition from punched cards to OCR/on-line input thus providing a swifter turnaround,

- the provision of formal plausibility controls upon initial processing of the data,

- the provision of logical linkage between an unrestricted number of diagnoses, therapies, complications and modifiers to all categories,

- the requirement of an obligatory verification of all medical information before acceptance for further processing and storage,

- the provision of an error correction procedure without the necessity for reprocessing of the source document,

- the provision of checkpoint facilities so that in cases of system breakdown the restart procedure should be clearly defined and lead to neither data duplication nor data loss.

This paper considers some of the experiences gained with the new system from usage and organizational aspects.

Medical aspects

The basic medical documentation within the Hannover Medical School prior to the system re-design was characterized amongst other things by the following aspects:

- the medical data, which, apart from admission and discharge information and information regarding risk-factors, consisted almost exclusively of diagnoses and came in the main from services oriented towards internal medicine,

- the codification was performed using the original version of the 'general' coding system KDS (Klinischer Diagnosenschluessel, IMMICH) without taking into account the particular requirements of individual disciplines,

- no verification by medically qualified personnel or the doctor-in-charge was carried out either of the data recorded or the codes used,

- it was only possible to correct erroneous administrative data.

Due to a new conception of the medical record cover-sheet (2) in conjunction with a complete re-design of the processing and storage procedure (5,6) there has been an evident alteration in the characteristics mentioned previously:

a) The question as to whether the co-operation of the services oriented towards internal medicine was the result of an under-developed awareness of the surgical disciplines with regard to basic documentation, or whether their lack of participation was due to a limitation in the system regarding their special requirements, cannot retrospectively be satisfactorily answered. We have noted, however, a definite change in the spectrum of departments making use of the system, which now allows the recording of diagnoses, therapies (mainly surgical) and complication information, along with their medical

inter-relationships. This alteration (4) came about through an
increase in the number of departments making use of the central
documentation service, mainly on account of the incorporation of
surgically-oriented disciplines (*=denotes services incorporated
since re-design):

Internal Medicine
    gastro-enterology
    cardiology
    nephrology
    pulmonology (*)
    rheumatology
    metabolism disturbances
Surgery
    heart-surgery (*)
    thoracic and vascular surgery (*)
    abdominal and transplant surgery (*)
    urology (*)
Paediatrics
    pulmonology
    nephrology (*)
    cardiology
Psychiatric and Neurological Medicine
    neurology (*)
    neuro-surgery (*)
Ear-Nose-Throat Medicine
    for adults
    for children
Radiology
    radio-therapy
Ophthalmology
    ophthalmological surgery
Dental Hospital
    dental surgery

As can be seen from the following analysis (Fig. 1), the
disciplines named make the main use of the possibilities offered
for the documentation, along with diagnoses, of therapies,
complications and certain modifiers, and that such possibilities
appear to be a basic necessity for documentation in the surgical
disciplines, the ear-nose-throat service and, to a lesser ex-

tent, in ophthalmology and radiotherapy.

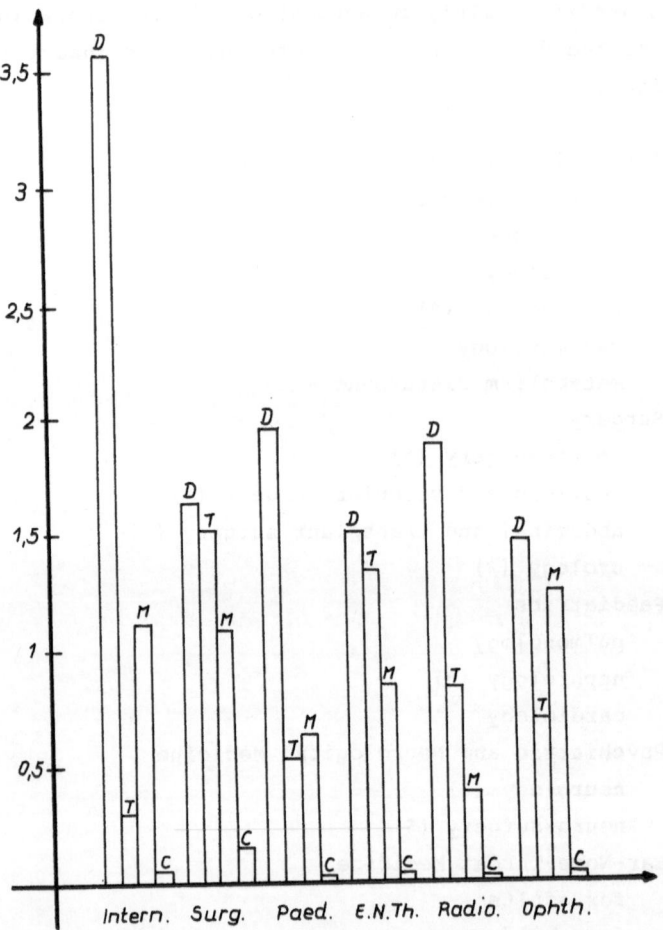

Fig. 1: Average number of diagnoses (D), therapies (T), modifiers (M) and complications (C) per medical record cover-sheet per discipline.

	D	T	M	C
Intern. Med.	3.59	0.31	1.13	0.05
Surgery	1.64	1.56	1.10	0.14
Paediatrics	1.99	0.55	0.66	0.04
E.-N.-Th.Med.	1.52	1.36	0.86	0.04
Radiotherapy	1.90	0.81	0.41	0.01
Ophthalmol.	1.47	0.69	1.25	0.03

For the former the ability to document therapy would appear at least as important as the documentation of diagnoses, which, it is felt, justifies the necessary adaptation of the system to cater for this requisite.

b) In the past years there has been developed a wide variety of special codes that are in the main tailored to suit the individual requirements of a particular medical orientation. The basic medical documentation of the MSH takes this trend into consideration in that, for divisions with special codification requirements, the individual catalogue is adapted by means of expansion to and complementation of the KDS for the codification of diagnoses and complications. For the codification of therapies a vastly modified version of the general surgical therapy code (SCHEIBE/GOEGLER) adapted to the individual desires of the physicians is used, while for the codification of modifiers a self-designed code is used.

As a result of the increased desires of the physicians over the past few years for the development of detailed documentation systems the centralized medical documentation service has at its disposal a considerable codification spectrum. This covers 11,654 codes for diagnoses and complications, of which 10,300 (88.4%) are taken from the KDS and 1,354 (11.6%) were newly created. 1,062 codes are available for the codification of therapies, all of which could be considered as our own development.

An analysis of just over 2 years usage (1.11.75 - 1.12.77) considering the code spectrum actually used by the physicians for the documentation of diagnosis and therapy shows that:
For 70,064 diagnoses coded, 4,260 different numeric codes (i.e. 36.6% of the available spectrum) were used. Of these
    1,157 were used 10 and more times,
      334 3 times
      603 twice and
    1,286 once.
Thus 154 codes cover 50%, 524 75% and 1,282 90% of the requirements. Of the 4,260 different codes 3,640 are contained in the KDS and 618 in the catalogue developed in-house, i.e. 35.3% KDS and 45.6% in-house.

Over the same period 853 codes were used for codification of 30,194 therapies, this being 80.2% of the available spectrum. Of these

362 were used 10 and more times,

66 3 times,

85 twice and

146 once.

42 codes so cover 50%, 125 75% and 262 90% of the requirements.

The results given above are, of course, average values covering all documenting departments and do not show how the documentation tendencies of various services differ.

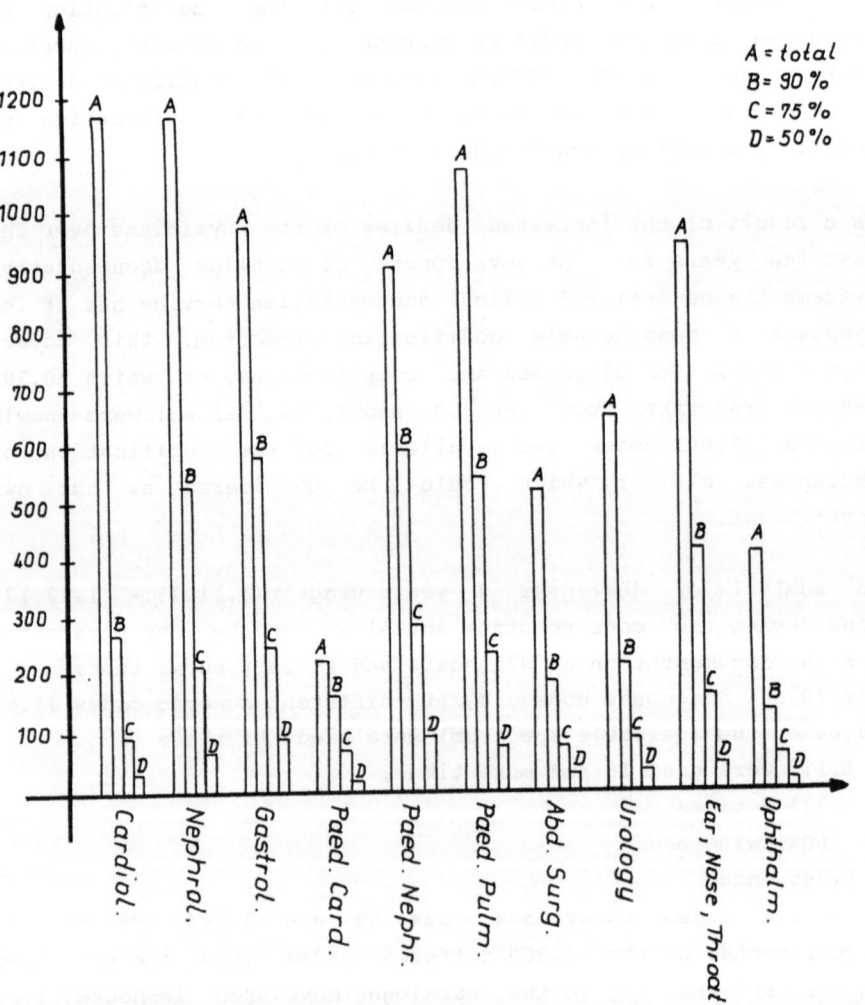

Fig. 2: Number of different codes used by the various services.

Although these differences have as yet not been satisfactorily explained we can here at least give a graphical overview of the implementation of the codes for diagnoses (Fig. 2).

If we consider urology and abdominal surgery (two departments for whom a specialized individually-oriented code-catalogue has been compiled) with regard to their use of already present and newly defined codes, then it can been seen that the necessity for general codification systems is under-estimated and that for the specialist systems over-estimated by the physicians.

	no. of codes in spec. catal.		no. of codes actually used	
	total	new	total	new
urology	376	219	649	179
abd.surg.	291	36	513	36

c) That the quality of documentation depends to a large extent on the completeness and accuracy with which the data are recorded is obvious. For this reason the MSH basic documentation places a great emphasis on data verification. If this verification is to be optimal it should be carried out both by the doctor-in-charge (to check the completeness and correctness of the recorded data) as well as by a medical expert with detailed knowledge of the code used (to check the codification used).

It soon, however, became apparent that a control by the doctor-in-charge could not in most cases be carried out, due mainly to the increase in his work-load and was for this reason discontinued. This was substituted for by control by a medically qualified person having intimate knowledge of the documentation system. This person is, of course, not in a position to decide whether the information is based on a erroneous diagnosis, if incorrect associations have been recorded or if information regarded as insignificant has been omitted. He can, however, locate inherent documentation and codification errors, these being as frequent as those formal errors located by the automatic information processing system (such as typing errors, digit interchanges, incorrect date sequencing etc.). Approximately 20% of all records processed contain errors of which (as has been stated) about 10% are formal errors and 10% intrinsic documentation/codification errors.

d) Inter-related with the verification concept is the correction procedure. The given system provides simple procedures for the correction of <u>all</u> the data. Furthermore, we expected due to feedback given upon introduction of this correction system to achieve a teaching effect upon the medical record librarians, though this cannot statistically be ascertained. The frequency of errors varies constantly - the percentage of inherent errors against total errors increasing from 46.2% to 55.1%,while formal errors have decreased from 53.8% to 44.9% - but the total percentage containing errors has remained constant. It has to be considered here also that over the past two years new departments have been constantly incorporated into the centralized medical documentation service, so that the medical record librarians are forever having to adapt to new requirements and new terminology.

To measure the acceptability of this documentation system we used two criteria:

1) the number of medical records passing through the central documentation department. In 1977, approx. 27,000 patients were admitted for in-patient treatment. In the same year the centralized medical documentation service coded 19,000 in-patient histories. It is expected that this difference will be reduced in 1978 since as of 1.1.78 the neurological and neuro-surgical wards have also been incorporated.

2) the number of retrieval and evaluation requests. In 1977, about 60 selection runs were prepared for the answering of 38 individual research enquiries, in addition to routine overview frequency statistics and on-line requests (8) for purposes of patient-care, since the basic documentation data were stored in the integrated patient-data base of the MSH (7) and the facility is provided for cross-evaluation of these data in conjunction with those acquired by means of various MSH application systems (laboratory values, ECG reports, administrative data). The exact number of such requests has not been monitored so far.

Organizational aspects

1) Although the system was designed to allow for both OCR and on-line input , to our suprise it was found that little or no use has been made of the on-line facility, the underlying reasons behind this tendency being probably:

   - that the OCR acquisition is independent of machine response time, terminal location and system up-time, and

   - that in the case of data loss (due to system failures such as e.g. a head-crash) no repeated data acquisition is necessary.

2) The system recovery procedure was initially based upon the provision of error recovery routines with mnemonic names alluding to the routine (and procedure name) being executed at the time of breakdown (e.g. for a breakdown after BASIS1 STEP2 the error recovery routine to be started would be BAS1E2). In spite of the simplicity of this procedure it was found impossible to completely cut out errors due to human factors - though through the process of obtaining file security copies the effect of such errors was minimised - and the error recovery procedure has therefore been automated by the creation of a tracking file that restarts at the appropriate point upon resubmission.

3) Through the increased acceptance of the necessity for and re-cognition of the advantages of a system for basic medical documentation, there has been voiced the desire for specialized documentation compatible with the general basic documentation and for such purposes an interface has been realized that caters for specific data acquisition (e.g. a limited code spectrum entered over OMR forms) with incorporation into the system for basic documentation and the resultant facilities for verification, correction and evaluation.

The continuously increasing usage of the retrieval system indicates that the re-designed system meets the need for both clinical and research work. At the moment we have started projects to study how

the SNOMED concept can be used in this typ of system and whether
identical semantic areas can be covered.

References

|1| Holthoff, G.: Aufbau einer multidisziplinaeren, zentralisier-
ten Medizinischen Basisdokumentation. Dissertation,
Tieraerztliche Hochschule Hannover, 1976.
|2| Holthoff, G., Moehr, J.R., Tramp, H.J., Reichertz, P.L., Sau-
ter, K., Zowe, W.: Aufbau, Routineeinsatz und Weiterentwicklung
einer computergestuetzten Basisdokumentation fuer die
Medizinische Hochschule Hannover, Teil 1: Krankenblatt,
Dokumentation, Mikrofilmverfahren. In: Reichertz, P.L. (Hrsg.):
Medizinische Informatik 1975 (Springer, Berlin, Heidelberg, New
York, 1976) 19-32.
|3| Holthoff, G., Moehr, J.R.: Die Bedeutung der klinischen Ba-
sisdokumentation fuer Information und Kommunikation im
Krankenhaus. Der Krankenhausarzt,<u>48</u>, (1975) 276-282.
|4| Von Gaertner-Holthoff, G.: Use and Utilization of the Cata-
logue of Diagnoses Created for the Medical Units of the Medical
School Hannover. Paper presented at the 4th European Conference
on Medical Records, Heidelberg, 20.-23.3.1978.
|5| Pocklington, P.R., Holthoff, G.: Die operationelle Durchfueh-
rung der medizinischen Basisdokumentation im MSH. In:
Reichertz, P.L. (Hrsg.): Informationssysteme in der
Medizinische Versorgung (Schattauer, Stuttgart, New York, 1977)
467-485. 467-485, 1977.
|6| Pocklington, P.R.: The Necessity for Requirements and Basic
Design of a General Data Interpretation and Evaluation System.
In: Anderson, J., Forsythe, J.F. (eds.): <u>Medinfo '74</u>, (North
Holland Publishing Co., Amsterdam) 411-418, <u>1975</u>.
|7| Sauter, K., Hill, R.D., Reichertz, P.L.: Data Base Concept of
the Medical System Hannover and the Analysis of Patient Data.
In: Anderson, J., Forsythe, J.F. (eds.): <u>Medinfo '74</u>, (North
Holland Publishing Co., Amsterdam, 1975) 399-409.
|8| Weingarten, W., Sauter, K., Weigelt, D., Reichertz, P.L.: The
Patient Information System and its User Reaction. Journee
d'Informatique Medicale, Toulouse/France, 3.-7.3.1975,
(IRIA,Paris 1975) XIV1 - XIV15.

EXPERIMENTS WITH MEDICAL DIAGNOSTIC SYSTEMS

J. Janecki, H. Kokott
Medical Academy
Warsaw, Poland

Application of computers in assisting medical diagnosis (computer aided diagnosis) has a long tradition (1). Nevertheless, there is a limited number of papers published which deal with optimization of this type of diagnostic system (2,3). At present, the process of medical diagnosis is still little recognized, and it is difficult to prematurely evaluate which computer system would serve best here, and which selected input parameters would be optimal for these purposes (4).

Our aim was to check what influence changes of certain parameters has on the efficiency of a simple system of differential diagnosis.

1. RESULTS OF APPLIED DIAGNOSTIC SYSTEM

Our system (5) was exclusively based on quantitative results of laboratory tests. They were the results obtained in two groups of patients with chronic liver diseases (up to 27 tests, from which were selected 10 for differentiation of 13 diagnoses in 128 patients and 19 tests for differentiation of 8 diagnoses in 158 patients) and also a group of patients with acute surgical diseases of bile-ducts and gallblader (up to 37 tests for differentiation of 4 diseases in 88 patients). The diagnostic criterion, forming the reference system for the set of results in each patient was definite clinical diagnosis, based mainly on histopatholo-gical findings or on the results of intra-operation surgical examination. All patients were hospitalized in specialistic wards in clinical hospitals.

On the grounds of statistical elaboration of laboratory results it was possible to establish in multi-dimensional space areas equivalent to each particular diagnosis, in which every dimension corresponds with one of the tests. These diagnostic areas were characterised by a mean value standard deviation of each test in a given diagnosis. Following the construction of those areas the probability of points attach-ment, corresponding with results obtained in each patient to proper diagnostic areas was checked (reclas-sification). Those values of probability were the comparative base in the evaluation of results obtained during further experiments. This was the method used for each of the three separate groups of patients, but the third, surgical group, was worked out slightly different from the others. This group consisted of 62 patients who had undergone many tests and 26 others on whom the number of tests was considerably smaller. The indentification of diagnostic areas was carried out on data taken from the larger group. Having checked up the relevancy of each patient's affiliation to the appropriate diagnostic areas the remaining 26 patients were tested in a similar way. This procedure helped to verify the universality of previously estabilished areas.

At this stage this diagnosis was taken into consideration, to which the computer attributed the high-est probability, irrespective of the value of this probability. If the computer recognition corresponded to the clinical diagnosis — the result was considered correct. But, if the computer indicated a different disease then that of the clinical diagnosis, the result was considered as incorrect. A wrong diagnosis by the computer was titled as "false positive". An unrecognized correct diagnosis by the computer was titled as "false negative" diagnosis. Tables I, II and III present the obtained results in all three groups of patients respectively.

In the first group (Table I) one of the diagnoses was neither " false positive" nor " false negative".

Table I

What is more interesting is that, this diagnosis was based exclusively on histopathological findings and, therefore, the precise accuracy of the computer aided diagnosis based only on the results of laboratory tests was quite unexpected. Patients with the next five diseases were always qualified by the computer correctly, but the same diseases were recognized incorrectly in some other patients. The remaining 7 diseases were sometimes recognized as both "false positive" and "false negative". The accuracy in diagnoses of some diseases was very low; for example, 9 times in 34 patients with cirrhosis inactiva, but the same diseases were also rarely recognized as "false positive" — cirrhosis inactiva in only one patient. However, other diseases were quite often recognized as "false positive", for example, in 7 patients the computer recognized falsely collagenosis hepatis and in 2 out of 6 patients with this disease the computer recognized some other disease. Such differences results rather from the character of diagnostic area of particular diseases, thus from scattering of test results in all patients with these diagnoses.

In the second group of patients (Table II) in spite of the fact that there were more diagnostic parame-

Table II

ters (19 instead of 10), fewer diagnoses (8 instead of 13), and more patients (158 instead of 128) — the accuracy of recognitions was worse. That was why our attention was drawn to the limited clear cut of the basic differentiating criterion in this branch of medicine, namely the histopathological findings. The studied diseases are often particular stages of the same pathological process, and therefore their close differentiation is very subjective.

In the surgical group (Table III) the general accuracy of diagnosis was the best, which was one of the

Table III

reasons, that this group was taken for further studies. The accuracy of qualification of 26 patients, which were not used in the construction of a proper diagnostic area, was also relatively high (21 for 26 cases). From the medical point of view the high accuracy of computer recognition of acute suppurative cholangitis was surprising, since this disease is clinically very difficult to diagnose (6).

2. EXPERIMENTS WITH DIFFERENTIATING SYSTEMS

The second stage of our research was based on the fact, that we limited the number of tests, changed their composition and, afterwards, checked up the changes in accuracy to recognitions of the proper diagnoses. Since we were concerned with the exact designation of differencies, we evaluated the average percentage probability of affiliation to the correct diagnostic area and not the number of patients with correct diagnosis.

The influence the number of tests had on the accuracy of diagnosis was our first concern. In the first group of patients we differentiated their diagnoses by haphazardly choosing 4 biochemical parameters. The obtained results were bed and considerably much worse than the results obtained following differentiation based on 10 parameters chosen by the computer. In the third group of patients we reduced the number of tests to 10, which were also chosen by the computer. The results were limited accuracy of all diagnoses, namely in particular diseases from 93.4% to 88.9%, from 89.6% to 62.8%, from 81.6% to 64.8% and from 85.0% to 81.6%. Further observations concerning the influence of the amount of data on the efficiency of diagnosis were carried out during studies on the third problem.

The second problem was the question, whether the computer choice of differentiating parameters gave better results than the choice based on other criteria. Such a criterion was, for example, the simplicity of determination of laboratory tests. We have carried out the differentiation based on 9 such simple tests and compared the results with differentiation based on 10 tests chosen by computer. The mean results were decidedly worse, namely in particular diseases 85.6% instead of 88.9%, 57.3% instead of 62.8%, 49.7% instead of 64.8% and 59.1% instead of 81.6%. Such great difference could not be justified by the fact that the "optimal" set covered 10 tests and "technically simple" set covered 9 tests.

The third study concerned the diagnostical possibilities depending on the degree of complication of tests. All examinations, which were carried out on the patients in the third group, were divided into four degrees of complications of laboratory technique: 9 basic tests, 8 comparatively simple, 3 complicated and 17 highly specialistic tests. The mean probability degree of obtained correct diagnoses based on an increasing number of more and more complicated tests is presented in Table IV. As illustrated,

Table   IV

the greater range of tests in each disease improved the average probability of correct diagnosis. For comparision the results obtained from 10 tests chosen by computer are also shown. Analysing the results of every stage of the diagnosis in each patient we noticed that sometimes (15%) an increase in the number of tests lowered the degree, sometimes greatly, of correct diagnosis.

The final problem results from pure practical and medical circumstances. It concerns an attempt at differentiating diseases on the basis of the degree of intensity of certain pathological processes. The initial study was carried out on our surgical group of patients. From the results of tests at our disposal we selected three groups, taking into account those disorders which could be controlled by those tests. Those disorders were liver or kidney disfunction and inflammatory process. There were respectively 9, 13 and 9 such tests done. Table V presents the mean degree of accuracy of correct diagnoses, based on

Table   V

each group of tests. In two diseases a comparatively high differentiating power of tests connected with one of the chosen pathological processes was observed. In the remaining two diseases, however, this phenomenon was considerably less marked which made the differentiation impossible.

3. DISCUSSION

The differential-diagnostic system applied by us (5) was very simple, but we obtained with its help results, which were sometimes surprisingly accurate. This indicates high potential possibilities contained in applied mathematical methods for medical differential-diagnostic process.

Great differences in accuracy obtained during the reclassification (7) of patients with various diseases could suggest the non-homogeneity of certain diagnostical group and less precision of diagnostic definition. Analysing the results obtained in the second group of patients our attention was drawn to the limited objectivity of diagnostic criterion which we used in the research, namely histopathological findings. On the other hand, the high diagnostic accuracy in the third group seems to justify a higher value of clinical surgical diagnoses. It may be very likely that clustering analysis will make better differentiation of individual diseases possible, not only based on morphological, more subjective results, but also on the complex of biochemical parameters (7, 8).

The experimets which we carried out during the second stage of our study were mainly aimed at explaining the problem of selecting diagnostic parameters quantative and qualitative alike. This choice is now occasional depending on the technical possibilities of the laboratory but, subjective anyhow, and on the experience and wishes of the doctor.

The larger the amount of information the higher probability of accurate diagnosis is a well-known statement. However, practically it is important to ascertain those simple tests by which it would be possible to determine the disease with a satisfactory differentiation probability. But it is also true, that using information without selecting it may lead to low diagnostic accuracy. In our studies this phenomenon was linked up with some non-specific tests in certain diseases. This prompted us to pay closer attention to optimization of selection of diagnostic tests (4) and, on the other hand, to consider carefully the possibility of a more physiopathological approach to computer diagnosis. Disease does not always strike a person who was previously copletely healthy. The experienced doctor can easily distinguish which deviations from normal are connected with the basic illness, and which ones are caused by the accompanying diseases. Computer aided diagnostic systems, in general, do not take such possibilities into consideration. Apart from insufficient clear cut boundaries of each disease, which in our case were often stages of the same progressing physiopathological process, these very symptoms of the accompanying diseases could blot out the boundaries of the diagnostic areas, thus reducing the accuracy of computer diagnosis. It seems to us that this could be avoided by considering a limited set of laboratory tests and by an initial selection of these tests, taking into account the symptoms of injuries to certain organs, disturbances of some metabolic processes or the occurance of certain pathological states. We hope to undertake this appro-

32

ach to computer diagnostics in our next study.

LITERATURE REFERENCES

1. Brodman K: – Diagnostic decision by machine. Med. Electronics, 7, 1960, 216
2. Fraser P.M., D.A. Franklin: – Mathematical models for the diagnosis of liver disease.Quart. J. Med., 43, 1974, 73
3. Lively W.M., S.A. Szygenda,– Modeling techniques for medical diagnosis. Computer Biomed. Res. 6, Ch. E. Mise 1973, 393
4. Janecki J.: – Computer selection of differential diagnostic parameters; in: Information systems for patient care, North Holland Publ. Comp. 1976, 401
5. Kokott H.: – Model matematyczny medycznej diagnozy roznicowej. Paper for magister's degree, WAT, Warsaw, 1975
6. Welch J.P., G.A. Donaldson:– The urgency of diagnosis and surgical treatment of acute suppurative cholangitis. Am. J. Surg. 131, 1976, 527
7. Solberg H.E., S. Skrede J. P. Blomhoff. – Diagnosis of liver diseases by laboratory results and discriminant analysis. Scand. J. Clin. &Lab. Invest. 35, 1975, 713
8. Winkel P.: – Patterns and clusters – multivariate approach for interpreting clinical chemistry results. Clin. Chem. 19, 1973, 1329

Diagnoses made by computer \ clinical	Fibrosis periportalis	Hiperbilirubinaemia post hepatitidem ac.	Sclerosis hepato-portalis	Cirrhosis post-alkoholica	Hepatitis chronica persistens	Steatosis alkoholica	Neoplasma hepatis	Cirrhosis biliaris primaria	Hepatitis in dec. collagenosi	Cirrhosis activa	Hepatitis chronica activa	Cirrhosis inactiva	Hepatitis reactiva	False positive
No.	5	10	7	4	3	3	6	7	6	9	27	34	7	
Fibrosis periportalis	5													–
Hiperbilirubinaemia post hepatitidem ac.		10										4	1	5
Sclerosis hepato-portalis			7				1	1	1			1		4
Cirrhosis post-alkoholica				4					1			1		2
Hepatitis chronica persistens					3						1	4		5
Steatosis alkoholica						3					1		1	2
Neoplasma hepatis							5	1			1	1		4
Cirrhosis biliaris primaria								5			3			3
Hepatitis in dec. collagenosi									4	1	2	3	1	7
Cirrhosis activa										5	2	4		6
Hepatitis chronica activa										2	15	6	1	9
Cirrhosis inactiva											1	9		1
Hepatitis reactiva									1		1	1	3	3
False negativa	–	–	–	–	–	–	1	2	2	4	12	25	4	50

Table I

Comparison of computer—made and clinical diagnoses in the first group of patients (128 persons)

Diagnoses made by computer	c l i n i c a l	Neoplasma hepatis	Cirrhosis hepatis	Hepatitis chronica activa	Hepatitis in cirrhosim vertens	Sanus	Hepatitis chronica persistens	Hepatitis toxica	Hepatitis reactiva	False positive
No.		18	25	15	10	16	18	32	24	
Neoplasma hepatis		12	2			1	2	1	5	11
Cirrhosis hepatis		2	16	4	2		3	3	5	19
Hepatitis chronica activa		1	4	9	1		1	4	1	12
Hepatitis in cirrhosim vertens				2	6	1		1		4
Sanus		1	1			9	1	2		5
Hepatitis chronica persistens						1	9	4	3	8
Hepatitis toxica			1				2	15	3	6
Hepatitis reactiva		2	1		1	4		2	7	10
False negative		6	9	6	4	7	9	17	17	75

Table   II

Comparison of computer—made and clinical diagnoses in the second group of patients (158 persons)

Diagnoses made by computer	clinical	Acute suppurative cholangitis	Cholecystitis	Icterus mechanicus	Cholangitis	False positive	Acute supp. cholang. (small group)
No.		16	16	15	15		26
Acute suppurative cholangitis		15	1	2	1	4	21
Cholecystitis			13	1	1	2	3
Icterus mechanicus		1	2	11	4	7	2
Cholangitis				1	9	1	
False negative		1	3	4	6	14	5

Table   III
Comparison of computer—made and clinical diagnoses in the third group of patients (88 persons)

Type of tests	No.	Acute suppur. cholangitis	Cholangitis	Icterus mechanicus	Cholecystitis acuta
basic	9	85.6	57.3	49.7	59.1
+ simple	17	86.5	60.7	72.1	84.1
+ complicated	20		76.9	79.6	
+ specialistic	37	93.4	89.6	81.6	85.0
computer chosen	10	88.9	62.8	64.8	81.6

Table   IV
Mean accuracy (in %) of computer diagnoses depending on the number and type of tests

Disease	Tests			
	total number	indicating on		
		inflammation	kidney failure	liver failure
	No. 37	9	13	9
Acute suppur. cholangitis	94	83	61	67
Cholangitis	90	42	54	66
Icterus mechanicus	82	46	45	55
Cholecystitis acuta	85	45	47	81

Table V

Mean fitness (in %) of computer diagnoses obtained with the help of pathophysiological groups of laboratory tests

AN ONLINE, INTERACTIVE, INFORMATION SYSTEM
FOR KIDNEY TRANSPLANTATION

Q P Lansbergen

Data Processing Department

University Hospital Leyden

Eurotransplant Leyden

One out of every 10.000 persons in Europe suffers from an endstage renal disease.
Only during the last ten years has kidney transplantation been an alternative to
haemodialysis.
The first kidney transplantation was performed in 1954, in Boston, between two
identical twins. In The Netherlands the first transplantation with a cadaver donor
kidney was in 1967 in Leyden.

A complication of the transplantation of an unrelated kidney is the rejection of
the transplant by the immunological system of the patient himself.
Although much is still unknown, some factors have been shown to play an important
role in the prolongation of the survival time of the kidney. These are the blood
and tissue types of the donor and recipients, the presensitisation of the recipient
by pregnancy, blood-transfusions and former transplantations. Sometimes this
sensitisation can be shown in the blood of the patient to be directed against a
specific tissue type.

In 1967 Eurotransplant was founded. Dialyses, tranplantation and tissue typing
centres in Austria, Belgium, Germany, The Netherlands and a part of Switzerland
co-operate in this organisation to exchange cadaver donor kidneys.
Patients, suitable for renal transplantation, are registered with ET (Eurotransplant). When a donor kidney becomes available, the pool of patients is searched
and the best-matched patients are selected for transplantation. The pool is
necessary because the chance of finding a complete match between random donor and
recipient tissue types is much less than 1 per thousand.

After transplantation donor and recipient data are stored on magnetic tape. By
means of half-yearly questionnaires the doctors in charge are asked about the
functioning of the kidneys and if the patients are still alive.
This information enables ET to do retrospective analyses, based on the method of
actuarial survival curves, about the influence of various factors on the graft
survival. The results are used to evaluate possible changes in treatment and
selection criteria.

To facilitate all these activities ET makes use of two different computer con-

figurations, namely:
- a dual configuration based on PDP 11/45 computers of the University Hospital in
  Leyden
- a configuration based on an IBM 370/158 computer of the Leyden University
  Computer Centre.

The registration and selection of kidney patients is implemented on the PDP 11/45's.
These computers have extensive online database facilities and provide a round-the-
clock service, seven days a week.
Also, besides terminals and displays, a link to the public telex network is supported.
The IBM 370/158 is used to register the transplantations done under auspices of ET,
and to run the analyses of the graft survival.

The kidney patient registration and selection system

All administrative and medical data of the kidney patients registered with ET are typed in centrally, using a visual display unit. In dialogue with the computer the information is entered, checked and corrected if necessary before it is added to the database.

Whenever a donor kidney becomes available the computer does a fast search through the file of patients waiting for transplantation after the matching parameters have been typed in. Within a minute the 30 best-matched patients are selected.
The regional tissue typing centres have remote access to the database via a chosen link in the public telex network. Privacy is assured by the use of assigned centre numbers and a linked password.

Global system structure

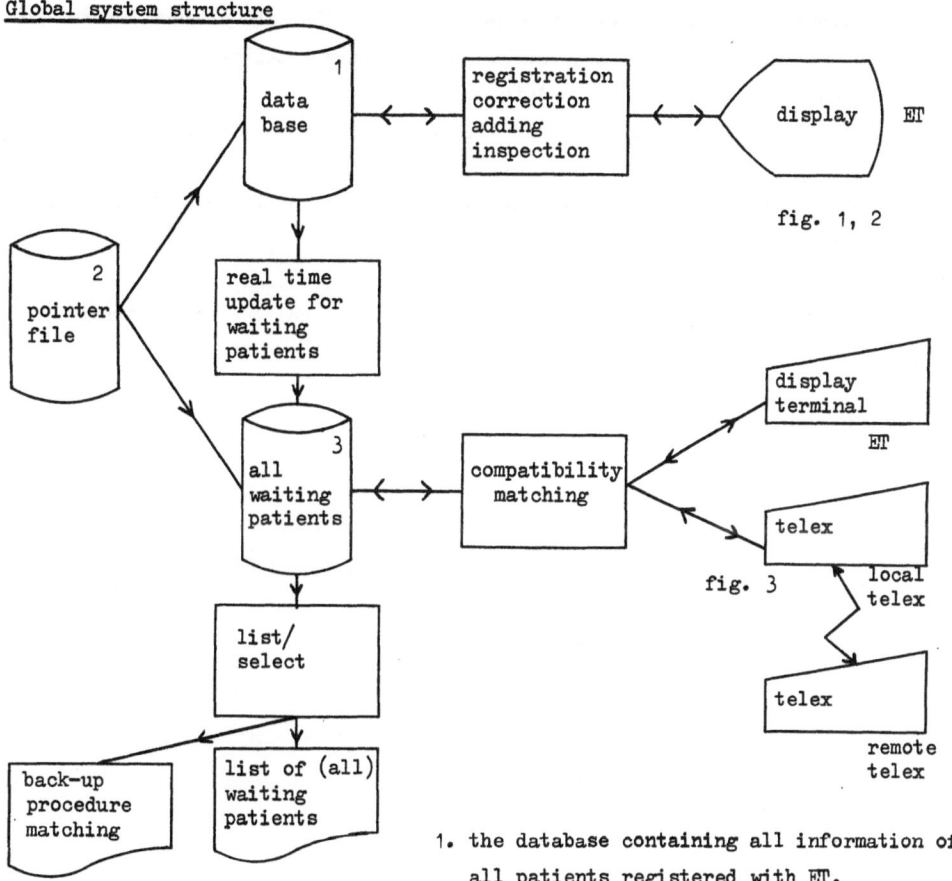

fig. 1, 2

fig. 3

1. the database containing all information of all patients registered with ET.
2. the file of all patients waiting for transplantation, containing a summary of the information in the database.
3. A pointer file to identify all kidney patients and all those who are waiting for transplantation.

The following functions can be distinguished:
- online registration of the kidney patients
- online input of blood and tissue type
- online input of medical data such as blood-transfusions and antibodies
- online inspection of all data recorded in the database
- online selection of the 30 best-matched patients
- printing lists of patients, selected and sorted on various criteria
    i   to do the matching by hand
    ii   as a checklist for the transplantation centres
    iii for management purposes.

Conclusions

An online database provides an efficient means of recording all patient information. Because data is entered online, in dialogue, and checked immediately it has a high quality. The data is also kept up-to-date constantly.
By maintaining, automatically, a file of all waiting patients a fast search is possible.
This concept permits flexibility with regard to expansion of items of information as well as adaptation of the selection algorithm.

Per 1-6-1978 this system is also used for patients who require a cornea transplantation.

The kidney transplant registration system

All kidney transplantations, done under the auspices of ET, are recorded on
magnetic tape residing at the IBM 370/158.
Administrative and medical data of the donor and the recipient are written down
on punch-forms. Periodically these forms are punched on cards, which are added to
the file on tape.
Twice a year the computer prints the questionnaires for the doctors in charge to
update the information about their transplanted patients.

The main kind of analysis on this data is based on the method of constructing
actuarial graft survival curves. For visual aid printed plots are supplied.
The influence of various factors on graft survival is determined by selecting
various subclasses.

Global system structure

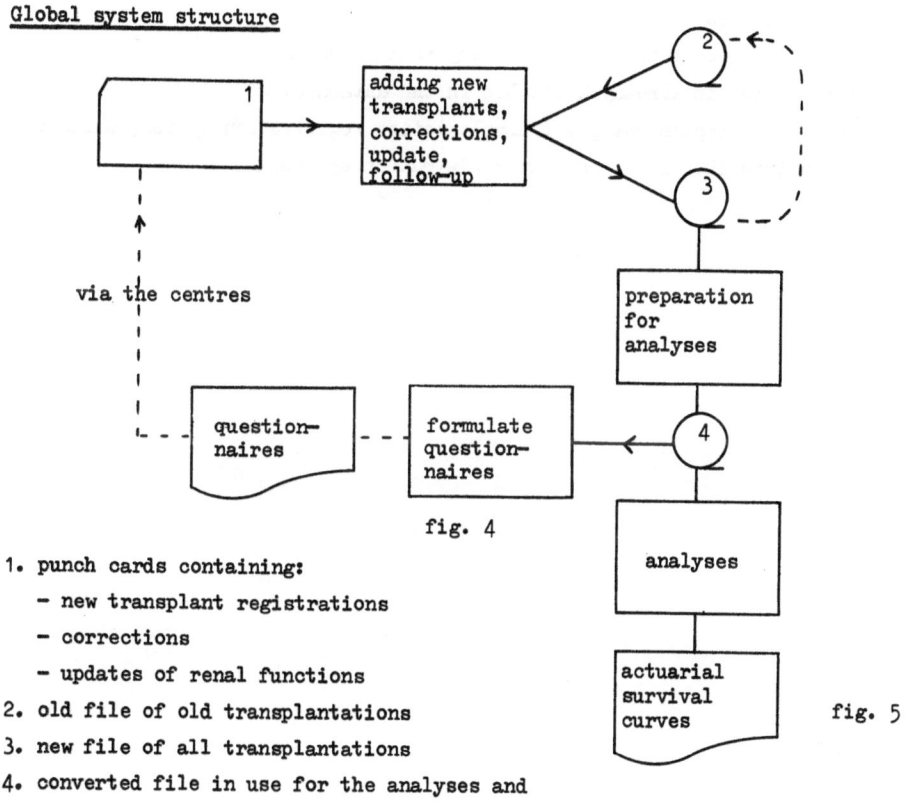

fig. 4

fig. 5

1. punch cards containing:
   - new transplant registrations
   - corrections
   - updates of renal functions
2. old file of old transplantations
3. new file of all transplantations
4. converted file in use for the analyses and
   the questionnaires

Conclusion

The need for a transplant registration system is evident. ET wants to know not only the results of all transplantations but also to control and, if necessary, to change the selection parameters. It is a helpful tool in sorting out the problems in the intricate rejection mechanism.

However, it is essential to have the full co-operation of all doctors participating in kidney transplantations.
To motivate their co-operation ET periodically sends them actuarial analyses performed on all the patients transplanted in their centre.
By keeping the questionnaires as short as possible, and by asking the information only on still functioning grafts ET tries to prevent demotivation.

ET is not satisfied with this system for the following reasons:
- the administration is time-consuming
- the system is batch-oriented, so it is easy to make mistakes
- patient information is already available in the database.
Therefore, ET is now implementing a transplantation registration system, which will be incorporated into the kidney patient registration system.

```
25-04-78 EUROTRANSPLANT SUPPLEMENTORY    RECORD DD:26-07-77    fig. 1
    NAME.....:                         NR...:5897
    BIRTHDATE:31-05-45   SEX:M          AZLNR:9215767
------------------------ EUROTR   PATIENTS -------------------------
( 1)CELLNR...:4589702           ( 2)NR.BLDTRF:
( 4)DIAL.CNTR:GZ                ( 3)NR.PREGNY: 0
( 5)TYP..CNTR:LB                ( 7)COUNTRY.C:NL
(10)WAITNGLST:Y                 ( 6)DIAL.DATE:
(11)URGENCY..: 2                ( 8)DEATHDATE:
(14)PAT.INTRN:Y                 ( 9)WITHDRAWL:
(12)DIAGNOSE.: O OTHER
(13)REMARKS..:


25-04-78 EUROTRANSPLANT TYPING            RECORD DD:27-03-76
    NAME.....:                         NR...:5897
    BIRTHDATE:31-05-45   SEX:M          AZLNR:9215767
------------------------ EUROTR   PATIENTS ------------------------
(2)ABO:O
(3)RHD:+
(1)HLA:
                                    BB              BB
        AA    A  A AAAAAA    BB    WWBBB   BBBB B   44BBB
        WWAAAWAAWAWWWWWW    BWWBBB11WWWBBWWWWWBWBBOOWWW 7BBCCCCCC
    AAAA2212231212333334BBB14411155133112452233..445SBWWWWWWWW
    1239340564189901236357824534512689781902757012123VE46123456
PT.: +-+-----.---------..-++------------.,--------..--.--.-+......
GTM:                                                         M
GTP:                                                         P


25-04-78 EUROTRANSPLANT SCREENING         RECORD DD:
    NAME.....:                         NR...:5897
    BIRTHDATE:31-05-45   SEX:M          AZLNR:9215767
------------------------ EUROTR   PATIENTS -------------------------
                        6                 1       2     3  4  5
R#              LAB,COEF              SERUMNR  BLDATE SCNRTC ST%
------------------------------------------------------------------
    1:B15,4                                   08-08-77          25
    2:                            0355248 13-06-77 535NH     2
    3:                            0355247 18-04-77 533NH     2
    4:                            0355246 14-02-77 531NH     2
    5:                            0355245 13-12-76 519NH     0
    6:                            0355243 02-08-76 514NH     0
    7:                            0355242 31-05-76 511NH     0
    8:                            0355241          504NH     8


COMMAND(SP,TY,SC,TR,):
PATIENT-KAART(J/N):
```

```
25-04-78 EUROTRANSPLANT WAITING LIST      RECORD DD:   fig. 2
   NAME.....:                          NR...:5897
   BIRTHDATE:31-05-45  SEX:M           AZLNR:9215767
------------------------- EUROTR  PATIENTS -------------------
NAME.....:                        SEX......:M
                                  BIRTHDATE:31-05-45
DIAL.CNTR:GZ                       BLOODTRNS:
DIAL.DATE:                         PREGNANCY: 0
URGENCY..:2                        SCR.DATE.:08-08-77
ANTIBODY%: 25                      XMT.DATE.:
ABO+RHD..:O    +
HLA PHENOTYP...:A1   A3   B7   B8   BW6
HLA MAT-HAPLO..:BW6
HLA PAT-HAPLO..:BW6
ANTIBODIES(HLA):B15
```

```
AZL                                                          fig. 3
BOS-PRODUCTIESESSIE AZL VERSIE 21-04-78 ST 188
RUN:CO
DATUM:25-04-78
TIJD:13:29
USERNR?:206
WACHTWOORD?:
WELKOM, LAATSTE GEBRUIK 25-04-78, 13:28, STATION 188
MATCH DEMO


EUROTRANSPLANT MATCH: EUROTR


(1)HLA:A1,A3,B7,B8
(2)ABO:O
(3)RHD:


CORR:
NUM.  NAME   CT U CM ABGHLA-TYPE                    ANTIBODIES
   OXXXXXXXX      15   O A1,A3,B7,B8,BW6,BW6

FULLHOUSE IDENTICALS
  489XXXXXXXX AL 2 15 00 A1,A3,B7,B8,BW6,BW6
 5897XXXXXXXX GZ 2 15 20 A1,A3,B7,B8,BW6,BW6        B15
 7693XXXXXXXX HO 2 15  O A1,A3,B7,B8,BW6,BW6
 4966XXXXXXXX KL 2 29 OA A1,A3,B7,B8,BW6,BW6
 8149XXXXXXXX AR 2 18  B A1,A3,B7,B8,BW6,BW6
 8243XXXXXXXX LG 2 18  B A1,A3,B7,B8,BW6,BW6        A9
 1811XXXXXXXX LM 3 15 00 A1,A3,B7,B8                A26
 6858XXXXXXXX MR 3 15  O A1,A3,B7,B8
 6484XXXXXXXX KS 3 18 1B A1,A3,B7,B8,BW6,BW6
 6670XXXXXXXX ES 3 18  B A1,A3,B7,B8
 7975XXXXXXXX MR 3 18  B A1,A3,B7,B8,BW6,BW6
 8152XXXXXXXX EB 3 29  A A1,A3,B7,B8,BW6,BW6


HIGH URGENT PATIENTS
 8134XXXXXXXX      0  5  O A1,B8,BW6
 1953XXXXXXXX TI 0  9 9A A1,B8,BW6,BW6              A2,A29,B7,
                                                   CW2
 2023XXXXXXXX TI 0  6 9B A1,B8,BW6,BW6              AW32,B37
 8174XXXXXXXX      0 10  ABA1,B8,BW6
 5438XXXXXXXX BN 0  2  B A1,A3,B17,BW35
 6402XXXXXXXX HO 0  0 00 A9,A10,A25,B8,B18,BW6,BW6
 7786XXXXXXXX HO 0  4  O A2,AW19,A29,B7,B12,BW4,BW6
 8240XXXXXXXX FM 0  1  ABA2,A11,B8,BW35,BW6,BW6,CW4
 2108XXXXXXXX DB 0  0 60 A3,A9,B12,B12,BW4          B37
 6567XXXXXXXX UW 0  0  O A1,A28,BW35,B40,BW6,CW3,CW4
 6867XXXXXXXX ML 0  0  O A3,AW19,AW32,B13,B17,BW4,BW4
 7837XXXXXXXX      0  0  B A3,A10,A26,B14,BW6
 4199XXXXXXXX WA 0    30 A28,AW19,AW30,B13,B27,BW4,BW4  A9
 6177XXXXXXXX UW 0  0 00 A9,AW19,AW30,B5,BW22,BW4,BW6,
                                                   CW3,CW4
                                                   AW30
 8045XXXXXXXX      0  6  O A2,A11,B5,B12,BW4,CW4
 8237XXXXXXXX ES 0  2  O A2,B12,B27,BW4,BW4


1 MISMATCHES, 1 ON A AND 0 ON B
 7165XXXXXXXX DA 1  8  O A1,A9,B7,B8,BW6,BW6
 5647XXXXXXXX EN 2  8 00 A2,A3,B7,B8,BW6,BW6
 5815XXXXXXXX ES 2  8 00 A2,A3,B7,B8
 6720XXXXXXXX ES 2  6  O A1,B7,B8,BW6,BW6
 7014XXXXXXXX MA 2  2  O A3,A10,A25,B7,B8
 7579XXXXXXXX HO 2 14 00 A1,A2,B7,B8,BW6,BW6
```

PLEASE RETURN THIS PAGE(S) TO:

EUROTRANSPLANT
ACADEMISCH ZIEKENHUIS   GEB. 23
RYNSBURGERWEG 10
LEIDEN   2401
THE NETHERLANDS

fig. 4

NR ETNR	NAME	BIRTH D.	DIALYS.ID	TRNSPL.D	FUC	IINR	RJ. DATE YY-MM-DD	FC	D. DEATH YY-MM-DD	DC	:REM
101:2756		25-03-14	72-04-04	74-06-10	LB	2635	—	—	—	—	:* F
102:2954		53-04-19	72-10-20	74-06-14	LB	1528	—	—	—	—	:••
103:1876		43-12-02	70-08-08	74-06-29	LB	1546	—	—	—	—	:••
104:3993		47-04-06	73-08-08	74-07-11	LB	1627	—	—	—	—	:••
105:4234		27-02-03	74-01-01	74-08-09	LB	1574	—	—	—	—	:••
106:4552		54-02-27	74-01-28	74-08-17	LB	1740	—	—	—	—	:••
107:4439		47-07-22	74-01-19	74-08-21	LB	1734	—	—	—	—	:••
108:4655		30-07-20	74-01-25	74-09-03	LB	1718	—	—	—	—	:••
109:2031		44-03-10	70-12-12	74-10-14	LB	1692	—	—	—	—	:••
110:3511		32-02-01	72-01-01	74-11-25	LB	1883	—	—	—	—	:••
111:4200		29-04-30	73-11-11	74-11-28	LB	1878	—	—	—	—	:••
112:4028		23-07-11	74-07-02	75-01-01	LB	2447	—	—	—	—	:• F
113:0500		28-09-17	68-10-10	75-01-09	LB	1824	—	—	—	—	:••
114:2460		47-07-05	72-01-01	75-04-17	LB	2006	—	—	—	—	:• F
115:4390		43-10-20	74-08-08	75-04-25	LB	1905	—	—	—	—	:••
116:4962		33-04-01	74-10-10	75-05-12	LB	1956	—	—	—	—	:••
117:4633		49-12-23	74-06-06	75-05-13	LB	1952	—	—	—	—	:••
118:3636		30-10-31	73-02-02	75-05-31	LB	1910	—	—	—	—	:••
119:4902		37-11-22	74-08-06	75-06-01	LB	1906	—	—	—	—	:••
120:3063		40-05-16	72-11-01	75-06-15	LB	2098	—	—	—	—	:••
121:5139		46-07-14	73-12-23	75-08-12	LB	2171	—	—	—	—	:••
122:2169		55-02-28	71-06-01	75-08-29	LB	2204	—	—	—	—	:••

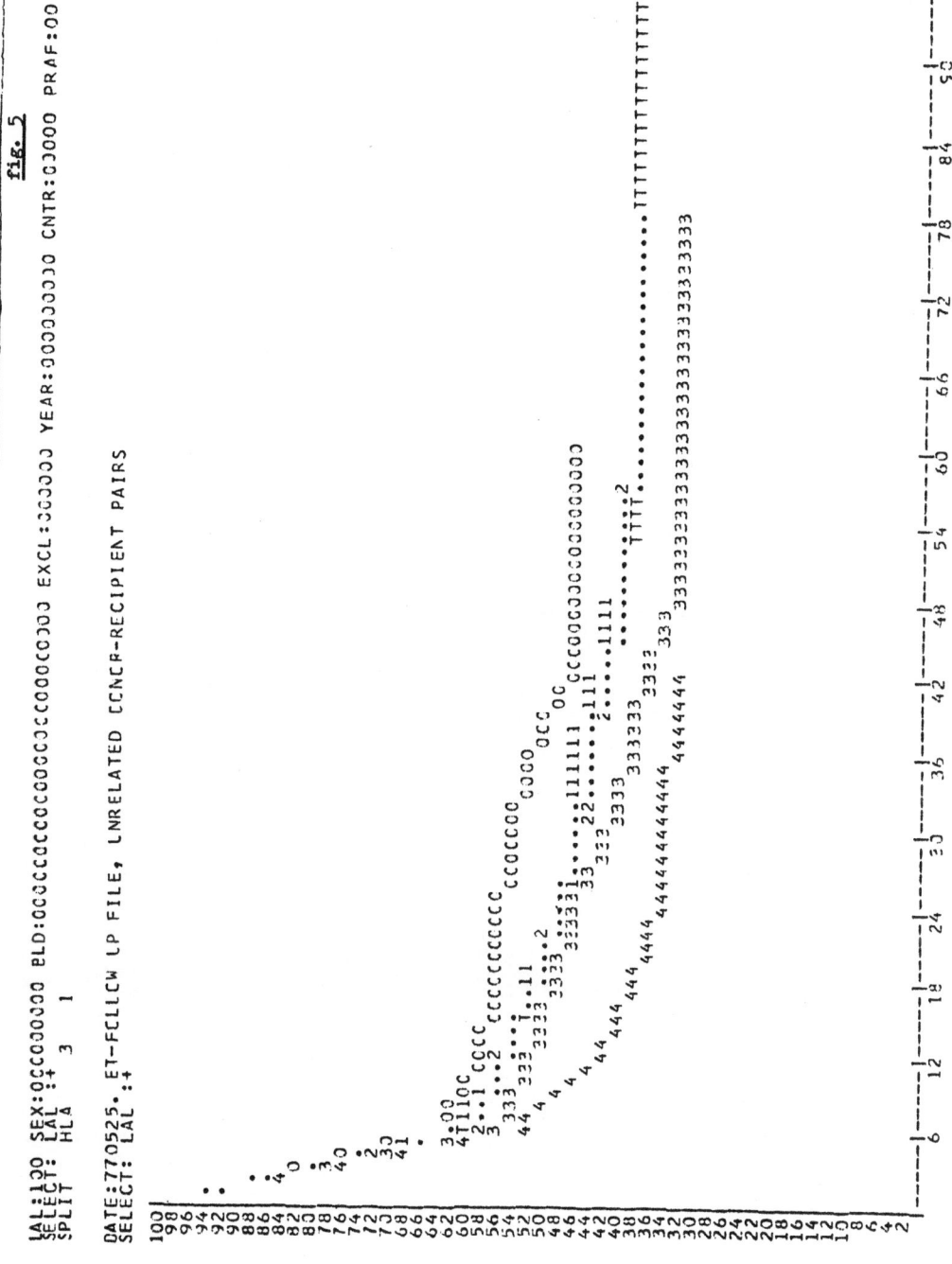

fig. 5

MFS - A USER-ORIENTED SYSTEM FOR DIAGNOSTIC DATA MANAGEMENT

E. Guidotti - R. Arrigoni
Centro Diagnostico Italiano
Milano, Italy

INTRODUCTION

Centro Diagnostico Italiano (C.D.I.) is an outpatient clinic operating in the health care field since the beginning of 1975.

At C.D.I.'s the flow of medical data is supported by the computer in several departments: Preventive Medicine (Multiphasic Health Check-up), Hormonal Contraception, Radioimmunology, Clinical Lab, Cardiology, and others.

But the activity performed by the computer in the first two of them is of special interest for this paper, as it is based on the use of a special package of programs, which will be dealt with here in detail. This package is called MFS (Medical data Filing System), and has been successfully in operation at C.D.I. since September 1976.

HEALTH CHECK-UP APPLICATION OUTLINE

Fifty out of the ca. 600 patients showing every day at C.D.I. are given a comprehensive multiphasic health check-up.

The patient fills at home a history questionnaire by checking with a pencil the mark-sense cards embedded in the questionnaire booklet. When the patient shows at C.D.I., his history is checked by a professional nurse, who also fills a second level questionnaire, according to the patient's needs; the mark-sense cards are torn-off and sent to the computer department. While the patient is given the tests which will be mentioned later, the computer processes the history information collected, by carrying out a thorough logical evaluation (formal and medical) on it. A summary report is then printed with warnings for data inconsistencies or omissions.

In the meanwhile the patient is driven by the nurse along the check-up circuit, including several steps: blood drawing, x-ray examinations, ECG, tonometry, vision, audiometry, spirometry, blood pressure, etc.

The patient is then given a physical examination by a doctor, who also corrects with him any inconsistency shown on the history printout.

The computer then loads functional tests results (coded on mark-sense cards by the nurse), x-ray findings (coded by the radiologist

on mark-sense cards), physical examination findings (coded by the
check-up doctor on mark-sense cards) and lab results.
When all data are available, the computer goes through them with an
overall logical evaluation and prints a final report.

HORMONAL CONTRACEPTION APPLICATION OUTLINE

In the Hormonal Contraception Department, up to twenty patients per
day are given a sort of screening based on some lab tests, on a very
detailed medical history questionnaire and on a physical examination.
The computer processes the information read from mark-sense cards ac
cording to a very sophisticated medical logic aimed at organizing
and grouping the data collected according to their relevance in six
pathological areas of specific interest. What the gynaecologist receives from the computer is so a list of warnings for potential or
real risks connected with the use of the "pill", rather than a print
out of raw data.
Moreover, for each warning a degree of likelihood is printed, accord
ing to the significance of the symptoms (or reference data) available.

DESCRIPTION OF MFS

As said before, the software supporting the applications above is a
generalized system called MFS, designed for collection and reporting
of medical data.
One major objective set in the design of this system was to build a
package which could be easily tailored to the requirements of several different applications, and which would allow the user to perform
easily frequent revisions on them.
This requires that:
1) exchanges of information between user and computer can be program
   med easily, no matter which is the channel of communication (mark
   sense or punched card, keyboard, CRT screen, printed report) and
   which is the mode of operation of the computer (batch or interactive);
2) the user-programmer must be involved as little as possible in the
   details of information recording on mass-storage media (records
   layout and physical organization of archives).
It was so decided to implement a package including a certain number
of generalized programs, capable of performing some typical repetitive tasks, which often require revisions (like history-taking, re-

porting in natural language, decision support/medical logic).
These programs are written in a machine-oriented language (Assembler) in order to achieve maximum execution efficiency. The medical
content, the phraseology and the logic of a certain application can
so be specified by the user on special coding forms, with moderate
programming effort, as to time and skill required.

Through the use of such generalized programs an unskilled programmer can access the patient data base (both in input and in output)
simply by specifying the symbolic names of the variables interested.
In case that special-purpose programs are needed (performing functions different from those of the generalized programs above, like
statistical evaluations of data, etc.), input-output routines for
accessing the patient data base are available. These routines can
be invoked by a skilled programmer implementing his programs in one
of the usual languages (Assembler, COBOL, PL/1).

After nearly two years of operation, it can be said that this package meets the requirements of:

- flexibility and ease of customerization (as specified above);
- compactness, as it can be operated with good performances in a
  small or medium size computer;
- ease of operation (as through a tracing facility, the system continuously monitors the data being collected for each patient; the
  activities of logical evaluation of data and printing of reports
  for each patient are so automatically triggered by the availability of the information needed).

Customerization, revisions and operation of the system can be done
through the use of the system facilities:

- Data description language (DDL): at system generation, through the
  DDL the user can make a description of the data to be managed (in
  terms of Data Items and Segments), specifying symbolic names and
  attributes. A Dictionary is so built.
- Compilers/Drivers: Driver is a program capable of performing a repetitive task on data not in a rigid way, but according to the
  user's specifications; Compiler is a program which translates the
  user's specifications into a Control Table which becomes part of
  the system and is looked up by the right Driver at execution time.
  In the user's specifications, input/output of data to the database is performed by specifying the symbolic names stored in the
  Dictionary.

At present Drivers/Compilers are implemented for four basic functions:

- Data acquisition through cards or card-image transactions.
- Reporting in natural language (either on-line on a terminal print-
  er, or in batch mode on a line-printer).
- On-line interview (according to a branch-tree logic) and Data Base
  inquiry.
- Decision support.

Generation and operation of an application with MFS are carried out
according to the following steps:

1. Generation of the Dictionary of all data items involved.
2. Generation of all Control Tables with fraseology, input descriptions, report outlines and video frames description.
3. Patient registration, to be done any time a patient requests services. The patient is assigned an ID. His data are recorded on
   the Patient file, and his requests are recorded on a control file,
   called Activity file.
4. Data collection, processing and reporting. These activities are
   carried out by the right generalized programs using the right
   Control Tables. Every time the operator feeds input data, the
   execution of the right programs is scheduled automatically by the
   system by comparing the type of data available at the time with
   the type of data expected for each patient.
   The Activity file is continuously updated in order to reflect exactly the status of the information required for each patient.

As to the data base structure, Data Items are grouped into Segments,
and Segments are recorded on mass-storage in fixed-length blocks.
Data for a patient are thus kept in a variable number of blocks link
ed together.
At registration of a new patient, a unique medical record number is
assigned by the system. As Segments may have many occurrences for
the same patient, data about subsequent visits of a patient are integrated in the patient records chain, which is accessible either by
medical record number or by patient name, sex and date of birth.

M.F.S. PERFORMANCES

The package runs in an IBM 370 system operated under DOS with the
support of C.I.C.S. for the on-line functions. The largest batch
program requires a 36 kb partition.
The largest C.I.C.S. task requires < 10 kb.
MFS has been in operation in C.D.I. since September 1976, and the
data of more than 15,000 patients have been processed so far.

To give an idea of the complexity of C.D.I.'s installation, the following figures should be considered:

- the check-up History Questionnaire for Males includes about 1000 items (of the boolean type;   i.e. YES/NO);
- the Female Questionnaire, about 1200 items;
- the Hormonal Contraception Questionnaire, about 500 items;
- codification of x-ray findings (chest, spine, teeth, breast) is done through the use of about 800 items (boolean);
- 200 items are required to handle numerical results and free texts;
- physical examination findings are coded through the use of about 500 items;
- logical evaluation of data collected is performed by checking each item against others related to it. This requires that each item is touched at least three times as an average for each patient;
- codification of the output ("the conclusions") of logical evaluations has required the definition of more than 2000 auxiliary items (boolean).

Notwithstanding such complexity, customerization (i.e. tailoring of MFS to the requirements outlined above) has required an effort of only a few months of clever but unskilled programmer.

Frequent revisions have also been carried out since then, in terms of changes of fraseology and logical evaluation rules, and addition of new Data Items to the Dictionary.

Up to 70 patients per day are registered in the system, and their huge amount of medical data are forwarded to the computer from the various departments (Radiology, Cardiology, Laboratory, etc.) any time in the two to three days following the patient encounter.

The computer, through the use of the tracing facility, automatically carries out the different stages of logical evaluation at the right moment, requests correction of inconsistent codifications, and prints provisional and final reports when all data required are available. All this is done very simply from an operational point of view, as the computer operator is relieved from the tedious task of sorting and clustering documents per patient before loading data into the computer and scheduling the various processing steps required.

AN ATTEMPT TO EVALUATE THE CONTRIBUTION

OF COMMON LABORATORY FINDINGS : AN EXPERIMENT

IN NEUROLOGY

J.L GOLMARD (1) - C. DEROUESNE (2)

B. ASSELAIN(1)- M. BERNADET (1)

R. SALAMON (3)- F. GREMY   (1)

1 - Groupe de Recherches U 88 - INSERM

   91, boulevard de l'Hôpital - 75634 PARIS CEDEX 13

2 - Clinique des Maladies du Système Nerveux

   Hôpital de la Salpêtrière

   47, boulevard de l'Hôpital - 75634 PARIS CEDEX 13

3 - Département d'Informatique - Université de Bordeaux II

   146, rue Léo Saignat - 33076 BORDEAUX CEDEX.

1.   INTRODUCTION

    This work describes an experiment to assist differential diagnosis in
Neurology. It seeks to furnish an evaluation of the contribution of the commonly
used laboratory tests in a retrospective study.

2.   DATA

    The medical records used came from the archives of two departments:
- Clinique des maladies du systeme nerveux, Hopital de la Salpetriere,
  Paris.
- Clinique Neurologique - Hopital de L'Hotel-Dieu, Rouen.
    The only criteria for the selection of records was the necessity of an
established diagnosis supported either by histology-pathology or concordance of
clinical and paraclinical findings.
    The totality of Neurological disorders was grouped into 31 different
diagnosis. These were chosen so as to make each of them correspond to a specific
behaviour (1,5).

    The medical data are divided into 4 chapters:
    The first three chapters represent the clinical examination:
    Evolution of the disease from the first symptom to the first
neurological examination.
    Personal and family history
    Physical examination (general and neurological).
    The fourth chapter includes the common laboratory tests i.e. Biological
tests (blood count, blood urea nitrogen, plasma proteins and sodium potassium,
chloride, wasserman test)
    X-rays of the skull
    X-rays of the spinal column. Lumbar puncture results (cytology,
wasserman reaction, proteins in the cerebrospinal fluid (CSF). Opthalmic
examination of the retina.
    These data correspond to 160 items. For each of them, three responses are
possible; yes, no or missing information (3,8)

    Methods
    A bayesian method, applied to decision making (5,6) permits the
calculation of the probability of each of 31 diagnosis as a function of a given
symptomatic profile. The results can be calculated in an interative way, and so

it is possible to know for example the results obtained by taking into account only the first three chapters, or the first three chapters and a laboratory test.

The comparison between these two results permits the assessment of the contribution to the diagnosis of the laboratory test considered. But what we call a result consists of 31 numbers which are the probabilities of each of the diagnoses. Criteria must be found to summarise this information in the best way.

I First analysis method

If we consider that the answer by the computer is the diagnosis with the higher probability, the result may be true of false (remember that the true diagnosis presented by the patient is known). Then we can choose as a criteria the number of errors, by default or by excess, that are corrected by the laboratory tests.

Nevertheless, this method cannot find the contribution of the laboratory tests in the following case. Let us suppose that the diagnosis 1 is the true one, and that, before the test is taken into account, the result is the following one:

$$p(D1) = 0.50 \qquad p(D2) = 0.45$$

When the test is taken into account, the result becomes:

$$p(D1) = 0.99 \qquad p(D2) = 0.01$$

The first method of analysis does not permit the finding of a useful investigation, even though it seems obvious; the diagnosis is certain after the investigation, it was beyond the bound before it. To be able to include the usefulness of the laboratory test in this case we decided to improve the analysis by adding a second method.

II Second analysis method

We call the "true diagnosis" the diagnosis which is actually presented by the patient and "reckoned diagnosis" the diagnosis with the highest probability before the laboratory tests are taken into account. The reckoned diagnosis can therefore be true or false.

To be useful a test must increase the probability of the true diagnosis. So the second criteria will be the difference before the considered test is taken into account. Practically, the results are shown by diagnoses: the criteria is the mean of the differences of probability determined from all the patients having this diagnosis.

But an investigation is also useful when it permits the correction of errors by excess, i.e. to eliminate the "false positive" areas. The corresponding result, with this method is the diminution of the probability of the reckoned diagnosis when this one is false. It is easy to see that this second analysis method cannot find the share of the laboratory tests in all cases. That is the reason why we choose finally to present the results obtained with the two methods simultaneously. None is indeed better than the other, and it seems to us that they complement each other.

We shall not talk here about other frequently used methods which are based on the entropy or ċosts (or utility). Other works based on these methods are on going (about utility, 2,4)

3.   RESULTS

Our results are based on 548 fits. We cannot here give all the results, only examples.

I   Results about the whole set of diagnoses and the whole set of tests

2219 tests have been made:
527 biological tests
427 X-ray of the skull
400 EEG
357 opthalmic examinations of the retina
339 lumbar puncture
169 X-ray of the spinal column
When these investigations were not taken into account, the results were:
409 right diagnosis (74%)
the mean probability of the true diagnosis being 0.68
When the investigations were taken into account:
435 right diagnosis (79%)
the mean probability of the true diagnosis being 0.76
So the laboratory tests have permitted the correction of 26 diagnoses
which is 85 tests for each diagnoses.
These figures lead immediately to two conclusions:
1. The mathematical model appears valid : 79% of good results
2. The diagnostic contribution of the common laboratory tests is low.

II Results of each test for the totality of diagnosis (1,7)

With these results we can evaluate the usefulness of each laboratory test for a given illness. When the two methods agree, the lumbar puncture and the EEG had a better rating than the other tests.

III Results for each diagnosis and each test (1)

1. Spinal cord compression : 52 patients
    The results when the tests are not taken into account are:-
    5 mistakes by default
    20 mistakes by excess
    the probability of the true diagnosis is 0.94
    the probability of the reckoned diagnosis when it is false is 0.80
    The lumbar puncture:-
    amends 3 mistakes by default
    adds 1 mistake by excess
    increases the probability of the true diagnosis by 0.03
    lessens the probability of the reckoned diagnosis by 0.05 when it is false.

2. Cerebral haemorrhage from an aneurysm (16 patients)
    When the tests are not taken into account, we find:-
    2 mistakes by default
    6 mistakes by excess
    the probability of the true diagnosis is 0.77
    the probability of the reckoned diagnosis when it is false is 0.66
    The lumbar puncture:-
    corrects no mistake, either by default or excess
    increases the probability of the true diagnosis by 0.14
    increases the probability of the reckoned diagnosis by 0.08 when it is false.

4. DISCUSSION AND PERSPECTIVES

1. About the data.
    We shall not discuss the problems of the choice of risks and diagnosis or the representatives of our sample, these problems have been discussed elsewhere (3,6)

2. About the methods.

The method which consisted of considering only the diagnosis with the highest probability obviously lacks some shrewdness. We have seen cases in which it was insufficient. Nevertheless it gives, with little calculation, an idea of the diagnostic interest of the tests.

The last result given (haemorrhage by aneurysm) gives an example of the usefulness of the second method of analysis. However, this method does not use the whole information contained in the result of the Bayes formula.

The use of both the methods is a compromise which seems to us sufficient to evaluate the diagnostic contribution of the laboratory tests. We are thinking of combining these results with those obtained by methods based on the measurement of entropy of utility.

It is not sufficient to be aware of the inflation of the laboratory tests. Our objective in the near future is to propose a viable diagnostic plan adapted to each patient. The theoretical solution for this difficult problem is being worked out.

6.   CONCLUSIONS

We have presented in this paper methods for quantifying in an objective manner the contribution of common laboratory findings to effective diagnosis. It appears now that overall this contribution is small. Steps will be taken to compare results with those obtained by other methods, and to determine, when confronted with the clinical profile of a patient, the order and number of laboratory tests necessary to achieve a good diagnosis at the lowest cost.

REFERENCES

1- J.L. GOLMARD - Intérêt diagnostique des examens complémentaires usuels en Neurologie. Medical thesis, 1978, PARIS XIII.

2- B. ASSELAIN. Le concept d'utilité dans la décision médicale : à propos d'une expérience en Neurologie. Medical thesis, 1977 PARIS VI.

3- R. SALAMON. Aide à la décision et enseignement médical : à propos d'une expérience en Neurologie. Human biology thesis, PARIS VI.

4- B. ASSELAIN, C. DEROUESNE, R. SALAMON, M. BERNADET, F. GREMY. The concept of utility in medical decision aid : example of an application. In SHIRES D.B. et WOLS H. MEDINFO 77, 1 vol. North Holland. Publishing campany, AMSTERDAM 1977.

5- C. DEROUESNE et R. SALAMON. Contemporary teaching of Neurology. Teaching neurological behaviour to general practitioners : a fresch approach. Medical education, 1977, 11, 28 - 31.

6- R. SALAMON, M. BERNADET, M. SAMSON, C. DEROUESNE, F. GREMY. Bayesian method applied to decision making in Neurology. Methodological considerations. Meth. Inform. Med. 1976, 15, 174 - 179.

7- R. SALAMON, J.L. GOLMARD, C. DEROUESNE, F. GREMY. Reflexions à propos d'un essai d'utilisation de l'informatique pour l'aide au diagnostic étiologique en Neurologie. Incidences pédagogiques de cette expérience Nouv. Presse Méd. , à paraître.

8- M. BERNADET, R. SALAMON, F. GREMY. Utilisation de l'algébre ternaire dans l'analyse des données médicales. Compte rendu de l'Académie des Sciences. Séance du 5.01.76. Tome 282, Fascicule n° 1, 135, série D.

ARTIFICIAL MEDICAL LANGUAGES, A SOLUTION FOR CLINICAL NEEDS
IN DOCUMENTATION. EXAMPLE USING REMEDE SYSTEM

M. de HEAULME
Groupe de Recherches U 88
Méthodologie Informatique et Statistique en Médecine
91, bd de l'hôpital, 75634 PARIS cedex 13

I. CLINICAL NEEDS IN DOCUMENTATION

It seems clear today that two distinct goals are pursued when clinicians' requests in data processing are discussed :

1. Systems for analyzing fully normalized data

Such systems require data collection by questionnaire. This way of doing implies enumeration of the possible cases having to be indexed. Diversity of medical descriptions is so broad that this way leads to indefinitely increase the questionnaires when the aim is to collect any relevant data on any patient admitted in a medical center. If these questionnaires are not devoted to specific data collection of relatively small sets, corresponding systems become more and more heavy, expensive and finally unefficient.

On the contrary, if they are only limited to specific data collection, they cannot satisfy clinicians' documentary needs. Most of them only provide data concerned with patient administration, or particular clinical research.

The formal reason is that the way of data representation using questionnaires proceeds by enumeration, while each patient associates signs, symptoms, treatments, etc ... according to his own way. There are always other features to describe not contained in the normalized questionnaire form.

2. Systems for describing any kind of "interesting" data

This way requires languages capable of combining words in "sentences" appropriated to each description, just as   is done in natural language. Systems of this type better deal with medical documentary purposes but it must be kept in mind that they have dropped one degree of normalization : as long as sentence - making is a free act, nothing guarantees that some clinical information will be reported by the same data, contrary to what could be possible when questionnaire technique is used.

But here the purpose is not to provide direct data analysis or some management computation. It is only to allow retrieval, or any kind of complex interrogation on the information pool provided by the medical system in spite of its sparsity. At this step, clinicians don't require to prove or to conclude yet, but only to perform investigations on what is where, to get an aid in assumption-making before testing relevant hypothesis, or merely to explore their data in a non-directive way.

Physicians know exactly these "documentary" needs which are fully integrated in their daily activity. Of course, better normalization could also be obtained if all users had to respect the same description pattern.

Any medical record request contains a part of such documentary needs, more or less explicit and implemented. Many actual questionnaire systems cannot entirely satisfy clinicians on this point.

The same needs in data representation concern at least two other documentary fields : medical specialized bibliography and documentation in aided diagnosis.

- specialized bibliography concerns restricted fields, contrary to aims assumed by general systems as Medlars or Erxcepta Medica.

In specialized fields, the aim is to provide complete content analysis of reports describing medical litterature, including sometimes lecturers' critics. It could be the case for a service which wants to manage its own bibliography as it often occurs, or for a speciality, a medical society, etc ... which wants to offer its members the possibility to interrogate all the papers concerned with it.

- The purpose of aided diagnosis documentation is to refresh users' memory about diseases, or to select diseases corresponding to a set of symptoms or of bio-medical signs. It doesn't involve any mathematical procedure in order to determine diagnoses, which can only be done in specific fields. This documentation system serves to remind facts about any disease as it is currently done by physician looking for medical books.

In these fields (medical records, specialized bibliography, documentary aid) the same functions are requested :
- to be able to describe any kind of situation relevant to the field (patient, papers, diseases)
- to provide content analysis as complete and precise as possible.

Finally, it seems that medical recording and retrieving activity requires a two-step system involving two different functions : a non specific "documentary" one, and a specific one requiring questionnaire utilization.

Using natural language for clinical documentation must first be discussed because of its possible immediate availability. But :
- natural language processing is not sufficiently developped yet when context is too large. Specialists still say "not before many years" (6) meanwhile we have to give solutions to physicians today.
- Even if natural language analysis becomes efficient, it is not sure that it would be a convenient tool for medical descriptions. Most often the medical way of thinking is fuzzy and proceeds by analogy or intuition, while computers require definite sets of data and proceed step by step by deduction. According to all authors, medical informatics will not develop itself, without medical education of thinking capable of highlighting precise facts and their articulations. The use of natural language too easily escapes this necessity. On the contrary, artificial languages

force physicians to reflect on what and how they are indexing information, while
they construct sentences still easily processable by computers.

Consequently interrogation of data indexed by artificial language is much
more sensitive and specific, as much as it is required for providing precise and
pertinent content analysis. This fact is very important in the medical field :
- 'silence'is not tolerable in Medicine, because it could imply dangerous decision,
  contrary to current purposes in general bibliography.
  Formal silence due to the system nature disappears with artificial languages which
  are logical themselves. Silence due to human defaults will always remain particula-
  rily due to the fact that physicians very often interrogate computers with implicit references coming from their medical background. But this kind of silence
  could never be reduced unless the computer is a doctor itself.
- Noise also cannot be important because clinical documentation is linked to the
  physicians' daily activity. Physicians proceed step by step in interrogating, pre-
  cising one idea or going to another one. They have not and they cannot check each
  retrieved record, even more if answers concern several hundred or thousand records.
  Thus the remaining noise must be as little as possible in medical interrogation
  systems.

Another condition of medical acceptability is the simplicity and the power
of interrogation commands.

Many requests necessitate a great amount of elementary commands leading to
long time of typing with possible errors and computer-time consuming. Complex command languages would not be so effective at the present stage of medical education.
Nevertheless, sophisticated but simple commands working as "macro-commands" are
very requested. For example, research of criteria combinations is a basic medical
request, and must be typed in a simple way.

Such commands are easily constructed with artificial languages as it can
be seen in the REMEDE example.

Summarizing the considerations above, we may point out :
a. an activity which concerns a broad descriptive field and a great variability of
   description, not suited with techniques using a priori possible enumerated cases.
b. the necessity of a precise text content analysis by computer processing
c. a low rate of silence and noise
d. a problem of users' mind education
e. the practical possibility to write future documents in a convenient way, which is
   not always possible. In the general bibliography source, documents have already
   their definite form in natural language
f. the disposal of macro commands for current requesting

These conditions concern each field of what is called by us "clinical documentation" and leads to choose artificial languages as a tool for pertinent description and powerful interrogation.

Two remarks must be still made :

- Since clinical documentation is implicated in the daily medical routine, systems
  must work in conversationnal mode
- Such systems are able to be implemented only if the cost of the elementary transaction (=one update, one interrogation, etc ...) remains very low, because they
  are used in an iterative way

These facts reinforce once more the choice of artificial languages which
processing may be very efficient in comparison to natural language processing.

II. ARTIFICIAL LANGUAGE SPECIFICATIONS IN CLINICAL ENVIRONMENT

If artificial languages are chosen, practical solutions have to be found for
their construction in order to avoid difficulties inherent to natural language.

2.1. Semantic properties

The goal is to escape the semantic variability. It is imperative to squeeze
this variability leading to the fact that same things are not called by same labels,
or that one same label could design different things. Medical words are tremendously
sensible to the field in which they are used, to the medical background of each physician, to the different medical schools of thinking, to the last conception in no-
sography, etc ...

Systems which would take into account such variability would be immediatly
submerged by the flow of personal connotations. Then, forcing physicians to use a
clear and well accepted design of each medical term appears to be a basic rule. Such
a duty is more or less easy to obtain concerning facts and "hard" information such
as signs, symptoms, topographies, bioclinical results, etc ...

The classical difficulty is to find a thesaurus organisation reflecting the
semantic links between terms. It is clear to day that such general organisation is
tremendously complex, if it does exist. But finding simple thesaurus organization is
quite possible if each semantic class of terms is lexically separated. In this case
each class follows its own rule or arrangement following the precision of each term
without respect to the others. The problem is only to know if a small number of term
classes is sufficient, as it seems to be the case in Medicine (1, 2, 3, 4, 5).

Ambiguous terms or "school wording" must be rejected and replaced by an exact
description. For example, "Freyberg disease" must be reported as "Aseptic osteone-
crosis of 2nd metatarsus". This way forces physicians to report their concepts into
simple factual terms, which is a great benefit for their self-education and considerably facilitates the data processing.

Finally, there is a match between the natural way of doing of the physician
when using notions quicker and more effective to be used at the data collection step,
and the data fiability of details they want during the interrogation step. When the

problem is clearly explicited to physicians, semantic solutions are available if they   accept self-education.

2.2. Syntaxic properties

Syntaxic operators have to link terms in such a way that sentence-making is never ambiguous in respect to the semantic content of each term. As long as sentences contain only one term of each semantic class, no problem occurs because the mutual links are univocal. But this way of writing is very long because it leads to repetition of same terms. However, mixing terms of the same class without syntax introduces noise and silence, as it has been seen above (3) .

The problem is also here to define convenient links according to the medical description needs. As for the number of semantic classes, these syntaxic operators must be in small number to be acceptable.

Some of them are easily found as genitive operators, causal operators, coordination operators, etc ... An example of such a set of syntaxic operators is presented in REMEDE.

These operators must obey formal properties for being convenient to artificial languages.
- they must represent a logical relation, which doesn't necessarily mean a boolean one. It is a condition for keeping a univocal meaning to the computer processing (3).
- the general grammar must be factorisable, in the sense that a complex sentence involving multiple-brackets (or any paired syntaxic operators) must contain exactly the same information as a set of simple sentences merely coordinate each others.

This makes sense as well for physicians who have not to be bothered by complex sentence-making, as for programmers during sentence scanning.

These two conditions seem to be enough for designing the needed language. The construction of the whole properties of such context calculable languages would necessitates more formal studies.

2.3. Temporal syntax

Capability of collecting dated events and of making interrogation is a necessity in Medicine as long as disease is a story.

Including temporal conditions in a grammar could lead to very complex situations. Two kinds of conditions have to be performed :
- on dates or delays, i.e. on numbers. They will be called "cardinal conditions".
- on the rank of events, called "ordinal conditions". Each of them are well known.
  The great difficulty is to mix them in a simple way of writing command languages, and to find efficient ways of processing them.

Formally, introducing temporal conditions does not raise special difficulties

as long as they also are themselves logical expressions. However, they are typically
context dependent. Example on how a temporal grammar could be implemented is given
in section III.

2.4. Technical aspects

Some technical effectiveness is required in clinical situation.

- Clinicians must definitely be able to work in conversational mode. This is due not
  only to the fact that clinical documentation needs are integrated to the medical
  routine, but also to necessity of providing quick and correct validation. It is
  easily obtained if staff secretaries are able to immediatly ask physicians for
  some difficulties and to correct records before information is lost. Samely, diagnostic documentary aid has sense only if it is immediatly available.

- It is harder to find efficient solution to the fact that context sensible sentences
  must be entirely examined before deciding if they answer to   a question. It means
  that the classical techniques of interrogation programming and data bases designing
  have to be adapted, because they usually use only boolean computation in their
  retrieval processing.

III. EXAMPLE WITH REMEDE

REMEDE, designed in 1973, is only an example of what could be a "complete"
language. Even it is only a subset of such a language, many current services are
already able to be requested in the actual version (1, 2, 3).

Only 8 classes of terms and 9 operators are used and quickly learnt. Try
to understand the following text (fig. 1). Even without education, it is quite
understandable.

a. semantic classes are : events (hospitalisation, consultation, arteriography,
   operation, ...), signs and symptoms, topographies, etiologies, treatments, bioclinical examinations, results.
   Synonyms could be defined. Thesaurus are printed by hierarchical or alphabetic
   rank.

b. operators are :

   <   linking terms to topographies
   >   linking terms to etiologies
   *   treated by
   =   results (of a treatment or a bioclinical examination)
   %   between (fistulae, anastomosis, ...)
   /   end of a sentence
   ,   and
   ( ) delimiting expressions
   :   event (hospitalisation, operation ...)

—   links adjectives to terms

c. <u>Dates are reported between</u> " "

    "date"   ponctual date

    "date-" begining date

    "-date" ending date

    "date-date" period

d. <u>adjectives can be defined</u>. Some of them, called "modifiers" are

    L   left

    R   right

    B   bilateral

    ?   doubtful

    ↑   certain

    N   negative (absent)

    C   complicated

        Free comments between (   ) are allowed anywhere.

        The report text is headed by a questionnaire defined by each user and able to contain any kind of normalized data.

        Records are created, updated and validated in conversational mode (1, 2, 3). Practically, secretaries know very quickly the current labels, and are able to rectify terms misorthographied by physicians.

        Thus physicians are not bothered by frequent thesaurus consultation. Dictated reports are being experienced in surgery. Success in surgery application would be ofmajor importance, for surgeons traditionnally meet great difficulties in data collecting. Today, REMEDE supports reports in rheumatology, cardiology, and vascular surgery (8000 reports indexed).

        Applying REMEDE to diagnostic documentary aid is being tested. Specialized bibliography has been fully studied in urology.

        Interrogation requires new facilities :

a. usual boolean prepositions OR and NO must be added

b. selections on tabulations must be able to be commanded on headings

c. interrogation of data events requires new syntax. Dates have the same representation as in text. Duration is merely indicated by . followed by x Days, y months, z years.

    Begining or end of events must be defined. For example

    "B 0377-0677" means events having begun between March and June 1977 (included)

    ".6M2Y" means a duration of 2 years 6 months.

        Terms having to obey temporal conditions are between square brackets. Such expressions could be chained. For example :

pain <(knee, hip),   "B 0377-" [arthritis > traumatism]

means : pain of knee and hip appeared after arthritis due to a traumatism having begun since March 1977. Meanwhile :

".6M-" $\left[\text{pain} < (\text{knee, hip})\right]$, "B 0377-" $\left[\text{arthritis} > \text{traumatism}\right]$
add another condition on this pain duration (at least 6 months).

d. A last facility is very often required : let·the computer be able to find by
itself some combinations of terms. The actual REMEDE could provide such automatic research of combinations.

pain < (knee, hip) > COMB   would find any cause of pain of knee and hip.

Frequencies and percentages are printed by hierarchical rank of founded terms.

CONCLUSION

A four years experience of REMEDE has shown that artificial languages represent a practical solution to many clinical requirements in documentation processing.
Other original tentative show the same ability (4). Solutions could be efficient
and effective. For example, average time for one record consultation is around
5 milli-seconds cpu time with REMEDE, while programs could be easily implemented
on mini-computers disposing dynamic core allocation.

Effectiveness in medical education is an important aspect of such language utilization, strongly related to progresses in medical informatics. Another important
aspect is the fact that the same language which means the same maintenance and the
same user education is available for many different applications involving documentation.

Moreover, this type of medical description is transparent to national languages which also could be an important property today.

Finally, the way of artificial languages in clinical documentation processing appears as a global strategy able :

- to provide a physician-computer communication in any field concerned with clinical documentation

- to motivate physicians in computing usage and self education

- to develop a unic language for any medical documentation aim, which means a great
economy.

REFERENCES

1. de HEAULME, M., MERY, Ch. An artificial language for medical reports on computer
Proceedings of Medinfo 74, p. 935-941

2. de HEAULME, M., MERY, Ch. Physician-computer communication. Proceedings of
MEDCOMP 77, p. 323-338

3. de HEAULME, M., MERY, Ch. REMEDE : an artificial language for clinical documentation. Computational Linguistics in Medicine. North Holland Pub. Cy. 1977

4. COX, E.B. Towards a medical language. Proceedings of MEDINFO 77, p. 253-256

5. PRATT, A.W. : The use of categorized nomenclatures for representing medical
statements. Computational Linguistic in Medicine. North Hollan Pub. C° 1977

6. SCHNEIDER, W., SAGVALL, A.L. : Computational Linguistics in Medicine. North Holland Pub.   C°, 1977

Figure 1

Example of report

SLE   means "SYSTEMIC LUPUS ERYTHEMATOSUS

=N   means "normal"

=P   means "pathological"

"1073"   ARTHRITIS < (KNEE-B, WRIST-G, FINGERS-G), FACIAL ERYTHEMA, RAYNAUD   PHEN., FEVER > SLE

"0374"   (L.E. CELLS, ANTINUCLEAR ANTIBODIES) = + / NBC = - / PROTEINURIA = N / SLE ✖ STEROIDS

"120876-270876" HOSPITALISATION :

PLEURITIS, PERICARDITIS > SLE > TREATMENT STOP /

PROTEINURIA = + + GLOMERULITIS SLE / RENAL

BIOPSY = P [extramembraneous glomerulitis] /

SLE ✖ (STEROIDS, IMMUNODEPRESSIVE DRUGS) /

KLAUKON -

A microprocessor system for free text acquisition with automatic error checking

W.K.H. Sager, J. Dudeck, J. Kinnling

Abstract:

Using new concepts for documentation of medical data based on free text processing raises the problem of achieving error free texts. KLAUKON (Klartexterfassung mit automatischer Textkontrolle) is designed to acquire and check free text data during clinical routine without additional effort. The system is independent of any host computer because it is implemented on a stand alone microprocessor system. It is independent of application and evaluation by use of parameter driven interfaces at both the user and the host computer side. The software consists of 5 modules. In this article the system is introduced briefly with a more detailed discussion of the interface to the evaluating system.

1.   Introduction

The importance of free text data in the medical communication process has been discussed elsewhere /1,2/ and may not be repeated here. In fact free text can not be substituted by any artificial language in near future. But nevertheless its translation into a formalized language is necessary for most of the evaluations needed in scientific work. Doing this translation manually would restrict the number of documents and the number of facts coded. And as a consequence the number of possible questions is restricted too. To avoid these disadvantages a variety of concepts for free text analysis have been developed. Common to all known methods for syntactic and semantic analysis of textual data is the presupposition to work with error free input. This holds especially for those methods which are 'algorithm oriented' i.e. methods where the text is analyzed by an algorithm using a dictionary to handle a few exceptions only /3/.

In order to obtain error free texts highly qualified proof readers would have to reread the texts several times. But during clinical routine this additional intellectual effort is impossible to achieve for various reasons. On the other hand the revision may be done automatically or at least may be supported by automatic methods. This support is given by KLAUKON during the original set up of the document in realtime independent of a host computer. The reduction in prices of powerful microprocessor systems and the commercial introduction of text editing systems were further reasons to design KLAUKON.

2.   Objectives of KLAUKON

To avoid additional effort the documents for later evaluation should be derived from texts used in the common information flow of the hospital (e.g. surgical operation reports, reports on special inquiries, final reports etc.). The acquisition on machine readable medium should be done during the original set up of the document without a major increase in routine work.

The design of KLAUKON therefore was based on the following objectives:

-       Acquisition of textual data during clinical routine by unskilled personnel
-       System supported text revision during acquisition
-       Creation of machine readable and printed copies of the error free text
-       Acquisition of formatted data
-       Independence of a host computer
-       Flexible user interface for various applications
-       Flexible interface to a host computer for various evaluations

3.   The Hardware Concept

The hardware selected for realization of the concept is the microprocessor system TDV 2114 developed by Tandberg in Norway. This system was chosen because of its flexible hardware and its powerful software.

As shown in fig. 1 the hardware of our configuration of the TDV 2114 consists of

-       an intelligent display unit based on the INTEL 8080A with display, keyboard and 32 K RAM,
-       two floppy disc units as secondary storage and
-       a printer for local report writing.

The TDV 2114 in this configuration is used as a stand alone unit guaranteeing high availability. The connection to the host computer may be direct or using modems and a telephone line.

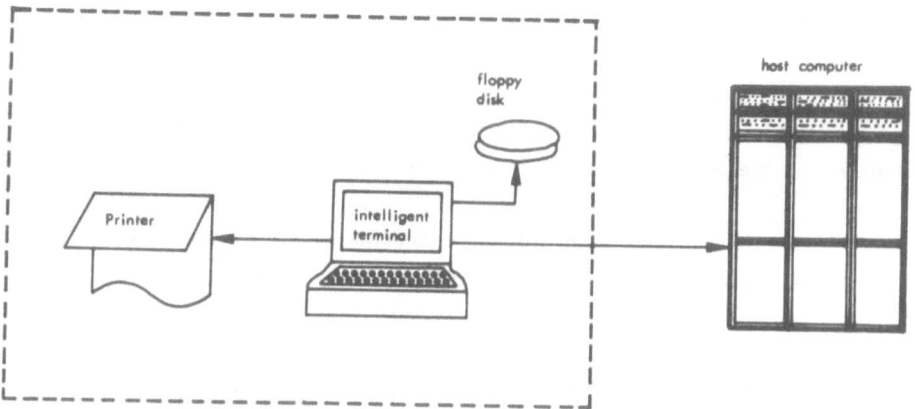

Fig. 1: Hardware Configuration of the KLAUKON
Free Text Data Acquisition System

4. The Software Concept

The software of KLAUKON is designed to run independent of the host computer. The connection to the host may be used for transmission and retrieval of the acquired data. As shown in fig. 2 the system consists of 5 program modules (represented as rectangles), 5 interfaces and 6 files. Four of the interfaces are designed for different user groups with restricted usage permission. In /4/ a detailed overview of the whole system is given. In this paper the 'Internal to External Mapping Generator' and the 'Output Module' are introduced. Brief outline of the 'Format Generator' the 'Acquisition' and the 'Dictionary Update' Module /5,6/ are for better understanding.

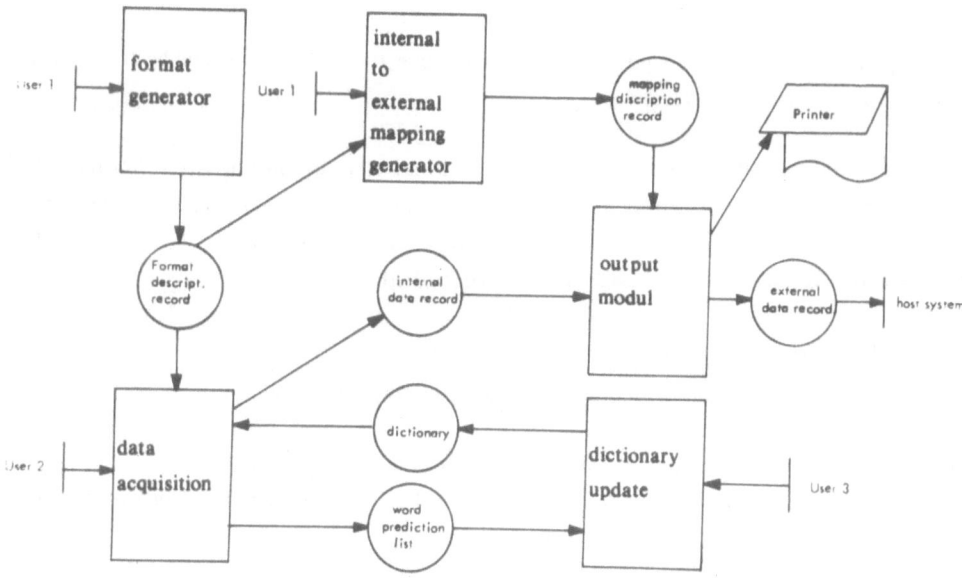

Fig. 2: Software Components of the KLAUKON
Free Text Data Acquisition System

4.1   The Format Generation Module

In the "Format Generation" module the format for data acquisition is initiated on screen in dialog by the system manager. By use of control characters type and length of data strings and display mode are defined. In KLAUKON we now provide 5 different field types:

1.   Protected fields in order to identify and terminate the unprotected fields
2.   numeric fields with specific entry checking
3.   alphanumeric fields with specific entry checking
4.   free text fields
5.   fields with predefined contents (constant field)

Each field may be displayed in one of 6 modes:

1.   normal intensity
2.   low intensity
3.   inverted video
4.   underlined
5.   blinking
6.   invisible

After definition the formula can be stored on the local floppy disc and may now be used to acquire data.

4.2   The Data Acquisition Module

During data acquisition the input is checked according to the field type and by the specific routines as defined in the formula .

Free text is checked in parallel with typing to avoid time of waiting after finishing the input. Checking is performed by analyzing word boundaries and searching each word in a dictionary stored on floppy disc. If the word is found in that dictionary it is assumed to be correct. If it is not found two cases can be distinguished

a)   There may be a typing error in the word.
      In this case the typist may correct it and it is checked again.

b)   The word may be correct but not yet included in the dictionary.
      In this case the typist will confirm the word causing its entry in a word-prediction-list.

Checking the input in parallel with typing requires quick access methods to the dictionary. This was achieved softwarewise by taking advantage of the interrupt features of the 8080 microprocessor, and the DMA feature of the I/O system.

The dictionary-file is stored on one floppy disc and is organized as a B-tree /7/ that provides:

- Quick access
- Easy expansibility
- Easy handling of variable length data and
- Maintenance of the lexicographical order.

By applying these techniques the checking is quick enough to keep up with the quickest typists.

The capacity of one floppy disc allows about 9000 word entries. This is enough if one creates several dictionaries each one for a restricted terminological area. For instance one subject area could be reports on surgical heart operations. This restriction is easy to achieve by combining formula , dictionary and word-prediction-list. In KLAUKON this combination is done by storing these files on the same floppy disc.

After the typist has ended the input or when the screen is filled the system gets into the 'Correction Mode'. The cursor is automatically positioned to the words not found during acquisition. The word must not be left before it is corrected and found in the dictionary or before it is confirmed and included in the prediction list.

After all words which were not found, are worked off the cursor may be moved freely over the screen for further corrections. Like before each modification will be notified and controlled by the system.

When acquisition and correction are finished, the data are stored on floppy disc in an internal format.

The 'Data Acquisition' module is designed to be used by non trained personnel. To prevent errors or confusion the typist is always informed about the program status and possible actions in a status line. Illegal actions are prevented by the program.

4.3   The Dictionary Update Module

The dictionary-update is based on the word-prediction-list and is done by an expert in the actual area. By this solution the dictionary is improved during the application period of the system and in principal no previous dictionary set up is needed.

According to our experience the rate of words which are correctly written but not found decreases very fast. It was less then 15 % after the first 200 reports on surgical heart operations or final reports. The size of the dictionary then was about 4000 entries in both cases.

4.4   The Output Module

The internal format of the data record is transformed to an external (application system oriented) format by the output modul. Like in the data acquisition module this program   is controlled by a set of parameters which is defined in the 'Internal to External Mapping Generator' module.

According to these parameters the fields of the internal data record may be

-    rearranged
-    separated to form two or more output fields
-    copied or
-    skiped partially or completely.

In any position a string or hexadecimal constant may be inserted in the output record. The output device is selected at runtime and may be a file on the local floppy disc, the host computer, or the local printer. When storing the data on floppy disc or transmitting them to the host computer an ASCII to EBCDIC conversion may be applied.

4.5   The Internal to External Mapping Generator

The parameter set for the output module is defined on screen in dialog starting with a refined representation of the input fields. To construct this representation the program analyzes the format description record (input format), creating one display line for each input field found. This line consists of the following fields:

1.	Line-type identifier
2.	Field name in the input format
3.	Current No. of the input-field
4.	Type of the input-field
5.	Length of the input-field
6.	Current No. of the output-field
7.	Length of the output-field

For a line which is created from the format description record the line type identifier is 'X'. After the input format is analyzed and the according lines are displayed on screen the system is waiting for input in field 6 and 7 of the first line.

This input may consist of a two digit decimal number or an alpha control code. In the first case the input field represented by this line is inserted into the output record in the relative position given by the decimal number. In the second case a new line is inserted on the screen in front of the current line where the line type and the line format correspond to the requested control code.

In the following the provided control codes and their meaning are outlined:

K	-	Definition of an additional constant field.
		The constant may be input as an ASCII-string or as a hexadecimal number. More than one constant may be specified in one line separated by a comma. The defined constant is inserted into the output record in the position specified in the current field number of the output field of this line.

R	-	Start of a repeating part of the parameter record.
		Control parameters enclosed by the 'R' and 'E' statement are repeated until the number of times specified in the 'R'-statement or the input field is exceeded.

E	-	End of a repeating part.

F	-	Continue with a non exceeded input field.
		If the length of the output field is smaller than the length of the input field the remaining part of the input is transferred to an output field specified in the 'F'-statement. If no F-statement is given the remaining part is skipped.

C   -   Copy an input field.

The input field specified in the C-statement by the current number is duplicated and inserted into the output record at the position specified in the 'C'-statement.

S   -   Skip characters in input field.

The specified number of characters is skipped in the input field specified by current number.

L   -   Delete an input field.

The appropriate input field is skipped completely.

Y   -   End of form.

The end of the refined representation is marked by a 'Y'-line. In addition it is used to append statements behind the last 'X'-line.

After finishing the definition part the program creates a compressed 'mapping description record' which is stored on floppy disc.

5.   Conclusions

Making use of a powerful but low cost microprocessor system we tried to solve the data acquisition and verification in a host computer independent solution. The independence is achieved by the design of flexible, parameter driven interfaces at the input and output side of the system. Using these interfaces KLAUKON may be connected to most of the free text processing systems providing error free texts with a minimum of additional effort.

References

/1/   Röttger, P.
       Informationstheoretische Aspekte medizinischer Routine-Befundmitteilung
       Symp. Klartextanalyse in der Medizin, Wien 1973, Siemens-Unterlagen

/2/   Wingert, F.
       Klartextverarbeitung in der Medizin
       in: Wingert, F. (Hrsg.) Klartextverarbeitung, Springer Verlag, Berlin 1977

/3/   Siemens
       CONDOR
       Siemens Datenverarbeitung München

/4/   Sager, W.K.H, J. Dudeck, J. Kinnling
       KLAUKON: Klartexterfassungssystem mit automatischer Textkontrolle.
       Systembeschreibung
       Inst. f. Med. Stat. u. Dok., Univ. Gießen (in Vorbereitung)

/5/   Sager, W.K.H., H.A. Michel
       Ein Konzept zur intelligenten dezentralen Erfassung formatierter Daten
       Vortr. Frühjahrstag. GMDS-GI d. FB Med. Informatik, März/April 1977, Gießen

/6/   Sager, W.K.H.
       Ein Programmsystem zur prüfung von Klartextdaten in der dezentralen Daten-
       erfassung
       in: Wingert, F. (Hrsg.) Klartextverarbeitung, Springer Verlag, Berlin 1977

/7/   Bayer, R., E. Mc Creight
       Organization and Maintenance of Large Ordered Indexes
       Acta Informatica 1 (1971)

FREE TEXT ANALYSIS: AN ATTEMPT TO SOLVE
THE DOCUMENTATION PROBLEM

G. Gell

Universitätsklinik für Radiologie (Prof. Dr. E. Vogler)

A-8036 Graz, Auenbruggerplatz 9, Austria

Medical documentation

Medical documentation is the storage of medical data with the possibility of subsequent selective retrieval according to medical criteria. As an example one
might ask for the retrieval of all cases where a histologically verified Ewing
sarcoma had been treated by irradiation. To achieve this, the medical information must be collected and stored in a suitable form, i. e. it must be classified
and coded in such a way that each item of information is tagged by unique and
unambiguous descriptors(indexing). If these descriptors are stored in a computer,
retrieval procedures can be programmed without great difficulties.

Despite the great interest in documentation, as yet virtually no integrated hospital information system (with documentation of all relevant medical data from all
departments) has been successfully inplemented. There are several reasons:
cost, problems of organisation, technical difficulties, the "soft" nature of medical data etc. One of the major obstacles is, however, a psychological one: lack
of interest and involvment from the part of medical and paramedical personnel
because of a poor "personal" cost - benefit relation of work in general documentation leads to incomplete and unreliable data. The exact documentation of
medical information (the indexing) is tedious and boring but requires in depth
knowledge of the subject and therefore can't be transferred to administrative
personnel. The benefit of documentation for the patient by a later scientific
evaluation of the stored data eventually leading to better diagnosis and treatment
is not obvious and too abstract and theoretical to provide for sufficient motivation.

One can try several methods to solve this problem:

Convince medical and paramedical personnel of the importance of documentation and the necessity of complete and reliable data collection. This should
be part of training programs but is unlikely to produce results in the near future.

Train and hire special documentalists for indexing. From the point of
view of documentation this is a possible solution (Koivisto (1976) reports that
documentalists were much better in coding radiologic reports than radiologists),
but it is very expensive and would be difficult to "sell" to governments and
hospitals.

Confine documentation to fields and projects, where phisicians are really
interested. This is done and shall be done successfully for special projects and
studies but it is no solution to the general problem.

Devise procedures and means which allow for the collection of data as a
byproduct of the medical routine without additional work for medical personnel.

Free text analysis attempts a solution of the documentation bottleneck by the last
of the listed methods.

Free text analysis

Free text analysis extracts the relevant information from texts in plain language
like radiology reports and is therefore especially suited for medical fields where
already most of the information is put routinely into written form (radiology,
pathology etc.). The task of classifying and coding (indexing) is left to the computer.

In our system (AURA, Gell, Oser, Schwarz 1976) the radiologic reports are
dictated as usual and written on special devices with display monitor and keyboard which produce together with the printed report for the ward a second,
computer - readable copy on magnetic tape cassettes. The display is operating
off-line without need of a direct connection to the computer.

From the cassettes the complete text of the reports is transferred into the computer and (with the omission of purely descriptive parts) stored on magnetic
tape. Indexing is performed with the aid of a so called thesaurus, a word list
where each word carrying a medical significance is connected with the appropriate descriptors which are appended to the report. A simple grammatical

analysis is done to detect negations. An easy to learn language was developed for retrieval. It allows the formulation of search requests using medical terms, logical operators (and, or, not) and brackets. One can ask for retrieval looking for clerical information (name, age, sex of patient etc.) for descriptors or simply for words or parts of words in the text or for any logical combination of such criteria.

The system is operational since 1970 in the central radiology department of a 3000 bed hospital. All reports from angiography, urography, mammography, computer-tomography and other special investigations are routinely processed. As an example we have a complete file of over 30 000 angiograms comprising all examinations from the last 15 years. This file was built by inserting old reports from the archive; with   free text analysis, this is only a typing problem. In the department for pathology a similar system is installed (Gell, Becker, 1973)

The stored information is used for

     individual retrieval for scientific research (case finding)

     regular production of statistical information about the workload of the department, the number of different examinations etc.

     regular distributions of feedback information to the radiologists working in the department.

With feedback information we mean the linking of information about the same patient from different sources. As on example the radiologist who performs computed tomography of the head gets the results of previous or subsequent angiographic examinations of the patient. A link with the department of pathology provides histological information from biopsies for patients where mammography had been performed (Härringer et al., 1977)

Free text: advantages versus disadvantages

The original decision to develop a free text documentation system had several reasons and of course depended on the available resources at that time. We had bad experciences with manual coding systems in radiotherapy and pathology, which had proved unviable because doctors did not like to code (or, when under pressure, produced garbage data). This was supported by similar experciences abroad. The available hardware within the department could not support an on-line system for automatic generation of reports (cf. below). So we had to develop a system complying with the following restrictions:

> no extra work for radiologists or typists,
> data collection must be off-line.

The only solution therefore was free text analysis (at that time we knew only few instances of free text systems in pathology - Röttger et al , 1969, Lamson et al, 1965 and radiology - Barnhard and Long, 1966). An overview on free text systems in radiology is given by Gell, 1978.

Retrospectively we may try to summarize advantages and disadvantages.

Advantages: Documentation is a relatively cheap byproduct of the normal operation of the department without additional load for doctors or typists.

> Data collection may begin at an early stage of the project, even when the software is not finished.

> Old reports from the archive can be included easily.

> One can start with a very simple retrieval on a look-for-words basis.

> Since the original text remains stored, it may be reanalized when more sophisticated programs become available. Changes in the system do not cause a loss of data - in the contrary, data become more accessible.

Disadvantages: The quality of retrieval depends on the clarity and conciseness of the dictated texts. The system does not enforce precise diagnostic decisions (as automatic reporting systems do - this is however of doubul value).

> Most disadvantages consist in the lack of possible benefits of other

systems: no reduction of typing work, no speeding up in the delivery of reports, no standardized diagnoses etc.

It is more and more understood, that manual coding is not a suitable way to do routine documentation with the exception of either very specialized fields with a few clear alternatives (cytology for example) or for very unspecific overall statistics, again restricted to few possibilities. Manual coding is only feasible, if the codes are short and may be remembered by heart.

The only alternative to free text systems are, at least in radiology, automatic report writing systems like SIRÉP(Siemens) or RAPORT (Gen. Electric) whose primary motivation are economical considerations (saving typists, fast and accurate billing etc.) not documentation. The general idea of these systems is, that the radiologist himself operates a terminal or marks a sheet. Items, describing possible radiological findings are displayed, the physician marks the pertinent points and the computer produces automatically from this information the text of the report which is printed immediately without need of a typist. Usually these methods are considered to be less convenient for the radiologist than free dictation. These systems are successful if there is a severe shortage of typists or if typists are costly and doctors are concerned about costs (as they are in private practice).

Experciences

We shall not give results of retrievals (for example frequencies of examinations or diagnoses) but our general expercience of the "consumer reactions" that is the acceptance of the system by the user.

First lesson: everybody is interested to get information, nobody wants to be involved. Especially in the environment of a university department with a high personal fluctuation it is difficult to get cooperation e. g. for creating a thesaurus for automatic indexing. In fact, the system depends entirely on the DP-specialist of the clinic. It was,however,easy to convince all radiologists to adhere to some (quite loose) dictating rules).

<u>Second lesson</u>: the retrieval requests to the system were less frequent and of a much simpler type than anticipated. Most questions ask for case finding, usually with quite simple criteria (for example: to find all instances of malignancy discovered by mammography; all cases of mass in the kidney etc.). This sets off for the lack of a thesaurus, since this kind of retrieval can easily be accomplished by a look for words. So with the exception of angiography, where a thesaurus had been constructed by two interested radiologists who have now left the clinic we use only word search which proves to be sufficient for most of the questions.

<u>Third lesson</u>: the most urgent demand is for feedback information. Paradoxically, the radiology-department, whose main task is to produce information, has itself a lack of information. Except for selected cases, the examining radiologist is not automatically informed if his diagnosis was confirmed or falsified by subsequent results - but he wants these data! So the most enthusiastic response to AURA was met, when the system could provide this type of service: as an example, providing mammographists automatically with histologic data, if a biopsy or an operation is performed; linking computer tomography reports automatically to angiographic results.

Summing up our experiences we may say that free text analysis is a viable way to medical documentation, requiring only a minimum of involvment on the part of medical personnel. A large data base is more important than very sophisticated retrieval procedures. Most important is the possibility to link otherwise unrelated medical information about the same patient together.

References:

Barnhard H. J., Long J. M., 1966. Computer autocoding, selecting and correlating of radiologic diagnostic cases. Am. J. Roentgen. 96, 854 - 863

Gell G., 1978. Free Text Analysis of Radiologic Reports. In: Considerations
about the use of computers in radiodiagnostic departments. The British Institute
of Radiology, Rep. No. 14, 41 - 50

Gell G., Becker H., 1973. Klartextanalyse pathologischer Biopsiebefunde mit
Bildschirmabfrage. Meth. Inf. Med. 12, 10 - 16

Gell G. Oser W., Schwarz G., 1976. Expercience with the AURA Free-Text
Documentation System, Radiology 119, 105 - 109

Härringer M., Becker H., Schober G., Gell G., Schneider G., 1977.
Computerized interclinical cross-check of radiological and pathological data.
Med. Inform. 2, 141 - 149

Koivisto E., 1976 personal communication

Lamson G. B., Glinski B. C. Hawthorne G. S, Soutter G. C., Russel W. S.,
1965. Storage and Retrieval of Uncoded Tissue Pathology Diagnoses in the
Original English Free Text Form, Proceedings of the 7th IBM Symposium,
411 - 426

Röttger P., Reul H., Klein I., Sunkel H., 1969. Die vollautomatische Dokumentation und statistische Auswertung pathologisch-anatomischer Befundberichte.
Meth. Inf. Med. 8, 19 - 26

A SURVEY OF DEVELOPMENTS IN MEDICAL RECORDS AND INFORMATION

SYSTEMS IN THE UNITED KINGDOM

A L Rector
D H H Metcalfe
L Hallam
A D Clayden
Department of Community Health
University Hospital & Medical School
Nottingham, England.

INTRODUCTION

Under the auspices of the King Edward's Hospital Fund for London, the authors have carried out an extensive survey of "Innovations in Medical Records in the U.K." A large portion of this work involved studying computer-assisted medical record systems of a variety of types, although the survey extended much wider and included both manual and semi-automated methods of data recording and analysis. Both the hospital and general practice services were included, as well as a large number of projects aimed at improving the coordination between the two. Systems already adopted as routine throughout the Health Service, such as the child health systems, were arbitrarily excluded as extensive references and comparative data are available elsewhere.

The results of the survey are compiled in an extensively annotated Gazetteer which has been published by the King's Fund.[1] However, a number of important themes emerged from many discussions and analyses during the survey.

The automated systems which we investigated might best be divided into five categories:

1) The large, hospital information systems which have matured to the degree that they manipulate a considerable amount of patient data, usually originating either from the laboratory, the pharmacy, or the nurses' notes, only rarely from the physicians themselves;

2) Systems for high dependency medicine, that is intensive care, cardiac care, neonatal intensive care and renal dialysis, in which large volumes of data about each patient are generated, and must be summarised to be easily absorbed by the doctor;

3) Systems for outpatient clinics, ambulatory and primary care with varying degrees of emphasis on the research or service aspects of the project;

4) Large scale registers and follow-up systems designed to provide services on a regional or national basis but not yet part of the standard services of the DHSS as a whole (e.g. thyroid follow-up);

5) Systems intended primarily for research which do not affect the normal process of making clinical notes.

A summary of the numbers of projects investigated in each group is given in Table 1.

With a few notable exceptions, the large hospital projects are concerned primarily with administrative data, and the projects for the collection of data for clinical research affect the medical record hardly at all. Our effort was therefore concentrated on the middle group of projects, and especially those for outpatient and primary care. There are many notable successes in this group, but there were also certain problems which recurred with distressing regularity.

TABLE 1
NUMBERS OF AUTOMATED SYSTEMS INVESTIGATED

1.	Hospital Information Systems of varying degrees of sophistication	17
2.	High Dependency Medicine	7
3.	Outpatient:	
	Maternity	6
	Hypertension	4 (1 multicentre)
	Diabetes	4
	Misc. (Glaucoma, Surgery, etc.)	7
	Accident and Emergency	5
	Primary Care	8
4.	Registers and Follow-up Systems	8
5.	Research orientated systems	20

Of the automated systems investigated, three have been identified since the original Gazetteer was prepared, and a number appear in more than one category.

COMMON DIFFICULTIES

The most important problem continues to be establishing adequate procedures for collecting and validating data prior to its entry into the system. It is not possible to require the discipline which is usual of those who record information in a commercial organisation. This is essentially a political problem, but its consequences must be faced and taken fully into account in the design of any system.

It is extremely important that the personnel collecting the data be involved during the design of the system. They should receive early and regular feedback from the system. More important still, they must feel that the system does something for them. The experience with the consultants' response to the Hospital Activity Analysis provides a classic example of the difficulty of generating enthusiasm for collecting data which they know will be unavailable for nearly two years and then only in printouts in which the consultants frequently fail to find the items of interest to their own service.

Important aspects of the data collection methods of a representative sample of the projects investigated are given in Table 2.

Many of the most successful projects have required someone to function as a data editor, screening the information before it is input. Usually this is a clerk, secretary or nurse, but the Switch system in Glasgow has found it desirable to use medically qualified persons for this task.[2] Whatever the formal qualifications of the individuals involved, the crucial factor in their success is that they be given sufficient access to the doctors collecting the information and sufficient backing to be able to insist that information be collected correctly.

One of the most attractive ways to improve the quality of the data collected is to integrate the data collection process into the routine process of producing the clinical notes. Where the episode of care is well defined and predictable, as in most obstetric care, this can be done by using special booklets which are left in the paper record to serve as the clinical notes but which are structured so that at the end of the episode they can be used as input documents to the information system.[3]

Where, as in most other medical specialties, the episode is less well defined or the users wish to use the data in the system before the end of an episode of care, there are two possibilities. One copy of the record booklet may be left in the notes and a second taken as input documents. This is relatively unusual, although simple and often effective. The more common approach is to use the computer to produce summaries from the data collected. The summaries then serve as the clinical notes. The primary difficulty with producing summaries in this way is that relatively rapid turn-around (usually under 48 hours) is required between the information being collected and the summary printed. Otherwise the information is likely to be unavailable when needed and the normal functioning of the medical records department seriously delayed. Direct, on-line, data entry has been used

TABLE 2

DATA CAPTURE TECHNIQUES EMPLOYED FOR A SAMPLE OF PROJECTS

Special Forms: Most research-orientated records projects use specially designed forms for data capture. These include:

a) King's College Hospital Diabetic Clinic Project;

b) King's College Hospital Glaucoma Records System;

c) Edinburgh Royal Infirmary Breast Clinic System;

d) The Oxford Record Linkage Study;

e) The Scottish Automated Follow-Up Register;

f) The Welsh Automated Follow-Up Register;

g) The Oxford Community Health Project;

h) University of Southampton, Department of Primary Medical Care Demonstration Health Centre Records System;

i) Tayside Master Patient Index.

Record Booklets: a) St. Thomas' Hospital, Computerised Obstetric Records System;

b) The Aberdeen Maternity Register;

c) The Oxford Obstetric Data System;

d) Royal Sussex County Hospital Paediatric Information System.

Record Booklets + Summaries: a) The Multi-Centre Hypertension Records System;

b) St. Thomas' Hospital Diabetic Clinic Project;

c) Western Infirmary Switch System, Glasgow.

Direct Entry by Health Professionals: a) Health Services Research Centre, University of Birmingham Medical School;

b) Wythenshawe Hospital Patient Data Display System;

c) Queen Elizabeth Hospital Major Computer Project;

d) The London Hospital Experimental Computer Project;

e) Exeter Community Health Project;

f) Ninewells Hospital Ward Computer Project.

Bar Codes: a) North Staffs. Hospital Centre Computer Project.

Mark Sense Forms: a) St. Thomas' Hospital Cardiology Records System;

b) Royal Victoria Hospital Cardiology System;

c) Charing Cross Hospital Computer Project;

d) St. Thomas' Hospital Experimental Computer System.

Dictated: a) The Nottingham General Practice Computer Project.

by only a relatively few projects. Its cost is dropping rapidly, but at the time
of the survey remained the province of the largest and most expensive projects.

Attempting to integrate data collection and the routine production of clinical notes
has also too frequently led to collecting more data than can reasonably be processed
or used. There is a real and fundamental dilemma. One may collect as much information as possible in order to provide immediate information on patients and in the
knowledge that it is not always possible to predict crucial variables for research
in advance. Alternatively, one may elect to collect only that information known to
be of particular relevance. The first approach has the advantage of making it easier
to establish uniform procedures and provide information which is immediately useful
clinically. However, the second strategy is usually less expensive, easier to manage and more likely to be able to make use of standard software packages. It is
usually to be preferred for smaller projects. The Switch system[2] and the Cannies-
burn orthopaedic projects[4] provide good examples of successful applications of
these two respective philosophies, both implemented by the same team. The difficulties in many other projects stem from the fact that they fall between these
two philosophies, collecting more data than they can manage, and experiencing all
the difficulties of the first type of project while reaping few of the advantages
of the second. Over-ambition has been the most common error in medical computing
since its inception, and it continues to plague many otherwise well thought out
efforts.

One source of this over-ambition is the feeling, still widespread, that once a computer based information system is installed in a clinic, all the problems of mounting clinical research will evaporate. The difficulties of using routinely collected
data for most areas of research are insufficiently appreciated. It is not just that
there are problems of data collection, but also that it is not practical or cost
effective to perform the type of precise measurements routinely in clinic which are
needed to answer many sophisticated clinical questions. Information systems may be
a prerequisite for much research and may provide certain types of epidemiological
data. They are not a panacea nor an excuse to ignore the careful design of clinical trials.

Difficulties in the technical implementation continue to be a problem for many
projects. There are still relatively few systems analysts and programmers available with extensive experience in the medical field. The complexity of the medical
environment, its differences from commercial data processing, and the heterogeneity
of medical data are too frequently not appreciated. The necessity that systems be
developed on the assumption that there will be more errors in the data than in commercial or scientific applications is frequently ignored and the checks provided

inadequate.

Flexibility and adaptability are still all too often given insufficient priority. It is crucial that analysts understand that no matter how carefully the original design was drawn up, changes after implementation will be the rule rather than the exception, because patterns of medical care are always changing. A more basic problem is that it is extremely difficult for doctors and others in the health service to specify exactly which functions would be most useful, or even which methods will work, until they have some experience of a system.

Lack of documentation, especially among the smaller projects, is still common. Without documentation, modification and transferability are very difficult. Whilst an impressive literature accumulates on methods and problems of transferring systems, practical examples within the Health Service remain relatively rare. Lack of documentation is certainly not the only problem of transferability, but among the smaller projects in the U.K. it is of considerable importance. For example, the expansion of the Scottish Automated Follow-Up Register for thyroid disease has been seriously hampered in this way (A.J. Hedley, S. Jones, A.L. Rector, personal communication, 1977).

Finally, there is a very serious problem which may be unique to the organisation of computing facilities in the U.K. or may be more widespread. Smaller applications usually use the computer facilities either of the local University or of the Regional Health Authority. Neither is normally equipped to deal with the special problems of medical records or to give the applications the level of priority they require for success. There are exceptions, but most University Computing Centres are orientated primarily towards scientific computing and have poor facilities for handling even moderately large input and output loads or for data manipulation. Furthermore, academic centres shut down for considerable periods between academic terms. The Regional Health Authority Computing Centres, on the other hand, must make the administrative functions of their Regions their major priority. It is virtually impossible for any system to achieve the level of service required to be integrated data collection into the standard clinical note taking procedures using either of these alternatives unless very unusual arrangements are made and clear understandings arrived at in advance.

There are also serious questions concerning the propriety of keeping identifiable medical data on University machines because of the difficulty ensuring that confidentiality will be adequately protected. Legal limitations are already in force in some countries and will probably soon exist in the U.K.

NEW DEVELOPMENTS AND TRENDS

Despite the persistence of many problems, we found many projects about which we
were very pleased and trends which we believe to be important. Of these, five de-
serve special mention.

1) The maturation of some of the large hospital information systems to the point
    where they manipulate considerable amounts of medical as well as administrative
    data.

2) The growth of systems for review and monitoring of patient care.

3) The enthusiasm on the part of users who are not primarily computer orientated
    towards a number of systems. More importantly, evidence that the data collec-
    ted is affecting policies and practice.

4) The demonstration of the possibility of mounting modest projects quickly and
    comparatively inexpensively using MUMPS on a 'bureau' basis.

5) The growing success of automatic encoding schemes.

One of the great potentials of computer assisted systems which has been recognised
from the beginning but only recently achieved is the reduction of human errors in
patient care, especially errors in drug prescribing. The Queen Elizabeth project
in Birmingham currently provides the most extensive example in this country of how
this might be done by checking prescriptions at the time they are ordered. The
Oxford Drug Monitoring Project and related efforts demonstrate one route by which
a much more intensive level of monitoring might be instituted on a larger scale.[5]
The recently announced plans to computerise the Prescription Pricing Authority will
make this type of monitoring simpler and more practical. The authors are engaged
in a project still in its early stages which seeks to provide immediate checks in
the level of the general practitioner's surgery.

The long-term follow up of patients known to be at special risk is a growing problem in a mobile population. When the potential consequences of a condition are
largely preventable given adequate follow up, as they are in glaucoma, for instance,
not to provide that care is a serious failure of the medical system. When the risk
is partly iatrogenic, as it is in patients who have been treated for hyperthyroidism,
it may well be thought to approach negligence. Follow up registers which form one
vital link in providing adequate preventive services are spreading, but their
progress is disappointingly slow.

The definitive evaluation of the Manor Hospital project which provides a 'bureau' service to those wishing to use MUMPS to implement small applications throughout a considerable region is not yet complete. However, the list of the project's accomplishments is already impressive. Much scepticism has been expressed over the possibility of non-professionals writing their own applications, even in such systems as MUMPS. The Manor Hospital project appears to be showing that with a modest degree of help from two full time programmer/analysts, a wide range of significant applications can be mounted in a relatively short time. Given the new implementations of MUMPS itself in which the 'balanced tree' system makes the physical file structure independent of the logical data structure and in which the language is standardised and made easier to use, the scope for this type of application should be greatly increased. The rapid progress of the projects at the Royal Marsden[6] and University College Hospital provides additional evidence of the effectiveness of MUMPS as a tool for medical applications. The value of easily used interpretive languages is further reinforced by the dramatic success of the small hospital administration system at Southend-on-Sea.[7] This was written in Basys, a fully interpretive derivative of Basic with very powerful string handling facilities.

Encoding diagnostic and other statements into computer readable form is one of the most time consuming and error prone tasks in many medical information systems. Three different 'families' of automatic encoding system are in use in the U.K. today:

1) The systems developed out of SWITCH in Glasgow[2];
2) The systems developed out of Kodiac by Greenwood[8] and being brought into routine use in the Oxford region by Gill[9] and in primary care by one of the authors.
3) The systems for coding of histopathology data adapted by Coles[10] at Northwick Park Hospital.

All these systems offer real aid in reducing the repetitive effort of coding common diagnoses and procedures. They allow systems to be designed which provide most of the advantages of free text data entry over the more usual highly structured self-encoding forms without sacrificing the greater ease of analysis and storage of coded data.

Finally, although the problems of evaluating the effects of these systems on the outcome of care has not been solved, many of them are generating both enthusiasm and actual change in behaviour among the doctors and other health care workers using them. The Exeter Community Health Project has demonstrated that given an adequately convenient interface, at least one group of doctors is willing to type their notes directly onto terminals. Furthermore, they will use the information gathered to change or improve practice procedures in preventive care, immunizations and other areas.[11] The St. Thomas' Hospital obstetric system data has lead to significant changes in policy concerning certain categories of at risk women and low birth weight babies.[12,13] Conversations with a number of junior doctors at the London Hospital and the Queen Elizabeth Medical Centre in Birmingham, admittedly informal, indicated wide acceptance and frequent vigorous approval of the computer system if only because it saves them much rushing between wards and form filling. The Oxford Community Health Project has whetted the appetites of a number of the participating doctors to a point where the project can no longer expand its services as rapidly as they would like and they are looking for ways either to upgrade the system or obtain more sophisticated alternatives.

Ultimately, it must be this kind of support from doctors and other health professionals who use the systems which will provide the incentive for further developments. As the cost of hardware falls and the sophistication of the software available improves, user backing and results which users believe important will become the main determinants of how far and how rapidly progress is made. That there is now strong support in many quarters, despite many problems and much hostility elsewhere must be the most hopeful single finding of the survey.

REFERENCES

1. METCALFE, D.H.H. et al (1977) "Innovations in Medical Records in the United Kingdom." King's Fund Project Paper, No. 16 (256 pp.).
2. KENNEDY, F. et al (1968) "SWITCH - A system producing a full hospital case-history on computer. Lancet, 2, 1230.
3. SOUTH, J. and RHODES, P. (1971) Computer service for obstetric records. Brit. J.Med., 4, 32-5.
4. LISTER, G.D. (1975) The development of clinical records for plastic surgery and their computer storage. Brit.J.Plast.Surg., 27, (1), 47-58.
5. SKEGG, D.C.G. et al. (1977) Use of medicines in general practice. Brit.Med.J., 1, 1561-3.
6. MILAN, J. (1977) A data base system for cancer research. Proc.MUMPS User Group Europe, September.
7. KENNEDY, T. and FACEY, P.V. (1973) Experience with a mini-computer based hospital administration system. Int.J.Man-Machine Studies, 5, 327.
8. GREENWOOD, R.M. (1972) Kodiac, a system for disease coding by a medium-sized computer. Int.J.Biomed.Comput., 3, (2), 123-34.
9. GILL, L. (1977) Personal communication.
10. COLES, E.C. and SLAVIN, G. (1976) An evaluation of automatic coding of surgical pathology reports. J.Clin.Pathol., 26, 621-5.
11. SPARROW, J. (1977) Personal communication.
12. HAERI, A.D. et al. (1974) A scoring system for identifying pregnant patients with a high risk of perinatal mortality. J.Obs.Gynaec.Brit.Com., 81, 535-8.
13. NALDRETT, J. (1976) Personal correspondence.

COMPUTERIZATION OF THE MEDICAL RECORD OF THE GENRAL PRACTITIONER : SYSTEMATIC
REGISTRATION AT EACH CONTACT PATIENT - GENERAL PRACTIONER.

Dr. J. Heyrman M.D.

I. INTRODUCTION

Belgium is one of the countries with a parallel-offer to the population of general
practice and specialistic care, without obligatory referral to one another. Our two
year investigation about the possibilities to centralise all medical data around the
patients links up with the fact that one may expect that the use of similar registration systems by the GP and the specialist can prevent a little bit the problems of ,
information gap, double-use or even loss of medical data.

II. OBJECT OF THE INVESTIGATION

A. Investigate on what conditions the computerized data collection, which has been
used for several years in the university hospital Gent, can also be made practicable
in general practice. The basis of this data collection is the systematic registration of each contact patient-GP.

B. See what kind of service the computer can offer to the GP so that implementation
is attractive and financially defendable.
We were in search for input forms that should link up as accurate as possible with
already existing practice routine. We built up some experience with a computerized
recall-system for the follow-up of chronical patients (diabetic, Hypertension), to
remind them the date of the next control visits, and to instruct them about the
preparations they have to make (blood sample on empty stomach, etc.).
Systematic administration and practice analysis made it possible for the GP to have
an insight in the way of running his practice, and if necessary to ameliorate this.
In this paper I would prefer to focus on the way of adapting continuous data collection to the specific needs of daily general practice.

III. SET-UP

During two years all items as noted down in a commonly used belgian family-file-
system, were coppied on a specially purpose-developped form. In the first phase
of the investigation, this form was studied carefully, and was adapted several times

till it was as adequate as possible. Then the input was done into the already working COMPADOS system of the university hospital Gent. In future this copying should be avoided when using a direct terminal or by replacing the traditional family file by this input form.

IV. REGISTRATION OF ADMINISTRATIVE AND MEDICAL DATA

Three types of forms were used:
- the ID form or introduction form
- the PAF form or Patient Antecedent Form as a general data base
- the VP form as registration file for each contact patient - GP

1. For each not yet registered patient, a number of essential administrative data were noted on the ID form : name, adress, date of birth, code of the medical record.
As the medical record code was composed by the rank-number of the family file, and a code number according to the place in the family, a list was made up of this record-code compared with the national person-code. This national code should become the common denominator to integrate all data of one patient, which will be registered under this number by the several medical disciplines.

2. The PAF form was developped by the WVVH and used as data-base. Some hundred questions about former illnesses of the patient himself and of his relatives, provide a computerized summary of the antecedents and of the risks he has for certain illnesses, devided into three grades, according to the gravity.
A serious problem in implementation of this form consists in the fact that most patients couldn't fill out such a form in the waiting-room. They had to think about it carefully, sometimes ask their relatives, so that it had to be taken home. Only 35 % of the forms were returned.

3. The VF form is the central document because the daily input of each contact patient-GP is done by this form. After a trial-period this classification was used:
   a) section 1: reason of contact
      Why does this contact take place? Most of the time this is the subjective complaint of the patient. Sometimes the complaint is formulated by the GP. Here was also noted whether it was a new or a control contact. This is important for the incidence/prevalence studies which can be done on the material.

b) <u>section 2 : objective examination</u>

Here the result of clinical or biochemical examinations are noted.

c) <u>section 3 : conclusion</u>

Generally this is the start of the action. Mostly this will be the diagnosis, sometimes provisional, sometimes tentative, but always the GP's conclusion at the end of the examination.

It can also be a description or a preventive act (e.g. general check-up).

It is clear that "reason of contact" and "conclusion" may often be identical especially when talking about preventive care or control visits. Therefore some administrative conventions were introduced so that one wouldn't have to write down the same thing twice. (e.g. B code, K and O code)

d) <u>Section 4 : treatment</u>

e.g. pharmaca, information, kinetherapeutic exercise, etc.

In order to minimize the workload of the registration two conventions were introduced: - only new treatments were noted

- because the other treatments were supposed to go on, one had to mention the duration of the treatment (e.g. **antibiotics** for 8 days)

e) <u>section 5 : control and referral</u>

Here the control scheme or the referral to specialists was noted.

We have to mention here that the letter of the specialist, resulting from this referral, was noted on a similar form, mostly in sections 2, 3 and 4.

Under the heading "control" the follow-up scheme, for e.g. diabetics, can be coded. This meant the start of the recall-system. As mentioned above a computerized service can send off letters to people who need intensive medical care, stating when they have to come in for control, what preparations they should take (stay sober, first go to the oculist, etc.). There were eight different kinds of follow-up schemes for diabetics. The most simple was the DR1 scheme (= for people under 40 who risk to get diabetic). It sends off letters every five years and asks the patients to come to the GP's office to have an oral glucose tolerance test. The most complex was the DIL scheme (for patients with Diabetes Insulent Dependant with Lipid disturbance). In this case letters were sent off every month with an adapted list of instructions.

As all items were divided among these five sections, a simple and uniform basis scheme was found. A sheet of paper of 15 to 20 cm showed large enough to contain all information of one contact. These sheets were held together in handy blocs of 50.

V. WHAT HAVE WE LEARNED IN CONNECTION WITH THE MEDICAL RECORD OF THE GP BASED ON CONTACT REGISTRATION ?

It isn't possible to go into all methodological and technical aspects we tried to consider. Maybe we can formulate our experiences and expectations as a hypothesis regarding the trend computerization in general practice should take, based on our tow-years experience.

1. The computerized information is only a part of the family file, it will remain necessary that the GP keeps a record with individual notes or remarks.

Not all notes the GP makes are equally important. Certain items are only temporaryly of use : the first formulation of a complaint (e.g. a tentation in the belly) is hardly ever a relevant diagnostic item (e.g. the GP will ask the patient how are his belly cramps, the patient will remark that it weren't really cramps but more a tention in the belly).
Other notes are nothing more than personal considerations of the GP. When made hard to objective parameters they are falsified. In spite of their subjectivity and vagueness they make up the essential basis for psycho-social or behaviour therapy. These casual remarks are probably the way to get accustomed to the personal way of functionning in this field.
At the start of the experiment we had hoped to realise a complete computerized GP file. Afterwards we realised that this is a utopia. For future computer area, we need a GP record system with working sheets for daily notes, and well defined places and ways of registrating data that are easy computerized. This has to be done so that a practice assistant can refer this data to the informatic systems. Computerize all GP notes is waste of time and money.

2. In order to importance the items that should be computerized are ; the conclusions, the treatment, the follow-up scheme and the objective examination.

a) The survey of the conclusions form a kind of permanent problem list. In this field the computer can add essential possibilities, to the manual problem oriented records.
   - the GP gets informed about former episodes of illness mostly gradually or fragmentaryly; a computer however can file these episodes chronologically. Moreover it is easy to establish the links between the different conclusions.

which is the result of previous conclusions, etc.
- surveys of similar diagnosis from different patients are a unique starting
  point for individual medical auditing.
- listing the conclusions and refering to a common national person-code, form
  the essential basis of an integrated persons-record with all information
  coming from the GP as well as from the specialist. Of course the use of
  secrecy clues is an absolute necessity on this material.

b) Pharmacological surveys are important because keeping in mind long term treatment, interferred as it is by periodical acute treatment, is quite a task for
   the GP.
   Here the computerization could bring in two important renovations :
   1) based on the PAF-form the computer for the moment gives already a complete
      list of pharmacological intolerance, derived from the personal and family
      history and the resulting risks. Adding to this the new intolerance and
      ideosynchrasives, certain alarm procedures could be introduced when pre-
      scribing certain medicine.
   2) An overall patient record with mention of the chronical medicine and into-
      lerances information coming from and accessible for several doctors would
      beyond doubt be an important step ahead.

c) The recall-systems for follow-up can be enlarged for a limited amount of
   chronical illnesses schemes.
   1) Actually we only have experience with a diabetes follow-up, which worked
      successfully.
   2) When having different schemes working together (e.g. diabetes - hypertension -
      geriatric) it will be important to have an eassly adaptable programmation in
      order to get a more or less equal workload for each control-set.

d) Regarding the objective information it is mostly the biochemical parameters which
   are important. In this field there is quite some double or triple use.
   1) For the time being we only have experience with the manual looking up.
   2) When using a computerized overall patients record it would be of great impor-
      tance to find common standards for the averages of biochemical investigations
      from different laboratories.

3. For the input of the data the computer will have to adapt itself to the GP.
   e.g. establishing a synonym-list, and not the other way, by forcing the GP to
   use a computer code.

   The COMPADOS system was a diagnostic scheme based on three diagnostic aspects :
   1. description of the disturbance (e.g. inflammation)
   2. definition of the localization (e.g. liver)
   3. definition of the etiological agens (e.g. virus disease)

In view of translating the input items into a code, lists of synonyms must be
drawn up, and should be adapted continuously. It is essential that the GP can
use his own terms for the input. The output information will have certain medical diagnostic terms but this seems no disadvantage. Nevertheless two nuances
are introduced. First it is possible to registrate the grade of certainty, although we hardly ever used it ourselves, because it seems very difficult to
clear out the grade of certainty in general practice. Secondly the origine of
the diagnosis is an important nuance that is also printed out. The diagnosis
"gastritis" made by a radiologist refers to the morphology of the gastric folds,
made by a GP it refers to a clinical state, made by an internist it indicates
the absence of a gastropic demonstrable ulcus.

Adaptations to the practice routine of the GP must be possible. The two GP's
in our investigation at the end of the contact, the other wrote it down during the
contact as he went through the different sections of the examination. This
made it necessary to make the sections "reason of contact", "objective examination" and "conclusions" exchangeable. Computer registration systems have to
offer the possibility of adapting the system to these habits.

4. An on-line terminal is essential for an easy computerization of the GP's medical record.
   - in a first phase, when only the conclusions would be brought in permanently
     it is difficult but still possible to work with forms that are regularly
     printed out and sent by mail.
   - the follow-up schemes get very rigid when they can't be adapted. Here the
     availability of an on-line terminal becomes more important. The slightest
     disorganisation in e.g. the diabetes, showed in our case great confusion
     about the date of sending the next recall letter for control. A periodical
     if possible daily on-line possibility to adapt the scheme would be a step
     ahead.

- when treatment surveys are introduced, a terminal screen on the consultation
  desk must be available, because the information must be checked continuously
  with the patient to be reliable.

CONCLUSION

It has shown to be possible to make a promising start for an easy and well adapted
computerization, especially purposed for the registration of each contact patient-
GP.
Because the basis system is the same as used in the university hospital setting,
easy integration can be expected.
The system asks quite an investment: a 1/4 time assistent per GP is necessary for
the input of the information and another 1/4 time for the permanent adaptation
of the system possibilities towards the GP, his habits, synonyms and routine.
Therefore it will be important to pay a great deal of attention to the elaboration of the computer service-aspects, which can make the investment worth while
for the GP.

THE PROVISION OF DATA PROCESSING FACILITIES FOR MEDICAL PRACTITIONERS

L.R.Neal, Brunel University, Uxbridge, Middlesex.

There is an increasing awareness amongst medical practitioners of the role
that computers can play in the various areas of their work. Computers are being
increasingly used in business data processing and their acceptance in medical work
is growing all the while. Computing costs, particularly of equipment, are
continually falling and any enterprise which entails handling large amounts of
information will be looking to see how a computer can help.

However, a computer can only be of use if it faithfully represents the
working of the particular 'system' that is required. Such systems can range from
the administration and running of a complete hospital to a simple computer
program that adds up a few numbers. To put any large system on a computer requires
the employment of professional computing people such as systems analysts and
programmers and the effort for a large project is measured in man-years of work.
Anyone coming into contact with such a scheme will not have to concern himself too
much with the detailed working of the computer(s) involved. On the other hand the
average medical practitioner is unlikely to have met such a beast. Even for the
much simpler systems that he will need, he does not know where to turn for
computing facilities and advice on their use.

A few practitioners have taught themselves computing, a few happen to
benefit from the side effects of a large computing project, and a few have contacts
with neighbouring colleges and universities. However for the average hospital
consultant or general practitioner such help is virtually non-existent. The basic
problem is, of course, resources, with money allocated to medical computing having
been mainly used for large scale research projects. Some computing facilities are
provided at a regional level but the present state of the art in computing means
that a physician cannot hope to make use of this without considerable help from
computing 'experts' and such help is generally not available.

We continue to discuss the sort of help that could be provided at a
reasonable cost. There are three main areas that would benefit from the use of a
computer

1) the administration of the enterprise
2) help with research problems
3) help in determining long term trends

As for the administration, the usual approach is to change from a manual
filing system to one that stores the information on a computer. One or two
medical and dental group practices have already completely computerised their
records. Once this has been done then all scheduling of appointments and monitoring of work loads can be controlled by computer programs. There is increasing use

of computer equipment in office administration - the time is rapidly approaching when commercial systems will be offered at attractive enough prices for more and more group practices to consider the investment worthwhile. Reports on pilot schemes are regularly given (1,2). It should be borne in mind that the actual equipment is only part of the cost - again professional advice should be sought to ensure that the system you end up with is the one you really want at that price.

We will now turn to a more mundane level and discount the expensive 'on-line' operational use of computers. Let us consider what help can be given to the medical practitioner who would like to collect data for later perusal. Since 1967, the Department of Computer Science at Brunel University has been involved in helping consultants at nearby hospitals with data processing problems. These have ranged from one-off research investigations to the gathering of data on an on-going basis for future research and planning. From these experiences it is possible to define the general steps that have to be taken in such investigations and to consider alternatives that minimise the cost of each project. It is possible to divide the process into four parts - problem definition, data capture, data validation and data processing. We will discuss each of these in turn.

Problem definition

It may seem like stating the obvious but the objectives of any project should be clearly determined at the onset. Once this has been done the scope and amount of data required for later analysis can be determined. Too often either too much is collected on the premise that 'it might come in useful' or alternatively some data needed for a vital criterion at a late stage of the project is found to be missing. In practice, however, it is not easy to anticipate what might be required. In the field of survey analysis the objectives can be clearly defined at the beginning. In medical research the way ahead only becomes clear by studying the results of previous consultations of the data.

Data Capture

In every case the data to be collected on the computer will be a subset of the total amount of data associated with each patient. Only rarely will one be in the happy situation of collecting data for operational use in a form that can then be input straight into the computer. The usual situation one is faced with is the problem of designing a pro-forma for the project in question and extracting the necessary data on to this form from the larger set of data in, say, a patient's medical record.

In simple exercises it is possible to condense the amount of information stored by coding the various alternatives that can happen to an individual. This together with some basic numeric data such as data of birth, height, weight, etc. will suffice for many projects. In this way it was possible to condense the major facts about each birth in a maternity unit into 80 characters which could then be put onto just one punched card ready for computer input. Increasingly though, consultants are requiring the facility to enter complete messages in English into the computer. Work using computer languages that can handle such problems such as MUMPS (3) and CODIL (4), is becoming extensive.

One important aspect regarding pro-formas is that of the confidentiality of the information. This can be adequately covered by duplicating non-sensitive data using carbon copies of the form and ensuring that sensitive data never leaves medical hands. Alternatively each page of the pro-forma can be split into two by a vertical perforation. The left hand side of each page contains printed information that can be quickly ringed as appropriate. The right hand side contains boxes for the corresponding codes and only this part of the document ever passes out of medical hands, it being impossible to identify an individual from the codes without access to a master list.

Once the forms have been designed and filled in, several alternatives present themselves depending on the money one is prepared to pay. Still the cheapest method of transferring the data into a form ready for computer input is the punch card. It is still relatively cheap for punch girls to read the coded characters of the forms and to punch holes in 40 or 80 column cards. The next step, in order of cost, would be for the forms themselves to be 'read' directly by mark sensing devices. The main difference is that, instead of having just one box with a character written in it that is then punched, we have a box for each of the alternatives. The appropriate one is ticked and the presence of a mark in that position is then sensed by electronic equipment. Finally, if one has lots of money and also a great bulk of data, then one can consider key-to-magnetic disc systems which transfer the characters directly into a medium acceptable to the computer. It is also possible to have systems that portray the schema of the form on a visual display unit and to fill it in using a keyboard and/or light pen. This does away with the need for the paperwork of the form but is more expensive as the 'online' use of a computer is involved.

Data validation

The results from the computer system will only be as reliable as the accuracy of the data input in the first place. The data validation phase is thus crucial for the success of the project. Possible sources of error are
1) medical records having been filled in incorrectly
2) errors in transcript from source records to the pro-formas
3) punching errors from the pro-formas onto the punch cards.
Whilst it is impossible to ensure 100% eradication of errors it is possible to have validation programs on the computer that can carry out various checks. Numeric data can be checked to ensure that the numbers entered are reasonable,

i.e. bounds can be put on such things as height and weight to pick out and
query the exceptional cases that usually arise from punching errors. Coded
information can again be checked to see if it falls within the correct bounds for
that case. An important source of checking is to make use of redundant information
to check for logical errors. Also various other logical checks can be used to
ensure that the right data is associated with the right patient, for example,
it is highly unlikely that a limb that has been amputated will receive further
radiotherapy treatment. Finally for small projects of the order of a few hundred
records it is well worth carrying out a 10% hand check of the data from computer
printouts.

Data Processing

Having got some data inside a computer what does one do with it? Analysis
and investigative computer programs now have to be used to gather together the
information that satisfy the original objectives of the project. The facilities
used will depend upon those available and also on the complexity of the problem.
On the one hand it is relatively easy to write a simple FORTRAN program to add up
and tabulate a score of alternatives - on the other hand the problem might entail
the use of some very sophisticated statistical techniques and, unless one is to
re-invent the wheel, access to one of the existing statistics software packages
becomes necessary. These are only usually available on very large university
and government computers. The best known of these packages such as SPSS, GENSTAT,
BMD, are referenced in (5).

The advantage of using a statistical package is that all the mathematics
and statistics involved have already been worked out and programmed, together with
a set of routines for presenting results in a meaningful way. All the programmer
has to do is to put his data in a form that the package will accept and to provide
the necessary parameters and requests from the package for the query in question.
Unfortunately such packages are not easy for the layman to understand and the
effort would only be worthwhile if use can be made of the package on several
occasions.

For some years the only other alternative was for the medical practitioner
to find a friendly FORTRAN or COBOL programmer and to persuade them to write the
appropriate programs. FORTRAN and COBOL have been used because programmers of
these languages are generally thicker on the ground than those of other languages.
There is however an increasing awareness that medical problems have their own
peculiarities which the conventional scientific and business languages do not
conveniently handle. Languages such as MUMPS are becoming increasingly popular
for medical work (6), the advantage here being that this language is built to
handle text as well as numeric and coded information.

However, even such languages still require the medical practitioner to become a programmer in the conventional sense if he is to use the language himself. Attempts are, though, being made to make computers directly usable by unsophisticated users (11). A research project by one of my colleagues at Brunel University is described elsewhere at this Congress (4). The objective here is for the non-expert user, with a relatively small amount of data, to be able to input this to the computer and ask questions of the collection without the need for detailed computer knowledge.

To illustrate the above points we will briefly look at four of the projects undertaken at Brunel.

Maternity records

This is an on-going project of ten years standing (7) that gathers a certain amount of data from every birth at Hillingdon Hospital Maternity Unit. The original system was card based and written in FORTRAN although later work in COBOL has 'packaged' the data input, validation and investigative programs. The form used is badly designed from the viewpoint of confidentiality and a sense of 'lets collect the data - we are sure it will come in useful' was evident. The complete data for each mother and child can be put onto 1 punch card and approximately 3,000 per year are accumulated.

Soft tissue sarcoma project (8)

This involved a much smaller population having a comparatively rare type of sarcoma - 266 cases in all gathered together over a 20 year period. However each patient has a considerable amount of information associated with him/her. In some cases up to ten treatments and assessments for recurrences and spread of the cancer were accounted for. Programming for this project was done in FORTRAN. A feature of the project is the way the results were presented in a visual form for easier interpretation by the consultant (9).

Myocardial infarction project

The main points of this project are described elsewhere at the Congress (4). The new language CODIL is being used for this work and hopefully the consultant and registrars involved will be able to program enquiries of the system themselves.

Accident and Emergency Unit

Here the problem is the detection of long term trends for planning purposes. In the present manual system 55,000 patients per year are treated but very little information can subsequently be gathered concerning their visit to the unit. A revised entry card has been drawn up (10) containing the necessary data for trend analysis and a one-tenth sampling of the population is in progress. The circumst-

-ances dictate that patients are not pestered by unnecessary questions, and the present work loads on the clerk and the nurses again means that the amount of data collected must be kept to a minimum. Test data has been run through the SPSS statistical package and further statistical work will be carried out when sufficient live data has accumulated.

Conclusions

Experience in the present work suggests that if computing facilities are to become more widely available to the average medical practitioner then improvements in the following areas will have to take place:

1. The production of cheaper computer configurations, both hardware and software, to aid research, planning and administration at local levels. The hardware requirement will be the most easily achieved as costs in this area continue to fall with the advent of microprocessor based systems. Very shortly, for a few thousand pounds, configurations will be available that have a reasonable amount of backing store and a usable programming language.

2. However, because of lack of training and time, medical practitioners will still have difficulty in making good use of these relatively cheap systems without expert help and advice. More research is needed in the area of communication between the computer and the non-expert user. Until the computer is easier to use, only the enthusiast will find time to undergo the necessary discipline and thus gain the benefits.

3. Until the above ideal situation is arrived at, then the only practical solution is to expand the computing teams that medical practitioners can turn to for advice and help.

To sum up, the present gap between the computer and the doctor who wishes to use its power needs closing by both sides - by the computing profession in providing better and easier techniques for the non-expert user and by the medical profession in accepting that education about the use of computers is an essential part of every practitioner's training.

References

1. E.MEDDINGS & P.FOLEY, Development of a computer based information system for cumulative patient profiles in a family practice setting, p457, MEDINFO 77 Shires/Wolf, editors, North-Holland (1977).

2. D.STIMSON, G.CHARLES, C.ROGERSON, A problem-oriented information system for a primary care group practice, p464, MEDINFO 77   Shires/Wolf, editors North Holland (1977)

3. Book of MUMPS, Compiled by Joan Zimmerman, MUMPS User's Group, 700 South Euclid Avenue, St. Louis, MO 63110, USA (1977)

4. C.F.REYNOLDS, Using CODIL to handle poorly structured clinical information Proceedings of MIE 78, Cambridge (1978)

5. L.R.NEAL, The computer handling of medical information for research purposes, MEDINFO 77 p651, Shires/Wolf, editors. IFIP. North-Holland (1977)

6. D.HALL, Experience of transferring an integrated hospital administration system from CODSYL Data Base to a standard MUMPS file structure, Journées d'Informatique Médical, Proceedings of Symposium on Medical Informatics, Toulouse (1978)

7. W.L.BLUNDELL, A computer based approach to the organisation of Hillingdon Hospital Maternity Records, Master of Technology dissertation, Brunel University (1972).

8. D. STAMELOS, Medical computing and the Mount Vernon project on soft tissue sarcomas, Master of Philosophy thesis, Brunel University (1975).

9. L.R.NEAL, Computer techniques for retrospective analysis, MEDINFO 74, Anderson/Forsythe, editors. IFIP North Holland (1974)

10. F.JAMA'N, The computer handling of records in the Accident and Emergency Unit of Hillingdon Hospital, to be presented as a Bachelor of Technology dissertation, Brunel University (1978).

11. L.HIRSCHMAN & R.GRISHMAN. Fact retrieval from natural language medical records, p247 MEDINFO 77, Shires/Wolf, editors. IFIP North Holland (1977)

SATISFYING THE INFORMATION NEEDS OF THE GENERAL PRACTITIONER FOR

IMPROVED PATIENT CARE

M. G. Sheldon,
General Practitioner,
69, Oxford Road,   Banbury

INTRODUCTION

The General Practitioner requires a constant flow of information from various sources in order to keep himself up-to-date, to provide his patients with appropriate advice and therapy, and to refer them to other agencies when indicated.   Post-graduate education is provided to assist the attainment of those goals but it may not always be directed towards the needs of the individual practitioner.

Information retrieval pertinent to practice management, patient care and audit of clinical care can only be collected within the practice itself.   There have been many advances in recent years in the provision of data necessary for improvements in practice management.   Many practices now have age/sex registers and recall facilities to maximise the effectiveness of all members of the primary health care team.

Problem orientated notes and a diagnostic index provide the G.P. with more detailed and more readily available knowledge about his patients so that a more positive approach may be taken in clinical care.

Audit of performance is possible, especially with the use of encounter forms which record all consultation details and enable analysis of the effects of therapeutic intervention by the doctor.

Previously all of this information retrieval and analysis has been done manually either by the doctor himself or by members of his ancillary staff. As in other fields of activity it is now being realised that mechanical analysis of information greatly increases the range of activities which may be pursued.   With the increasing use of computers it is now possible for the average non-academic practice to routinely collect and analyse pertinent information on practice activities thus facilitating the delivery of a higher standard of clinical care.

PRACTICE MANAGEMENT

For an efficient use of resources a general practitioner needs a basic practice register, an age/sex register, "at risk" registers, a postcode register (or similar means of identifying the area of residence of his patients), a recall system for chronic conditions, and facilities for screening various sub-groups of patients. Without a large amount of perserverence and the available number of man-hours the maintenance of all these registers is virtually impossible if mechanical aids are not used.

Many practices have a high turnover of patients as well as a fair proportion of patients who change their name, address and occupation during each year. Computerised practice registers will allow a single entry to be accessed to all registers at the same time so turning a very difficult task of register maintenance into a fairly simple one. The analytical powers of the computer can then be used to provide listings of sub-groups of patients for everyday use.

CLINICAL PATIENT CARE

It seems unlikely that the written clinical record will be replaced in the forseeable future. Much of the recorded information is of use for only a short period of time. Many consultations take place away from the surgery and so the records must be portable. The amount of storage needed to contain all of the medical record would be expensive with present technology.

There is, however a place for the computer in providing summaries of clinical data which have been collected for other purposes. Thus a problem list may be produced to go into the record from the information collected to create a practice diagnostic index. Similarly morbidity and drug data can be summarised to provide on one sheet an account of all doctor-patient interactions over a period of time.

A therapeutic index listing of all patients on particular drugs will be of use to monitor side-effects and adverse reactions.

A simple recall system with the facility for identifying defaulters will aid the management of chronic diseases. Screening of sub-groups of the practice is facilitated by the production of lists from the practice register and the computer can print addressed labels at the same time.

Providing a print-out of the computer details of each patient to go in the record envelope enhances data accuracy as frequent reference to the details by health care workers will identify inaccuracies and so enable corrections to be made.

AUDIT

Audit has become a fashionable topic of conversation but satisfactory methods of clinical audit in general practice are rare.   The importance of audit is not its performance but the changes in behaviour which result.   One well tried method of clinical data collection is the use of encounter forms to record morbidity and therapeutic or other intervention at every doctor-patient contact.   Analysis of this data is extremely difficult without a computer.

Auditing of clinical care has been achieved in our practice and can lead to more appropriate prescribing, a reduction in consultation rates per illness episode and quicker recovery for the patient.

METHODS AVAILABLE

(a)   FOR INFORMATION COLLECTION

Most of the information has to be obtained directly from the patient either by the doctor or his ancillary staff.   The efficient use of registration sheets, patient questionnaires and clinical summary sheets will assist this process and lead to greater degrees of accuracy in the data collected.

The collection of consultation data may be best achieved using encounter forms where a carbon copy of the prescription is produced to which the doctor adds other clinical details.   The data collection is completed by a procedure for including important items of information from letters and investigations which come into the practice without a consultation taking place.

With little additional ancillary staff this complete data collection system can be maintained indefinitely in any practice.

(b)   FOR DATA ANALYSIS

Traditionally all data was analysed by manual methods which with the volume of data created is so time-consuming as to virtually prohibit its use.   Occasionally small amounts of data are more suitably sorted by hand without resource to mechanical measures but in the majority of cases some form of mechanisation will be needed.

Much useful work can be done with batch-processed methods using a large central computer. The Oxford Community Health Project has maintained this service to approximately 30 practices for several years. The main limitations of this system is a slow turn-round of data leading to less accurate registers which are of limited use when they are more than a few months out of date. Confidentiality also becomes a problem when large amounts of sensitive clinical data are handled by a remote computer.

All recent work has pointed towards the dedicated, on-site, micro or mini-computer as the ideal answer to these information needs of the General Practitioner. Machines at a suitable price with the necessary software to satisfy these information handling needs are now available.

CONCLUSIONS

More attention should be paid to the clinical information needs of the general practitioner. Efficient methods of data capture backed by the analytical powers of a dedicated small computer owned by the G.P. could improve most aspects of patient care in general practice.

It is my belief that the cost would be amply justified by the improvement in practice management and patient care. General practice is no longer a cottage industry but the front-end of a vast health services structure with a large investment in terms of money and people. Antiquated methods of handling the problems in general practice do a dis-service to the patients, the G.P.'s and all other workers in the health service. Efficient information handling systems should be created at this, the main point of contact between patients and the health service.

INFORMATION PROCESSING IN RESEARCH AND ROUTINE NUCLEAR CARDIOLOGY

Cornelis N. de Graaf, Peter P. van Rijk and O Ying Lie
Institute of Nuclear Medicine
Utrecht, The Netherlands

1. INTRODUCTION

Nuclear Medicine is the application of radioactive material to the diagnosis
and treatment of patients and the study of human disease. It is a rapidly
growing specialism, mainly because its diagnostic tools are not agressive and
non-invasive. It can be divided into two fields: the in-vitro techniques, by
which samples of blood, urine, etc. are examined after incubation with radioactive materials, and the in-vivo techniques, by which not only the spatial
distribution of radioactive tracer, but also its variation in time can be
externally measured. Nuclear Cardiology is one of the in-vivo techniques and
provides the assessment of essential cardiac parameters such as cardiac output,
ejection fraction, intracardiac shunting etc., while wall motion abnormalities
and coronary perfusion defects can also be visualized.

1.1. Gamma camera imaging

In general only the stationary detector devices are suitable as imaging equipment, and this for practical purposes limits us to the use of the gamma camera.
(Fig. 1.).
A gamma camera transposes a three-dimensional distribution of radioactivity into
a two-dimensional picture, which is interpretable. In the system two units can
be distinguished, namely the detector head and the control circuitry (Fig. 2.).
Gamma rays emitted by radioisotopes first pass through a collimator. This
collimator, consisting of thousands of channels ("holes") in a lead plate,
absorbs all but a small fraction of gamma rays coming from a well-defined derec-
tion. At the exit side of the collimator this results in gamma rays impinging
on a thallium activated sodium-iodide crystal.
Gamma rays are absorbed, partly or totally, by the crystal and give rise to
scintillations. The brightness of a scintillation is proportional to the
absorbed energy. The NaI(Tl) crystal is viewed by a hexagonal array of 37
or more photomultiplier tubes. Each scintillation activates the photomulti-
pliers differently depending on local geometry with respect to the origin of
the scintillation.

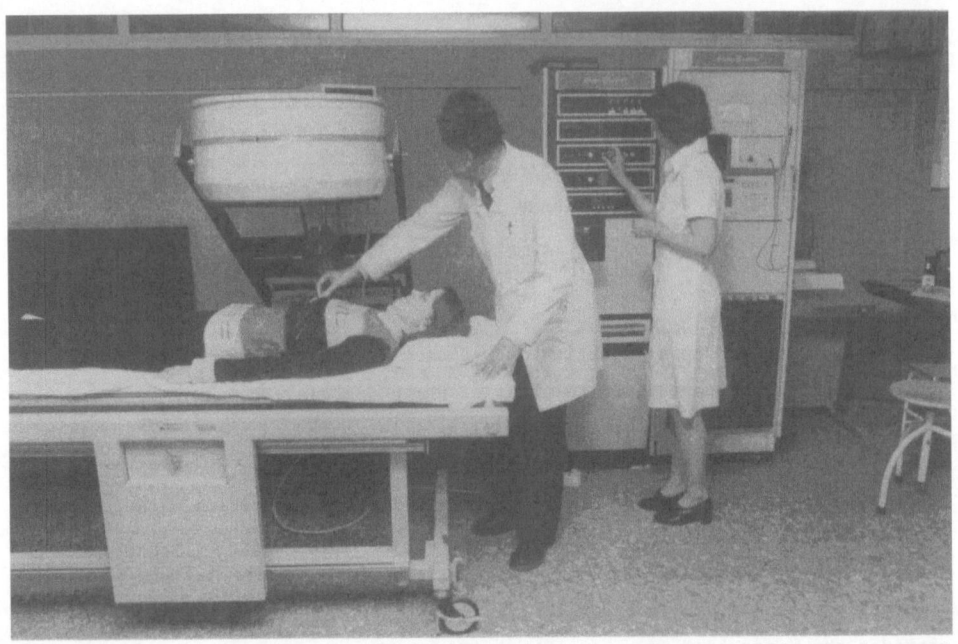

Fig. 1. Set-up of gamma camera. The physician positions the patient under the camera head previous to measurement. The technician sets the controls of camera console and computer.

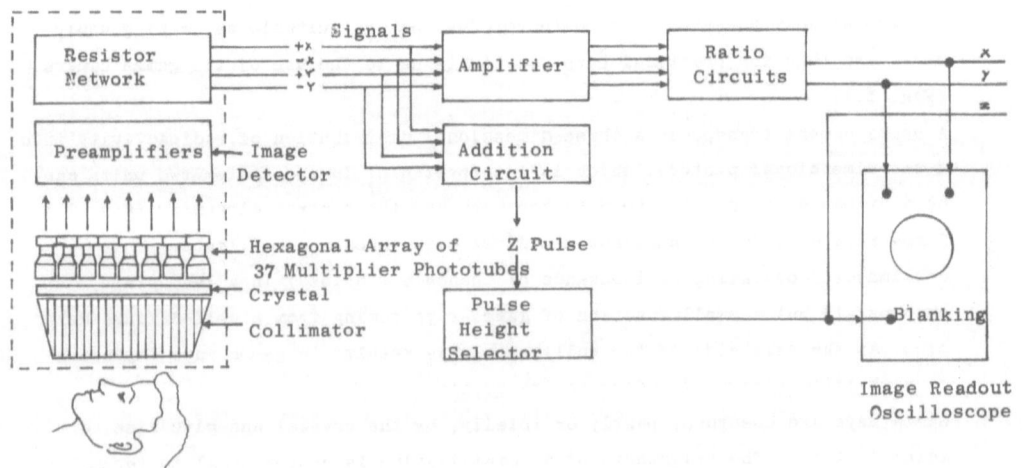

Fig. 2. Scheme of gamma camera measurement

After amplification,the output signals from the photocathodes pass through pre-
amplifiers and a resistor network, which produce four signals (+x, -x, +y, -y)
containing information on the position of the scintillation and the absorbed
energy of the gamma ray. Within the control circuitry the signals are again
amplified and sent, via a ratio circuit, to the plates of an oscilloscope. From
an addition circuit a third signal (Z) which is proportional only to the
brightness of the scintillation, regardless of the origin, is applied to the
input of a single-channel pulse-height selector, of which the window is adjusted
to accept only the totally absorbed unscattered gamma rays from the photopeak.
Unwanted signals due to scattering of gamma rays in the object or detector head
are thus eliminated. A true output from the pulse-height-selector unblanks the
beam of the oscilloscope, resulting in a point flash of light on the screen.
An optic camera placed in front of the screen collects all these flashes on a
common X-ray film. After developing, a two-dimensional projection of the
three-dimensional distribution of radioactive material is obtained. X, Y, and
Z-signals are also led to the ADC-system of a computer for further processing.
Although the gamma camera enables us to image the distribution of basically
chemical or biochemical compounds in the human body, and therefore provides
us with functional rather than morphologic information, its imaging characteristics are not perfect. The modulation transfer function (MTF) yields an effective spatial resolution of 6 to 12 mm. Furthermore the images are distorted by
inhomogenity effects at the sites of the photocathodes, and contain Poisson
distributed noise due to the statistical nature of radioactive decay.
Computer-enhancement of the images may be carried out using high-emphasis
filters for refining the resolution, low-pass filters for rejecting noise [1],
and inhomogenity correction by multiplication by the inverse of the response to
a uniform flat radioactive source ("flooded field"). In some commercially
available cameras a built-in inhomogenity correction is carried out by a microprocessor.

1.2. Collimators

Collimators may be of various design. There are collimators for low energy
(e.g. ^{99m}Tc, $E\gamma$ 140 keV), medium energy (e.g. ^{131}I, $E\gamma$ 364 keV), and high
energy (511 keV) gamma-emitters. High-resolution collimators have low efficiency, whilst high-sensitivity collimators produce images with low resolution.

Since most of the cardiac investigations are "dynamic studies" (studies in time) where high resolution is not essential, in most cases high sensitivity collimators are applied in nuclear cardiology. When the collimator holes focus on one point, a converging or diverging effect can be achieved. A collimator especially designed for cardiac studies (Fig. 3) consists of two

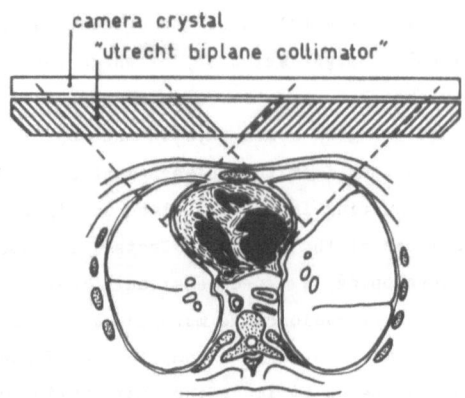

Fig. 3. Measurement with a biplane collimator

semicircular parallel-hole collimators facing each other with a slant of 40° relative to the camera axis, so that biplane studies can be performed [2]. This is facilitated by the fact that the heart is a small organ in comparison with the size of the detector.

1.3. Computer acquisition

In the majority of nuclear cardiac studies further computer-processing of the information is needed. A typical data collection system [3] is comprised of two-ramp-type analog-to-digital-converters (ADC) and a mass-storage operating system with display facilities (Fig. 4). At the acquisition part of the system the X- and Y-signals from the camera are converted into 6 to 8 bits [4] at a maximum rate of 0.5 to 1.5 MHz, while the blank/unblank signal ("Z") activates the sampling circuitry and direct-memory-access (DMA) transfer of the information (mostly as a 16-bit word) to the acquisition memory. This mechanism of storage is known as "list mode" acquisition, since all events - counts interspersed with timing information - are stored sequentially in memory and are blockwise dumped into a mass memory.

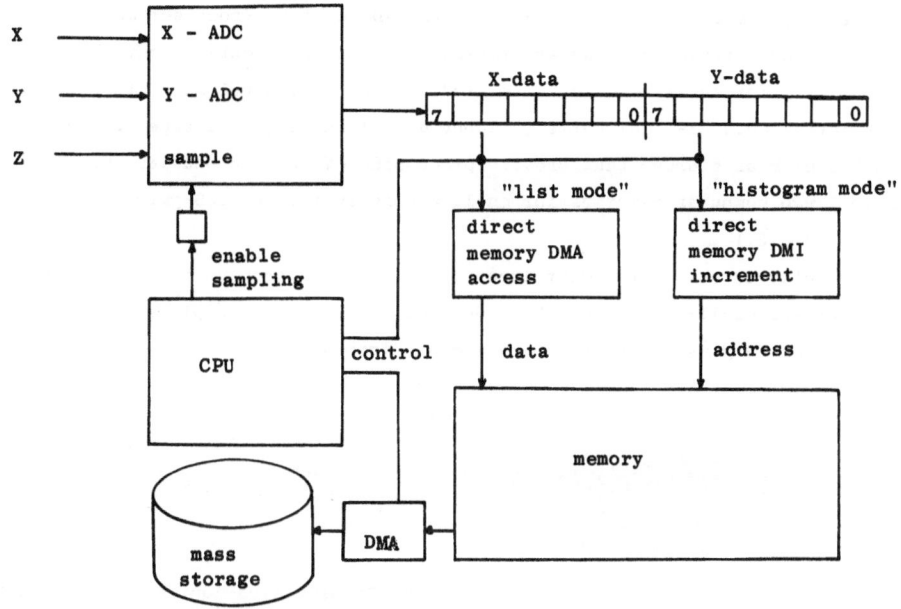

Fig. 4. Scheme of computer acquisition

An alternative method of acquisition is the "histogram mode" or "frame mode",
where DMA is replaced by direct-memory-increment (DMI). The DMI hardware calculates under initial CPU-control the memory-address of a location to be
numerically incremented by 1, so that an image of the counts-distribution is
directly built-up in memory. Both modes have their advantages. List-mode
acquisition usually gives more flexibility in off-line processing, and histogram-mode facilitates higher acquisition rates. Fast ADC's (typical dead time:
1 μsec) are required to avoid serious data losses during routine dynamic
studies. For example, during cardiac first-pass studies where 10 mCi of
$^{99m}TcO_4^-$ are rapidly injected, the data rate of photopeak events is 40,000
counts per second during 2 to 3 seconds of the study. A dead time of 20 μsec
would lead to 62% data loss. At list-mode acquisition, data transfer rate to
the mass storage memory is the limiting factor: steady state transfer rates
range from 10 kHz for magnetic tape units to 30 up to 250 kHz for moving-head
discs.

1.4. Storage and display

Some manufacturers are at present bringing dedicated nuclear medicine computer
systems on the market, which show a wide variety in performance and price.

Commercial systems generally consist of an ADC-system, processor and storage medium, and interactive display station. Most of them contain software packages especially for analysis of cardiac studies. The most usual mass storage media are moving-head disc, diskette ("floppy disk") and magnetic tape. Systems with slow mass storage that provide processing of cardiac studies, usually have large computer memories for on-line construction of ECG-gated studies (section 8.3.).

The display is one of the most important pieces of hardware in the system. The refresh oscilloscope and the video monitor have wide application, for display of 64 x 64 to 256 x 256 matrices ("frames").

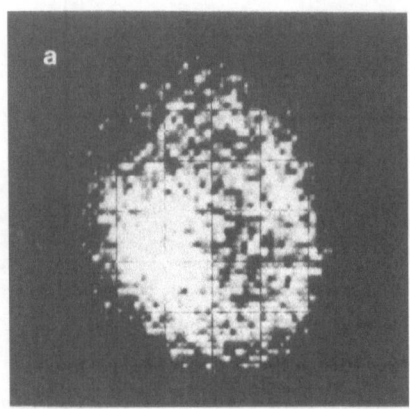

Fig. 5. Display hard-copies of a thallium image: a. polaroid picture from refresh oscilloscope; b. electrostatic plot; c. electrostatic plot after low-pass filtering

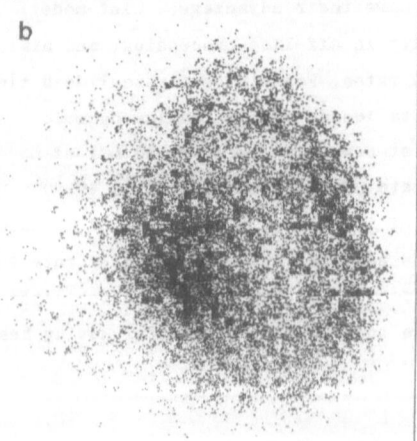

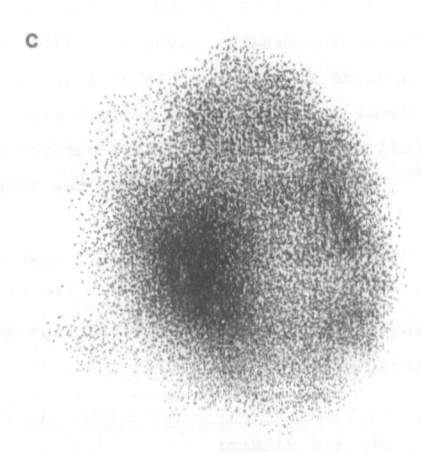

Colour displays, mostly offered as an option with the commercial systems, facilitate superprojection of different images, and some observers prefer colour-coded isocontour display to the ordinary grey-shade. In nuclear cardiology, display-units should be capable of showing at least 12 successive frames per second in endless-loop flicker-free movie format.

Hard-copying is mostly carried out by taking polaroid pictures from a screen. In some systems an electrostatic plotter is an option, although even a line-printer can be applied with character-coding of grey-shades.

Fig. 5 shows a polaroid picture (a) from a refresh oscilloscope displaying a raw 64 x 64 frame of a ^{201}Tl scintigram, together with (b) the same frame plotted with an electrostatic plotter, where each pixel (picture-element) is coded as an 8 x 8 matrix of randomly distributed dots, facilitating 65 pseudo-grey-shades. Fig. 5.c. shows the same frame after low-pass filtering with a two-dimensional segmental least-squares polynome operator.

2. STATIC MYOCARDIAL IMAGING

Over the last ten years, progress resulting from clinical, pathologic and epi-demiologic studies has led to a better understanding of the natural history of coronary artery disease (CAD). A wide variety of radiopharmaceuticals are being employed; they reflect the various pathofysiologic manifestations of CAD that affect blood flow through the coronary arteries, with consequent alterations in myocardial function. Currently most of the traditional radiopharmaceuticals for imaging of myocardial abnormalities such as ^{43}K, various Cs and Rb-isotopes, all as monovalent ions, are replaced by ^{99m}Tc-pyrophosphate (TcPYP) and ^{201}Tl^{+}.

2.1. TcPYP myocardial scanning

TcPYP (like some less frequently applied ^{99m}Tc-compounds) is deposited into the damaged myocardial cells and is therefore used as a scanning agent in cases of acute myocardial infarction (AMI) [6]. However, there is no uptake in ischaemic areas nor in scar tissue, i.c. old infarcts. In selected patients, suspected of having AMI, in whom a reliable history cannot be obtained, or the usual diagnostic tests (electrocardiography - ECG -, iso-enzymes distribution, etc.) have not been helpful, a TcPYP infarct scintigram may contribute important diagnostic information [7].

TcPYP - being a commonly used bone imaging agent - shows in an anterior scan
of a control person, only the sternum and ribs (Fig. 6). In AMI patients these

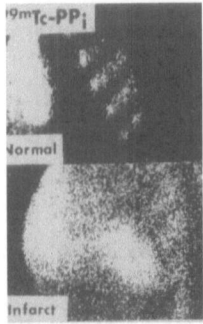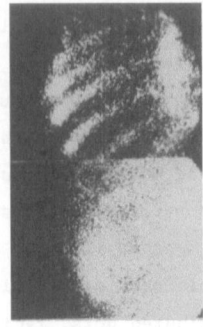

Fig. 6. Anterior and left-lateral
TcPYP images of normal person and
patient with infarct [34]

structures may partly obscure the infarct. Attempts have been made to mathematically remove rib-contributions from TcPYP images [5]. The energy contribution
of the rib structure in the anterior TcPYP image is contained over a narrow
frequency band, while the energy distribution of an infarction is more uniformly
spread over the spectrum. A digital band-reject filter successfully removes
the ribs from the image, although operator intervention is needed to enter
filter coefficients.

2.2. Static Thallium scanning

$^{201}Tl^+$ is taken up by the heart muscle cell in the same way as potassium ions,
but is released at a much slower rate. Thallium images of the heart therefore
reflect the distribution of the metabolism of the myocardium, and also show
the perfusion of the heart muscle tissue [8]. Lesions - less perfused areas or
areas of necrotic tissue - will show up as "cold spots" (Fig. 7,8). Since
the actual distribution of lesions is three-dimensional, images in more than
one projection should be made for accurate localisation of infarcts. Due to
limitations of radiations hazards, only a small amount of ^{201}Tl (in the order
of 2 mCi) can be administered, which results in a low count rate. Also the
target/non-target ratio (tissue vs background-tissue uptake) is rather low
- 2:1 -, so that the signal-to-noise-ratio of Tl-images is poor compared to
images of ^{99m}Tc labeled agents [9].

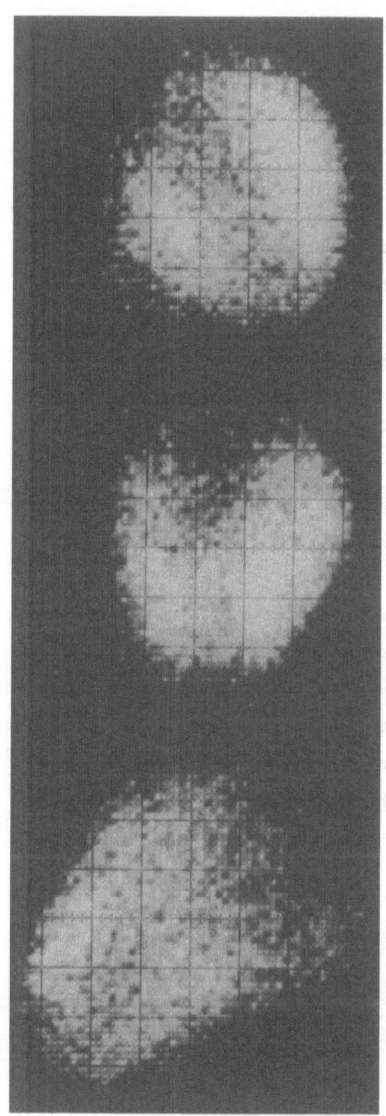

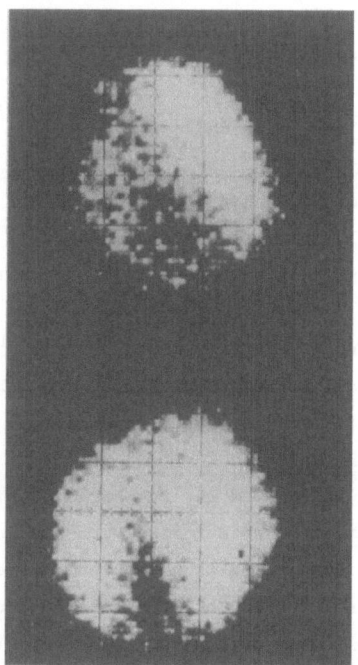

Fig. 8. Anterior and left-anterior-oblique ^{201}Tl-images of patient with anteroseptal infarct

Fig. 7. Anterior, left-anterior-oblique and left-lateral ^{201}Tl-images of normal person

Thallium imaging covers a wider range of clinical indications than TcPYP scintigraphy, such as AMI, stable and unstable angina, and old infarcts. Stress scintigraphy - after injection of ^{201}Tl during excercise - can be applied for the differentiation between old infarcts and ischaemic areas.

Static Thallium-images generally do not need further image processing apart from noise filtering.

3. QUANTITATION OF INFARCT SIZES

Several methods have been proposed for infarct sizing from TcPYP scans. The apparently most successful technique [5] outlines the boundary of the infarction by an edge detection technique, so that a measure of the size is expressed as cm^2.

These, and other experimental studies [10] [11] suggest that the size of an acute myocardial infarction, measured from the TcPYP scan, does correllate with the size of the scintigraphic abnormality. These studies, however, have been performed in dogs.

In human TcPYP studies, in which the size of inferior or subendocardial infarctions estimated by serum enzymes was compared with the size of scintigraphic abnormalities, results have been less encouraging. This can be explained by the variable perfusion of infarcts, and the complexity of geometry of the infarct. There is no way of applying edge detection algorithms to ^{201}Tl images in order to quantitate infarct size. Any attempt to determine the area of decreased activity depends solely on human subjectivity. However, it seems possible to measure relatively small changes of the infarct size in the follow-up of one patient [12]. This technique works as follows (Fig. 9): On the basis of an outline of the left-ventricular myocardium, drawn by the observer, a thinning algorithm is applied to select a skeleton with high countrates over the image.

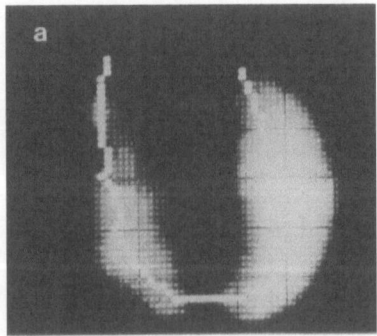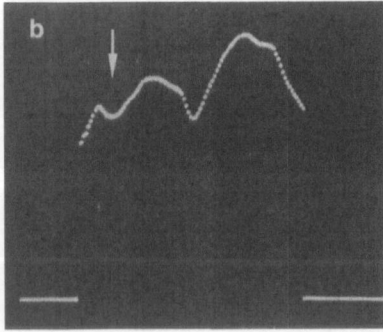

Fig. 9. Pseudo-sizing of infarcts in ^{201}Tl images: a. filtered LAO30 ^{201}Tl image of patient with high septal infarction, together with structure skeleton; b. skeleton profile, the infarcted area is represented by the inclination in the left part of the profile (arrow)

These areas in the image represent regions of the myocardial wall that show
most changes in countrate in the case of varying perfusion and can reproduci-
bly be relocated in the actual myocardium. A sensitive parameter of the extent
of the infarction can be achieved by measuring the distance of the inflection
points of the inclination the infarct causes in the skeleton profile.

4. COMPUTED TOMOGRAPHY

Transverse section tomography can be carried out for either transmission or
studies [42] [44] [46]. However, for the latter photon attenuation correction is required. There are also several possible beam configurations, and the reconstruction algorithms which are derived for the parallel beam configuration,
are after modification also applicable for other configurations.
Because of the beating of the heart, data collection should be carried out with
the ECG gating technique (chapter 8). It is necessary that the projections for
one reconstruction must be measured at the same phase of the heart beat. The
projection frames are obtained as described in section 8.2., by updating the
data each time the phase occurs.

4.1. Reconstruction methods

The analytical reconstruction methods are based on Radon's formula [13]:

$$\mu(r,\phi) = \frac{1}{2\pi^2} \int_{-\frac{1}{2}\pi}^{\frac{1}{2}\pi} \int_{-\frac{1}{2}1}^{\frac{1}{2}1} \frac{\partial p(s)}{\partial s} \cdot \frac{1}{r\sin(\phi-\theta)-s} \, ds \, d\theta$$

where the projections (Fig. 10) are given by:

$$p(s) = \int \mu(r,\theta) \, \vec{d\ell}$$

This can be solved by direct integration, series expansion, or the widely used
convolution. The inner integral represents a convolution, and discrete approximation of the convolution function gives the various convolution reconstruction
methods. Another solution to the problem is by using the matrix equation method

$$p(k) = \sum_{i,j \in k\theta} w(i,j)\mu(i,j)$$

$$\underline{P} = W\underline{X}$$

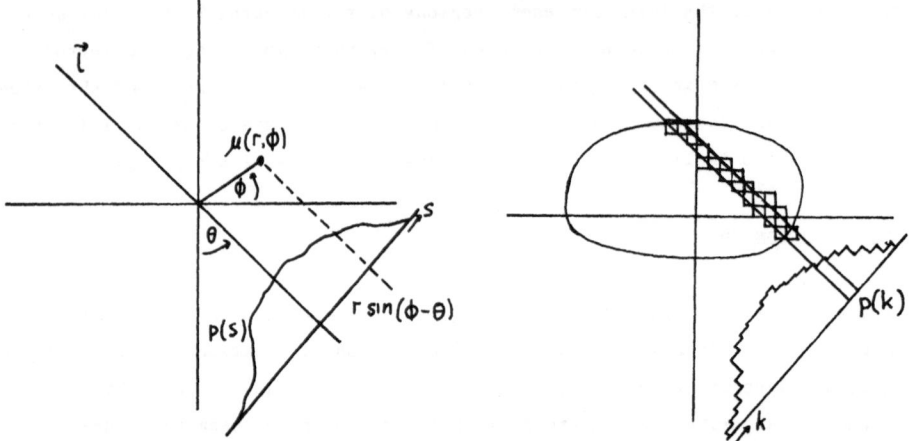

Fig. 10. Tomographic projection   Fig. 11. The weighting elements

W is the geometrical weighting matrix (Fig. 11). Due to the large size and defectiveness of the matrix W, it is preferable to apply iterative solution methods instead of direct inversion.

Some methods are:

- ART and SIRT which approach the minimum norm solution.
- The weighted or unweighted iterative least-squares method.

Amongst these reconstruction methods, the convolution methods seem to be the most attractive ones. Furthermore, it is not difficult to modify the function for other beam configurations. Attenuation correction can also be carried out during reconstruction. However, if the field of view is limited, then the iterative methods are preferable.

4.2. Attenuation correction

The transmission measurements (Fig. 12) are given by:

$$I(k) = I(0) \exp\{- \sum_{i,j \in k\Theta} w(i,j)\mu(i,j)\}$$

and the projection values will be:

$$p(k) = \ln I(0) - \ln I(k) = \sum_{i,j \in k\Theta} w(i,j)\mu(i,j)$$

Conjugate views are equal to each other:

$$p(k;\Theta) = p(K-k;\Theta+\pi)$$

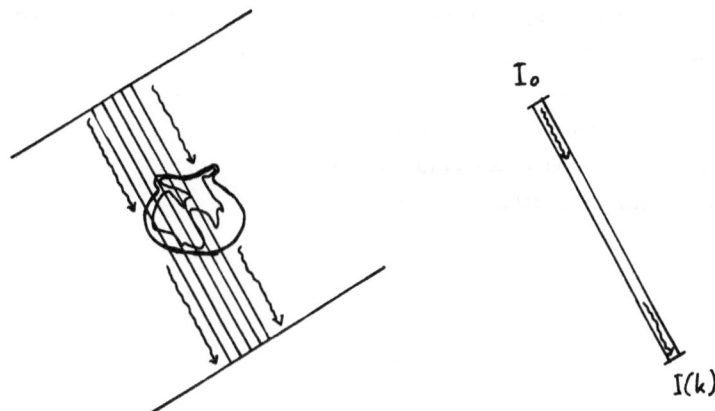

Fig. 12. Transmission study

In the case of emission studies (Fig. 13), the measured projection values do not
represent the linear sum of activity densities. Conjugate views are not identical.

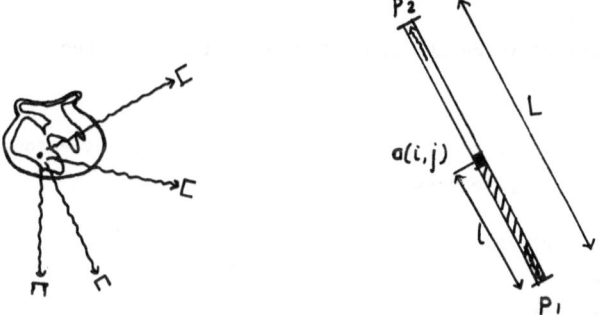

Fig. 13. Emission study

$$p(k;\theta) = \sum_{i,j \in k\Theta} a(i,j) \exp\{-\Sigma\ell(i,j)\mu(i,j)\}$$

$$p\{K-k;\theta+\pi\} = \sum_{i,j \in k\Theta} a(i,j) \exp\{-\Sigma(L-\ell(i,j))\mu(i,j)\}$$

where $\Sigma l(i,j)$ is the path length between the element $a(i,j)$ and the detector,
and $\mu(i,j)$ are the attenuation coefficients along the path.

Attenuation correction can be applied before, during, or after reconstruction, usually by application of the conjugate projections p_1 and p_2 or reconstruction values a_1 and a_2 of conjugate projections.

The following are some correction formulae:

1. Before reconstruction: projection compensation.

   a. Simple geometrical or arithmatic mean:

   $$p = \sqrt{p_1 p_2}$$

   $$p = \frac{p_1 + p_2}{2}$$

   b. Weighted mean [14]

   $$p = \frac{\sqrt{p_1 p_2} \cdot \exp\{\mu \tfrac{1}{2}1\} \cdot \mathfrak{t}\mu \tfrac{1}{2}1}{\sinh\{\mathfrak{t}\mu \tfrac{1}{2}1\}}$$

   and derived [45]:

   $$p = \frac{\tfrac{1}{2}(p_1 + p_2) \cdot \exp\{\mu \tfrac{1}{2}1\}}{\cosh\{\mu (\tfrac{1}{2}1 - \ell)\}}$$

2. During reconstruction:

   a. Iteration method to be applied after each iteration step [1 3]

   $$a = a' e^{\mu k}$$

   b. Convolution methods to be carried out for each pair of reconstructed values from conjugate views [14]:

   $$a = \sqrt{a_1 a_2} \cdot \exp\{\mu \tfrac{1}{2}1\}$$

   or [45]:

   $$a = \frac{a_1 \cdot \exp(\mu \ell) + a_2 \cdot \exp\{\mu (1 - \ell)\}}{2}$$

3. After reconstruction:

   $$a = a' \cdot \frac{1}{M} \Sigma \exp\{\mu \ell\}$$

It is clear that correction method 2. will give the best results. The other two methods would result in over- or under-compensation for some points. The values of the absorption coefficients $\mu(i,j)$ can be estimated by transmission reconstruction or by a phantom study. The most appropriate way is by using its typical value.

As the statistical properties of scintigraphic data are rather bad, multi-plication of conjugate views should be avoided. It is preferable to use the arithmetic mean above the geometric mean.

4.3. Beam configurations

There are several beam configurations: parallel ray configuration (Fig. 14), equal ray length fan beam (Fig. 15), planar detector fan beam (Fig. 16), and circular ring configuration (Fig. 17).

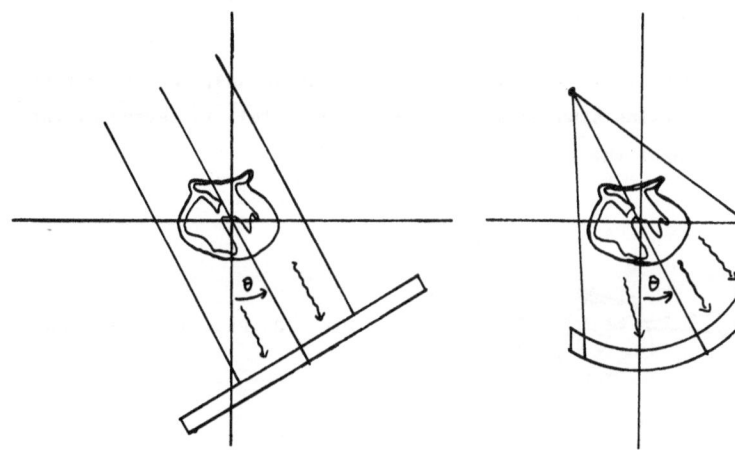

Fig. 14. Parallel ray   Fig. 15. Fan beam

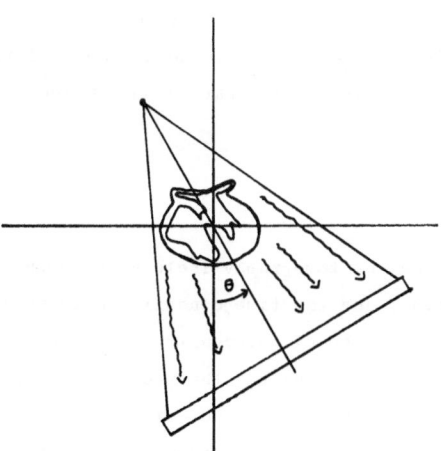
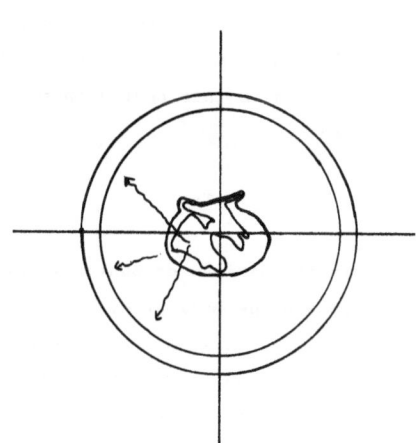

Fig. 16. Fan beam   Fig. 17. Circular ring

It is possible to perform reconstruction after reordening the rays into a
parallel configuration. This can only be done after all projections have been
taken. Due to the finite angle increments, there will be some missing values,
and these must be approximated by their neighbouring points.
It is better to derive a set of transformations which represents the relationship to the parallel beam configuration. Furthermore similar to the parallel
beam reconstruction method, a convolution function can be calculated. In this
case it will be impractical to apply the matrix equation method, because of
its complexity related to the calculation of the geometric weighting matrix W.

4.4. Positron emission

As a result of the statistical properties of scintigrams, the measurement-time
required makes routine studies mainly impractical. This is caused by the
poor transmission of the lead collimator.

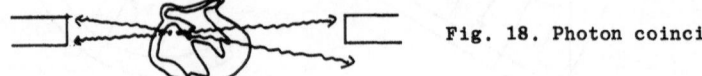

Fig. 18. Photon coincidence

By the use of positron emission, the collimator is effectively replaced by
an electronic detecting system, which detects the 180° coincidence annihilation
photons. With this photon energy, there will be no attenuation correction
needed.

4.5. Concluding remarks

Basic limitations of photon transverse section tomography include the need
to rotate the patient or move the detector, and the time-consuming mathematical
operations required. Furthermore, the resolution of the constructed images
is limited due to poor statistics in the projections and the poor intrinsic
resolution of the gammacamera. Nevertheless, the performance of a transverse
section emission tomography system may compete with the X-ray attenuation
tomography devices ("CT-scanner"), because of its price and the nature of

the information achieved.

With multi-crystal ring detector systems some of the limitations are overcome, althrough the application of positron emitters involve the near presence of a cyclotron.

5. FIRST-PASS STUDIES

From the first pass of thoracical circulation after intravenous bolus injection several clinically interesting parameters can be achieved. The technique is relatively simple. A gamma camera is positioned to record from the leftanterior-oblique-40° (LAO 40) projection. After injection into the antecubital vein, during approximately 20 sec. data is recorded in either list-mode or histogram-mode, 1 to 5 frames per second.

Most frequently applied radiopharmaceuticals are $^{99m}TcO_4^-$, ^{99m}Tc labeled red blood cells (TcRBC), and ^{99m}Tc labeled human serum albumin (TcHSA).

5.1 Cardiac output

Apart from the LAO-40, also the RAO-30 view can be applied for cardiac output measurement. The framing rate should be at least one per second.

After the first pass measurement the patient stays in the same position under the gammacamera for 10 min., after wich an aquilibrium image is made.[15,16]

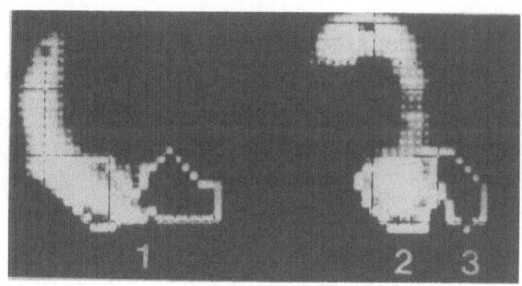

Fig. 19. Biplane first-pass study: right heart phase; also using the phase of LV filling, ROI have been drawn for:
1. LV + RV at RAO;
2. RV at LAO;
3. LV at LAO.

Fig. 19 shows an example of cardiac output measurement in both the RAO and the LAO view employing the biplane collimator. Regions of interest (ROI) are drawn - by using a lightpen - over the left and right ventricles in the LAO view, and over the combined left (LV) and right (RV) ventricles in the RAO view.

In practice a single ROI over the entire heart, either in LAO or RAO, is satisfactory.

Fig. 20 shows that there is a good correlation between the LV + RV curves for RAO and LAO. The area below the first passage heart curve is determined (p counts), either by extrapolation, of by gamma function variate fitting (see section 6.1).

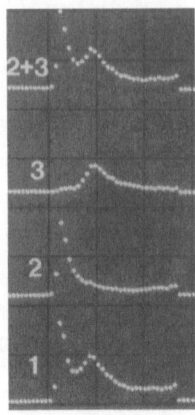

Fig.20. Curves 1, 2 and 3 from the ROI of fig.19. The sum of 2 and 3 is almost identical to 1.

Futhermore the countrate in the same ROI is measured at equilibrium, scaled to counts per minute (q cpm). Finally the blood volume (V dm^3) is determined by dilution measurement of the injected material by means of a blood sample or, in case of $^{99m}TcO_4^-$, it is determined seperately.
The cardiac output is now simply calculated as: $CO = \frac{V.q}{p}$ dm^3/min.

Note: Cardiac output measurement can also be carried out by using a well-positioned single scintillation probe instead of a gamma camera. Correlation of the results of the radioisotope determination of cardiac output with the conventional test (catheterization dye dilution) is very close, r = .95.

5.2. Ejection fraction

To determine the ejction-fraction by means of a first pass study, the gamma-camera is positioned in LAO-30 or LAO-40 projection, to obtain a clear separation of RV and LV in most patients. Better seperation of LV and left atrium can be obtained by the 10° craniocaudal modification.[15]
Acquisition, after intravenous bolus injection of 10 mCi $^{99m}TcO_4^-$ (TcHSA or TcRBC if a follow-up equilibrium study is to be performed), is done in list mode, so that the framing rate (number of images per second) can be determined at off-line analysis.

Fig. 21 shows curves obtained from a ROI over the LV. Initially a framing rate of 5 sec. was chosen in order to determine where the peak activity of the LV-curve was reached.

Notice also that from this curve the initial integral for cardiac output measurement can be calculated. A second series of frames of 40 msec. intervals is made corresponding to the peak activity of the LV. From the curve that is generated, using the same ROI, the LV ejection fraction can be calculated as the average of the relative fall-off ratios for a selected number of heart beats, it is advisable to perform a correction for blood background in the lungs by subtracting a curve obtained from a crescent shaped ROI around the LV ROI. If necessary the ejection fraction of the RV can be calculated also in the same way. There exists a good correlation between the radionuclide and contrast techniques.[17] [18]

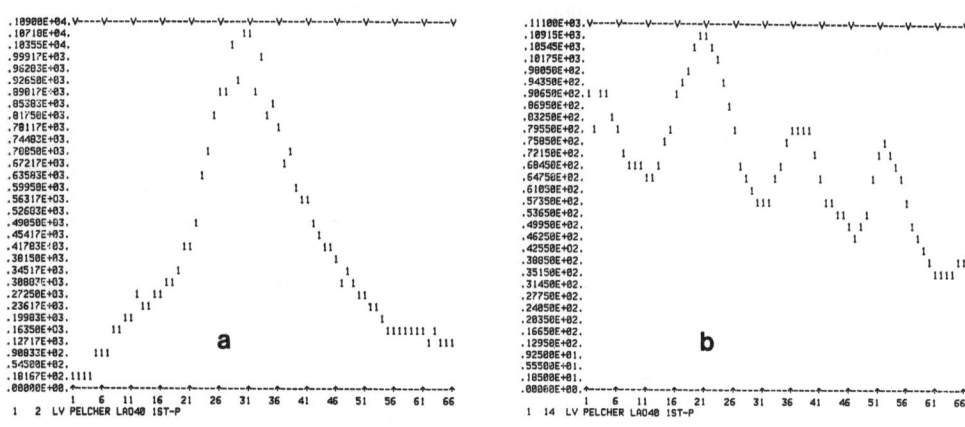

Fig.21. First-pass LV curves at:
a. 5 sec./frame; b. 40 msec./frame.

6. SHUNT DETECTION

The most commonly used methods for left-to-right intracardiac shunt detection and quantitation, oxymetry and dye- or ascorbinate-dilution, involve cardiac catheterization. Several techniques based on the radioisotope first-pass study have been investigated. Currently, in the favourised analysis techniques are based on gamma function variate least squares fitting of the timeactivity curve of the lung. [19] [20]

Right-to-left shunts are more difficult to quantitate.

The most accurate method is to administer ^{99m}Tc-microaggregates or - micro-
spheres intravenously, and to measure the activities over both lungs and the
rest of the body. The inverse ratio of these figures gives the magnitude of
the right-to-left shunt.

6.1. Gamma fitting

In most cases the injection technique involves puncture of the jugular vein
or an intravenous catheter into an arm vein in order to obtain as abrupt an
injection as possible, wich is essential for accurate quantitation. If a
deconvolution algorithm takes part in the analysis procedure (section 6.2.),
simple injection into the antecubital vein can be applied, wich is preferable, as most of the shunt patients are infants.
The first-pass study is performed as described in previous sections, with
10 (or less) mCi ^{99m}TcO$_4^-$, and succesive frames are created of $\leq$ .25 sec.
time-intervals (fig. 22).

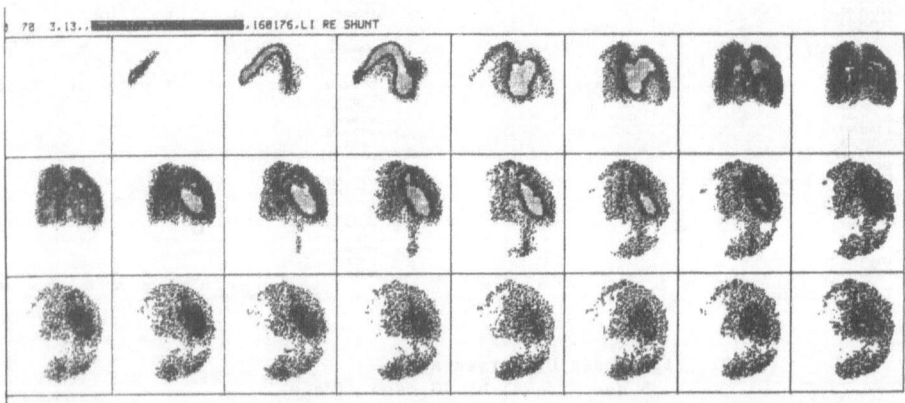

Fig. 22. First-pass study framed at 25 sec. intervals,
first 12 seconds. Each picture in this figure is the
sum of 2 consecutive frames.

The total duration of the study should be >15 sec. Fig. 23.a shows a frame
during the phase when most of the activity is in the lungs. A ROI is chosen
so that it covers only lung tissue (i.e. part of the right lung) and serves
to create the lung time-activity curve (defocused points in Fig. 23.c).
Tracer curves obtained from vascular beds are fairly well described by gamma
function variates of the form:

$$y(t) = A(t-\tau)^\alpha e^{(t-\tau)/\beta}$$

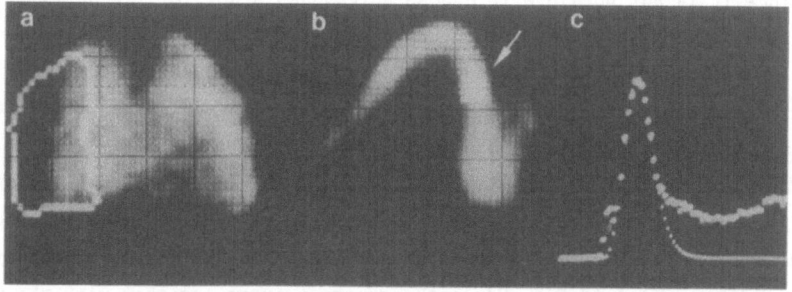

Fig. 23. Left-to-right shunt quantitation: a. lung ROI; b. superior
vena cava ROI (arrow); c. lung curve (defocussed), and
gamma fit to pulmonary peak (focused).

By fitting a curve following this model to the peak interval of the lung
curve (focused points in Fig. 23.c), an approximation is obtained of the
lung curve in the case of no shunting and no systemic recirculation were
present. The fitting algorithm should be iterative, since the gamma variate
equation cannot be analytically minimized because of the presence of
parameter τ [21]. Most commercial systems lack an iterative gamma fitting,
so that τ is to be set interactively.

6.2. Deconvolution

At the time the activity reaches the lungs, the bolus is already spread
considerably, even after jugular puncture, so that the lung curve $y(t)$
should be described as the convolution of the spread function $p(t)$ and
the vascular response of the lungs upon injection into the pulmonary
artery $f(t)$:

$$y(t) = \int_0^t p(s) f(t-s) ds$$

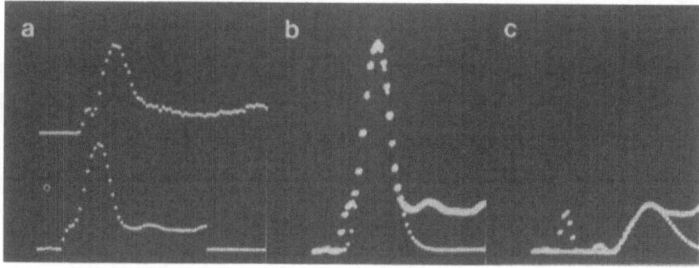

Fig. 24. Curves related to deconvolution and shunt quantitation.

Since it is not possible to choose a reasonable ROI for the pulmonary
artery, a ROI of the superior vena cava (Fig. 23.b) is taken as an estimate.
Deconvolution of the measured lung curve upon the superior vena cava curve
will therefore not give the true lung response, but has been proven to make
injection into the arm possible, instead of into the jugular vein [21].
Fig. 24.a shows the lung curve before (top) and after (bottom) deconvolution.
The shunt contribution is already clearly to be seen . Fig. 24.b: the
deconvolved lung curve (defocused) and the gamma fit to the pulmonary
peak (focused), and Fig. 24.c: the subtract curve together with the gamma
fit to the shunt contribution. The ratio of the areas of the two gamma fit
curves is the magnitude of the shunt.

7. IMAGING WITH INERT GASES

The need to calculate regional myocardial blood flow has led to the evaluation
of numerous radionuclides and radiopharmaceuticals. The group of diffusible
soluble radioactive gases (e.g. Xenon-133, Krypton-81m) gives satisfactory
(semi-) quantitative results. When an inert gas dissolved in solution is
presented as an intraarterial bolus it will be proportionately distributed
into the myocardium according to its solubility in the extracapillary
compartments. This distribution, however, is transient, and comparitive
perfusion levels can only be measured in the early phase of the study. The
gas diffuses rapidly into the pericapillary space and equilibrates with the
intravascular contents. The equilibrium time varies according to the specific
solubility of the different tissues. After the early phase of the inert gas
study, a washout occurs at exponential rates which are characteristic of
the exchange rates of the various extravascular compartments. The inert gas
in the venous blood is rapidly excreted by the lungs; thus only a small
amount of radioactivity recirculates.

7.1. Xenon-133

A bolus of ^{133}Xe dissolved in saline is rapidly injected into the main stem
of the coronary artery. The radioactivity in the myocardium is detected by
the gamma camera and data are collected by a computer system. When the
study is completed, wash-out curves from different regions of the myocardium
are constructed, and the clearance rate constants of the tracer are
calculated by mono-exponential analysis.
Using the Kety formula: $F = k\lambda/\rho$ where k is the clearance rate constant,

λ is the blood/myocardium partition coefficient for ^{133}Xe (0.72) and ρ is
the specific gravity of the tissue (1.05 g/cm^3). The myocardial blood flow
F (cm^3/100g.min) in the different regions can be calculated. There are
however methodological problems. In the Kety formula only one clearance
constant is assumed, but it is well known that ^{133}Xe has a high lipid
solubility and diffuses rapidly from the myocardium into the epicardial fat
during the initial phase of the wash-out, and is held up there. Therefore
the curve is altered from the start of the wash-out [39] and regional differences
in ^{133}Xe wash-out curves may be related to varying degrees of epicardial
fat. Recirculation of the indicator through the organ is assumed to be
negligible since, as a result of its low blood/air partition coefficient,
it is rapidly cleared from the circulation during its first passage through
the pulmonary capillaries. Animal experiments [40] have shown an average
error of 16% when no background correction was applied on data from regions
of infarction.

It has also been stated that a three-compartment model gives more accurate
results [41]. The presence of tails in the wash-out curves was not explained,
neither by the nonmyocardial background nor by inhomogeneous spatial perfusion
patterns. Several suggestions were made to explain that the departure of
inert gas wash-out curves from those of a single exponential model may be
caused by the already mentioned epicardial fat storage, collateral flow,
nonhomogeneous tissue structures, etc.

The use of Xenon-133 for calculation of regional myocardial blood flow can
provide only semiquantitative information, however, it can give important
diagnostic and pathophysiologic information.

7.2. Krypton-81m

^{81m}Kr has a half-life of 13 seconds. This radioactive inert water-soluble
noble gas emits a 190 keV gamma ray and is produced at a constant rate by
spontaneous decay of Rubidium-81 in an ^{81}Rb-^{81m}Kr generator delivery system.
The generator is eluted by 5 percent dextrose in water and infused intra-
arterially, directly into the aortic sinus.

The ^{81m}Kr travels through the vascular bed and after transit, the gas diffuses
rapidly into the extracapillary spaces. The third process is that of distribution between the accessible extravascular compartments, according to
pressure and diffusion, and is a slow process compared with the first two
movements.

This results in a scintigraphic image composed of both the vascular and

extravascular compartments. However, due to the rapid decay, the contribution
of the extravascular space is low. Therefore an observed heterogeneity in
the picture mainly reflects a difference in perfusion.

Theoretically the two compartments (intra- and extravascular) may be differentiated by the relative rates of wash-out of the vascular and extravascular
^{81m}Kr activity. If the ^{81m}Kr infusion is interrupted, the fraction of the
total activity which is derived from intravascular activity, will be rapidly
washed out. The extravascular components will wash out at slower rates.
After correction for decay, each component of the wash-out curve is extrapolated back to the time of interruption of ^{81m}Kr delivery, and the value of
either fraction may be obtained by subtraction of its zero intercept from
the total activity [47] [48].

Except for the detection of myocardial heterogeneous perfusion at high
countrates and calculation of exchange time in the tissue compartment, the
method has additional advantages in allowing repetition of experiments
after brief intervals, entirely free of any residual radioactivity. This
includes the testing of the effects of vasoactive drugs, pacing, physiologic
gating and reversible or irreversible injury.

8. ECG-CODED STUDIES

An alternate means of obtaining information about ejection fraction, which
at the same time provides access to other physiologically and clinically
interesting cardiac parameters, utilizes a physiological trigger and the
gamma camera, so that images are recorded during specific phases of the
cardiac cycle [22] [23]. This system has several advantages: images can be
recorded at high statistical quality; multiple projections are obtained
after a single injection of radioactive material; and regional wall motion
changes can be detected, both by applying ^{99m}Tc and ^{201}Tl.

8.1. Acquisition technique

There are perhaps as many data collection protocols for ECG-code studies
as there are nuclear medicine institutes and departments where these studies
are done. At the authors' institute, 2 mCi of ^{201}TlCl, or 20 mCi of ^{99m}TcO$_4^-$,
^{99m}TcHSA or ^{99m}TcRBC are administered intravenously to the patient (or in
case of transmission imaging or tomography a flooded-field phantom with 20
mCi ^{99m}Tc is applied), and the camera is positioned according to the type
of study and the clinical indication. In most thallium and

technetium studies the biplane collimator (section 1.2) is used. Three
ECG-leads are connected to an ECG trigger device. After the radiotracer
becomes uniformly distributed throughout the patients blood pool, scintigraphic data, the ECG trigger pulses and 10 msec clock ticks, coded into
digital words and inserted into the list-mode data stream, are collected
for approximately 1000 heart beats (Fig. 25). Data is collected either on
magnetic disc or tape, or in some cases is processed on-line (see section
8.3).

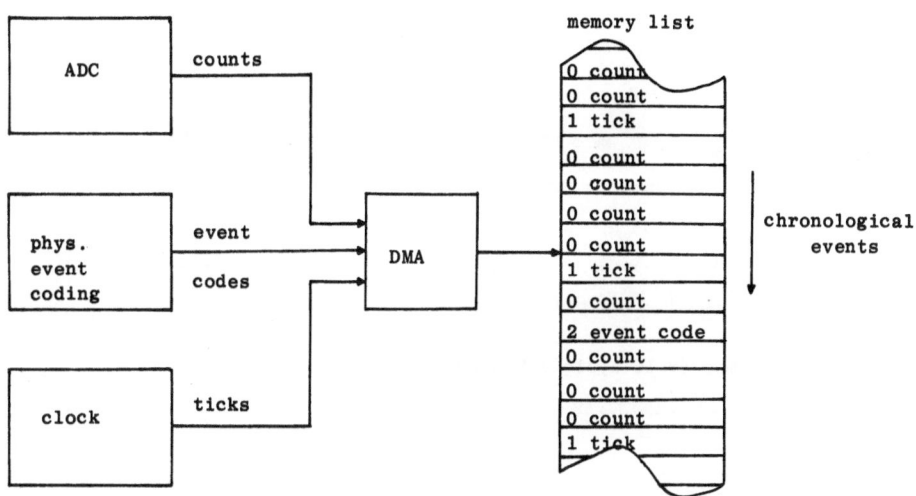

Fig. 25. Scheme of acquisition in the case of an ECG-coded radioisotope
study. Camera counts, R-wave trigger codes and clock ticks are
sequentially stored into memory.

8.2. Processing

The usual way of processing ECG trigger code list mode data is the high
temporal resolution construction technique (HTR) [24]. All counts detected
in the first time slice of 10 msec (or multiple of 10 msec) following
every detected R wave are sorted by their x, y coordinates into their proper
spatial location in the first picture matrix. All counts detected from the
second time slice following every detected R wave are sorted into the second
picture matrix. This process is continued untill all counts in the raw data
file have been sorted into their correct locations in the appropriate
picture. Some construction programs employ an initial scan of the data file
for build-up of an R-R interval spectrum and the rejection of irregular

heart beats. At the authors' institute the high phase resolution (HPR)
construction technique [25] is applied. This method consists of subdividing
each cardiac cycle into a fixed number of intervals of variable length
rather than a variable number of intervals at fixed time-offsets. R-R
intervals deviating from the modal heart cycle duration by more than 20%
are rejected, as are also their two successors. List mode counts contain
7 bit x and 7 bit y information at recording, corresponding to 128 x 128
matrix resolution, whereas processing is carried out in the same resolution,
but with 64 x 64 matrices zoomed-in on the heart.

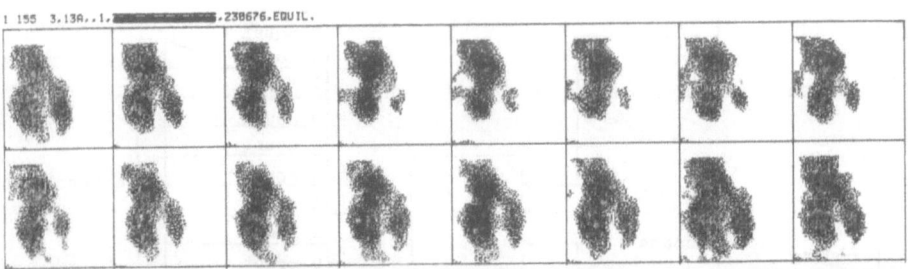

Fig. 26. Frames of 16-cycle TcHSA heart beat.

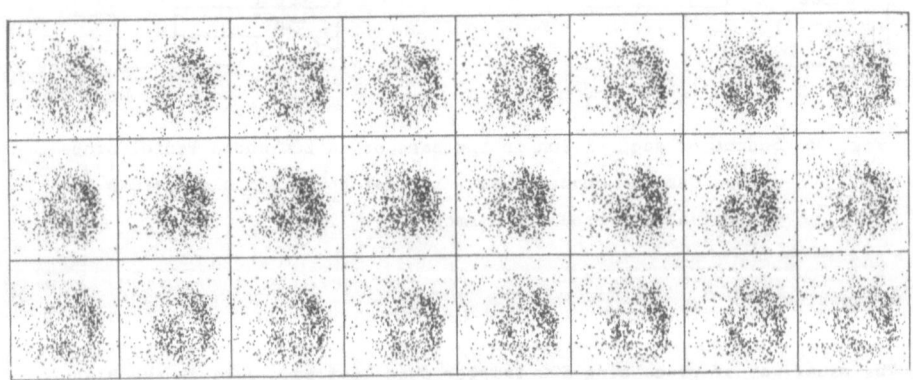

Fig. 27. Frames of 24-cycle ^{201}Tl heart beat.

Fig. 26. shows a 16-cycle TcHSA heart beat after construction with the HPR
technique. The first frame (top left) is approximately at end-diastole,
while end-systole is in frame number 6 (6th frame of top row). The last
frame (bottom right) precedes the first one in the cycle. Fig. 27. shows a
similar sequence of ^{201}Tl images in a 24-cycle heart beat. It should be
noticed that the statistical properties of the thallium cycle are much

inferior to those of the TcHSA cycle.

8.3. Simultaneous acquisition and processing

The processing of a trigger-code study, as described in the previous section involves a great number of accesses to the background memory. The NIH group (Bethesda, Md. USA) has therefore developed a minicomputer software system to perform HTR construction on-line [26]. The idea behind a real-time on-line construction system is, that histogram-mode acquisition of gated studies requires several independant sequential data collections to span the average cycle, or, at higher temporal resolution, requires extensive mass storage and retrospective processing before the gated image sequence is available for the user. In section 8.4. it will be pointed out that the display of

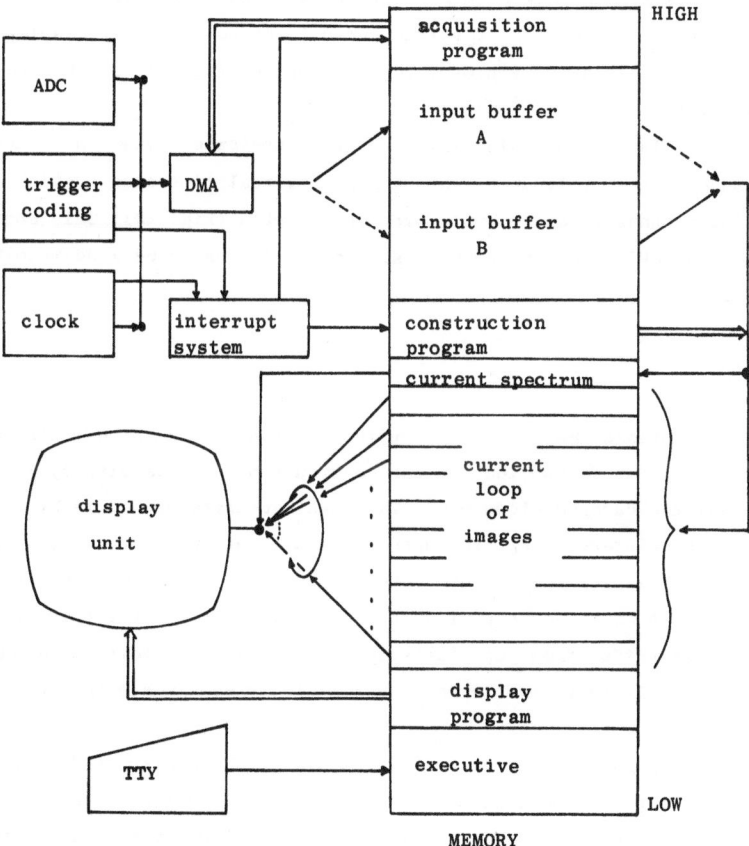

Fig 28. Scheme and memory map of a real-time system for on-line
cardiac cycle film display.

the image sequence from the average cardiac cycle in a dynamic periodic
format would be potentially advantageous, since the cardiac cycle is a
periodic process. These considerations led to the development of a system
that combines the advantages of both the list and histogram data-acquisition
modes simulaneously with endless-loop movie format display of interim results
in real-time. Fig. 28. shows a scheme of such a system. Data-counts, trigger
codes, and clock ticks are acquired in list mode via DMA to two memory
buffers, while these buffers at the same time are input for the constuction
program that creates a memory-resident span of images. These programs work
on a buffer swapping basis: if acquisition takes place into buffer A,
buffer B is processed, and the reverse. At each heart beat also the frequency
spectrum of R-R interval times is updated by the construction program. In
spare memory cycles, the intermediate contents of the span of images can be
displayed in endless-loop movie format at the speed of real heart rate. In
variants of this system, all acquired buffers are dumped to background
memory; ROI are drawn for the LV volume curve to be concurrently displayed;
retrospective processing is employed to overcome the fall-off at the end
of the cycle; etc.

At the authors' institute a distributed nuclear medicine system is in use [27],
where - amongst other software - the package for real-time construction of
ECG-code image spans is distributed over three CPU's (Fig. 29). This approach
facilitates the HPR construction of a span of 24 frames in 64 x 64 resolution
pseudo on-line.

8.4. Wall motion

It should be mentioned here, that apart from an equilibrium study, also a
first-pass study can be applied for the construction of a cardiac cycle
frame-span of the cardiac blood pool. The least accurate method is by
establishing a software triggering upon the maxima of the LV curve (Fig. 21.b).
Using ECG-leads, a usual HTR or HPR construction as is described in the
previous sections can also be applied to first-pass data. First-pass frame-
spans generally suffer from low statistics, and from a considirable amount
of background activity in the lungs, compared to frame-spans obtained from
equilibrium studies.

To visualize wall motion, the results of an HTR or HPR constructed series
of frames are displayed on a screen in endless-loop film format, simulating
the real-time beating of the heart. At some centers the perimeters of the
left-ventricular blood pool are outlined (e.g. are drawn by lightpen, or
constructed by an edge-detection algorithm), mainly because the processing

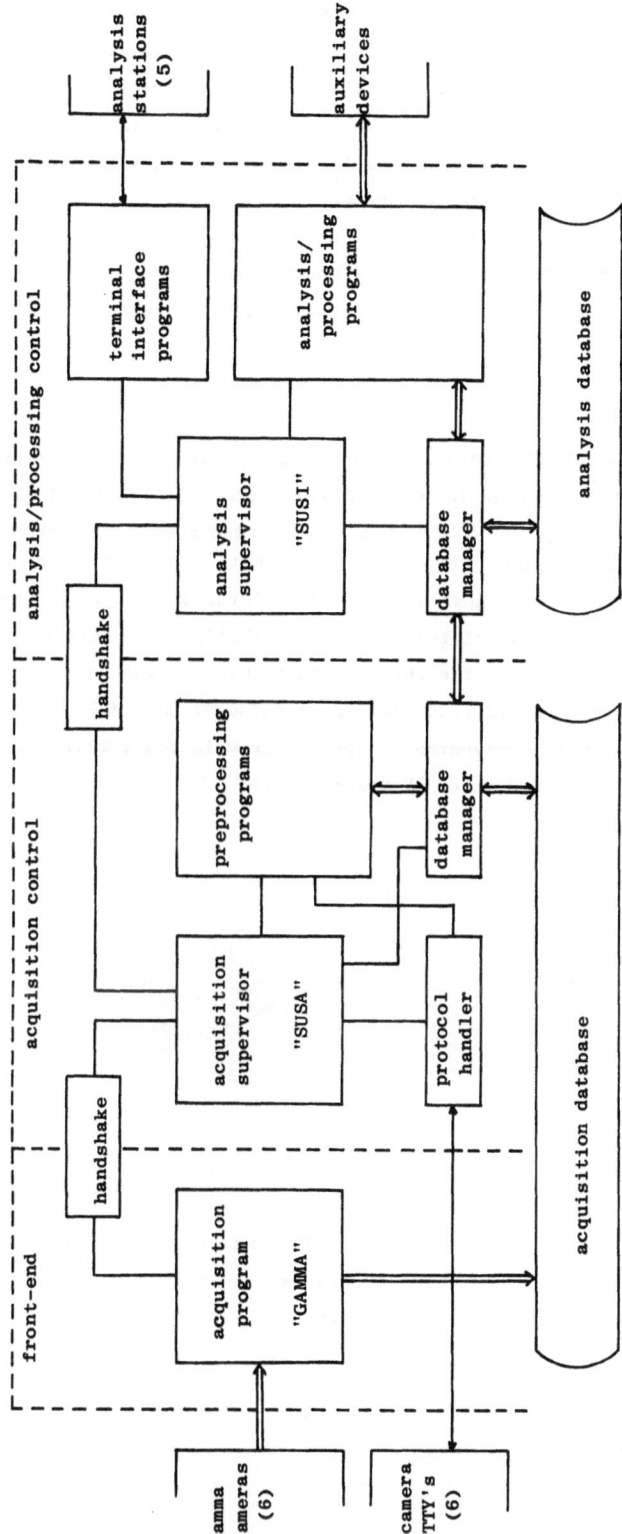

Fig. 29. Software scheme of the nuclear medicine system developed at the authors' institute. Acquisition, processing and analysis are distributed over three computers.

technique used involves construction of ED (end-diastolic) and ES (end-systolic) images only [28]. The analysis of these outlines is similar to that of contrast angiograms [29]. However, visual examination of a film of gated cardiac cycle frames is superior to these semiquantitative analyses [30], especially when the heart is viewed from two directions simultaneously, e.g. by application of a biplane collimator [3].

Since a large number of heart diseases is associated with wall motion abnormalities, the techniques described in this section are very useful in non-invasive screening of out-patients, and acutely sick patients [31].

8.5. Ejection fraction

Another major aspect of ECG-coded studies is the construction of the LV volume curve, in order to calculate the LV ejection fraction. A ROI is drawn over the LV at ED (Fig. 30.a), and a crescent-shaped ROI is chosen for background determination. These ROI give, together with the cardiac cycle frames, the curves as shown in Fig. 30.b. After background correction the ejection fraction is calculated as $\{A(ED)-A(ES)\}/A(ED)$, whereas $A(t)$ is the corrected LV curve. At the authors' institute a method of "moving" ROI has been developed (Fig.31): LV ROI are created at ED and ES, and a set of intermediate ROI is computed by spatial translation techniques, in order to achieve a better defined LV volume curve.

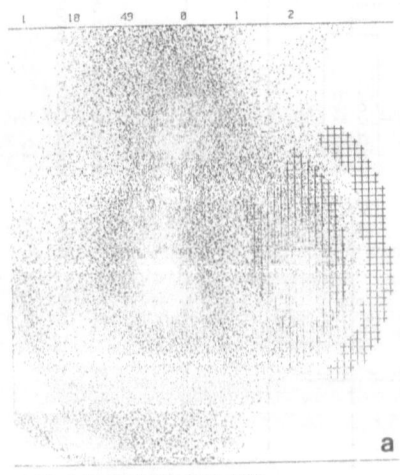

Fig. 30. End-diastolic frame of a TcHSA cardiac cycle with ROI for the LV and background (a), and related curves (b).

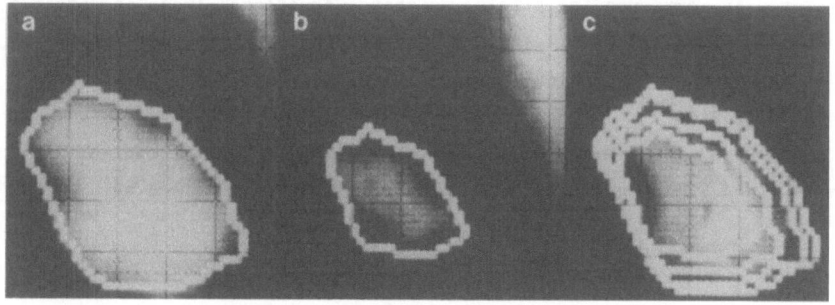

Fig. 31. End-diastolic (a) and end-systolic (b) frames of a
TcHSA cardiac cycle, together with lightpen drawn outlines,
and (c) an intermediate frame with four out of a set of 16
computed intermediate outlines.

As mentioned in the previous section, most practically applied construction
techniques produce ED and ES images only. The ejection fraction can be
calculated in a similar manner as described above.
The comparison of LV ejection fraction between radionuclide equilibrium
studies and contrast angiography gives a correlation coefficient of approximately .9 [30] [31].

9. FUNCTIONAL IMAGING

The concept of functional imaging in nuclear medicine was introduced as
early as 1969 [35]. By definition, a functional image is an image of the
spatial distribution of a functional parameter. This is in contrast to a
static scintigraphic image, which represents the spatial distribution of
radioactive material.
A functional image is constructed from data contained in a series of frames
in a background memory, or, e.g. in the case of an ECG-code study, a cardiac
cycle frame-span. This set of data can be thought of as a three-dimensional
structure of pixels with dimensions x and y for spatial coordinates and t
for the temporal coordinate. Each pixel x, y, t contains the number of counts
that were measured at position x, y in the camera field of view, at time t,
and during a time-interval Δt.
Apart from regarding the structure as being a sequence of frames, one can
also consider it as a set of parallel time-series, or time-activity curves,
one for each x, y location. As is generally the case with scintigraphic curves,
these can be fitted to a model, depending on the radiotracer used, and the
imaged biological structure. Parameter values obtained for all x, y locations

can be stored in corresponding pixels, so that a functional image is obtained, which can be treated and displayed in the normal way. For each different parameter that can be calculated in the fitting to a model, one functional image can be created.

Wash-out analysis of the myocardial blood flow using ^{133}Xe is a typical example (section 7.1). Generally, wash-out curves can be modelled by:

$$y(t) = \sum_{k}^{n} C_k e^{-\lambda t}$$

where n is the number of "compartments", C_k are initial occupancy parameters, and λ_k are wash-out rate parameters. In the case of two compartments, there will be four parameters: C_1, C_2, λ_1, and λ_2, and there-fore four possible functional images can be created, although only the λ_1 image may be of clinical interest [36] [37].

Functional images related to wall motion can be obtained from nearly all radioisotope cardiac investigations [38], such as first-pass, TcHSA, TcRBC, ^{201}Tl studies, etc. Fig. 32. shows a biplane TcHSA study of a normal patient. The end-diastolic image (Fig. 32.a), out of the 24-cycle HPR constructed frames-series, gives a clear separation of the right and left ventricles in the LAO view, wilst RV and LV in RAO are superimposed. A functional image (Fig. 32.b) was constructed by "downslope" analysis during the systolic phase (frames 1 to 9 out of 24), that is, in each of the 4096 pixel curves of 9 elements, the disappearance rate of activity was approximated by linear least-squares fitting, and these values were restored into a pixel-matrix to be displayed. A special algorithm (FUIM), developed at the authors' institute, is able to perform this operation in 1.2 sec within a 12K background partition of a 16-bit minicomputer. Fig. 32.c shows the result of the same operation, zoomed-in on the left ventricle.

In more specific applications [38] the downslope functional imaging can be carried out in narrow bands of the systolic phase, to obtain a better spatial resolution. In cases of wall motion abnormalities distortions of the horse-shoe pattern will be observed, while also early systolic hypokinesia can be traced.

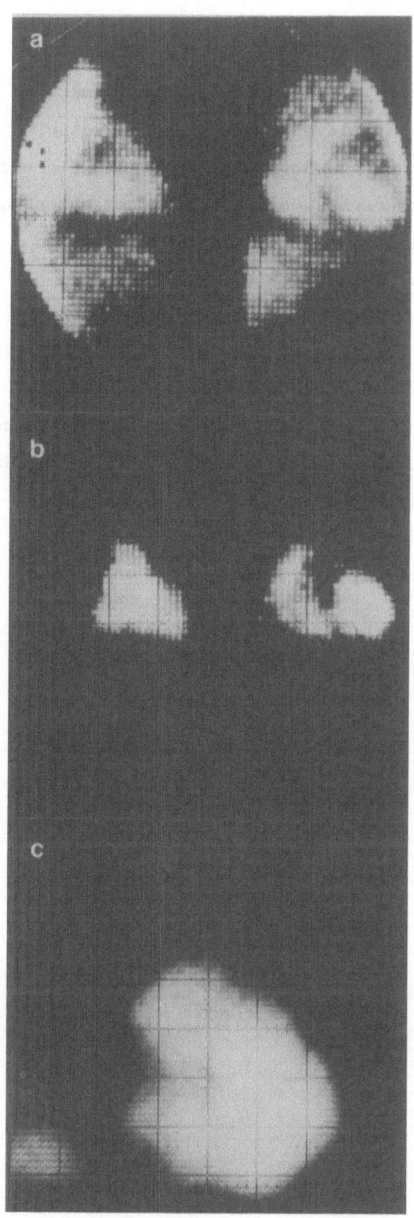

Fig. 32. End-diastolic frame of a biplane TcHSA cardiac cycle (a); downslope image computed over the entire systolic phase (b); and (c) the picture of (b) zoomed-in on the left ventricle.

10. DISCUSSION

The greatest potential role of nuclear cardiology in the future is in the identification of the high-risk patient. It plays a role alongside other non-invasive procedures, such as ultrasound, phonocardiography, and electro-cardiography [49]. In the last few years there has been a rapid development of nuclear medicine instrumentation, especially in the field of information processing equipment, leading to bedside examination of critically ill patients, i.e. in the coronary care unit. Systems, as described in section 8.3, can nowadays be miniturized to be incorporated together with the gamma camera into a mobile unit.

In routine nuclear cardiology the current trends are towards fast processing of clinical studies, using dedicated microprocessor systems with low flexibility, commercially available as "turn-key" systems.

New developments in radiopharmaceuticals and instumentation, however, will still make it necessary that the research centers should carry on with their general purpose computers, in order to implement and test elaborate information processing techniques [50].

11. REFERENCES

1. Pizer, S.M., Todd-Pokropek, A.E.: Noise character in processed scintigrams. Information Processing in Scintigraphy, Ed: Raynaud, Orsay (Fr): 1-16 (1975).
2. Van Rijk, P.P., de Graaf, C.N., Jambroes, G: The Utrecht biplane collimator. Proc. 2nd Congr. Eur. Soc. of Nucl. Med., London: 45 (1978).
3. Budinger, T.F.: Clinical and research quantitative nuclear medicine system. Medical Radioisotope Scintigraphy, IAEA Vienna 1: 501-555 (1973).
4. Erickson, J.J., Brill, A.B.: Quantitative approach to determination of minimum digital resolution in digitized camera images. J.Nucl.Med. 11: 317 (1970).
5. Stokely, E.M., Parkey, R.W., Lewis, S.E., et al: Computer processing of ^{99m}Tc-phosphate myocardial scintigrams. Information Processing in Scintigraphy, Ed: Raynaud, Orsay (Fr): 164-173 (1975).
6. Bonte, F.J., Parkey, R.W., Graham, K.D., et al: A new method for radionuclide imaging of myocardial infarcts. Radiology 110: 473 (1974).
7. Marcus, M.L., Kerber, R.E.: Present status of the ^{99m}Technetium pyrophosphate infarct scintigram. Circulation 56: 335-338 (1977).
8. Strauss, H.W., Harrison, K., Langan, J.K., et al: Thallium-201 for myocardial imaging: relation of thallium-201 to regional myocardial perfusion. Circulation 51: 641-645 (1975).
9. Hamilton, G.W., Trobaugh, G.B., Ritchie, J.L., et al: Myocardial imaging with intravenously injected Thallium-201 in patients with suspected coronary artery disease. Am. J. of Card. 39: 347-354 (1977).
10. Stokely, E.M., Buja, L.M., Lewis, S.E., et al: Measurement of acute myocardial infarcts in dogs with ^{99m}Tc-stannous pyrophosphate scintigrams. J. Nucl. Med. 17: 1 (1975).
11. Botvinick, E.H., Shames, P., Lappin, H., et al: Noninvasive quantitation of myocardial infarction with technetium-99m pyrophosphate. Circulation 52: 909 (1975).
12. Jambroes G., de Graaf, C.N., van Rijk, P.P.: Quantitation of the myocardial thallium image and objective border detection of myocardial infarcts in a heart model and in patients with myocardial infarction. Proc. Conf. Computers In Cardiology, Rotterdam (1977). In Press.
13. Radon, J.: Bestimmung von Funktionen durch Integralwerte. Ber. Saechs. Akad. Wiss. Leipzig. Math. Phys. kl. 69: 262-277 (1917).
14. Budinger, T.F., Gullberg, G.T.: Three dimensional reconstruction in nuclear medicine by iterative least squares and Fourier transform techniques. Report LBL-2149 Univ. of California, Jan. 1974.
15. Weber, P.M., dos Remedios, L.V., Jasko, I.A.: Quantitative radioisotopic cardiography. J. Nucl. Med. 13: 815-822 (1972).
16. Alazraki, N.P., Schelbert, H.R., Verba, J.W., et al: Utilization of the radionuclide cardiac angiogram for determination of cardiac output and ejection fraction. J. Nucl. Biol. and Med. 19: 127-134 (1975).
17. Hecht, H.S., Mirell, S.G., Rolett, E.L., Blahd, W.H.: left-ventricular ejection fraction and segmental wall motion by peripheral first-pass radionuclide angiography. J. Nucl. Med. 19: 17-23 (1978).
18. Alderson, P.O., Bernier, D.R., Ludbrook, P.A., et al: Serial radionuclide determination of the ejection fraction with 99mTc labeled red blood cells. Radiology 119: 729-730 (1976).
19. Thompson, H.K., Sturmer, C.F., Whalen, R.E., Melutosh, H.P.: Indicator transit time considered as a gamma variate. Circ. Res. 14: 502 (1964).
20. Maltz, D.L., Treves, S.: Quantitative radionuclide angiocardiography. Circulation 47: 1049-1056 (1973).

21. De Graaf, C.N., van Rijk, P.P., Harinck, E.: A non-invasive technique
    for quantitative detection of cardiac left-to-right shunts by least-
    squares gamma variate fitting of deconvoluted radioisotope dilution curves.
    Proc. Conf. Computers in Cardiology, St. Louis USA (1976), IEEE 76CH1160-
    1C: 275-280.
22. Strauss, H.W., Zaret, B.L., Hurley, P.J., et al: A scintiphotographic method
    for measuring left ventricular ejection fraction in man without cardiac
    catheterization. Am. J. Cardiol. 28: 575-580 (1971).
23. Green, M.V., Ostrow, H.G., Douglas, M.A., et al: Scintigraphic cineangio-
    graphy of the heart. Medinfo 1974: 827-830 (1974).
24. Green, M.V., Ostrow, H.G., Douglas, M.A., et al: High temporal resolution
    ECG-gated scintigraphic angiocardiography. J. Nucl. Med. 16: 95 (1975).
25. De Graaf, C.N., van Rijk, P.P.: High temporal and high phase resolution
    construction techniques for cardiac motion imaging. Medical Radionuclide
    Imaging, IAEA Vienna (1): 377-384 (1977).
26. Bacharach, S.L., Green, M.V., Borer, J.S., et al: A real-time system for
    multi-image gated cardiac studies. J. Nucl. Med. 18: 79-84 (1977).
27. Ephraïm, K.H., de Graaf, C.N.: Praxisgerechte DV-anwendung im nuklearmedi-
    zinischen Betrieb. Nuklearmedizinische Praxis und Forschung (ISBN
    3-921550-05-X) 3: 49-61 (1977).
28. Schad, N.: Nicht invasive Darstellung der Wandbewegung und Schlagvolumen-
    verteilung den linken Ventrikels nach Myokardinfarkt. Fortschr. Röntgenstr.
    124: 201-206 (1976).
29. Hecht, H.S., Mirell, S.G., Rolett, E.L., Blahd, W.H.: Left-ventricular
    ejection fraction and segmental wall motion by peripheral first-pass
    radionuclide angiography. J. Nucl. Med. 19: 17-23 (1978).
30. Strauss, H.W., Pitt, B.: Common procedures for the noninvasive determination
    of regional myocardial perfusion, evaluation of regional wall motion and
    detection of acute infarction. Am. J. Cardiol. 38: 731-738 (1976).
31. Pitt, B., Strauss, H.W.: Myocardial perfusion imaging and gated cardiac
    blood pool scanning: clinical application. Am. J. Cardiol. 38: 739-746 (1976).
32. Steele, P., Kirch, D., LeFree, M.: Radionuclide angiocardiographic measure-
    ment of left ventricular volume and ejection fraction. Chest 69:
    672-676 (1976).
33. Qureshi, S., Wagner, H.N., Alderson, P.O., et al: Evaluation of left-
    ventricular function in normal persons and patients with heart disease.
    J. Nucl. Med. 19: 135-141 (1978).
34. Perez, L.A., Hayt, D.B., Freeman, L.M.: Localization of myocardial disorders
    other than infarction with 99m-Tc-labeled phosphate agents. J. Nucl. Med.
    17: 241-246 (1976).
35. Kaihara, S., Natarajan, T.K., Wagner, H.N., et al: Construction of a functio-
    nal image from regional rate constants: J. Nucl. Med. 10: 347 (1969).
36. Price, R.R., Brill, A.B., Graham, T.,et al: Analysis of cardiac function
    and regional myocardial blood flow using radioisotope and radiographic
    images. Information Processing in Scintigraphy, Ed: Raynaud, Orsay (Fr):
    136-163 (1975).
37. Natarajan, T.K.: Image display and analysis system in cardiovascular nuclear
    medicine. Cardiovascular Nuclear Medicine, Ed: Strauss, et al, St. Louis USA:
    52-64, (1974).
38. De Graaf, C.N., van Rijk, P.P., Jambroes, G., Green, M.V., Line, B.R.,
    Bacharach, S.L., Bailey, J.J.: Functional imaging in nuclear cardiac studies.
    Proc. Conf. Computers in Cardiology, Rotterdam (1977). In Press.
39. Maseri, A.: Regional myocardial blood flow in man-evaluation of drugs.
    Cardiovascular Nuclear Medicine, Ed: Strauss, St. Louis USA: 163-180 (1974).

40. Stokely, E.M., Parkey, R.W., Bonte, F.J.: Regional myocardial perfusion studies. Dynamic Studies with Radioisotopes in Medicine, IAEA Vienna 2: 305-315 (1974).

41. Stokely, E.M., Nardizzi, L.R., Parkey, R.W., Bonte, F.J.: Regional myocardial perfusion data with spatial and temporal quantization. J. Nucl. Med. 14: 669-676 (1973).

42. Herman, G.T., Johnson, S.A., Lakshminarayanan, A.V., et al: An algorithm for on-line real-time reconstruction of the intact heart. Computers in Cardiology, IEEE 75CH1018-1c: 115-119 (1975).

43. Keyes, W.I., Chesser, R., Undrill, P.E.: Transverse-section emission tomography. Medical Images: Formation, Perception and Measurement. Publ.: J. Wilcy & Sons: 51-67 (1976).

44. O Ying Lie: Digitale reconstructie van een object vanuit zijn projecties, met toepassing in de nucleaire geneeskunde (Digital reconstruction of an object from its projections, with application in nuclear medicine. Dutch with English summary), M.Sc.thesis, Technical University Delft, The Netherlands. (1976)

45. O Ying Lie: Attenuation correction for emission reconstruction, and fan beam convolution methods. Internal report, Institute of Nuclear Medicine, Utrecht, The Netherlands (1977).

46. Ter-Pogossian, M.M., Cox, J.R., et al (Ed's): Reconstruction tomography in diagnostic radiology and nuclear medicine. University Park Press (1977).

47. Kaplan, E., Mayron, L.W., Barnes, W.E., et al: Continuous radionuclide generation. II. Scintigraphic definition of capillary exchange by rapid decay of ^{81m}Kr and its applications. J.Nucl.Med. 15: 874-879 (1974)

48. Mayron, L.W., Kaplan, E., Colombetti, L.G., et al: A minigenerator for the production of ^{81m}Kr and its application. Int.J.Nucl.Med.Biol. 2: 40-42 (1975).

49. Wagner, H.N.: The development of cardiovascular nuclear medicine. Cardiovascular Nuclear Medicine, Ed: Strauss, St.Louis USA: 1-5 (1974).

50. Nootschap, G.: Is nuclear medicine helpful in clinical diagnosis? Annual Lecture Societas Nuclearis Trajectinus (Utrecht, 1978). In Press.

IMAGE ANALYSIS IN HISTO-CYTOPATHOLOGY

L. Arnould, Cl. Fiévez, M. Fiévez,
J. Hustin, L. Koulischer, M. Donnay,
J. Hamels, Y. Gillerot, P. Courtoy,
J.P. Cosyn.

Institut de Morphologie Pathologique,
Loverval, Belgium

O. Abstract.

An image analyzer is described (Quantimet 720 System 20) and its role
in histology and cytology is presented with four different examples of
measurements : epithelium thickness, liver steatosis, microdensitometry
and lymphocyte stimulation. The stress is laid on the way of using the
machine and on its advantages rather than on the interpretation of the
results.
A lot of slides will be shown during the presentation of this paper.

1. Introduction.

Since the early 70's, automated image analysis has become a more and
more used tool in the histology and cytology laboratories. The six
"Automated Cytology" conferences organized by the U.S. Engineering
Foundation (1), and the congresses and symposia organized by the International Society for Stereology (2,3), regularly made a balance between
the increase of these new technics and their applications.
This paper is not at all a general survey in this field : it intends
to demonstrate the role an automated image analyzer can play in an institution such as ours, mainly oriented towards routine, histopathology
(50,000 biopsies/year), cytological cancer screening (18,000 smears/
year) and cytogenetics (4,000 karyotypes/year).
The machine and the methods will be presented with four examples, but
the medical interest of the results of these works will not be discussed here.

2. The image analyzer.

Our machine is a Quantimet 720 System 20, including a PDP 11/05 mini-computer with 32K of central memory and two disk-cartridges.(4)
It is a very complete one in which we find the usual working diagram of this kind of systems.
The microscope, supporting the TV-scanner, is provided with a program-mable scanning stage of 5 microns steps.
The "detector" makes the first selection of the image features we want to look at, by using the image contrast and by fixing grey levels on a linear scale between black and white.
A second detector, the "digitizer", working on a logarithmic scale, allows densitometric evaluations.
Image modifications, called "erosion" and "dilation", are possible with two "amenders" and these, connected in series, realize also more com-plex operations called "opening" and "closing", as we shall see further.
With the "image editor" and its light-pen, we can accept or reject some parts of the field by drawing on the TV-screen. This manual operation is of course slow but it is sometimes very useful.
Other modules do the measurements and also realize the interfacing with the computer. This computer plays a double part :
- it makes the measurements complete by setting the histograms, compu-ting statistical data, storing results on the disk, etc.;
- it makes the system automatic : from the general program, we can build up different routines for different applications, but we can also write our own programs, here in Basic language.

3. Endocervical epithelium thickness.

While the effects of hormonal contraception on the endometrium have been extensively studied, little attention has been paid to the modi-fications of the endocervical epithelium under the influence of synthe-tic steroids.(5)
Usually the pathologist takes PAS-stained specimens, with a strongly stained epithelium, but this is not convenient for a good detection by the machine, even after erosion and dilation of the image.
Anyway, we still need to use the light-pen for selecting areas of in-terest and we prefer to draw these areas directly on the image of a HES-stained slide, where the basal cellular membrane is clearly seen.

We draw the epithelium thickness at some places : the machine takes the mean of the measurements and stores the results.

Afterwards, the statistical work takes into account these measurements and also the age of the patient, the type of contraceptive, the duration of contraception and the day of the menstrual cycle.

But there is an important problem : this "mean thickness" is certainly not the true thickness in the 3D-space, because most of the histological sections are not perpendicular to the epithelium. On the other hand, this "mean thickness" corresponds to what the observer is seeing and to the sizes he is familiar with, and this is important.

Similarly we shall see that the diameter of the projected image of a cell nucleus is more significant for the human eye-and-brain than the nuclear volume. Anyhow we have stereological models to calculate this true mean thickness.(6,7)

This situation is quite frequent in histology : it is not always possible to realize an automatic detection of the objects to be measured, but as the measurements and the following statistical handling are automatic, there is a tremendous time profit by comparison with older methods.

4. Liver steatosis.

The volume of hepatic biopsies is generally too small to allow a biochemical determination of the stage of steatosis. And the pathologist appreciation on histological sections remains subjective, so we started to render it quantitative by doing morphometric measurements on these sections and by using stereological formulas.

With an adapted OsO_4 staining, lipid droplets look like black circles, isolated or in clusters, on a light background : the situation is theoretically favourable, even if the smallest droplets detection is questionable.

Stereology gives us the basic formula : $V_v = A_A$: the volume fraction (of lipids in liver) is the area fraction (of black circles in the section).(8,9,10)

But, on one hand, the droplets clusters have often non-convex shapes, what makes the general formula invalid, and on the other hand, it is important to distinguish between micro- and macrodroplets. For both reasons, we must be able to set up a granulometry of these droplets.

The machine performs it by an "opening" procedure. By gradually eroding and dilating again the droplet profiles, we gradually remove bigger and bigger droplets from the detected image, and the black area decrease at each "opening" step represents the area occupied by the removed black circles : so we can set up a "lipid area" distribution in terms of droplet size, but still in two dimensions.

There is now a new important question, when we plan to go to three dimensions : the section thickness, in general 5 microns with paraffine embedding. Theoretically, it should be zero !

We can try to use corrections, but choosing the right formula is not so easy -should it exist- and the calculations become quickly heavy. We can also try to make that thickness negligible by using semi-thin sections, for instance 0.5 micron with Epon embedding.

This work has been presented in a preliminary state (11) and it is still in progress, in both directions : corrected formulas and semi-thin sections.

5. Microdensitometry.

In many cases, we tried nuclear size measurements on different tissues, for instance on the renal glomerulus. It is quite easy to perform it, but we often lack reference values for estimating pathological variations and more, for these karyometric measurements, the variability of tissue-processing conditions is problematic.(12)

On the other hand, here is a routine example of nuclear measurements where our Quantimet brought an appreciable contribution to the physician's diagnostic.

The densitometer is working here on the whole TV-image : we can get, at once, integrated or mean optical densities histograms for all the features selected by grey value, by shape, by size or also by drawing with the light-pen.

In this case, we had to certify the presence of a genetic anomaly in abortus products we received already fixed. As the karyotyping was thus impossible, we tried a specific DNA analysis on thick sections. Standard Feulgen staining gives a good nuclear detection : with the light-pen, we select regions in maternal and foetal tissues and DNA histograms are obtained immediately.

This procedure allowed the "histological demonstration" of triploïdy or mosaïc, when tissue culture was not possible (infection) or when there was no growth at all.

6. Lymphocyte stimulation.

This last example shows the power of these image analyzers and the tremendous amount of information you can get from them, in a very short time.
It is not necessary to recall what is the lympocyte stimilation test or lymphoblastic transformation test.
If the so-called "flow-systems" present an evident interest in this case (13,14,15), it is also interesting and very useful to face the automation of the usual slides interpretation.
The first measurement we thought of is of course the apparent dia-meter or the apparent area of each smeared nucleus, what is made, qua-litatively, by the observer.
The second is, like the flow-systems, the DNA content, what is impos-sible to the human eye.
And a third immediate measurement, close to the visual impression, is the staining intensity, the "grey" of the nucleus, what is in some way related to the area and DNA content.
It is also possible and interesting to analyze the chromatin structure (16,17) but we don't make it at this time.
The definite advantage of the machine in this case is speed : for in-stance, you can get 10 histograms (diameter, area, DNA content, mean optical density, form factor, etc.), including conditions on the nuclei to be measured (small, medium-sized, rather light, 4n-DNA, etc.), in one scan on the slide, typically in 5-6 minutes and on 3000-4000 lym-phocytes ! Autofocussing is the most time-consuming operation...
Area and DNA histograms give a good description of the slide but a li-mit between unstimulated and stimulated lymphocytes is not evident.
On the other hand, the machine can easily show you that already medium-sized and lighter nuclei are not yet in the S-phase thanks to their DNA content, and such refinements explain a discrepancy between a too simple measurement and the human diagnostic.
By the way, what are, in objective and physical terms, the human cri-teria...?
An interesting finding is, when we ask the machine to select, in a first scan, truly circular (shape factor) and small (area) features, where the unstimulated lymphocytes must be, we can see, on a "grey" (mean

optical density = DNA content/area) histogram, the peak of these unstimulated darkest ones but also a group of lighter ones, clearly distinct, which must be taken as stimulated.
Now we could have an objective criterion, automatically measured : we
could use it in a selctive count.
Comparison is actually made with radioactive markers measurements, for
validating our method.

7. Conclusion.

These four examples where chosen to present different applications and
ways of working of an automated image analyzer in the field of histology and cytology.
We are also using it in autoradiographic grain counting (18), in bone
study, in metaphase finding and also, without the microscope, to look
at photographic and radiographic pictures, where an artificial contrast
enhancement is always possible.
An important fact is that using such systems often requires a specimen
processing different from what meets the human eye satisfaction, for
instance section thickness, new stainings, no counter-stainig sometimes, a better spreading in cytology, etc.
There is a lot of work to do here, and we need to define new standards,
and then to use them.
An other point is to carefully select the best criteria and the best
measurements, among the fantastic flow of data you can get from the
analyzer.
This beautiful machine remains a machine, with of course its speed, its
power, but also with its limitations, and even its defects.

8. References.

1. Proceedings of Automated Cytology V (Pensacola, Florida, Dec. 9-15,
   1976), Ed.: B.H.Mayall, Special issue of J.Histochem.Cytochem.,
   25:7(1977).
2. Proceedings of the 4th Int.Congress for Stereology (Gaithersburg,
   Maryland, Sept. 4-9, 1975), Ed.: E.E.Underwood, R. de Wit, G.A.
   Moore, National Bureau of Standards Special publication 431 (1976).
3. Proceedings of the 2d Eur.Symposium on Quantitative analysis of mi-
   crostructures in Material sciences, Biology and Medicine (Caen,
   France, Oct. 4-7, 1977), Ed.: J.L.Chermant, Special issue of Practical Metallography, 8(1978).
4. Cambridge Instruments, Melbourn, Royston, Hertf. SG8 6EJ, U.K.

5. R. Mingeot, C. Fiévez, Obst. Gynec. 44:1(1974)53.
6. E.R. Weibel, B.W. Knight, J. Cell Biol. 21(1964)367.
7. H.J. Gundersen, T.B. Jensen, R. Osterby, Pract. Metallog. 8(1976)320.
8. E.R. Weibel, G.S. Kistler, W.F. Scherle, J. Cell Biol. 30(1966)23.
9. E.E. Underwood. Quantitative Stereology. Addison-Wesley (1970).
10. J.P.A. Baak, J. Oort, G.M. Bouw, L.A.M. Stolte, Europ. J. Obstet. Gynec. Reprod. Biol. 7:1(1977)43.
11. P.J. Courtoy, L. Arnould, J.P. Cosijn, Pract. Metallog. 8(1976)334.
12. J.P.A. Baak, P.C. Diegenbach, Europ. J. Obstet. Gynec. Reprod. Biol. 7:1(1977)33.
13. L.S. Cram, E.R. Gomez, C.O. Thoen, J.C. Forslund, J.J. Jett, J. Histochem. Cytochem. 24:1(1976)383.
14. M. Cassidy, C. Yee, J. Costa, ibid. 373.
15. Z. Darzynkiewicz, F. Traganos, T.K. Sharpless, M.R. Melamed, Cancer Research 37(1977)4635.
16. J. Rowinsky, M. Pienkowski, J. Abramczuk, Histochemie 32(1972)75.
17. S. Beucher, F. Meyer, Centre de Morphologie mathématique, rue St Honoré, 35, 77305 Fontainebleau, France. To be published.
18. J. Hustin, L. Arnould, Proceedings of the 2d Int.Symposium on Endo-metrial cancer and Related topics (London, March 30-31, 1977), Ed.: M.G. Brush, R.G.B. King. Tyndall-Bailliere, in press.

9. Acknowledgements.

We wish to thank Dr R. Mingeot and Dr R. Weckhuyzen (Clinique St Michel, Brussels) and Dr L. Rondelez (C.G.T.R., Montigny-le-Tilleul) for their collaboration in parts of these works.

COMPUTER SIMULATION OF MONOCHROMATIC X-RAYS

Gabor T. Herman, Ph.D.
Department of Computer Science
State University of New York at Buffalo
4226 Ridge Lea Road
Amherst, New York, U.S.A.

ABSTRACT

We investigate how one can estimate from the total attenuation, p, of a polychromatic x-ray beam what the total attenuation, m, of a monochromatic beam would have been along the same ray.

1. INTRODUCTION

The aim of computed tomography is to assign to every point inside the body a number which is specific to the tissue occupying that point. A suitable candidate for this number is the x-ray attenuation coefficient of the tissue. A difficulty arises due to the fact that the x-ray beam used in computed tomography consists of photons at different energies. (Such x-rays are called polychromatic.) Because the attenuation at a fixed point is generally greater for photons of lower energy, the energy distribution (spectrum) of the x-ray beam changes (hardens) as it passes through the object. X-ray beams reaching a particular point inside the body from different directions are likely to have different spectra (having passed through different materials before reaching the point in question) and thus will be attenuated differently at that point. This makes it difficult to assign a single value for the attenuation coefficient at a point in the body.

A possible solution to this difficulty is to assign to the point the attenuation coefficient of photons at a particular energy. If we used x-ray beams consisting of photons only at that single energy (such x-rays are called monochromatic), beams from different directions would be attenuated in the same way at a fixed point. Reconstruction of such attenuation coefficients is a well-defined aim of computed tomography.

Broadly speaking, this article addresses the following problem: Given the total attenuation of polychromatic x-ray beams through a body, can we give estimates of the total attenuation of monochromatic x-ray beams through the same parts of the body which are precise enough for diagnostically useful reconstruction of the monochromatic linear attenuation coefficients in the body? In other words, can we correct for beam hardening in computed tomography?

The importance of the problem of correction for beam hardening in computed tomography is reflected in the large number of publications that have appeared in recent years on this topic. While attempting to find and evaluate simple correction methods, the author of this article studied among others the publications of McCullough et al.[13], McCullough [12], Pang and Genna [14], Brooks and DiChiro [3], McDavid et al. [11], Tsai and Cho [19], Macovski et al. [10], Alvarez and Macovski [1], Berggren et al. [2] and Wickizer et al [20]. These articles have strongly influenced and in some cases even provided many of the ideas expressed below; however, these influences are so intermingled with each other and with the author's own work that no further acknowledgement will be made to the people listed above.

This article is a shortened version of Technical Report 129 of the Department of Computer Science at the State University of New York at Buffalo. That report contains derivations as well as an experimental example based on a cross section of the human thorax in [15].

2.   THE PROBLEM OF BEAM HARDENING IN COMPUTED TOMOGRAPHY

The aim of computed tomography (CT) is to obtain information regarding the nature of material occupying exact positions inside the body. In this section we describe the mathematical and computational procedures used for achieving this aim.

In computed tomography we have two sets of measurements:

(a)   calibration measurements, based on which we can estimate what the detector measurements would be if the object to be reconstructed were not between the source and the detector,

(b)   actual detector measurements with the object of interest in position.

We now discuss the method by which these measurements are taken. There is a region of space which during the calibration measurement is occupied by some homgeneous reference material, such as air or water. During the actual measurement, the object of interest is inserted into the reconstruction region, (partially) replacing the reference material. It is an important restriction that the object of interest does not occupy any point outside the reconstruction region. On the other hand, we allow the possibility of additional objects occupying fixed positions outside the reconstruction region during both the calibration and the actual measurement.

Thus our theory is general enough to handle different types of CT configurations, such as presence or absence of water bath (this is done by using water or air respectively as the reference material in the reconstruction region) or the presence or absence of filters and collimators between the source and the reconstruction region or between the reconstruction region and the detectors.

From the two sets of numbers produced by the calibration and the actual measurements, we wish to produce a third set, namely, the set of CT numbers for a cross section of the object under investigation. When the cross section is represented as an image, each CT number is the value associated with a pixel (picture element).

In vacuum all the photons which leave the source in the direction of the detector will reach the detector. When a material is placed between the source and the detector some of the photons which leave the source in the direction of the detector will be removed from the beam (absorbed or scattered). The probability that a photon gets removed depends on the energy of the photon and on the material between the source and the detector.

The linear attenuation coefficient, μ_e^t, of a tissue t at energy e is defined as follows. Let ρ be the probability that a photon of energy e, which enters a uniform slab of the tissue t of unit thickness, on a line perpendicular to the face of the slab, will not be absorbed or scattered in the slab. We define

$$\mu_e^t = -\ln \rho,$$

where ln denotes the natural logarithm. Note that the size of the linear attenuation coefficient is dependent on the unit of length used. For example, the linear attenuation of water at 73 keV is 0.19 cm^{-1}.

In what follows we shall be working with the relative linear attenuation at energy e. At any point of space, we define the relative linear attenuation to be $\mu_e^t - \mu_e^a$, where 't' is the tissue occupying the point of space during the actual measurement and 'a' is the tissue occupying the point during the calibration measurement. Since we assume that the exterior of the reconstruction region is constant during the two sets of measurements, the relative linear attenuation is zero for all points outside the reconstruction region for all energies. Note also that for all points inside the reconstruction region μ_e^a is the same, since the reference material is supposed to be homogeneous during the calibration measurement.

Now suppose that we are interested in a cross-sectional slice of the human body which is, say, 1.3 cm thick. We can subdivide this slice into small 1.3 cm long blocks with equal, square shaped cross sections. These blocks are usually referred to as volume elements, or voxels, for short. Roughly speaking, a CT number represents the average relative linear attenuation in a voxel. Since the relative linear attenuation itself is energy dependent, the above definition needs further clarification.

We would like the following statement to be true: "The CT number assigned to a voxel is a property of the tissue occupying the voxel and does not depend on the location of the voxel in the slice." This is obviously desirable for diagnostic purposes. Also, as we shall see below, the truth of the statement is assumed in the development of mathematical procedures for calculating CT numbers.

There are many possible ways of defining CT numbers so that the statement above is true. In this paper, we shall concentrate on one such definition, in which the CT number of a voxel is a multiple of the average linear attenuation of the voxel at a specified energy, which we shall denote by $\bar{e}$.

Suppose now that we have a monochromatic x-ray source with photon energy $\bar{e}$. For a fixed position of the source and the detector, let C_m be the calibration measurement (the number of photons counted by the detector before the insertion of the object to be reconstructed), and let A_m be the actual measurement (the number of photons counted by the detector with the object of interest in place). We assume that the duration of the calibration and the actual measurement are equal. We define the monochromatic ray sum, m, for this beam by

$$m = -\ln \frac{A_m}{C_m} \ , \qquad (1)$$

and we refer to the set of m's for all source-detector pair positions as the monochromatic projection data. Based on the physical and mathematical facts to be discussed below, we know the relative linear attenuation inside the slice at the given energy $\bar{e}$ can be accurately estimated from the monochromatic projection data.

In practice, the x-ray beam is polychromatic. Let C_p and A_p denote the calibration and actual measurement, respectively, for a particular source-detector pair position with the polychromatic x-ray beam. We define the polychromatic ray sum, p, for this x-ray beam by

$$p = -\ln \frac{A_p}{C_p} \ , \qquad (2)$$

and we refer to the set of p's for all source-detector pair positions as the polychromatic projection data.

Our problem is the following: For any source and detector position we can obtain p, but the reconstruction procedure requires m. The question naturally arises: Does p uniquely determine m? Unfortunately, except in unrealistically restrictive cases, the answer is "no".

A more pragmatic question is: Given p, can we approximate m well enough so that it leads to diagnostically useful CT numbers? There the answer appears to be "yes".

We now discuss the method for obtaining CT numbers from the monochromatic projection data. In practice, we apply this method using corrected polychromatic projection data in place of the (usually unavailable) monochromatic projection data.

In order to design an algorithm for obtaining CT numbers from monochromatic projection data, we first replace the problem by a simplified mathematical idealization of it. The simplifying assumptions we make in setting up the theory for reconstruction algorithms are: 1) slices are infinitely thin, 2) for any particular source and detector pair position, all x-ray photons travel in the same straight line (which lies in the infinitely thin slice). A consequence of the first assumption is that the distinction between voxels and pixels disappears. Indeed, since the slice is infinitely thin, it can be thought of as a picture whose grayness at any point (x,y) is proportional to the relative linear attenuation $\mu_e(x,y)$ at that point. For this reason the theory behind reconstruction algorithms has often been referred to as "picture reconstruction from projections".

Let L be the straight line which is the path of all the x-ray photons for a particular source-detector pair and let m be the corresponding monochromatic ray sum. Based on our definition of a linear attenuation coefficient, it can be proved that

$$m \approx \int_0^D \mu_e(x,y)\,dz. \qquad (3)$$

In this formula, $\approx$ denotes "approximately equal", and z is the distance of the point (x,y) on the line L connecting the source to the detector. Thus our problem is to calculate the values of $\mu_e(x,y)$ from estimates of its integrals along a number of lines, namely, from the monochromatic projection data.

In some sense this problem has been solved in 1917 by Radon [16]. Let ℓ denote the distance of the line L from the origin, let θ denote the angle made with the x-axis by the perpendicular drawn from the origin to L and let $m(\ell,\theta)$ denote the integral of

$\mu_e(x,y)$ along the line L. Radon has proved that

$$\mu_e(x,y) = -\frac{1}{2\pi^2} \lim_{\varepsilon \to 0} \int_\varepsilon^\infty \frac{1}{q} \int_0^{2\pi} m_1 \ (x\cos\theta + y\sin\theta + q, \ \theta) \ d\theta \ dq, \quad (4)$$

where $m_1(\ell,\theta)$ denotes the partial derivative of $m(\ell,\theta)$ with respect to ℓ. While the exact details of this formula are likely to be obscure to the nonmathematician, its implication should be clear: the distribution of relative linear attenuations in an infinitely thin slice is uniquely determined by the set of all its integrals.

This seems to indicate that the reconstruction problem has been solved since 1917. However, there are some practical difficulties in applying to computed tomography this mathematical solution to the idealized problem:

(a) Radon's formula determines a picture from all its line integrals. In computed tomography we have only a finite set of measurements.

(b) The measurements in computed tomography can provide only estimates of the line integrals of $\mu_e(x,y)$.

(c) Radon gave a mathematical formula; we need an efficient algorithm to evaluate it.

There has been a very great deal of activity in recent years to find algorithms which are fast when implemented on a computer and which produce acceptable reconstructions in spite of the finite and inaccurate nature of the data. For a very elementary introduction to this topic, see Gordon, Herman, and Johnson [6]; for a thorough survey of algorithms, see Gordon and Herman [5]. Information about recent developments in the mathematical and computational foundations of computed tomography can be obtained from the August, 1976, special issue of Computers in Biology and Medicine, devoted to "Advances in Picture Reconstruction - Theory and Applications", and in the recently initiated Journal of Computer Assisted Tomography. Specific devices and methods are described in [7,8,9,17,19].

3.   CORRECTION FORMULAS FOR BEAM HARDENING

In this section we discuss mathematical formulas which describe the nature of polychromatic ray sums and methods which may be used to find the corresponding monochromatic ray sums.

In particular, it can be proved that the polychromatic ray sum p approximates an integral of the form

$$p \simeq -\ln \int_0^E \tau_e \ \exp \ [- \int_0^D (\mu_e(z) - \mu_e^a) \ dz] \ de. \quad (5)$$

We now give a detailed explanation of the meaning of the symbols in Equation (5).

It is assumed that the source emits a polychromatic x-ray beam with photons at energies between 0 and E. We use τ_e to denote the ratio of photons at energy e which are detected during the calibration measurement to the total number of photons which are detected during the calibration measurement. Here we have adopted the somewhat non-standard notation of using τ_e to denote the value of a function of energy at energy e. We refer to this function as the detected spectrum during the calibration measurement.

D and z have the same meaning as in the last section, $\mu_e(z)$ is a function of two variables (the energy e and the distance z), whose value is the linear attenuation coefficient at energy e at the point z on the line L during the actual measurement. On the other hand, μ_e^a is a function of one variable only (the energy e), whose value is the linear attenuation of the reference material 'a' at energy e. Thus, $\int_0^D (\mu_e(z) - \mu_e^a)dz$ is the integral of the relative linear attenuation at energy e along the line L. The notation exp[x] is used to denote the exponential function of x. (Thus, $(\ln(\exp[x]) = x.)$

Note in particular, that the polychromatic ray sum depends only on the relative linear attenuations (at all energies between 0 and E) and on the detected spectrum during the calibration measurement.

Rewriting Equation (3) in the same notation we get

$$m \simeq \int_0^D (\mu_{\underline{e}}(\dot{z}) - \mu_{\underline{e}}^a)dz. \qquad (6)$$

Recall now that CT numbers are multiples of relative linear attenuations at a fixed energy $\bar{e}$; and that they are to be obtained from estimates of the monochromatic projection data which are themselves calculated from the experimentally obtained polychromatic projection data. The method of estimating the monochromatic projection data from the polychromatic projection data is the topic of the rest of our discussion.

We start with a theoretical discussion of a special situation.

Suppose that during the actual measurement there are only two types of material, a and b, in the reconstruction region (a is the reference material). Consider a fixed source-detector pair, and assume that the total length of the line L which goes through material b is B. From Equations (5) and (6) we get

$$p \simeq -\ln \int_0^E \tau_e \exp\left[-B(\mu_e^b - \mu_e^a)\right] de \tag{7}$$

and

$$m \simeq B(\mu_{\underline{e}}^b - \mu_{\underline{e}}^a). \tag{8}$$

Combining Equations (7) and (8) we get

$$p \simeq -\ln \int_0^E \tau_e \exp\left[-\frac{\mu_e^b - \mu_e^a}{\mu_{\underline{e}}^b - \mu_{\underline{e}}^a} m\right] de. \tag{9}$$

The important thing to observe in Equation (9) is that provided either $\mu_e^b > \mu_e^a$ for all energies between 0 and E or $\mu_e^b < \mu_e^a$ for all energies between 0 and E, its right hand side is a monotonically increasing function of m. (Note that τ_e is positive for all e.) Hence, given any value of p, there will be only one value of m which will make the two sides of Equation (9) equal. In practice we can use the plot of the right hand side of Equation (9) to correct for beam hardening; we simply find the value of m for which the value of the right hand side is the experimentally obtained polychromatic ray sum p.

Equation (9) was obtained under a rather restrictive assumption: there are only two different types of material between source and detector. If the organ we are looking at is a head inserted into a water bag, this assumption is not too badly violated, since the contents of the head are bone and material whose x-ray attenuation properties are not too dissimilar to water. Thus Equation (9) may be used for correcting for beam hardening in such a situation.

It has also been suggested that one may use Equation (9) to correct for beam hardening in a body scanner, assuming that the only two materials in the reconstruction region are air and water. However, one can do much better than the corrections provided by such an approach.

While the precise method based on Equation (9) must be considered to be unreliable because of the too restrictive nature of the underlying assumptions, the general approach suggested by it is very attractive: specify a function f(p) of the polychromatic ray sum p such that if we use f(p) as our estimate of the monochromatic ray sum m, then we get reasonably good reconstructions of the relative linear attenuations at the fixed energy $\bar{a}$.

Natural candidates for such a function are polynomials, i.e., functions of the form

$$f(p) = a_n p^n + a_{n-1} p^{n-1} + \ldots + a_2 p^2 + a_1 p + a_0, \tag{10}$$

where n (the order of the polynomial) is a fixed integer and $a_0, a_1, a_2, \ldots, a_{n-1}, a_n$ are fixed coefficients which need to be deter-mined so that f(p) provides an acceptable estimate of m for our purpose. There are two computational advantages of polynomial approximations to others (e.g., approximation by combination of exponentials): The coefficients are easy to calculate [4] and, once they are calculated, Equation (10) is easy to evaluate.

From our point of view, the strongest case for using poly-nomial approximation is its efficacy. Even using low order poly-nomials (n=2, at most 3), one can estimate the monochromatic pro-jection data from the polychromatic projection data in such a way that most of the degradation due to beam hardening is compensated for. In particular, quadratic polynomial correction (n= 2) gives a superior result to what can be achieved by assuming that the body consists of water alone and using Equation (9).

On the other hand, it is conceivable that in certain cases there is no single function f such that replacement of m by f(p) in the Radon inversion formula would lead to acceptable reconstructions. One may then be forced to use multiple correcting functions specific to the source-detector pair positions, or even an iterative correc-tion procedure such as the one demonstrated by Ruegsegger et al.[18].

4. CONCLUSIONS

Correction for beam hardening is usually necessary in com-puted tomography. Methods based on the assumption that there are only two different materials between the source and detector are in some cases inadequate. Correction procedures based on a quadratic poly-nomial fitted to a sample data set are inexpensive to obtain and use, and they lead to acceptable results.

ACKNOWLEDGEMENTS

The research of the author is supported by NCI contract CB53860 and NIH grants HL 04664 and HL 18968.

REFERENCES

1. Alvarez, R.E. and Macovski, A.: Energy-selective reconstructions in x-ray computerized tomography. Phys.Med.Biol. 21: 733,1976.
2. Berggren, M. J., Johnson, S.A., Greenleaf, J.F. Robb, R. A., Sturm, R. E., Herman, G. T., and Wood, E. H.: A method for se-lective tissue and chemical element three-dimensional recon-structive imaging from radiographic film and roentgen-video images. Image Processing for 2-D and 3-D Reconstruction from

Projections. Stanford, Ca., August, 1975; pp. MB2-1 - MB2-4.

3.   Brooks, R. A. and DiChiro, G.: Beam-hardening in x-ray recon-
     structive tomography. Phys. Med. Biol. 21: 390, 1975.

4.   Dahlquist, G. and Bjorck, A.: Numerical Methods. New Jersey,
     Englewood Cliffs, 1974.

5.   Gordon, R. and Herman, G. T.: Three dimensional reconstruction
     from projections: a review of algorithms. International Review
     of Cytology (eds. G. H. Bourne and J. F. Danielli). Academic
     Press, New York,N.Y., 1974; pp. 111-151.

6.   Gordon, R., Herman, G. T., and Johnson, S. A.: Image reconstruc-
     tion from projections. Sci. Am., pp. 56-68, October 1975.

7.   Herman, G. T., Lakshminarayanan, A. V., and Naparstek, A.:
     Reconstruction using divergent ray shadowgraphs. Reconstruction
     Tomography in Diagnostic Radiology and Nuclear Medicine (ed.
     M. Ter-Pogossian et al.). University Park Press, Baltimore, Md.,
     1977; pp. 105-117.

8.   Herman, G. T. and Naparstek, A.: Fast image reconstruction based
     on a Radon inversion formula appropriate for rapidly collected
     data, SIAM J. Appl. Math. 33: 511, 1977.

9.   Hounsfield, G. N.: Computerized transverse axial scanning
     (tomography): Part I. Description of system. B. J. Radiol. 46:
     1016, 1973.

10. Macovski, A., Alvarez, R. E., Chan, J. L., and Stonestrom, J.
     P.: Correction for spectral shift-artifacts in x-ray computer-
     ized tomography. Image Processing for 2-D and 3-D Reconstruction
     from Projections. Stanford, Ca., August, 1975; pp. MB1-5 -
     MB1-8.

11. McDavid, W. D., Waggener, R. G., Payne, W. H., and Dennis, J:
     Spectral effects on three-dimensional reconstruction from x-
     rays. Med. Phys. 2: 321, 1975; Correction for spectral artifacts
     in cross-sectional reconstruction from x-rays. Med. Phys.
     4: 54, 1977.

12. McCullough, E. C.: Photon attenuation in computed tomography.
     Med. Phys. 2: 307, 1975.

13. McCullough, E. C., Baker, H. L., Houser, O. W., and Reese, D.
     F.: An evaluation of the quantitative and radiation features
     of a scanning x-ray transverse axial tomography: the EMI scan-
     ner. Radiol. 111: 709, 1974

14. Pang, S. C. and Genna, S.: A Fourier convolution fan-geometry
     reconstruction algorithm: simulation studies, noise propagation,
     and polychromatic degradation. Reconstruction Tomography in

Diagnostic Radiology and Nuclear Medicine (ed. M. Ter-Pogossian, _et al_.) University Park Press, Baltimore, Md. 1977, pp. 119-137.

15. Pernkopf, E.: _Atlas of topological and applied human anatomy, Volume Two - Thorax, abdomen and extremities_. W. B. Saunders, Philadelphia, 1964.

16. Radon, J.: Uberdie bestimmung von funktionen durch ihre integralwete langs gewisser mannigfaltigkeiten. _Berichte Saechsische Akademie der Wissenschaften_ 69: 262, 1917.

17. Redington, R. W., Edelheit, L. S., Knutson, J. W., Berninger, W. H., Carlson, C. J., Ellis, G. W., Eisner, D. R., Eichelberger C. W., Garratt, P. M., Gittinger, N. C., Gordy, L. W., Henkes, J. L., Jr., Houston, J. M., LeBlang, A. S., Lynk, E. T., Puckette, C. M., Whetten, N. R., Barrett, D. M., Godbarsen, R., Herman, G. T., and Reese, D. F.: A computerized mammography system. Image Processing for 2-D and 3-D Reconstruction from Projections. Stanford, Ca., August, 1975; pp. MA3-1 - MA3-4.

18. Ruegsegger, P. E., Ritman, E. L., and Wood, E. H.: Performance of a cylindrical CT scanning system for dynamic studies of the heart and lungs. Proceedings of the San Diego Biomedical Symposium, San Diego, CA, February 1977, Vol. 8, pp. 143-157.

19. Tsai, C. M., and Cho, Z. H.: Water bath and averaging effect of attenuation coefficients in transmission tomography. Image Processing for 2-D and 3-D Reconstruction from Projections. Stanford, Ca., August, 1975; pp. MB3-1 - MB3-4.

20. Wickizer, R., Zacher, R., Krippner, K., and Liu, Y.: A comparison of some models of x-ray beam hardening. Application of Optical Instrumentation in Medicine V. Washington, D.C., September, 1976; pp. 276-282.

REAL TIME COMPUTATION OF PULMONARY MECHANICS

BY DIGITAL COMPUTER

Lorino, H., Brault, Y., Harf, A., Atlan, G., Laurent, D.
INSERM U 138 et Service Explorations Fonctionnelles
Hôpital Henri Mondor
94010 - Créteil (France)

The SYSCOMORAM system was built up around a mini-computer to process in real time signals sampled during ventilatory mechanics tests. The patient is sitting in an open body plethysmograph. The lung volumes are calculated from thoracic flow and mouth pressure recorded during the Pflüger's maneuver. Thoracic flow and transpulmonary pressure variations measured with an intra-esophageal balloon, are analyzed to get the static lung compliance. The forced expiration maneuver gives indications about the obstructive nature of the respiratory disorder. Results obtained since June 1977 are highly reproducible in volunteers, and show a satisfying agreement with those got by the standard methodology for both volunteers and patients.

INTRODUCTION

Assessment of lung function in adults allows the accurate evaluation of functional changes with various pulmonary disorders, as well as early detection of suspected lung and airways diseases. The description of some mechanical features of the ventilatory system belongs to the group of tests used to study routinely lung function in our Clinical Physiology department. Four to six patients undergo every day a series of tests using the body plethysmographic technique. Thanks to a joint project with Aerospatiale Company, a computerized system was developped to analyze flow and pressure signals in real time (10), as it had been done previously for cardiac catheterization data (3). Some laboratories already use a digital computer, often on a time-sharing basis, to process data collected by spirometry or plethysmography (5, 9, 11,14). SYSCOMORAM was made of a modular set of programs activated in real time, but quite suitable for off-line use; it is dealing with three functional tests : computation of actual lung volumes (6); analysis of forced expiration maneuver (1,2); estimation of static lung compliance (16). This paper describes the algorithms used and the results obtained both in volunteers and in patients.

MATERIALS

Transducers

The patient is seated in a total body plethysmograph, namely a 500 litres box in communication with room atmosphere via a screen opposing a linear resistance to the movement of air. Having applied a nose clip he breathes outside the box through a rubber mouthpiece. Considering lung structures to be homogeneous, the expression of differences in pressure accross each structure may be used to assess the distribution of stress. With differential pressure transducers (CH 5022 Schlumberger), one can measure :

- mouth pressure P_m at the airways opening
- thoracic barometric pressure P_b bearing on the chest, here inside the box
- alveolar pressure P_a , which equals P_m when mouth flow was interrupted
- pleural pressure P_{pl} : it is admitted that the variations of intra-esophageal pressure P_{es} correctly approximate intra-pleural pressure changes.

To measure P_{pl} a thin latex balloon is introduced through one nostril into esophagus, inflated with 0.5 ml of air and connected to an external pressure transducer. Gas flow at mouth V_m' is measured using a Jaeger Lily pneumotachograph (H 5112 Schlumberger transducer). Changes in the volume of thoracic cage and abdomen when the patient is breathing cause instantaneous changes of P_b, as measured by a H 5112 transducer. An analog circuit reproducing the box transfer function delivers thoracic flow V_t' as a calculated signal (8). Time integrals of V_m' and V_t' stand for variations of gas volume at mouth and thoraco-abdominal volume.

Every pressure signal is passed through a second-order analog filter (z = 0.7; cut off frequency = 30 Hz).

Computer

The T1600 mini-computer was equipped with a 40 K 16-bits words core memory, a floating-point operator, a 10 million bytes disk, a Wang magnetic tape, a MDS card-reader and a Logabax line-printer. The A/D converter can digitize up to 8 signals at frequencies ranging from 1 Hz to 150 Hz. The clinical laboratory was provided with a Tektronix 4010 graphics console. Programs were written in Assembly and PL 1600 languages, and split up into 3 K words overlay units.

After barometric pressure and subject's identity and height were entered, the patient undergoes three to five times each test, so that an overall result will be finally retained. The following functions may be activated by the technician: measurement of zero for each transducer; sampling and pre-processing of signals; optional display of the signals; processing of the signals, and display of the results; validation of the results; elaboration of the definitive results at the end of the test.

METHODS

Forced expiration

After having deeply expired, then inspired, the patient is asked to expire as rapidly as possible his intrathoracic gas. (Figure 1). Mouth flow rate V_m' and thoracic flow rate V_t' are sampled at 150 Hz for 30 seconds. After time integration three signals are analyzed : V_m', V_m and V_t. Maximal Expiratory Flow (MEF) is calculated from V_m', and the beginning of the forced expiration is located in the preceding second. Vital Capacity is calculated from both volumes as VC_t and VC_m. The program then calculates : the Forced Expiratory Volume in the first second of expiration (FEV_1); the Maximal Expiratory Flow, when the subject expired 50%, then 75% of his VC_t (MEF_{50} and MEF_{75}); the Mean Maximal Expiratory Flow between 25% and 75% of VC_t (MEF_{25-75}); the ratio FEV_1/VC_m. Others workers, such as Rosner (15) calculated slightly different parameters, which tend likewise to describe the shape of the V_t curve. The $V_m' - V_t$ curve is finally displayed, after its fraction posterior to the peak-flow was smoothed using an averaging technique. A further quantitative analysis of the descending part of this curve should be investigated, in order to relate some particular shapes to a specific physiopathological diagnosis. In a personnal communication Mead J. put forward a suitable method to describe the convexity of the MEFV curves, using the method of slope ratio analysis. Here an alarm code is simply displayed every time the patient expired less than three quarters of his Vital Capacity.

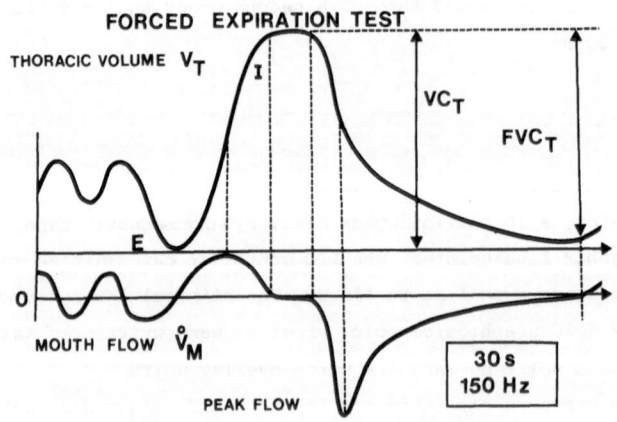

Figure 1. V_t' and V_m' signals are sampled at 150 Hz. The maximum of the flow rate, then the start of the expiration are located on V_m'.

Lung volumes

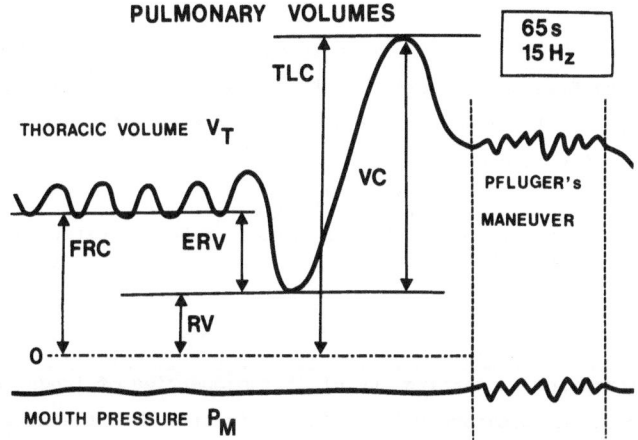

<u>Figure 2.</u> P_m-V_t points obtained during the panting maneuver
fit a straight line. This linear relation is
improved by using the P_m' and V_t' first derivatives.

The patient keeps breathing spontaneously for six to eight cycles, then he expires
and inspires maximally; the next expiration is interrupted for a few seconds at
about the end expiratory level. The patient is instructed to "pant" against the
mouth shutter by using his abdominal muscles, without blocking his glottis nor in-
flating his cheeks. P_m and V_t' signals are sampled at 15 Hz for 65 seconds. By analyzing the V_t curve, using a smoothed first derivative :

$$DER = V_t \ (i+4) - V_t \ (i-4)$$

the program calculates : Tidal Volume (TV), the maximum of which is called Vital
Capacity (VC); mean Respiratory Rate (RR); Expiratory Reserve Volume (ERV), and
the end expiratory volume level.

Then the so-called "Pflüger's maneuver" is located in time as a zone of noticeable
variations of P_m. By application of Boyle's law to the gas contained in the lungs
(4,6), one may write :

$$V_t = a + b. \ P_m$$

Therefore linear regression of V_t measurements over P_m measurements leads to the
calculation of the Thoracic Gas Volume(TGV)of the lungs :

$$TGV = |b| \ . \ (P_{atm} - P \ H_2O \ (37°C)). \ K_P/K_V$$

with   b = slope of the regression line

        $P \ H_2O \ (37°C)$: water vapor pressure at body temperature

K_p and K_V : pressure and volume calibration coefficients.
The quality of the linear dependence of volume over pressure is sanctioned by indication of the correlation coefficient (r). Actual values of pulmonary volumes are
finally derived from TGV : Residual Volume (RV), Total Lung Capacity (TLC) and
Functional Residual Capacity (FRC). Time integration of thoracic flow V_t' having
proved to generate frequently a drift of the volume baseline, the b parameter
was more accurately calculated by searching a linear relation between the first
time derivatives of V_t and P_m :

$$V_t' = a + b. P_m'$$

This equation proved to yield much higher values of the correlation coefficient.

Static lung compliance

Much of the information concerning the elastic properties of lungs can be derived
from the static volume-pressure curves. It is admitted that the difference between
P_{pl} and P_m pressures satisfactorily reflects P_{tp} transpulmonary pressure changes.
After the patient swallowed the esophageal balloon, he is instructed to breathe
spontaneously for 8 to 10 ventilatory cycles, then to perform a Vital Capacity
maneuver. The expiration which follows is then interrupted intermittently by closure
of the mouth shutter for about 4 seconds. The computer samples, at 15 Hz for 80
seconds, thoracic flow V_t' and differential pressure P_{tp}, as well as a marking
channel where square waves were generated during the no flow periods. (Figure 3)

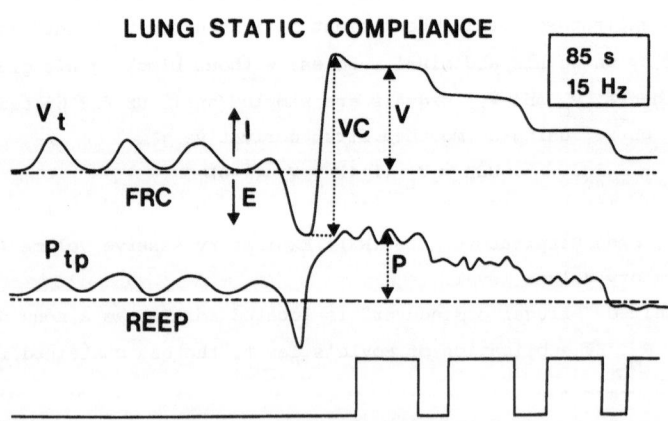

Figure 3. V_t and P_{tp} signals are sampled at 15 Hz; zero flow
instants are located in time thanks to square waves
generated manually on a third channel.

The computer calculates FRC and Resting End Expiratory Pressure (REEP) levels during spontaneous breathing. The last third of each of the 5 to 6 pressure steps is then analyzed to obtain an average value of static pressure (P); the corresponding average value of the volume step is calculated (V). In the presence of disturbances due to deglutition or esophageal spasms, the PV static level is discarded. The PV values are referenced to the resting end expiratory levels of this trial. At the end of each of 4 to 5 attempts, the PV points are displayed, each set being represented with a specific sign; the technician is thereby allowed to eliminate these sets which would stand aside from the general exponential trend. Those PV points which where finally validated enter the curve-fitting procedure. It is usually assumed that such static pressure-volume curves are S-shaped (16,12), and that the PV relation can be accurately expressed by an exponential equation, either above FRC (7,13,16) or on both sides of FRC (12), by using either relative (7,16) or actual (12,13) values of lung volumes. We considered that PV points standing above FRC could be fitted by :

$$V = B_1 + B_2 \exp (-kP)$$

To identify the B_1, B_2 and k parameters, we used the Newton-Raphson method, as it was worked out by Schroter (7). It consists in a Taylor series expansion of the non linear function : $V = f (P, k)$, then in an extension of the least squares method (here a two variables linear regression) to the solution of problems requiring iterative approximations. The procedure is stopped when k became stable enough; the following results are displayed : the curvature of the curve (k); the theoretical asymptote value above FRC (B_1); the compliance at FRC level ($C_0 = B_1 . k$); the position of the axis intercepts :

$$V_0 = B_1 + B_2$$
$$P_0 = (-1/k) \log (-B_1/B_2)$$

as well as the residual standard deviation (D).

DISCUSSION

Forced expiration

About thirty tracings were recorded on paper and analyzed manually by the technician. The differences between computer-derived and hand calculated results are significant for VC_m (P < 0.001), VC_t (P < 0.01) and FEV_1 (P < 0.001); but, as Rosner remarked (15), there are not clinically significant, since the mean difference equals : 110 ml for VC_m, 67 ml for VC_t, 69 ml/s for FEV_1, while the reading error can reach 50 ml. The differences are slightly significant for MEF_{25-75} (0.02 < P < 0.05), with a mean difference of 128 ml/s. They are not significant for MEF_{50} and MEF_{75}, with a mean difference of 70 ml/s. Therefore a satisfactory agreement was found between hand and computer measurements.

Static lung compliance

The value C_{om} of static compliance near FRC was obtained by hand calculation from an empiric best visual fit, as the slope of the chord between FRC and (FRC+600 ml) levels. Results obtained over a three months period in volunteer YB show only minor intrinsec variations of the curvature k and the asymptote value V_m. C_o and C_{om} values of compliance do not differ significantly, but the coefficient of variation is markedly lower for C_o than for C_{om}. That demonstrates the good reproducibility of this method. Ten cases were taken at random among the results obtained in patients since December 1977. C_o was found significantly higher than C_{om} (P < 0.1), which reflects the difference between the calculation methods. To test the fitting procedure we drew an off-line comparison between three curve-fitting methods : the present Newton-Raphson method, the simple Newton second-derivative method, and the one-variable linear regression method used by Pengelly (13). We found a perfect agreement between the two first methods, and a slight disagreement with the third one. The reduction of the overall variance attributable to the theoretical curve was nearly identical for the three procedures, while the coefficient of variation of the k parameter increased from 5% to 13% in the third case.

The degree of accuracy of our method is first depending on a reliable determination of the FRC-REEP frame of reference, at each repetition of the trial. The precision of the method is conditioned by a correct measurement of zero air flow pressure levels. The reason why repeated attempts can deviate from each other has still to be investigated; potential sources for error can be : change of the location or the gas contents of the balloon in the esophagus; cardiac artifacts; changes in esophageal tone; swallowing. If it is desired to include data below FRC in the study, a sigmoid model using upper and lower asymptotes must be used, and at least five parameters have then to be identified.

Lung volumes

Three types of experiments were carried out to check the computer method. First of
all a small pump was set up in the plethysmograph to provoke a periodic 0.05 liter
variation in the volume of a metallic cylinder, filled with 2.8 liters of air under
barometric pressure (4). Eight measurements yielded a mean value of 1.98 liter
with a standard deviation of 0.1 liter. Since the gas transformation can be considered as adiabatic, the actual estimate of the volume of the cylinder becomes 2.77
liters.

In order to check the within-subject reproducibility of the on-line computation
method, multiple determinations of the thoracic gas volume were done in five healthy
volunteers, over a period of several months. In subject HL for instance, 26 measurements yielded extreme values of 7.30 and 7.99 liters, a mean value of 7.69 liters
with a standard deviation of 0.19 liter. It must be noticed that the Pflüger's maneuver was executed at volume levels ranging from 3 liters to 6 liters. The technician computed the b parameter by dividing the volume change between two successive
zero flow points by the associated pressure change; about five consecutive such
"tidal volumes" yield the mean value of b. In volunteer HL, this method yielded
results ranging from 7.16 to 7.97 liters, with a mean value of 7.66 liters and a
standard deviation of 0.21 liter.

Then 120 tracings were selected in 50 patients by keeping only correlation coefficients better than 0.98, which eliminates most of improperly executed maneuvers.
The comparison between hand (h) and computer (c) calculation yielded the following
relations :

$$TGV_h = 0.972\ TGV_c + 0.111\ \text{liter}$$

with $\quad r^2 = 0.988$ and $S = 0.147$ liter

and

$$TLC_h = 0.973\ TLC_c + 0.106\ \text{liter}$$

with $\quad r^2 = 0.986$ and $S = 0.181$ liter

The mean within-subject dispersion of TLC values was found to be slightly lower when
using the computer method. These conclusions look comparable to those obtained by
Sykes (17), when using a barometric plethysmograph and a 200 Hz sampling frequency
in 10 emphysematic patients.

REFERENCES

1. Ayers, W.R., Ward, S.A., Weihrer, A.L., Abraham , S. and Caceres, C.A.: Description of a computer program for analysis of the Forced Expiratory Spirogram. I - Instrumentation and programming. Compt.Biomed.Res. 2 (1969) 207-219.
2. Ayers, W.R., Ward, S.A., Weihrer, A.L., Abraham, S. and Caceres, C.A.: Description of a computer program for analysis of the Forced Expiratory Spirogram. II - Validation. Comput.Biomed.Res. 2 (1969) 220-228.
3. Besse, P., Kubidjan, F., Legoff, G., Gouverneur, G., Bricaud, H., Desloges, M., Laurent, D.: Acquisition et prétraitement en temps réel des paramètres hémodynamiques pour la constitution en temps différé d'un fichier complet des malades cathétérisés. Proceedings of "Congrès d'Informatique Médicale",Toulouse,March 1974, 133-142.
4. Briscoe, W.A.: Lung volumes. in Handbook of Physiology, 1965,Respiration II, Amer.Physiol.Soc.Wash.,D.C., 1333-1355.
5. Dickman, M.L., Schmidt, C.D., Gardner, R.M., Marshall, H.W., Day, W.C. and Warner, H.W.: On-line computerized spirometry in 738 normal adults. Amer.Rev.Resp.Dis.100 (1969) 780-790.
6. DuBois, A.B., Botelho, S.Y., Bedell, G.N., Marshall, R. and Comroe, J.H.Jr.: A rapid plethysmographic method for measuring thoracic gas volume : a comparison with a nitrogen washout method for measuring functional residual capacity in normal subjects. J.Clin.Invest.3 (1956) 322-326.
7. Glaister, D.H., Schroter, R.C., Sudlow, M.F. and Milic-Emili, J.: Bulk elastic properties of excised lungs and the effect of a transpulmonary pressure gradient. Resp.Physiol. 17 (1973) 347-364.
8. Harf, A., Lorino, H., Atlan, G.: Capteur pléthysmographique corporel total : modélisation et traitement du signal de pression. Proceedings of "Colloque International sur les capteurs biomédicaux BIOCAPT" Paris, November 1975,vol.I,403-409.
9. Hoffer, E.P., Kanarek, D., Kazemi, H. and Barnett, G.O.: Computer Interpretation of Ventilatory studies. Comput.Biomed.Res. 6 (1973) 347-354.
10. Lorino, H., Atlan, G., Brault, Y., Harf, A., Boitaud, J. and Laurent, D.: Explorations fonctionnelles et études en mécanique ventilatoire assistées par le système SYSCOMORAM. Proceedings of "The International Symposium on Medical Informatics", Toulouse, March 1977, 219-232.
11. Moser, K.M., Torzewski, D.F., and Nubla, L.E.: Practical computer program for routine spirometric testing using the time-sharing concept. Dis.Chest 56 (1969) 92-97.
12. Païva, M., Yernault, J.C., Van Eerdeweghe, P. and Englert, M.: A sigmoïd model of the static volume pressure curves of the lung. Resp.Physiol.23 (1975) 317-323.
13. Pengelly, L.D.: Curve-fitting analysis of pressure-volume characteristics of the lungs. J.Appl.Physiol. 42 (1977) 111-116.
14. Rosner, S.W., Palmer, A. and Caceres, C.A.: A computer program for computation and interpretation of pulmonary function data. Comput.Biomed.Res.4 (1971)141-156.
15. Rosner, S.W., Palmer, A., Ward, S.A., Abraham, S. and Caceres, C.A.: Clinical spirometry using computer techniques. Amer.Rev.Resp.Dis. 94 (1966) 181-187.
16. Salazar, E. and Knowles, J.H.: An analysis of pressure-volume characteristics of the lungs. J.Appl.Physiol. 19 (1964) 97-104.
17. Sykes, T.W., Haynes, R.L. and Mc Fadden, E.R.Jr.: On-line determinations of lung volumes by plethysmography and digital computer. Amer.Rev.Resp.Dis. 115 (1977) 581-585.

THE COMPUTER IN THE FUNCTIONAL STUDY OF THE KIDNEY WITH RADIONUCLIDES.

Moreno-González J.,Martínez-Alonso J.R., Zunzunegui M.V.
Millan-Santos I., Chamorro J.L., Ortiz-Berrocal J.
Depto.Medicina Nuclear, Dpto.Bioestadistica. Clínica Puerta de Hierro
Madrid-35. SPAIN.

INTRODUCTION.

In this work, there is an attempt to improve results in the diagnostic evalua tion of renal studies methods that are routine in a Nuclear Medicine Depart ment. Our aim has been to carry out an automation of later processes after clinical studies.

The renogram reflects the activity variations (curves) detected in each kidney after the injection of an adequate material (1). These curves define the beha vior of the radioactive material within the kidney and its comparison with pattern curves will give the clinical diagnosis of the study (Fig.1).

The study of the beavier, in blood, of a tracer that is eliminated exclusively by the kidney permits us to sutdy kidney clearance and effective renal plasma flow (2). The method used is based on the application of a two compartmental model (3). In practice, it is reduced to adjust a series of points to a curve, the sum of two exponents whose slopes will define the constans that measures the variation of flow in the kidneys.

This work attempts to carry out a complete automation of all the later proces ses after the obtaiment of results in a renogram, with the goal of avoiding certain errors inherent to manual treatment of the data, making use of the characteristics of the computer for the obtainment of results and the creation of files. Among the different sources of error in a nonautomative treatment, and the following:

= The data obtained by external detective methods are affected by statistical fluctuantions that cause an error in these data (4).

= The original information corresponds, logically, to the presented activity in each kidney. Nevertheles, upon carrying out the study with external detec tors, (scintillation tubes or Anger camera), it is evident that it has recor ded par of the activity corresponding to an extrarrenal zone (5).

= The specific functions of accumulation and elimination, of great interest for the clinical evaluation of a renogram, are very bothersome to calculate by manual procedures.

= The manual method of calculation of the clearance and FPRE, is in general, slow and difficult, both for the doctor and for the clinician in charge of its realization.

On the other hand, taking into account the possibility of using a computer belonging to the department, we have taken advantage of its general characte ristics, in order to create a data bank of the studies (7),thus, reproducing or recuperating a specific study to define general diagnosis criteria, by means or statistical treatment of the filed data.

2. DATA PROCESSING.

The sistem consists of 20 programs stored on disks. One of them is the direc, ting program an the remaining ones carry out the different elementary informa tive processes (Fig.2). The system controls the dependency among then, with is

the order of executions and the number of times that the process is carried
out, using as a base the same information.
The definite file is on magnetic tape, not being directly processable on it,in
such a manner, that in order to carry out the treatment of the recorded infor
tion on tape, it is absolutely necessary to transfer this information to
the disk.

2.1. DATA INPUT.

The input of the information is separated into two processes:
= Identification of the patient.
= Measurements of time activity of the study in the three chosen zones.
The start of the automation of each study can beging (itself) indistinctly
with one process or another and the data is recorded in the RINON file (Fig.3)
The identification data contain information referring to the name of the
patient, referring department, name of the doctor in charge of the case, date
of the study, protocol corresponding to the Department of Nuclear Medicine,
location (of admittance and ambulatory) and specific conditions under which
the study was carried out.
The specific data of the study, corresponding to the variations of the radioac
tive tracer in the detection zones, can enter the computer in three different
ways, according to the following entrance paths:
= Directly, through an on line connection.
= Information perforated on paper tape by Tally rapid perforator (8 values of
activity in each record).
= Perforated on paper tape by a teletype (each record contains one value of
activity).
= The corresponding program makes these different forms of imput, homogeneous.

2.2. DATA PURIFICATION

The gross datta obtained directly with the activity detectors are influence by
different factors affecting the real renal curve.
On one had, the signal received and transmitted by the detection system is af
fected by statistical fluctuations of desintegration (noise). The reason for
the noise is due to the nature of the radioactive material, that is desinte
grated according to Poisson's probability. For this reason, it is of interest
to filter the obtained data. The technique used to suppress the noise are
called smoothing techniques.
On the other hand, we must take into account that upon utilizing external
detectors, on the renal areas, the values of activity received do not corres
pond exactly to the data of renal activity, that are definitely those which
define kidney behavior. Due to this, to carry out a renogram correctly,we must
to use a method that, according to a correct criterium, carries out the corres
ponding correction, subtrahending the value of the corresponding extrarrenal
activity in each step of the study (Fig.4).
The smoothing process used consists of transforming the value of activity
measure in each time, substituting it for the weighted medium, taking into
account the nearest, previous and posterior values:

$$X^1_i = \frac{X_i - 2 + 2X_i - 1 + 4X_i + 2X_i + 1 + X_i + 2}{10}$$

The correction method used for the subtraction of extrarrenal activity is as described by Hall and modified by Britton and Brown (9) with slight variations that affect the tecnical aspect of our equipment.

The initial hypothesis is that the extrarrenal activity curve is proportional to the precordial curve:

$$AE = K \times AP.$$

In order to the determine value of K, human sero albumin measured with I-131 which is not caught by the kidneys and circulates freely throught the blood. Under these conditions, the values obtained by the detectors placed on the kidney will correspond to those of the extrarrenal activity (Fig.5).

$$K = AE(t)/AP(t).$$

2.3. DETERMINATION OF PARAMETERS OF CLINICAL VALUE.

The corresponding processes included all of the calculation; this is necessary to obtain definite results of clinical interest. It comprehends the determina tion of accumulation and elimination in the long run, the analytical descrip tion of the net curves of the renogram for each kidney and its comparison among them, and the calculation of kidney clearance (Fig. 6).

among them, and

2.3.1. SPECIFIC DETERMINATION OF THE FUNCTIONS OF UPTAKE AND KIDNEY ELIMINATION

According to a widely accepted hypothesis, the uptake of the kidneys is propor tional to the integral of the clearance precordial curve, as in the following relationship:

$$\text{Uptake } (t) = m \int_{t_o}^{t} P(t)\, dt + C \qquad (1)$$

In order to determine the Up (t) function, it is necessary to know the cons tants of proportionality m and C.

Leave as is the fist part of the renal curve represents the variations of the amount óf Hippuran in the kidney before beginning its elimination through the urine, in this time interval the uptake curve coincides with the renogram curve since the elimination is zero.

The time interval in which the elimination can be considered null is from one to three minutes.

Following this, the values of m and C can be calculated as follows:

$$R(t) = m \int_{t_o}^{t} P(t)\, dt + C \qquad (2)$$

For $t = 1$ and $1 < t < 3$

Once m and C are determined, we can obtain the accumulation function.

Taking into account that the renogram curve measures the activity captured by the kidney less that which is eliminated, the function of the elimination is given as:

$$Elim (t) = Up (t) - R(t).$$

In Figure 7 the form of the results obtained in a sample can be observed. The elimination factor of isotope IRF is a point of clinical interest. It measures the percentage of uptake in the time t, which is eliminated in time $(t + \Delta t)$. (Fig. 15).

$$IRF = \frac{Elim (t + \Delta t) \times 100}{Up (t)}$$

2.3.2. <u>DETERMINATION OF PARAMETERS OF THE CURVE.</u>
The significance of the parameters that have been taken to describe, objecti vely, the renal curve, will be shown (Fig.8).

a) <u>Heights of interest in the renogram.</u>
The correspond with the activity presented in certain determined times.
They are those reached at fifty seconds (the value that is considered as ini tial height starting with the one that really begins the distribution of acti vity in the kidneys), at 2,5,12,15 and 20 minutes and the maximun height pre sented in the renogram.

b) <u>Times of interest.</u>
The characteristic times of the curve are the time of maximun activity (peak time), half time of the peak (time transpired from the peak time until the moment when the half maximal activity was reached) and the quarter time of the peak. Their values define for us the characteristics of the elimination.

c) <u>Relationships between parameters.</u>
They result from realizing the quotient between two parameters, previously calculated. The relationships calculated are the following:
= Height of the peak and height at 50 seconds.
= Height at 12 minutes and height at 50 seconds.
= Coefficient of accumulation or relationship between activities reached at 2 minutes, 50 seconds, with regard to the activity at 50 seconds.
= Coefficient of excretion or relationship between the maximal activity and the activity measured 10 minutes later.

d) <u>Angle of accumulation.</u>
It studies the first phase of the curve from when the radioactive material arrived practically at the kidney, until the elimination phase began.The accu mulation angle measures the variation of activity with respect to the time or the slope of this first phase of the curve. Its calculation is carried out considering it as an angle of a right triangle.

e) <u>Other parameters.</u>
The parameters previously described are calculated for each kidney indistinc tly and the program obtains, on the other hand, acomparative study of such parameters in each kidney as a percentage of the value from one another.

Other values that measure the common functioning of the kidneys are also calcu lated. These are:
= The mean values of the peaks.
= The relationship of the heights at 50 seconds between the two kidneys.
= The percentage of urine.

2.3.3. RENAL CLEARANCE .

Renal clearance of a substance is the relationship between the urinary output of that substance by the minute, and its concentration in the plasma.It repre sents the volume of the plasma that the kidney purifies completely during a fraction of time.

Is determination is based on a mathematical model that is adapted to the beha vior of the plasma and which is formed as the following compartmental system (Fig.9); in which each compartment has the following significance:

1. PLASMA.
2. EXTRAVASCULAR SPACE.
3. KIDNEY.

It is assumed that in equilibrium states the variations of the flow in the dif ferent compartments are constant and remain defined by the intercompartmental constants (K12,K21,KE).

We will utilize the notation R (R1,R2) to define the existing activity in each compartment that is proportional to the concentration of the tracer that, upon distributing itself uniformly,measures for us, indirectly, its volume. the analytic solution of the model is expressed in the following system of li near equations:

$$dR1/dt = K21\ R2 - (K12 + + KE)\ R1 \qquad (1)$$
$$dR2/dt = K21\ R1 - K21\ R2 \qquad (2)$$

The solution of R1 (a fuction that can be measured experimentally), depending on time, is the following:

$$R1 = a1e^{-r1t} + a2e^{-r2t}$$

Being:

$$r1\ .\ r2 = KE\ .\ K21.$$
$$r1 + r2 = K21 + K12 + KE.$$

In practice, the problem consists of calculating the intercompartmental con tant starting from a1, a2, r1, r2, that are the parameters that can be obtai ned by adjusting the curve to the experimental data. A new equation in needed that is obtained with the following hipothesis:

For t = 0, r1 = 1, R2 = 0, dR1/dt = -(K12 + KE) = -a1r1 - a2r2.

In conclusion:

$$r1 \cdot r2 = KE\ K21 \qquad (7)$$
$$r1 + r2 = K21 + K12 + KE \qquad (8)$$
$$a1 + a2 = 1 \qquad (9)$$
$$a1r1 + a2r2 = K12 + KE \qquad (10)$$

Whose solution is:

$$K21 = a2r1 + a1r1 \qquad (11)$$
$$KE = r1r2/a2r1 + a1r2 \qquad (12)$$
$$K12 = a1r1 + a2r2 - KE \qquad (13)$$

A parameter of great clinical interest is the effective plasmatic renal flow.
It is determined as the product of the volume of dilution by the constant KE.
The solution of the calculation of clearances (Fig.10) with a computer is
expressed as the realization of 4 processes:
= Adjustement of an exponential function to the experimental data.
= Determination of the interval of separation of the two exponential branches.
= Determination of the function that corresponds to the real values of
activity.
= Calculation of the intercompartmental constants and the effective renal
plasma flow.

Adjustment of an exponential function:
The problem consists of obtaining, starting with the experimental data, an
exponential function that we will identify, with the one obtained by means of
the study of the theoretical model. From there, the particular characteristics
of the system will be known in an immediate form.
In essence, then, the problem consists of adjusting a series of value pairs
(t_i, y_i) to the function:

$$y = A1\ e^{-r1t} + A2\ e^{-r2t}$$

The values of A1,A2,r1,r2, will analytically give us the desired curve and
from these values the calculation of the parameters that define the model
under study is immediate.
The linearization of the function to be adjusted can be carried out after the
formulation of a hypothesis that is completed in tracer Kinetics.
The assumption of an exponential function of two branches defined by a value
t_1 that separates two intervals: $t < t1$ and $t > t1$.
In the second interval ($t > t_1$),the influence of the first branch of the
curve is insignificant.

As in the following:

$$\text{For } t > t_1 \qquad y = A2\ e^{-r2t}$$

$$Lny = LnA2 - r2t.$$

That is a linear function, obtaining the values A2 and r2 by the general method of least squares linear regression:

For $t < t_1$

$$y = A1\ e^{-r1t} + A2\ e^{-r2t}$$

$$y - A2\ e^{-r2t} = A1\ e^{-r1t}$$

$$z = A1\ e^{-r1t}$$

$$Lnz = LnA1 - r1t$$

A1 are r1 are obtained the same way.

Determination of the separation interval of the two branches.

In renal studies, sufficient experimental points are generally obtained (generally 180, if measurements are taken every 10 seconds for one half our).In order to determine the time that separates the variation interval of the two branches,the previously described adjustment is done with the 25 first and 25 last exprimental points.

The intersecting point of the two branches will define for us, the separation interval of the two branches with which the definite adjustment of all of the points will be carried out.

Determination of the exponential function that corresponds to the real values of activity.

The study has been carried out with external detectors. The shape of the curve obtained, corresponds to reality, but a proportionality factor exists which must be calculated and corrected experimentally. To do so, two real points are determined, extracting two blood samples from the patient at different times of the study, measuring with a sample counter the value of the real activity obtained.

The curve that exactly measures the activity variation with time is a curve parallel to the one calculated starting from the data obtained with external detectors. However, the activity measuring curve passes through the time activity experimental values obtained by means of blood extraction.

The equation of the curve will be:

$$Y = B1\ e^{-r1t} + B2\ e^{-r2t}$$

The slopes of this curve are the same as the ones previously calculated, but the constants B1 y B2 differ from A1 and A2. Taking into account that this curve has to pass through the points X1,Y1,X2 and Y2, determined with blood extractions, the values B1 and B2 are obtained by solving a simple system of two equations with two unknow quantities.

Determination if the intercompartmental constants and effective renal plasmatic flow.
It consists of directly applying the formulas (11), (12) and (13).

2.4. OUTPUT.
The results obtained, the grafic representation of the curves of the renogram and an account and analytical evaluation of the study, are the conclusive processes of our system.
The calculation programs record the results with a control value in the magnetic disk, so as to check later if the previous calculations have been carried out and the results recorded on the disk (Fig.11).
In Figure 8, a picture with the semiquantitative parameters of the renogram curve can be observed. The value of each paramater is triple (right kidney, left and percentage of one to another). The value of the calculated percentage is given with a negative sign when the compared values present a higher value in the rigth kidney. On the other hand, we use the notation $$$$ when the parameter corresponding to the information received could not be determined.
The different used are represented graphically with a printer (Fig.5,7 and 12) or a plotter (Fig.13), optionally. The basic functioning of the programs consists in adapting the data of the curves recorded on disk to the corresponding scale.
Although the representation by the ploter is more perfect now that the discontinuation in the representation is insignificant, the slow functioning of our unit inclines us to use the printer in the grafic representations done in the routine of the report.
In the final account (Fig.14), a simple description of the study is presented as well, as the evaluation of certain parameters of clinical interest and a computer diagnosis of the patient.

2.4.1. VALUATION OF PARAMETERS FOR AUTOMATIC DIAGNOSIS.

So that the computer emits a diagnostic judgement with the results of the study, we have selected a series of paramaters that are evaluated in individual forms. This evaluation has been carried out by treating the results obtained with our experience with a computer, applying adecuate statistical methods and determining the corresponding intervals.

2.5. TRANSFER OF INFORMATION.

The processed study is recorded completely in an index of the disk file (RINON). This information may come directly with the input program, being modified and lengthened later with different processes of purification of data and calculation of results. The definite location of each study is materialized in a magnetic tape in which each study occupies a similar index upon utilizing its process on the disk.
Logically, two simple processes of transfer of the information to the magnetic tape have to be foreseen. The first one of them stores the information of a

newly processed study on the disk or, rather, will record again on magnetic tape, a study previously carried out on which new processes of purification of data or calculations of new results have been done. The other process trans fer renogram information from magnetic tape to the file on the disk on which all the calculation programs and presentation of results act, in order to make a new revision of stated studies.

REFERENCES.

1. WINTER, C.C.
   Radioisotope Renography. Williams and Wilkens Co., Baltimore. (1963).

2. BLAUFOX, M.D., POTCHEN, E.J., MERRIL, J.P.
   Measurement ofeffective renal plasma flow in man by external counting methods. J.Nucl.Med 8, 77, (1967).

3. TAUXE, W.N., MAHER, F.T., TAYLOR, W.F.
   Effective renal plasma flow: estimation from theoretical volumes of distribuition of intravenously injected I-131 orthoiodohippurate. Mayo Clin Proc 46, 524, (1971).

4. JOHNS, H.E.
   The physis of radiology. Charles C. Thomas, Publ., Springfield, Illinois. (1964), pp.536.

5. BRITTON, K.M., BROWN, N.J.G.
   Clinical renography. lloydLuke Ltd. London (1971).

6. BROWN, N.J.G. and BRITTON, K.E.
   A new method of separation of renalr and non renal components of the Hippuran renogram. In "Radioisotopes in the diagnosis of diseases of the kidneys and urinary tract". Ed.by Timmermans, L.,Merchie, G. Excerpta Medica. Amsterdam. (1969).

7. ORTIZ - BERROCAL,J., MORENO - GONZALEZ, J., MARTINEZ - ALONSO, J.R., and ZUNZUNEGUI - PASTOR, V.
   Automatización del estudio de la función renal con su valoración con ayuda de ordenadores electrónicos. III Congreso Nacional Informática. Madrid. (1975).

8. HALL, F.M. and MONKS, G.K.
   The renogram. A method for separating vascular and renal components. Invest Radiol 1, 220, (1966).

9. BRITTON, K.E. and BROWN, N.J.G.
   The clinical use of C.A.B.B.S. renography. Brit J. Radiol 41,570,(1968).

198

LEGENDS TO THE FIGURES.

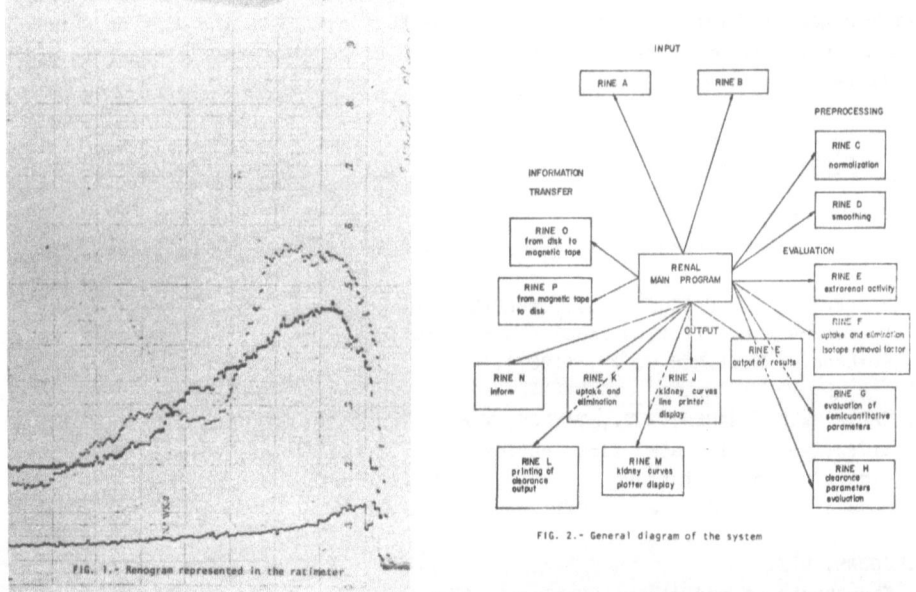

Fig.1.- Renogram in the ratimeter.   Fig.2.- General diagram.

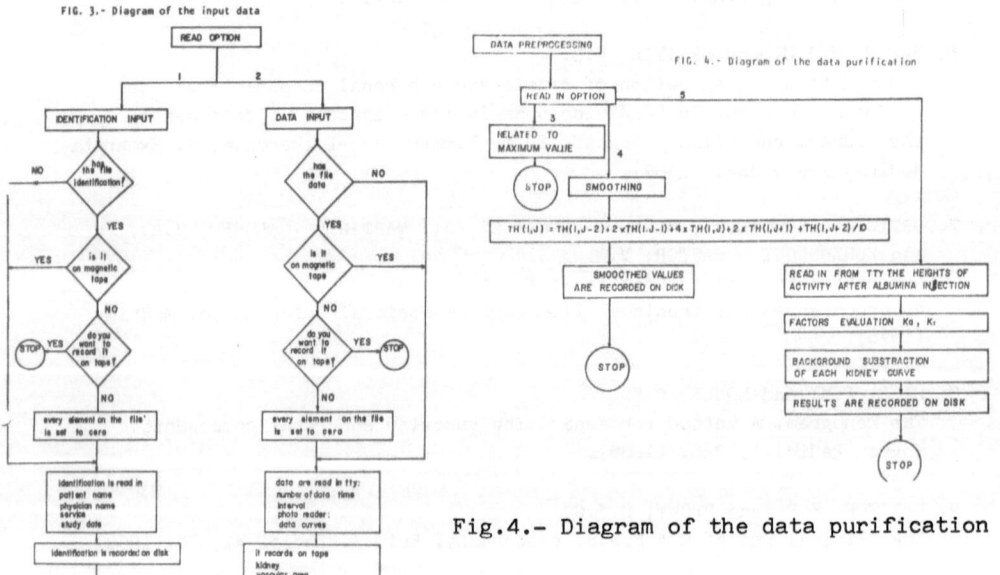

Fig.4.- Diagram of the data purification

Fig.3.- Diagram of the imput data.

FIG. 5a.-Graphic representation of the renogram, printer (form 1)

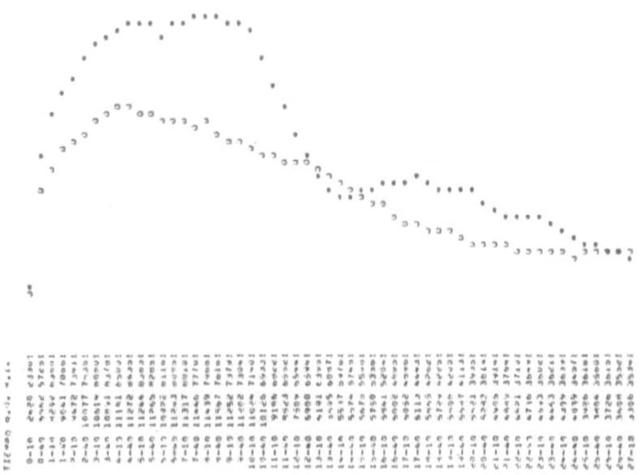

Fig.5a. Grafic of
the renogram (form 1)

FIG. 5b.- Smooth curves

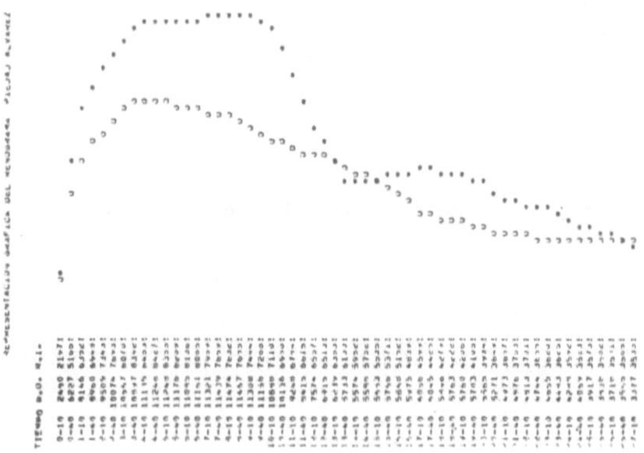

Fig.5b. Smooth curves

FIG. 5c.- Curves subtracted from extrarenal activity

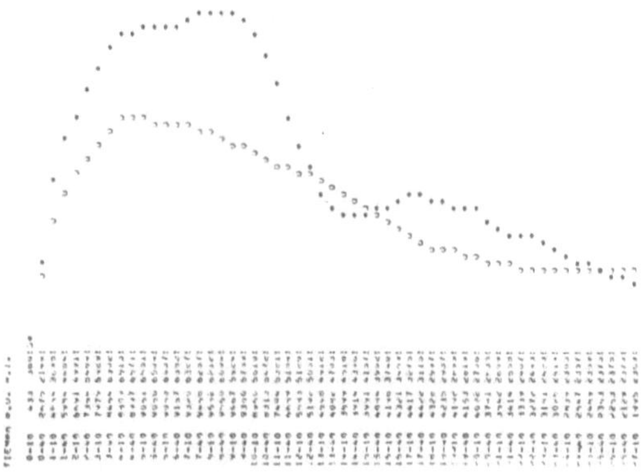

Fig.5c. Curves subtracted

Fig.6. Diagramm of
calculation process

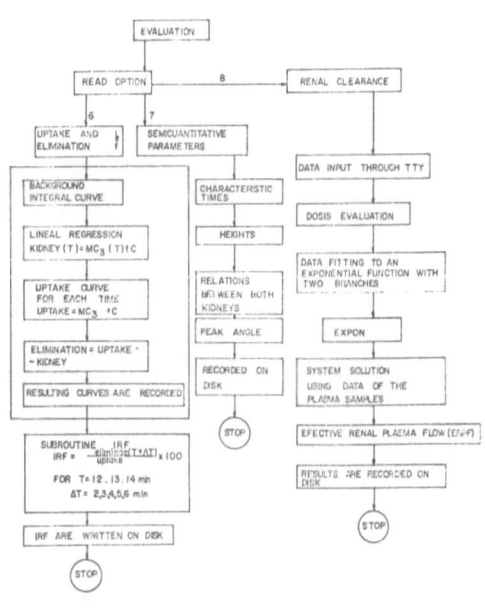

FIG. 6.- Diagram of calculation process

FIG. 7.- Impression of uptake and elimination curves

ESTUDIO SEMICUANTITATIVO DEL RENOGRAMA.
DATOS ORIGINALES

FIG. 8.- Description of the parameters, that objectively define the curve of the renogram.

	RIÑON DERECHO	RIÑON IZQUIERDO	COMPARACION
TIEMPO DEL PICO	[illegible] MIN.	[illegible] MIN.	[illegible] %
TIEMPO MEDIO DEL PICO	[illegible] MIN.	[illegible] MIN.	[illegible] %
TIEMPO CUARTO DEL PICO	[illegible] MIN.	[illegible] MIN.	
ALTURA TRES S.	[illegible] MM.	[illegible] MM.	[illegible] %
ALTURA DEL PICO	[illegible] MM.	[illegible] MM.	[illegible] %
ALTURA [illegible]	[illegible] MM.	[illegible] MM.	[illegible] %
ALTURA [illegible]	[illegible] MM.	[illegible] MM.	[illegible] %
ALTURA [illegible]	[illegible] MM.	[illegible] MM.	[illegible] %
ALTURA [illegible]	[illegible] MM.	[illegible] MM.	[illegible] %
ALTURA [illegible]	[illegible] MM.	[illegible] MM.	[illegible] %
RELACION PICO / ALTURA TRES S.	[illegible]	[illegible]	[illegible] %
RELACION ALTURA [illegible] / ALTURA TRES S.	[illegible]	[illegible]	[illegible] %
ANGULO [illegible]	[illegible] GRADOS	[illegible] GRADOS	[illegible] %
RELACION [illegible]	[illegible]	[illegible]	[illegible] %
COEFICIENTE DE ACUMULACION	[illegible]	[illegible]	[illegible] %
COEFICIENTE DE EXCRECION	[illegible]	[illegible]	[illegible] %

[illegible]

[illegible]

NOTAS

[illegible]

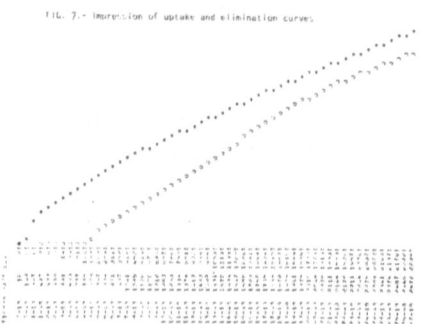

Fig.7.- Uptake and elimination curves. Fig.8.- Description of the parameters

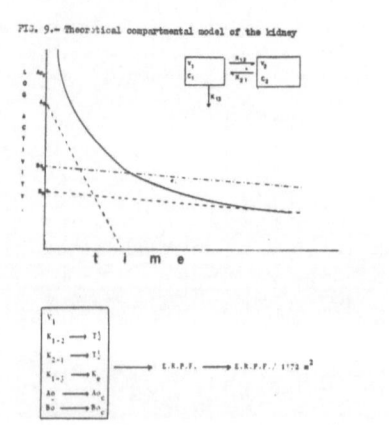

FIG. 9.- Theoretical compartmental model of the kidney

ACLARAMIENTO DE LOS RIÑONES

PARAMETROS DE LA CURVA (2 EXPONENCIALES)

A(1) = 262.135   K(1) = 1.107424
A(2) = 556.272   K(2)= .072800

PARAMETROS CALCULADOS

VOLUMEN DE DILUCION = 5795.47 C.C.

K21 = .776038
KE = .103607
K1 = .404190
K12 = .000002

ACLARAMIENTO FPR = 602.076

FIG. 10 Description of the clearance results

Fig.9.- Theoretical compartmental model. Fif.10.- Clearance results.

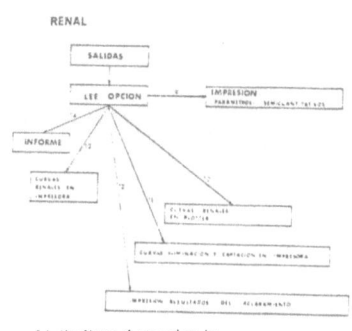

Fig.11.- Diagram of output of results.

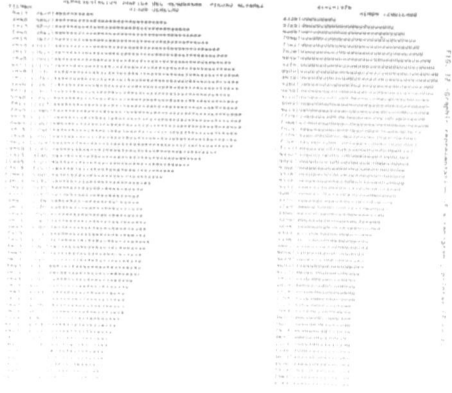

Fig.12.- Renogram printer (form.2).

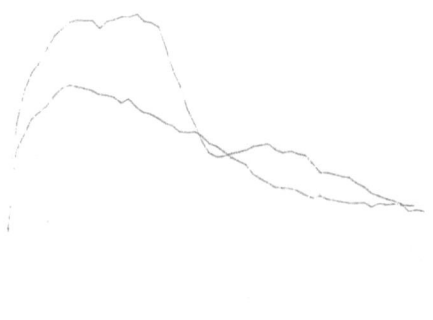

Fig.13.- Renogram. Plotter.

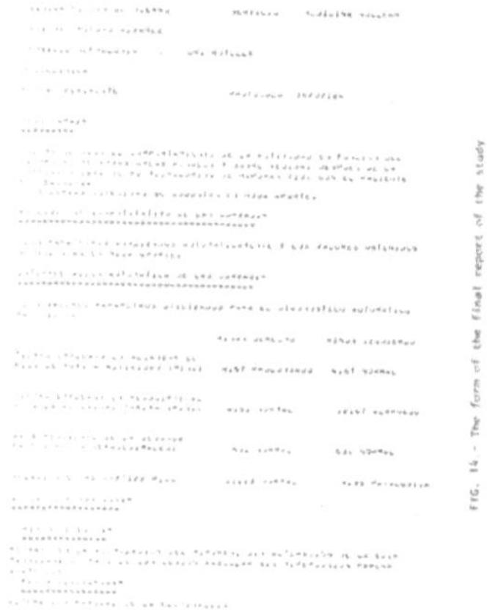

Fig.14.- Final report of the study.

	Riñón derecho (%)	Riñón izquierdo (%)
DT = 2	75,29	71,18
DT = 3	90,22	78,52
DT = 4	102,91	87,96
DT = 5 ,..............	109,93	97,10
DT = 6	115,19	105,39

Fig.15.- Results of the factors of isotope elimination.

Improvement of Programming Efficiency
in Medical Image Processing by a Dialog Language

G. Pfeiffer and K.H. Hoehne
Deutsches Elektronen-Synchrotron DESY

Abstract

A system for image processing in medicine should on the one hand provide an easy and safe application of proven methods of picture analysis. On the other hand a smooth path for improvements or new applications should be provided. It is argued that the required system and programming flexibility can be achieved by a dialog language, which in addition provides for a better transparency and documentation of the resulting software.

The system described consists of two languages, a high level problem oriented dialog language and a low level machine oriented programming language. The paper summarizes the high level dialog language. Particular features include specific interactive facilities, versatile display control and menu techniques, a powerful procedure concept and the use of default values and current representations of data types in procedures.

1. Introduction

Image processing is of growing importance among the variety of computer applications in medicine. Many applications have been published, mostly in Nuclear Medicine, Radiology or Cytology. In our laboratory we are presently developing a system for the analysis of X-ray angiograms[1]. The overall system is subdivided into three major parts, the

- system hardware,
- system software and the
- application software.

In this paper we will concentrate on our approach to an appropriate system software. A detailed hardware description can be found in ref. 2. An overall view of the hardware may be obtained from the block diagram in Fig. 1. An X-ray picture series taken from a standard TV-interface (50 frames/s) are digitized in real time (256 x 256 pixels/frame) under control of a host computer. The digitized images are transferred to a mass storage device for further investigation. Image presentation is done on a colour TV monitor with light pen, track ball and key board. Results of first applications are described in ref. 3.

The *system software* represents an appropriate abstraction level to hide special hardware pecularities from the user as well as to provide application oriented tools for interaction with the hardware components. From experience with a system we had previously developed which included the interactive analysis of scintigraphic images[4,5] we learned that the complexity of the man-machine interaction is a major problem in the design of a system for large scale application of image processing for use by physicians in a hospital. One has to face a double task:

- *Development* of algorithms for new applications. Typical problems are varying modes of data acquisition, filtering algorithms or methods of data presentation.

- *Integration* of proven algorithms into a system which must not only be operational in daily routine, but sufficiently flexible to be applied to new areas of scientific research. The system is constantly subjected to modifications. These may be changes to already available programs (e.g. modifying a smoothing algorithm) or even entirely new applications to be fit into the system.

As has been pointed out by Kupka[6], the underlying issue is that of *procedural* and *non procedural* problem solving. The former involves transformation of a special problem to a mathematical algorithm, which in turn is represented by a program in an appropriate programming language. Non procedural steps, on the contrary, are concerned with developing, testing or modifying algorithms and they imply last but not least system maintenance tasks such as adapting the system to changing demands.

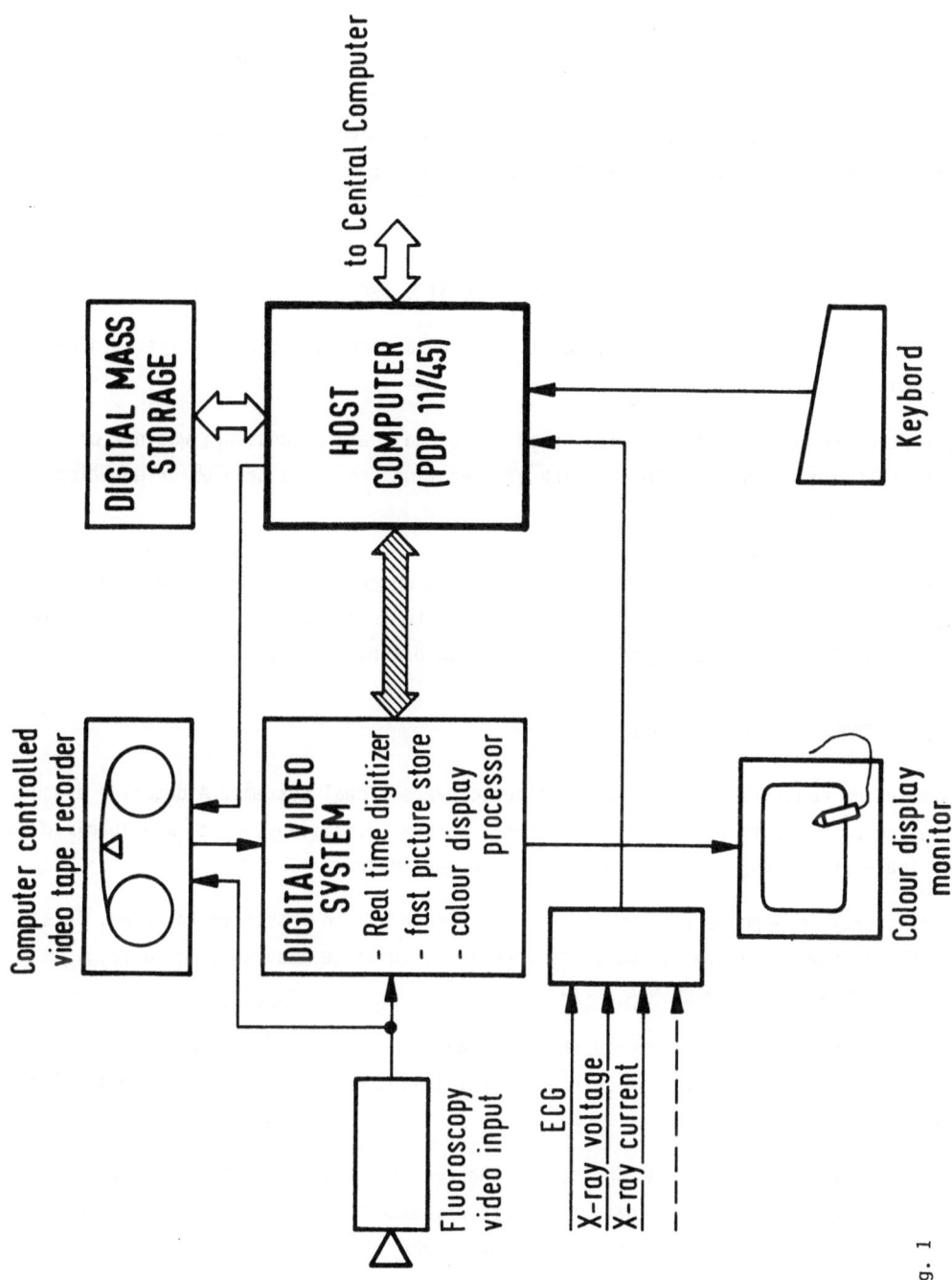

Fig. 1

In this respect we felt that a problem oriented, conversational high level language could improve programming and system flexibility in image processing.

Available dialog languages, which we investigated, proved to be deficient for our application in one or more of the following respects:

- Low efficiency due to interpretative execution.

- Lack of specific facilities for image processing (problem orientation).

- Restricted portability due to specialized hardware and to operating system dependencies.

In particular MUMPS, which is widespread in medical data processing, was not considered suitable, mainly due to its lack of execution speed and problem orientation for image processing.

In this paper we will describe a dialog language which has been developed from experience with an earlier version[7]. Its purpose is to contribute to the solution of at least the first two of the difficulties mentioned above.

2. Requirements to the language

Some design conditions are common to other conversational systems. A detailed discussion can be found in refs. 6 and 8. Further general conditions, which are specific to the image processing application, have to be considered:

- Efficiency - Response times must be short enough not to frustrate the user. This forbids interpretative execution of operations on large amounts of data (e.g. transformations of image matrices).

- Simplicity - Intricate concepts should be avoided in favour of simple and concise rules, so that untrained but interested physicians or technicians can use the language.

- Wide range of problems - A high level language may be inapplicable to some problems, e.g. acquisition of data from fast processes. Therefore, means must be provided to include applications outside the primary scope of the language.

- Wide range of users - A strict separation of routine and scientific use is in general not possible. The system has to satisfy users which only want to push buttons and users writing sophisticated application programs.

- Specific hardware support - The instruction sets of special processors with special memories must be accessible from the high level language.

3. System Concept

Fig. 2 shows the general structure of the system. Essentially it covers two different languages embedded in a common frame:

- a *low level* machine oriented programming language[9]

and   - a *high level* problem oriented dialog language.

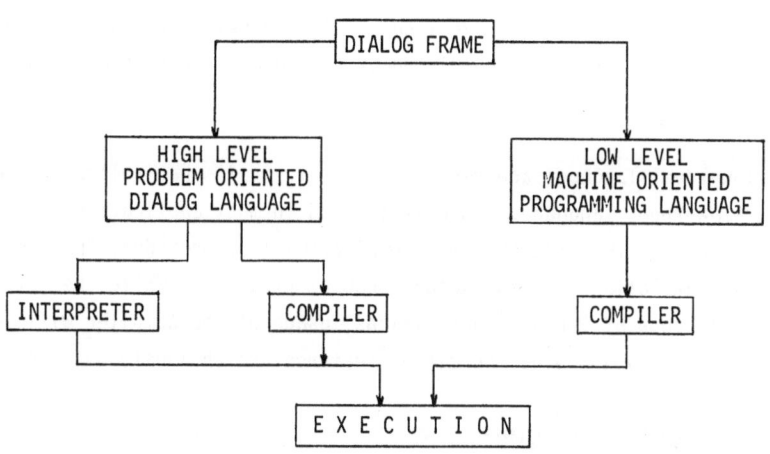

Figure 2: Structure of the Dialog System

The dialog frame consists of operations and data structures common to both languages.

The low-level language belongs to the class of PL360-like languages[10] and combines the style of a high-level language with the efficiency of an assembler language. It will be used when the application problem requires especially efficient code or explicit access to system hardware. In the dialog system the low-level language serves a double purpose:

- The system is *implemented* in the low-level language. Thus system modifications, which never can be totally avoided, are achieved more easily.

- Procedures of the low-level language may be *linked* to the high-level language during a dialog session. Thus in applications not suited to high-level programming one can switch to low-level programming. However, use of the low-level language still requires considerable knowledge of computer hardware. In practice, therefore, its use will certainly be restricted to experts.

Although the low-level language and the high-level language fulfill entirely different requirements, they have a set of common language constructs. In fact there
exists a subset of syntactic rules which have exactly the same definitions in both
languages. Essentially these are the rules for

- formulation of expressions and

- program control structures.

The common subset is limited on either side by the machine orientation as well as
the problem orientation of the respective language. Nevertheless the similarity of
the two languages can facilitate the rewriting of tested algorithms from high to low
level language.

Details of the low-level language are described in ref. 9. In what follows we concentrate on the *high-level* language, since it is used in most applications. To enhance efficiency, besides the interpreter a compiler will be provided. The user decides the mode of translation from the actual problem structure. While the interpreter offers the full scope of language definitions, usage of the compiler will impose
some restrictions of the user, e.g. the dialog features are obviously not available.

4. Elements of the High-Level Language

The most important language features are summarized below. More details are given in
ref. 7. Some concepts used in this language have been taken from other languages[8].

Declaration and Data Types

For numerical computing and string processing the data types BOOL, STRING, INTEGER
and REAL are available. Since our application is image processing, we provided the
problem oriented data types IMAGE and FRAME. A series of images in an angiographic
study is represented by a three-dimensional image in the language. Frames represent
rectangular or arbitrarily shaped areas of an image (e.g. a particular vessel in a
kidney might be an arbitrarily shaped frame). The frames may have one, two or three
dimensions.

By indexing images with frames one has access to sub-images. For example, from a
series of 200 images (256 x 256 pixels) a sub-series with a frame given by the parameters x = 10-200, y = 1-256, z = 20-100 could be extracted like

```
IMAGE[10-200,1-256,20-100]            or by using key words for axis orientation
IMAGE[%Z=20-100, %X=10-200, %Y=1-256] or just
IMAGE[FRAME]                          if FRAME represents the desired three-
                                      dimensional region.
```

Declaration of objects may be done implicitly from the context or explicitly by a
DECLARE statement, e.g.

        DECL I1,I2:IMAGE, X,Y,Z:REAL, TABLE[100]:INTEGER

User Defined Data Types

Users may define their own problem oriented data types, a feature well known and
appreciated from other programming languages. For example, the user could combine a
picture taken from a patient with his identification into a new structured data type,
called RECORD:

        STRUCT RECORD=IDENT:PERSON, ITEM:IMAGE
        STRUCT PERSON=NAME[10]:STRING, AGE[3]:INTEGER

RECORD itself is composed of another structured type, called PERSON and an object of
primitive type IMAGE. The components of the structured types can be accessed by numerical indices or by identifying names, as in the example IDENT, ITEM, NAME, AGE.

Current Variables

When working intensively with one object, e.g. trying a number of manipulations on
an image, it is awkward to refer to this object always by its name. Better practice
is to identify the object *currently* in use by a special symbol. Thus there may exist
a current representation of each data type, primitive or structured. It is identified by the type name and the character $, e.g.

        IMAGE$[FRAME$]+REAL$

means addition of the current real number to an area of the current image, defined
by the current frame.

Reserved Names

Some special purpose memories, e.g. two fast 256 x 256 8-bit memories for images are
part of the hardware. In the dialog language they are represented as pre-defined objects with reserved names. To avoid conflicts with user-defined names the special
sign '%' always must precede a reserved name. The hardware supplied image memories
for example are integrated into the language as

        %MEM1[256,256,1]and %MEM2[256,156,1]

of type IMAGE.

Control Structures

A well-proven set of control structures was selected for the system. Iteration is provided through a FOR, WHILE or REPEAT loop, conditional execution through an IF...THEN...ELSE, whereby the ELSE clause is optional.

Examples:

```
FOR 10 →IUPTO 100 → UP DO<STATEMENT>
IF IMAGEȢ → I<LEVEL THEN 0 → I ELSE IxI → I
```

The last example requires comment. An image is assigned to I. The condition will be tested for each element of image I and the THEN or ELSE exit is taken depending on the result of the test. Thus execution of the condition for an image involves implicit execution of a loop. The above statement squares each image element above a given threshold and zeroes the rest.

Case selection is performed by a sequence of IF...THEN... Statements, guarded by DOCASE...ODCASE, e.g.

```
DOCASE
    IF    RESULT EQ A THEN PRINT A
    IF    RESULT EQ B THEN PRINT B
    ELSE  PRINT 'FALSE'
ODCASE
```

The first TRUE condition is selected for execution.

A simplified loop structure allows iteration in an array without specifying any loop indices, e.g.

```
DECL ARRY[256]:INTEGER
LOOP ARRY[X] DO X → ARRY
```

Iteration is performed for all elements of the object ARRY. The dummy name 'X' is only used to identify the current index in each iteration step. This loop stores the numbers 1 to 256 in ascending order into ARRY.

Expressions

Expressions are evaluated strictly from left to right, without hierarchy of operators. Parantheses may be used to override this rule. Assignment also obeys these rules, as the example indicates:

$$XY \rightarrow LEVEL + (FPARM+100. \rightarrow X) \rightarrow XY$$

The result is LEVEL=XY and X=FPARM+100. and XY=LEVEL+X.

Procedures

Procedures are divided into two classes,

- Internal Procedures (PROC) and
- External Procedures (XPROC).

Internal procedures (referred to as procedure) are program modules generated inter-actively in the high level language. *External procedures* form the link between dia-log programs and low-level programs. Internal and external procedures are declared in a parallel manner. The handling of parameters is the same for both cases.

Depending on the context the user may select from several notations for the passing of parameters:

- *functional* notation

- *operational* notation, for up to two parameters

- *keyword*   notation, for selection of specific parameters

This is illustrated by the following procedure:

```
PROC SUB (FIRST,SECOND:IMAGE)
IF ABS(FIRST-SECOND) LT LEVEL THEN  0 → FIRST
RETURN
```

If applied to images belonging to an angiographic series this procedure would elimi-nate static regions, i.e. only dynamic changes above a given intensity level would be preserved.

The procedure may be called in one of the following equivalent ways:

```
SUB(I1,I2)
I1 SUB I2
SUB with FIRST=I1 & & SECOND=I2
```

Procedure SUB can be transformed to an external procedure by the declaration:

```
XPROC SUB(FIRST,SECOND:IMAGE): XSUB
```

where XSUB is an arbitrary name referring to an entry point in the low-level lan-guage.

Thus depending on the efficiency required, one may choose to generate either a procedure in the high-level language or an external procedure in the low-level language. External procedures turned out to benefit not only the user but also the system programmer. During implementation they are extremely useful in a kind of bootstrap procedure. Thus the language definition need not have contained any operations at all from the beginning. Only the general concept of procedures is provided in the syntax as well as the means to generate them. Just for convenience some primitive, hardware supported, operations like arithmetic operations on integers were, in fact, included. Other operations can be added as desired. In particular all input/output functions as well as most functions to control specific hardware have been realized as external procedures. This technique guarantees a flexible adaption of the system to changing requirements without changes in the dialog language itself.

Default Parameters

In routine applications one mostly uses a set of standard parameters which seldom need to be changed. These parameters could receive pre-defined values. Nevertheless, the option must be preserved to change these parameters in special applications. For that purpose one may assign default values of parameters in the procedure definition, e.g.

```
PROC CONTRAST(I=IMAGE$,LLEV=MIN(I),ULEV=MAX(I):INTEGER)
256X(I-LLEV)/(ULEV-LLEV) → I
RETURN I
```

Variation of the thresholds LLEV, ULEV yield a contrast enhancement of the picture. In a call of this procedure the parameters LLEV, ULEV may be omitted. Then the specified default values will be taken. If explicitly stated, however, they override the respective defaults.

This feature proves to be particularly useful when combined with current variables. In the example the current image is assigned to I as default value. Calls to CONTRAST now can be of the form:

```
CONTRAST
```

All parameters are used as default from the procedure definition.

```
CONTRAST(IM,LLEV=10)
```

Only ULEV is used as default.

Dialog Specific Features

The dialog specific facilities are characterized by:

- The concept of *direct* and *indirect* execution as first realized in the language JOSS[11] and adapted by many other dialog systems. Procedures (also called *PARTS*) are created by the user in indirect mode, using the edit facilities of the language, while in direct mode each statement is immediately translated and executed. This concept unifies the usually separate steps of program writing, editing and execution via a job-control language.

- *Interruption facilities* - Interruption of execution may be programmed via a STOP command or forced by a user interrupt. One can inspect and modify values of variables, execute other programs and finally resume execution.

- *Use of undefined variables* - Variables need not be declared in advance. The user must supply the missing information when the system prompts him. This feature is particular useful in program development and testing.

Image Presentation and Menu Technique

We have paid special attention to image presentation. The hardware contains an (X,Y) CRT display (16 grey levels) with a light pen and a TV display (256 levels of brightness, up to 512 shades of colours) for presentation of x-ray images, with light pen and track ball.

The dialog language offers various means of display control. Objects of any type may arbitrarily be added to or deleted from a *Display File*, using the commands *DPLAY* and *DCLEAR*, e.g.

        DPLAY IMAGE$,'KIDNEY ANGIOGRAM'

would issue the current image and the text at the present beam position, while the command

        DCLEAR IMAGE$(FRAME$)

would delete an area defined by the current frame from the image being displayed.

Menu technique is provided by the *DMENU* command followed by one or more items describing the menu, e.g.:

        DMENU 500,20,LTHRLD,'SUBTRACT LOWER THRESHOLD'

Command DMENU itself is not primarily included in the language definition. Rather the language has been extended by this external procedure.

The command issues the text string at position (500,20) on the screen. Pointing to the text with the light pen causes execution of the procedure LTHRLD. Menu creation is greatly facilitated by utilization of structured data types, as the following example indicates:

```
STRUCT MENU=X,Y:INTEGER, EXC:PART, IDENT[203]:STRING
DECL LOWTHR=500,20,LTHRLD,'SUBTRACT...':MENU
DECL UPTHR=500,40,UTHRLD,'ADD...       ':MENU
DMENU LOWTHR, UPTHR,...
```

The first statement declares data type MENU. The two following statements generate the objects LOWTHR and UPTHR. The DMENU command displays these items and leaves the system waiting for light-pen input.

5. Present State

The dialog language has been successfully implemented on a PDP11/45 computer, using the low-level language. To gain experience with the application software for the analysis of x-ray angiograms a stand-alone system PROFI11 [12] has been implemented concurrently.

Presently we insert the algorithms of PROFI11 into the dialog-language system. This is easily performed by using the external procedure technique of the dialog language.

6. Conclusion

The dialog language described is an attempt to provide an efficient, simple and flexible tool for image analysis, especially for medical applications. *Efficiency* of execution and *dedicated hardware* support is guaranteed by combining a high-level interpreter/compiler system with a low-level programming language. *Problem oriented* data types and a versatile display control are adapted to image processing. The needs of the casual user and of routine operation are met be supplying a set of standard functions triggered either by *menu selection* via light pen or by pressing *push buttons*. The dialog technique facilitates production and maintenance of programs by the experienced user.

References

1. K.H. Hoehne, G. Nicolae, G. Pfeiffer, W.-R. Dix, W. Ebenritter, D. Novak, M. Boehm, B. Sonne, E. Buecheler; An Interactive System for Clinical Application of Angiodensitometry; GI-Fachtagung, Digitale Bildverarbeitung, München, 1977.
2. G.C. Nicolae, K.H. Hoehne; Digital Video System for Real-Time Processing of Image Series; DESY report DV 78/2, Hamburg, 1978.
3. K.H. Hoehne, M. Boehm, W. Erbe, G.C. Nicolae, G. Pfeiffer, B. Sonne; Functional Imaging - A New Tool for X-Ray Functional Diagnostics; DESY report DV 78/1, 1978.
4. K.H. Hoehne, K. Dahlmann, W.R. Dix, W. Ebenritter, G. Pfeiffer, K. Harm, R. Month; A Decentralized Computer System for Processing of Information from Heterogenous Medical Applications; Proc. of the 1st World Conf. on Medical Informations (MEDINFO 74), Stockholm, 1974, 95 - 100.
5. K.H. Hoehne, H. Lipps, G. Pfeiffer, W. Ebenritter, C. Schneider, R. Montz, D. Novak; ISAAC - Ein System für die interaktive Szintigramm-Aufnahme und Auswertung mit einem Computer, DESY report DV 73/1, Hamburg, 1973.
6. I. Kupka; Conversational Languages and Structural Interactive Programming. Formal Languages and Programming (Aguilar, R., Ad.), North-Holland, Amsterdan, 1976, 43 - 64.
7. G. Pfeiffer, K.H. Hoehne; A Dialog Language for Interactive Processing of Scintigraphic Data; Proc. of the 4th International Conference on Information Processing in Scintigraphy, Orsay, 1975, 221 - 232.
8. M. Klerer, J. Reinfels (Eds.); Interactive Systems for Experimental Applied Mathematics; Academic Press, New York and London, 1968.
9. G. Pfeiffer; SIMPL11, eine einfache Implementierungssprache für PDP11-Rechner; DESY report DV 76/2, Hamburg, 1976.
10. N. Wirth; PL360, A Programming Language for the 360; Computers Journal of ACM, Vol. 15, 1968, 37 - 74.
11. J.W. Smith; JOSSII: Design Philosophy; Ann. Rev. Aut. Progr., Vol. 6, 1970, 183 - 256.
12. M. Böhm; PROFI11 - A system for Processing and Retrieval of Functional Images; to be published.

Addresses of the Authors

Dipl.-Phys. G. Pfeiffer,   Notkestraße 85, D2000 Hamburg 52

Priv.-Doz. Dr. rer. nat. K.H. Hoehne, Notkestraße 85, D2000 Hamburg 52

SYSTEMS SUPPORT FOR THE ROUTINE REQUIREMENTS OF CLINICAL NEUROPHYSIOLOGY

Peter R. POCKLINGTON, Leopold GUTJAHR, Helmut KUENKEL,
Peter NIETHARDT, and Peter L. REICHERTZ
Department of Biometrics and Medical Informatics
Department of Clinical Neurophysiology and Experimental Neurology,
Medical School Hannover,
D-3000 Hannover 61, Federal Republic of Germany

In five years of co-operative work there have been developed within
the Departments of Medical Informatics and Clinical Neurophysiology
of the Hannover Medical School a wide variety of projects that are
in various stages of implementation, the spectrum covering the
documentation and analysis of Electroencepholograms, Nerve
Conduction Velocity- and Electro-Myographic observations, along
with epileptic seizure documentation and trend analysis. Using
examples from the routine projects we comment on the experience
gained and draw conclusions as to criteria to be fulfilled by
information systems intended for routine clinical usage.

E.E.G. DOCUMENTATION AND ANALYSIS

A pre-requisite for the development of a program for automatic EEG
analysis is the presence of enough documented and analyzed EEGs
that are both clearly documented with regard to their relationship
to a variety of EEG characteristics, while also containing no
effects that could lead to a falsification of statistical values,
these conditions having a decisive influence on the characteristics
selected as suitable for automatic analysis.

In 1968, HELMCHEN et al. remarked on the desirability of EDP
support in the documentation of electro-encephalographic data |4|
and accordingly designed a data acquisition form using Optical Mark
Recognition (OMR) techniques.

A slightly modified version of this form was introduced for EEG
documentation within the Department of Clinical Neurophysiology of
the Hannover Medical School in 1971. The initial processing

routines contained no formal check routines for the medical consistency of the data recorded and a retrospective study carried out in 1972 |11| analyzing 6434 EEGs showed an error rate of up to 70% for those items recorded by the clinicians requesting that an EEG be carried out, with an error rate of between 5 and 15% for the recording of the visual EEG interpretation, for which the doctors carrying out the data acquisition were highly motivated and trained in the use of OMR forms. The introduction of the general optical mark reader form processing program AMAP |6|, the system design of which includes an obligatory consistency and completeness check routine for each medical application incorporated, resulted in the creation of an extensive error check routine taking into account the results of this previous analysis. By this means logical inconsistencies were detected upon initial processing of the form, so that failures in documentation could be corrected soon afterwards. The error rate was reduced by half upon introduction of this checking routine but we noted that, after this initial improvement, we were not able to achieve any marked further improvement. We noted also to our disappointment, that the corrections were made in order to pass through the check routine, without referring to the original EEG tracing, since this was, in most cases, already in the archive for recording on microfilm. As a consequence of the above we decided that the most satisfactory method of documentation would be by means of an interactive data acquisition system, the data being recorded directly while the original EEG tracing is at hand.

Accordingly, an interactive system was developed within the medical information system DIES (Data Interpretation and Evaluation System |8|) for the EEG documentation. The dialogue consists of a fixed set of frames for the recording of the background activity, followed by selected frames depending on pathological findings in the EEG (e.g. see Fig. 1a). Plausibility checks are provided for both intra-frame and inter-frame recordings so that only complete and logically consistent data are archived. The program generates a report containing a summary of the input, supplemented with the doctors observations that are noted in free-text format in the final frame.

Due to the development of both batch (OMR) and on-line (interactive display) systems (see Figs. 1a,1b), we are in a position to ensure continuity in documentation even in cases of severe system disturbance, the format of the records archived being identical for both systems.

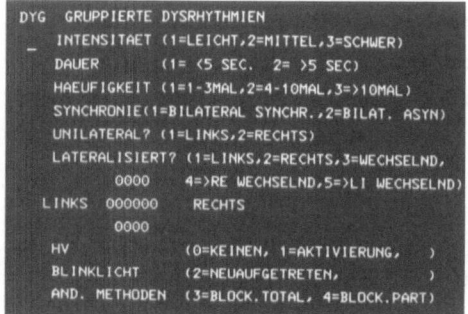 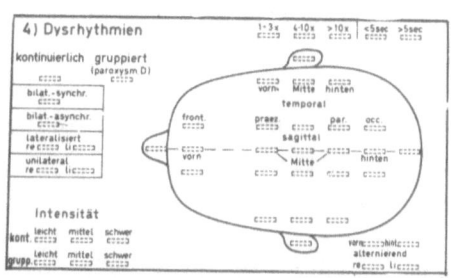

Fig. 1 EEG-Documentation by means of a) interactive display, b) OMR techniques.

In a further retrospective study an aspect of the documentation was checked that had, prior to the introduction of the automatic check routine, an error rate of 40%. Upon re-checking the documentation against the case-histories of the patients this error was reduced to 5%. A further check of error free records against the case-histories, however, resulted also in a 10% error, due to the physician recording plausible but incorrect findings on the OMR forms.

While recognizing the possibility for errors mentioned above and taking into account that the effects of inter- and intra-observer variations result in inherent uncertainties, the data undergo frequent analysis regarding questions of clinical interest. One of the interesting aspects considered was the likelihood of epileptic attacks given specific patterns in the EEG. From our extensive documentation (covering approximately 14000 first registered EEGs from Berlin and Hannover), we observed, for example, that, contrary to the traditional beliefs, the probability of epileptic attacks given a specific EEG pattern was only 63% |3|, i.e. it is not possible to draw highly reliable conclusions regarding epileptic seizures given this specific EEG pattern, and further diagnostic tools should be used before reaching any decision.

A suite of programs has also been developed to provide routine service information such as, for example, the identification information for EEG recordings displaying certain characteristics (for use by the project team researching into automatic EEG analysis), or, of a more administrative nature, a list of the EEGs evaluated for each physician, or those recorded by each EEG-technician.

NERVE CONDUCTION VELOCITY DOCUMENTATION AND ANALYSIS

Another problem in clinical neurophysiology that we considered concerns the diagnostic value of measurements of nerve conduction velocity. In this case, a project was designed in order to improve the accuracy and ease with which a founded judgement of the measured values could be made. Measurements of latency and distance are made at points determined by four coordinates - the stimulated nerve, the path measured (e.g. upper arm, thigh, etc.), the side of the body (left or right) and the type of conduction velocity (e.g. motoric, sensible or mixed). Of the theoretically 200 such points it was decided to establish norm values for those of most clinical relevance (i.e. those most frequently investigated) resulting in norm values for 1/3 of the points.

When describing functions and functional relationships on or about the human body it is, however, not sufficient merely to take into account a small number of variables (in this case the four co-ordinates). With respect to the measurement of nerve conduction velocities and related amplitudes it has been shown |1, 5, 9| that age, body-size, weight, sex and skin temperature also have major influences that have to be taken into account when analyzing the results.

For the first stage of the project an OMR form was designed that allowed the clinician to record all relevant data. In this case again rigorous completeness and consistency checks were performed on the data, and at this stage a report was generated containing

the data recorded and the evaluation thereof in prose form. While
this format was useful for data control purposes its clinical
acceptance was minimal.

After eighteen months of routine data acquisition the second phase
of the project was started, in which the data were analyzed in
order to obtain better estimates of the norm values, and to produce
reports in a format that would receive clinical acceptance.

The so-called independent factors, body-size, weight etc. correlate
amongst themselves. The degree to which the factors that have no
correlation to one another influence the nerve conduction velocity
is expressed by means of partial regression co-efficients that are
calculated using multiple regression techniques (see Figs. 2a,2b).

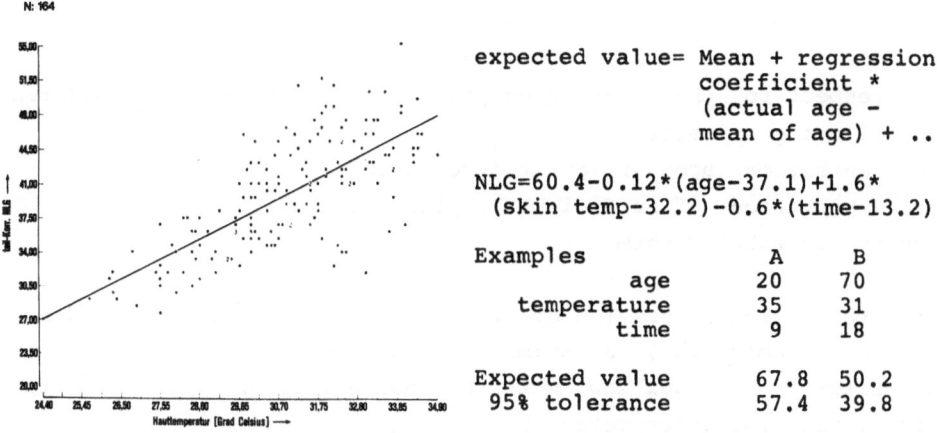

expected value= Mean + regression
coefficient *
(actual age –
mean of age) + ..

$NLG=60.4-0.12*(age-37.1)+1.6*(skin\ temp-32.2)-0.6*(time-13.2)$

Examples		A	B
age		20	70
temperature		35	31
time		9	18
Expected value		67.8	50.2
95% tolerance		57.4	39.8

Fig. 2a) Ulnar Nerve, Sensible, Hand
         Partial Regression between partially corrected sensible
         NLG of negative phase (dependant) and skin-temperature
Fig. 2b) Example of an equation using multiple regression
         coefficients

Apart from the time-of-day (that has a phasic influence on the
conduction velocity |2, 12|) the influencing factors are linear so
that the individual effects of the partial regression co-efficients
could be additively calculated with the result undergoing an F-test
as to its significance. If the F-test is significant the factor may
be considered to contribute to reducing the unexplained variance of

the conduction velocity. In order to clarify the relevance of this method consider the following (Fig. 2b):

Measurements were made at the same points on two patients. For a seventy year old patient examined at 6 p.m. the expected value was 50 m/s, while for a 20 year old patient examined at 9 a.m. the expected value was 67 m/s. The tolerance level for the younger patient was 57 m/s whereas that for the older patient was 40 m/s. This demonstrates that for the same areas of observation completely different values can only be correctly interpreted by taking into account the factors influencing the nerve conduction velocity.

The practical value of this project lies in the production of better estimates and an up to 40% improvement in accuracy for the areas under consideration and resultant improvements in the interpretation of the results.

With respect to the re-designed presentation format we considered the following criteria:
- concentration upon relevant information
- the provision of sufficient explanation
- output in tabular form

Prior to the interpretation of the recordings the report contains, for each examination, a summary of the patient's data and an explanatory text dealing with the abbreviations used and the methods used for interpretation.

EMG DOCUMENTATION AND RECORD LINKAGE

A further project for the Department of Clinical Neurophysiology covers the recording on OMR forms the results of EMG examinations and the routine provision of reports containing a summary of the findings in free-textual form, combined with their interpretation as entered using the Clinical Text Inquiry System |7| that functions as a sub-system of DIES.

Due to the inter-relationship of the examinations performed in the Department for Clinical Neurophysiology, (e.g. nearly all EMG examinations have an associated NCV) consideration has recently

been given to the question of record linkage to which end a general
header section has been designed (see Fig.3) for all Clinical
Neurophysiology applications as a pre-requisite to the production
of reports and analyses combining information from several disjoint
examinations.

Furthermore, the insertion of relevant sub-sets of the data arising
in the Department for Clinical Neurophysiology into the patient
data-base of the MSH allow for deeper analysis and interpretation
of these data in combination with data from other facilities within
the Hannover Medical School, e.g. over the Patient Information
Display System |10|.

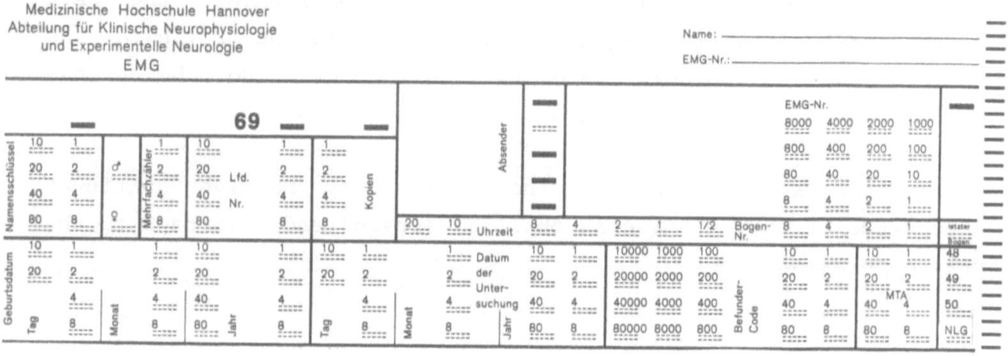

Fig. 3. Common OMR form header section for Clinical Neurophysiology
applications

CONCLUSIONS

In conclusion we would like to point out some of the features that
we consider to be essential for information systems that are to be
accepted in routine clinical usage:

- The incorporation as early as possible of extensive check
routines to improve data validity and integrity.

- Flexibility with respect to data acquisition. The user should be able to select the means of data acquisition most suited to his requirements as opposed to those of the computer system.

- Sufficient consideration must be given to the presentation of the results in a form clearly understandable to those not immediately concerned in the development of the system.

- There must be a constant dialogue between designer and user of any information system to ensure that difficulties are foreseen and taken care of before a wall of resistance has been allowed to be built up.

- In order to improve the reliability of the data interpretation, the data recorded should be reviewed and re-checked at sporadic intervals, this checking not being only restricted to obviously incorrect observations.

Information systems in medicine will only receive continued acceptance if they provide an obvious service and advantage to the user population.

REFERENCES

|1| Gutjahr,L.:
Normal Values of Neural Conduction Velocity.
Electroencephalography and Clinical Neurophysiology, 40 (1966) 203

|2| Gutjahr,L.:
Circadian Rhythm of the Nerve Conduction Velocity in Correlation to the Skin Temperature.
Presentation, Congress for Applied Chronobiology and Trends toward Chronotherapy.
Ravenna 17-19 October 1974

|3| Gutjahr,L., Machleidt W., Ferber G.:
The significance of 'Seizure Patterns' for the Diagnosis of Epilepsy
Der Nervenarzt, in press.

|4| Helmchen,H., Kuenkel,H., Oberhofer,G., Penin,H.:
EEG-Befund-Dokumentation mit optischem Markierungsleser.
Der Nervenarzt, 39 (1968) 408-413

|5| Lang,A.H., Bjorquist,S.E.:
Die Nervenleitgeschwindigkeit peripherer nervenbeeinflussender konstitutioneller Faktoren beim Menschen.
EEG/EMG 2-4 (1970) 162-170

|6| Pocklington,P.R.:
AMAP - A General OMR Form Evaluation Program
Meth. Inform. Med., 12 (1973) 211-222

|7| Pocklington,P.R.:
CTIS - Clinical Text Inquiry System
In: Reichertz,P.L.: Medizinische Informatik 1975,
Springer Verlag, Heidelberg (1976) 118-123

|8| Pocklington,P.R.:
The necessity for, requirements of, and basic design of a General Data Interpretation and Evaluation System(DIES)
In: Anderson,J., Forsythe,J.M.: Medinfo 74,
North Holland Publishing Co:, Amsterdam (1975) 411-418

|9| Wagmann,J.H.:
Maximal Conduction Velocity of Moto-ulnar Nerve of Various Ages and Sizes
J. Neurophysiology 15 (1952) 235-244

|10| Weingarten,W., Sauter,K., Weigelt,D., Reichertz,P.L.:
The Patient Information Display System and its User Reactions
Institut de Recherche d'Informatique et d'Automatique,
Communications des Tables Rondes XV1-XV15 (1975)

|11| Wingert,F.:
PAULA - Program zur Auswertung logischer Ausdruecke
Meth. Inform. Med., 12 (1972) 96-103

|12| Wyrick,W., Duncan,A.:
Within-Day Trends of Motorlatency and Nerve Conduction Velocity in Males and Females.
Amer. J. Physiolog. Med. 49 (1970) 307-315

On the Expression of Relations in Medicine: Linguistic Aspects

B.J. Kostrewski
Centre for Information Science
The City University, London EC1, UK

J. Anderson
Department of Medicine
Kings College Hospital, London SE5, UK

1. Introduction

The medical vocabulary has to encapsulate concepts for a variety of levels and
applications and the advent of computer processing has highlighted linguistic communication problems, firstly at the level of individual communication and recording
of disease and secondly across the artificial boundaries of related disciplines
(Anderson, 1968). The increased understanding of basic biological processes, applied
in conjunction with developments from other sciences has contributed to the complexity
of information and hence language at all levels of application. This, coupled with
the extended limits of medicine to embrace the Hippocratic concept of the 'total
man', has resulted in a vast terminology relevant to the practice of medicine.
Language based data in medicine has its main applications in patient care, medical
education , training and research.

1.1 Patient Care

Here medical records have a variety of applications
(i) The systematic recording of disease, its development, diagnosis, treatment and
progress.
(ii) As medical decision support.
(iii) As an educational aid.
The information in the medical record reflects the synthesis of information from a
variety of sources and, as such, is at the basis of all medical information systems.
Here, language standardisation has implications at the following levels:
(i) the interpersonal level - for the unambiguous definition of data of particular
significance in group practice for communication between doctors;
(ii) in mechanized systems, for the unambiguous retrieval of relevant information;
(iii) for the collection of statistical data for administrative, medico-legal and
planning purposes at local, regional, national and international levels;
(iv) for the collection of aetiological data for prevention and control.

1.2 Education

The aim in medical education is to enable the student to construct a cognitive framework within the bounds of what is known and to illustrate decision making
and problem solving. An unambiguous terminology is essential for framework formulation and for the definition of relations between data.

1.3 Research

Research need is highlighted at several levels; the analysis of patient records, to define research problems and theoretical research based on experimentation and creative endeavour and its documentation for subsequent storage and retreival.

2. Language Processing

Language information processing and transfer can be considered from the following vantage points:

1. subject related models;
2. semantic levels;
3. cognitive frameworks.

All three are interrelated both conceptually and by virtue of being language linked. However, in this paper we shall concentrate on 1 and 2, since 3 relates to a conceptual level which goes beyond language and reflects a process of abstraction. Ultimately of course, such abstractions have to be expressed in language but they are independent of any particular language; (this point would be disputed by Whorf (1956) who argued that our native language does influence our cognitive processes). However, with respect to standardised reference languages there is a danger that excessive rigidity could have a stifling effect on creative thought and precipitate a stagnant terminology. Here we define reference languages as structured, controlled vocabularies e.g. classification schemes and thesauri, embracing the terminology of a defined area of discourse.

3. Models and Reference Languages

It is now generally agreed that science does not only develop by the accretion of discoveries or 'truths' about the universe and the nature of life but that the framework which we impose on the perception of phenomena plays an important role in their interpretation. In the communication of phenomena we thus have the complex interaction of perception, model relation and language. The early cultures perceived a totality of the universe and at the time of Plato the world was conceived as a vast system of classified and hierarcharized sympathies. This approach is reflected in the divinatory nature of the early divisions of the universe. Thus the Chinese Yin and Yang is conceptually similar to the war and peace of Heraclean Ionism, and Emerodes love and strife, the relationship between the two major divisions being that of complementation. The link between the early and present day classifications is a tenuous one, since modern nomenclature and classification has been vastly influenced by Cartesian philosophy and reductionism and subsequent positivism which sought to establish proof of existence as the ultimate criterion of reality. Thus modern classifications and reference languages are very much entity orientated with a proliferation of terminology seeking to identify the ultimate or most specific.

The reductionist method has had a particularly strong impact on nomenclature in medicine. Firstly this approach decreased the capacity of the classificatory systems to reflect the dynamic state of interaction and transformation and secondly resulted in a proliferation of terminology with an accretion of synonyms and eponymous disease names. The latter are of particular importance to medicine since the conditions which they delineate, reflect a complex network of relationships. Relationships within defined classes of data tend to be reflected by the hierarchical classification establishing the similarities in terms of origin and structure rather than in terms of function and control. For example, in aetiological agents of disease their different structures are made plain but the functional relationships have to be contextually defined.

The concept of hierarchy appears to have been a construct of western philosophy, since the Japanese language has no word which can encapsulate this notion of domination and subordination (Heidegger 1959). The idea itself stems from Plato and Aristotle but the term was introduced by Pseudo-Dionysius in relation to priestly and angelic hierarchies. Hierarchical ordering in terms of reflecting degrees of similarity has been a connecting thread of the majority of classificatory systems and has had a strong influence in the structuring of the natural sciences. Such constructs impose a rigidity upon the classificatory framework.

Atherton (1965) suggested that any method of creating relations is a system of classification. Recently there has been an attempt to establish a more flexible faceted system, independent of a rigid framework but encapsulating the vocabulary of a well-defined universe of discourse. The limits are contextual and the relationships implicit by virtue of content.

A subsequent development has been the incorporation of an explicit syntactic structure. An example of such a system is SNOMED (Systematized Nomenclature of Medicine). Such syntactic systems allow for the unambiguous expression of an item of information but do not reflect an overall semantic structure. Their strength lies in their high degree of structure with respect to the reflection of functional classes within the framework of a defined application.

4. The Relationship Between Structure, Language and Reference Languages

The formulation of a model, based on metaphor,has become an accepted tool of scientific methodology. Such structures break away from the rigidity of accepting the existence of the ultimate reality and accept instead an interpretation based on the concept of models of reality and the establishment of relations between the model components. Such models are of necessity language based and should incorporate the appropriate vocabulary within the total framework.

Most of the linguistic work investigating the nature of semantics or meaning has been carried out on the language of everyday discourse where, in spite of a fairly loose framework, certain inferences and expectations are implicit. The inquiry into semantics is relatively recent and concentrates on natural text; work by Fodor and Katz (1964) being the earliest which is frequently cited. Semantics was seen as being an attribute of syntax and thus related to meaning at the sentence level. However, McCawley (1968) demonstrated with the sentence "My buxom neighbour

is the father of two" that syntactic sense may be semantic nonsense. Thus the semantic component of language must have some correspondence to reality or a fact as we
know it to exist. Such frameworks of reference are culture related and built up
during a life time.

This raises the question of the overall role of syntax in relation to semantics.
Moreover, syntax cannot be separated from the lexical components of the language,
and the extent to which specific meaning can be conveyed by any one particular
language is dependent upon the peculiarities of the language itself. Thus, such
time linked medical concepts as prognosis or pharmaco-kinetics could not be captured
in the Hopi (Indian) language which cannot convey the notion of time.

Specialist vocabularies serving a particular reference group can be considered
as being equivalent to the natural language of a particular culture or nation. In
the case of the specific vocabulary the frames of reference are more clear cut than
in everyday discourse and relate to the overall structural framework of the subject
under consideration.

The communication process is the underpinning of good medical practice. This
presents problems since, in making humanity its primary concern, it incorporates
two broad levels of language namely the everyday and the specialist terminology.
Each level is multi-faceted, reflecting national nuances at the patient/physician
encounter and the specialist vocabulary drawn from the multitude of specialities
now being applied to the practice of medicine. The distillation of this information
into an unambiguous reference language is essential for structural synthesis and
subsequent application. The adaptation of a reference language to the function that
it is intended to perform can be considered in systems terms. For example, what
are the linguistic structures needed to designate meaning at defined levels of
medical application?

5. Levels of Designation

These can be considered as reflecting the interaction of two linguistic
parameters:
1. The designatory parameter relates to the least meaningful unit of language whose
complexity is limited by context and the level of application.
2. Syntactic or combinatory parameter relates to the linguistic levels necessary
to effect meaning within contextual limits.

5.1 Designatory Levels

The emphasis is on meaningful combinations since, obviously, the less complex
the structure of the word string the greater the number of "meaningful combinations"
that it can enter into. Hence the introduction of the term 'designator' since this
implies an operational unit whose function is contextually defined. Designators
may be character strings such as prefixes and suffixes, keywords or compound phrases
which convey a particular notion. We have based this approach on the assumption

that in order to effect a specific structure we need to introduce the concept of exclusiveness of components and specificity of relations, which jointly interact to form a specific structure. Naturally the narrower the context in which designator is used the less complex is its structure.

5.2 Syntactic Levels

Syntax here is defined as that linguistic tool which allows the sequencing of linguistic units in a manner which will convey a particular meaning. We have based the following syntactic levels on the definition of Lamb (1966). These have been identified in relation to their application in medical language data processing.

1. The phonological level. Here the combinations of particular phonemes (symbols) to convey an identifiable combination. Thus MAMM- or MAST- while incomplete in themselves, identify terminology relating to the breast. Sense and nonsenses sequences are relatively easy to establish at this level.

2. The word level. Here a sequencing of symbols is used to denote a particular notion. Ideally such a sequence should be unique and unambiguous. However, this is also the level of synonymy and homonymy which can be seen as a breakdown of the linguistic system in terms of exclusiveness of components. A further elaboration of this level is the compound word which is particularly common in medical terminology and reflects synthesis within and between levels 1 and 2.

3. The phrase level. In medicine observations and conditions are frequently expressed as phrases, e.g. 'high blood pressure' or 'pain removing agent'. Subsequently the concepts conveyed by such phrases frequently become designated by a single word e.g. 'hypertension' or 'analgesic' respectively and thus become designators operating at level 2.

4. The sentence level. Here the sense and nonsense sequences are fairly clear cut. However, even when the syntax is incorrect, meaning can be discerned after a pause for reflection. This points out that there is reference to an overall framework, as does the fact that a sentence can be syntactically correct and yet meaningless. This is the level of Chomsky's innate "Generative Grammar" and since this is also the level of "Transformational Grammar", which can be considered as being equivalent to being a programming sequence appropriate to another language in order to effect the same function (meaning), this again points to reliance upon a reference model or structure.

5. The semantic level. Here syntax conveys the overall meaning that relates to a macrostructure which can be broken down into application linked substructures.

Ideally in a reference language a transformation sequence from one level of syntax to the next should be incorporated. Such transformations occur naturally and are quite clear cut at levels 1 and 2. In normal discourse level 4 to level 5 transformations are automatic, although the reference related mechanism through which this occurs is not fully understood. Different levels of syntax need to be incorporated into medical   reference languages for different applications. These

syntactic levels are seen as reflecting relations between notions and thus levels
of relations (as well as their associated notions) are also seen to exist.

6. Implications for Levels of Syntactic Relations in Reference Languages

At all levels of application the structure of reference languages should be
such as to both capture and reflect that complex amalgam of continuity and change
that is so characteristic of medicine. Levels 1 and 2 are concerned with the
synthesis of units identifying notions or components of notions. Into this category falls the straightforward formation of compound words by novel juxtaposition
of word strings to designate new meanings which the structure should be capable of
absorbing. Provided that the subject area is well defined, the contextual framework defines the limits of application of word strings and thus has an implicit
semantic framework equivalent to levels 4/5.

In mechanized processing the principle of meaningful unit of level 1 and subsequent syntheses to level 2 has been utilized by Wingert (1977), who segments the
suffixes, associated with particular word roots building up a network of monophemes
which can define the syntactic/semantic role (and thus within contextual limits to
simulate levels 4 and 5 with some redundancy). This approach results in a reduction
of dictionary and file size and also allows for direct translation between languages.

Level 3 represents the meeting point between every day language and its
translation into an unambiguous technical vocabulary; it reflects observation,
change, assimilation and progress. Level 4 involves the simulation of syntactically
sound statements at a high level of specificity which define a fairly specific
condition or mode of treatment. Such a framework is relatively easy to simulate
provided that the nature of relations between the components remains relatively
constant. It is important to appreciate that at this level the syntactic structure
reflects specific statements and not an explicit relationship to an overall structure.
Such systems are applicable to the encoding of patient records where specificity is
of paramount importance. In practice, unless operating in a specialist application
contextual limits at this level are difficult to define. Hence the designators
need to be unique, highly specific, and unambiguous; this results in a vast reference
language. SNOMED is an example of a reference language operating at this level.
Each statement relates to a medical incident. The drawback of such systems is that
they do not mirror the semantic structure relating to an overall event. Level 4,
the sentence level in natural language, is not the exact equivalent of level 4 in
reference languages since the latter encapsulates a wider range of concepts than
would be possible at the single sentence level. It is thus difficult to delineate
the point of transition from level 4 to level 5 in reference languages.

Semantic structures must of necessity be application related and reflect
different levels and facets of the overall structure of medicine and yet be autonomous within themselves. They should embody the characteristics of wholeness,

transformation and self-regulation inherent in systems in their own right and yet be capable of being incorporated in transformations to a higher level (Kostrewski et al 1978).

At the semantic level syntax is the most complex. Here the model structure and relations must be most accurately reflected. Moreover, in terms of both complexity of structure and diversity of representation it presents the greatest challenge. Semantic frameworks can be considered for a variety of levels both in terms of specificity of content and level of application. Model representation in reference languages at this level amounts to carrying out an analysis of the language of the field of knowledge, and identification of the manner of representation generally involves macrodata both in terms of volume and context.

The importance of model structuring and implications for processing language by computer have been stressed by Schank (1975). However, most of the work done has concentrated on literary text with implications for automatic translation and artificial intelligence, and while this applies to the processing of medical literature, this is only one type of a variety of medical data. A similar approach was taken by Pratt (1973) when deriving SNOP (Systematized Nomenclature of Pathology) which laid the foundations for SNOMED. Here it was not the full text that was being examined but phrases from pathology reports which already represented condensed and structured data. The identification of the linguistic devices used in the expression of relations resulted in a syntactically structured reference language. Another approach deriving a reference language from text was adopted by Wolf-Terroine (1972) who used statistical methods for word frequencey and co-occurence for the derivation of a reference language SABIR-C within the contextually defined field of cancer.

Elsewhere (Major et al 1978) we have presented a model for the representation of linguistic parameters as components of meaning based on Saussure's model of paradigmatic and syntagmatic linguistic parameters. We have shown the gradual shift from structures developed through primarily syntagmatic relations to their assimilation at the paradigmatic level. This can be seen as reflecting a new fixed position within the subject related model. Such synthesis, achieved through the concatenation of relations, can be seen at all levels of syntax, and it is the understanding of these processes that will give an insight into the nature of transformation relations between syntactic levels. Such linguistic models are an aid in the design of reference languages which require appropriate semantic power for their application. As yet we have insufficient understanding of linguistics to allow expression of total semantic structures.

The very complexity of such frameworks makes their simulation by appropriate reference structures exceedingly difficult. At this level medical reference languages have to perform a variety of functions embodying what is known about medicine and reflect a multifaceted set of relations. The diverse range of applications of language data at the semantic level includes education (the building up of the reference structures),patient records, collection of data for the delivery of health care at local, regional,national and international levels and the representation of library material. Each of these applications presents different demands on the capabilities of a reference language (Major et al 1978).

Patient records require specificity of expression both in terms of absolute accuracy of terminology and definition of relationships. This requirement is partially fulfilled by SNOMED which is capable of simulating syntactically correct structures of level 4. Thus in order to allow level 4 to contribute to the formulation of a semantic structure of level 5 (useful in education) a definition of transfer relations is needed. The collection of data for the delivery of health care requires a reference language with a broad inference structure both in terms of vocabulary and relations· The utilization of information gained from library data as well as patient care is an important aspect of scientific research; the nature of most modern research relates to the establishment of new relations within the model. Reference languages for such systems need a highly developed and flexible set of semantic relations to allow for heuristic interaction and to stimulate creative thinking.

7. Implications for Computer Processing

In human discourse relations are usually implicit. For computer processing they have to be made completely explicit. The simulation of levels of the human communication process represents an appropriate approach. Thus the simulation must recognize the contextual relationship.

Within the limits of present day technology several alternatives are available for the definition of relations in computerized systems handling language data. Firstly by the utilization of the contextual parameters of a language to delineate a specific area of discourse Within this framework the implicit relationships between entities become definable. Secondly the expansion of context, both in terms of application and coverage, demands a definition of relationships by the identification of the linguistic units involved and their expression. Within a rigorous scientific framework the linguistic devices used to express particular relationships are limited and hence can be defined and linked to a functional or relational indicator. Thirdly in larger systems both in terms of coverage and application the contextual parameter assumes wider dimensions, since at this level relations become multifaceted. Thus the contextual definition of relations is important. This can be achieved by partitioning and demands the definition of classes, ideally within a flexible framework.

References

ANDERSON, J. (1968) The Computer: Medical Vocabulary and Information. Brit. Med. Bull. 24 (3) 194-198.

ATHERTON, P. (1965) Classification Research. Proceedings of the 2nd International Study Conference. Copenhagen, Munsgaard.

HEIDEGGER, M. (1959) On the Way to Language. Harper and Row (1971). First published in German by Verlag Gunther Neske (1959).

KATZ, J. & FODOR, J. (1964) The Structure of Semantic Theory. In: The Structure of Language, J. Fodor & J. Katz (eds.), Prentice-Hall, Englewood Cliffs, N.J.

KOSTREWSKI, B., COOPER, D., ANDERSON, J. (1978) The Physician/Computer Dialogue, paper presented at WAMI Conference, Toulouse, March 13th - 17th.

LAMB, S. (1966) Outline of Stratificational Grammar. Georgetown Univ. Press, Washington D.C.

MAJOR, P., KOSTREWSKI, B. & ANDERSON, J. (1978) Analysis of Semantic Structures of Medical Languages. Part I. A Framework for the Semantic Power of Reference Languages. Medical Informatics (in press).

MAJOR, P., KOSTREWSKI, B. & ANDERSON, J. (1978) Analysis of the Semantic Structures of Reference Languages: Part II. Analysis of the Semantic Poser of MeSH, ICD and SNOMED. Medical Informatics (in press).

McCAWLEY, J. (1968) The Role of Semantics in Grammar. In: Universals in Linguistic Theory, E. Bach and R. Harris (eds). Holt, Linehart & Winston, N.Y.

PRATT, A.W. (1973) Medicine, Computers and Linguistics, Advances in Biomed. Engineering 3, 97-140 (Academic Press: New York).

SCHANK, R.C. (1975) Conceptual Information Processing. North Holland Publishing Company, Amsterdam.

WHORF, B.L. (1956) Language Thought and Reality: Selected Writings of Benjamin Lee Whorf, J.B. Carroll (ed) MIT Press Cambridge, Mess and Wiley, New York.

WINGERT, F. (1977) Morphosyntactic Analysis of Compound Word Forms in Computational Linguistics in Medicine edited by Scheider, W. & Sagvall-Hein, A.L.. North Holland Publishing Company.

WOLF-TERROINE, M., D. RIMBERT & B. ROUALT (9172) Improved Statistical Methods for Automatic Construction of a Medical Thesaurus. Methods Inform. Med. 11 (2) 104-113.

SOFTWARE OF DIALOGUES :
PHYSICIAN - COMPUTER - PATIENT

A.Brodziak
Gastroenterology Clinic of
Silesian School of Medicine
Computer Laboratory
Katowice, Poland

Direct dialogue between medical personnel and computer is becoming more frequent as a means of storing data in medical information systems. In some cases it is intended that the patient has direct contact with the computer terminal. One of the uses of computers in medicine is the automatic collection of data from the patient during the initial medical interview. Such interviews, though they cannot substitute a direct conversation with the doctor can be a valuable complement to collected data /it avoids forgetting certain important questions/. The procedure is not a burden for the doctor and does not take much time since the doctor only has to familiarize himself with the report printed out by the computer. The dialogue between patient and computer should satisfy the needs of the given medical centre. In other words, there should be the possibility of easy alteration by the doctor, or the hospital staff the questions to be asked. Up till now this has caused problems as the programing of a new version of the medical questionnaire has demanded a good deal of effort both from the computer scientists and doctors who prepare certain structured set of questions. This paper discusses the properties of the packet of basic programs which eliminate the necessity of writting new programs for every new interview or dialogue. The solution suggested is a system of programs which first of all collects from the doctor data about the interview, forms a suitable file of data, and then using this file is able to ask the patient questions.

Description of the anticipated transfer of information between physician, computer - scientist and computer.

To attain communication between the doctor and the computer, we propose to utilise four different mutually co - operating stage :

1/ The first stage of this requires the doctor to formulate the initial set of data using extremely simple notation /quasi - language/. The stage does not allow the direct introduction of the data set to the computer memory.

2/ The transitionary stage is action of the program, which accepts the notation formulated in stage 1 and "during the more difficult moments for the doctor" takes the initiative and imposes a dialogue during which the program demands essential detail.

3/ In stage there the initial phase of using the program, the doctor may need help from a computer programmer. The latter's function is, however, much simplified because of the existence of the initial notation. The reversal of roles may also take place at this strage. In other words, the writing of the initial structure and content of the dialogue specifies the problem to such an extent that the running of the program can be done by the computer programmer on the basis of the notation.

4/ The program mentioned in point 2, at the end of the run can on request print out the content of the formulated file. The print-out can be similar in format to the initial data set written by the doctor. The content print-out forms a kind of feed back of an information run.

The method of preparing the initial notation from the data.

Because of the speed with program runs, the doctor must be prepared to co-operate with the program by preparing the initial notation. The convenient way to prepare it is on sheets. For most interviews /medical questionnaires/ it is sufficient to anticipate the following elements of the notation.

1/ Line of standard text /'/

2/ Line of the text of the questions /trychotomic /*/ or numerical questions /+/ /. In the phase of the automatic collection of the interview, after displaying the question, the program must be stopped to anticipate the patient's answer.

3/ Data on necessary control of the logic the patient's answer to the question /C/.

4/ Data on conditional jumps /$/. These allow for the questions to be dependent on previous answers. For example, if a patient is male then the questions directed at females will be omitted. In other

words conditional jumps allow for a hierachical dendritic order of
the questions and texts.
5/ Data on unconditional jumps /S/.
6/ Terminator notation /E/.
Data of type C, S, Ø, E can be written by the doctor in natural
language. The introduction of the first symbols of these lines initiates the dialogue imposed by the program introducing data.

The organisation of programs and the description of their functioning.

The main part of the system is composed of two programs written in
FORTRAN. The first is used twice : 1/ For writing the structure and
report for the doctor. This program has built in basic functions
such as furnished by the standard program often known as an Editor.
In other words, it alternately makes use of two files on the disc
which remember the former and the new version of data about the structure of the interview. The writing of the structure of the interview
can therefore be carried out in stages. Files formulated by this program may be used by the second program conducting the interview with
the patient. The program remembers the data supplied by the patient,
prepares a report for the doctor and records the collected data in
a separate file. In the first phase it displays questions on the monitor enquiring on which peripheral the dialogue with the patient will
be carried out. In later phases, action of the program is observed
from that peripheral. At the end of the run it asks whether to prepare a report for the doctor. Then it enquires whether to memorize
the data in the "archival" file and finally whether there will be an
interview with a further patient.

A short description of the configuration of equipment used to run
the system and the checking of its functioning.

This system of programs was worked out for two types of hospital
information systems. The programs : LANDIA /from "language dialogue"/
and the DIAMAL /"dialogue avec le malade"/ written in FORTRAN run
firts on Texas Instruments 980 computer with a core memory size of
32 K words, equipped with disc memory units, basic terminal monitor

SILENT 700 ASR and with two displays. The equipment is in operation
in Centre de Calcul, Clinique de Maladies et de l'Encephale, l'Hospi-
tale Sainte-Anne, in Paris. The system discussed constitute a packet
of basic software independent of content of specific medical questionnaires. It can be run on the same installations for many different
purposes. At a later date I reconstructed this system on the basis
of the BASIC interpreter on the computer at the Gastroenterology
Clinic, the Silesian Medical School in Katowice. The computer terminals found in this Clinic are linked by telephone line with an ICL
computer of call size 128 K words, 28 bits. BASIC interpreter are
based on the GEORGE 3 operating system. The compiled programs allow
for the collection of completed questionnaires from the patient and
the collection from the medical personnel of data for the hospital
information system. The correctness of the program has been proven
by many test runs.

References.

1. Brodziak A.: Algorytmization of natural medical diagnostics. An
   approach to the electronic system indicating correct diagnostic
   procedure. Ann. Med. Soc. Pol. Sci., 1970, 5, 15.
2. Brodziak A.: Psychonika. Teoria struktur i procesów centralnego
   systemu nerwowego człowieka i jej wykorzystanie w informatyce.
   Wydział Nauk Medycznych Polskiej Akademii Nauk, Katowice, 1974.
3. Card W.J. i wsp.: A comparison of doctor and computer interrogation
   of patients. Int. J. Biomed. Comput., 1974, 5, 175.
4. Dreyfus J.F.: Presentation sur ordinateur de questionnaire aux
   malades psychiatriques : valeur de l'information recueillie.
   Memoire de fin d etudes en psychiatrie 1975, Paris, Faculte de
   Medicine Broussais - Hotel Dieu.
5. Gledhill V.X. i wsp.: A multilingual self - administered symptom
   history. Arch. Intern. Med., 1975, 135, 612.
6. Grossmann J.H., Barnett G.O., Mac Guire M.T., Swedlow D.B.: Evaluation of computer - acquired patient history. J. Amer. Med. Ass.,
   1971, 225, 1286.
7. De Heaulme M., Mery C.: REMAID - A artificial language for medical
   reports on computer. Proc. Medinfo, Stokholm, 1974.
8. Martin J.: Design of man - computer dialogues - published by Pren-
   tice - Hall. Inc. Englewood Cliffs, New Jersey, 1973.

<u>Formal Languages and their Semantics</u>
<u>Tools for the Application Programmer</u>

G Osterburg, K Schadewaldt

German Cancer Research Center, Heidelberg
Institute of Documentation, Information and Statistics
(Director: Prof.Dr.med.G.Wagner)

Introduction

The Data Processing Department of the Institute of Documentation,
Information and Statistics at the German Cancer Research Center,
Heidelberg, is concerned with maintaining the operating system,
advising the users, supporting their programming activities and last
but not least with the development of basic software. In the past,
this software was mainly used to establish different kinds of information systems [9]. During the course of our work, we had the following experiences with the so-called 'software crisis':

- insufficient program documentation
- unreliable programs
- time-consuming program testing
- problems with system extension
- uncompatible subsystems
- difficult system handling

These problems are well known and often discussed in the literature.

Application programmers usually encounter people who have no knowledge
of data processing. Those people are mainly interested in the easy
and secure handling of programs and do not care about the complexity
of program construction. Experience shows that hardly any user is
able to define the ultimate goals of his programs in advance. The
final product results from an intimate interaction between the user
and the programmer. Therefore, there is a strong need for better tools
to define and implement programs. About three years ago, feeling that
a good mathematical foundation would at least grant us deeper insight
into the nature of the problems mentioned, we began to study formal
language theory. As a result of our work in 1977, we completed a
'scanner generator', based on the theory of formal languages, and a
'parser generator', based on LL(1)-language theory [1,2].

The problem of planning and programming semantic routines corresponding to grammatical rules of a language has been approached with
the aid of the theoretical concepts of Goguen et al. [5,6,7]. As a
result, we implemented a generator for programs with the input language defined by a grammar [8]. This approach to software construction reflects the theoretical development from regular languages via
context-free languages to the semantics of formal languages. For the
user as well as the programmer a more natural strategy for constructing programs is the following:
At first it has to be specified what a program should do, what its
operations are and how they should be defined. Then the input language has to be designed and, finally, the result has to be implemented.
This strategy suggests a generating system which, based on the semantic definition of the operations, implements the intended program as
well as its syntax.

1. Generation of Scanners and Parsers

Normally, a compiler proceeds in two basic steps. At first, the
syntax of a source program is checked and the source program is
transformed to a derivation tree (syntactic analysis). According to
this derivation tree, the object module is generated in a second step
(code generation). Interpreters, in contrast with this, interpret
the given source input instead of generating code. This simple model
(fig. 1) can be used for most programs or programming systems.
Normally, the syntactical analysis is divided into lexical analysis
and parsing. The theoretical foundations are regular languages and
context-free languages, respectively [1]. Programs doing lexical
analysis and parsing are called scanner and parser. A scanner reduces
the input string to a sequence of tokens by replacing certain regular
character sequences, such as integers, real numbers, strings, and
keywords, by type. A parser analyses this sequence of tokens for
their structure, e.g. it checks if the input resembles a correct
arithmetical or logical expression. To explain the capabilities of
scanners, parsers, and their generators, we will give a simple
example:
Within any information system with inverted file and keyword catalog,
we need a retrieval program. The input should be any query built up
from the operations union (+), difference (-) and intersection (x),
applied to descriptors denoting the corresponding sets of the inverted file. The result of such queries should be printed by means of a

"print-command". Fig. 2 shows the generator input from which Scanner
and Parser - the complete program for syntactical analysis - can be
constructed. (Actually we use LL(1)-Parser, so the grammar of Fig. 2
is only an informal one. The grammar aforementioned can be transformed to an LL(1)-grammar by simple techniques [1]). The lexical
definitions specify (based upon regular expressions) the denotation
of descriptors and commands in a readable manner. The "IGNORE"-
construct forces the scanner to ignore any blank sequence, so the
user is free to type in his own input. According to the regular
definition, a descriptor starts with an alphabetic character
followed by any number (> $\emptyset$) of alphabetic characters or digits
(* - operation). The number in parenthesis after the token name
specifies the corresponding token type.

The syntactical structure of a query is defined by the (context-free)
grammar in Fig. 2. To decide whether a given input corresponds to
the syntactical rules of the grammar, each non-terminal (the names
enclosed between '<ℑ' and '>') - beginning with the start symbol -
has to be replaced by one of its right sides, as long as non-terminals
remain. It must be possible to reconstruct an input by such a derivation in order to be sure that the input is syntactically correct.
A derivation is represented by a sequence of numbers which represent
the rules applied. The task of finding a correct derivation or
rejecting the input as syntactically incorrect is done by the parser
constructed from the generator according to the grammar. The output
of each generator consists of an assembly language program, which
can be used as subroutine from PL1, FORTRAN, SPITBOL or ASSEMBLER.
The programs can be generated with some additional features mentioned
below. A complete description is contained in reference [3].

2. Semantics of Formal Languages

Scanner and parser are appropriate tools for performing syntactical
analysis of user input. The actions to be undertaken by the system
according to this input - the meaning (semantic) of the formal
language - have to be specified by additional semantic definitions.
The principle is to attach semantical meaning to each grammatical
rule, starting more or less abstractly, and then to refine it in the
form of a concrete program. The mathematical treatment of this
problem [5,6,10] is extremely complex and by no means completed,
although Goguen et al. [5] show an approach based on category theory

which comprises many existing special methods.

As an example of how to apply this theory ("initial algebra semantics"), a program will be constructed which, for a given systems language, performs the semantic actions, according to the derivation tree delivered by the parser. The basic idea is to assign to each non-terminal of a grammar a specific set of values and to view each grammatical rule as a function, the arguments of which are given by the non-terminals on the right side of the rule. That is, the range of such a function is given by the Cartesian product of the value sets of the right hand non-terminals, while the domain consists of the value set given by the non-terminal on the left side of a rule. In simplified manner,Fig. 3 shows the semantic definitions of the example shown in section 1. Rule 2, for example, can be interpreted as a constant (function with no arguments) which returns, for a specific descriptor, its corresponding member of the inverted file. The meaning of the functions seems to be quite clear, as well as the program code which implements this meaning (e.g. a program which performs the union or intersection of two sets of keys). Note that the mathematical semantics in Fig. 3 gives a precise definition of what is going on in the program. To define and implement the single functions operating on the value sets are the only tasks that have to be performed by the systems analyst and the programmer. The remaining portions of the program, e.g. those parts which control the correct evaluation of arbitrary complex expressions, can be generated automatically.

To demonstrate a complete and yet small example and also the flexibi-lity of the theoretical model, we will alter the meaning of the operations (Fig. 4). Let the symbols '+', '-' and '*' represent addition, subtraction and multiplication. Replace <descriptor> by <integer> in the grammar. Any expression accepted by this grammar can be viewed as an arithmetical one. The mathematical semantics is easily defined by the corresponding mappings from pairs of integers to the set of integers. In this case, the target language is PL1, so the code for each function consists of PL1 language statements. From this input the generator [8] constructs an executable PL1 program which,together with an appropriate parser and scanner, can be used as a rudimentary desk calculator. This concept has also been success-fully applied in a much more complex environment, while programming parts of interactive data base software [9].

3. Further Applications and Extensions

3.1. Generation of Interactive Systems

One further application suggested by the theories described in [5] is the construction of a semantic generator. We implemented a proto- type version of such a generator and described it in [4] (the imple- mentation is rather inefficient). The operations of the desired system and their abstract definitions now form the starting points. Those operations are the basic functions and can generally be easily implemented by small parts of program code. In a system containing such basic operations, the user is able to derive his own operations (including recursive functions) from the basic operations, to alter such derived operations, to store them or to execute them at any time. Errors, a big problem in many systems, can be handled in a very precise manner [7]. We believe - and some applications carried out give good reasons why - that generators of this kind provide effective tools for the application programmer.

3.2. Syntax Analysis again

Normally application programs are employed by inexperienced users. Therefore, there is a strong need for a reliable check of input by the program. This is done in a satisfactory manner by scanners and parsers. In principle, the parsing procedure is as follows [1]:

Each input symbol is looked up in a table. If the current input symbol is found in the table, it is shipped and the parser continues to search until no further input symbol is found. The parser actions are finished when "syntactically correct" is returned or an error is reported. In other words, the parsing tables contain exactly those symbols that are admitted as next input symbols in a specific state of the parser. This can be used to make operation easier for the user.

- menu display
  If the parser detects an error, it can inform the user - even if the input is incomplete - of all possibilities of correct continuation or completion of input.

- additional explanations
  In many cases, the rules of a grammar have an intuitive meaning, e.g. rule 1 of Fig. 1: "Enter a print command" or rule 2: "Enter a descriptor". It is possible to add additional explanations to

the rules. In case of error the generated parser prints out those explanations together with the menu. This feature allows the user to become easily familiar with the system language and its meaning.

- System levels

  In many software systems the system commands can be grouped together according to their meaning. Fig. 5 shows, in the form of a transition function, three different system levels (enclosed in circles). The arrows signify a transition from one level to another if one of the commands appended to the arrow is given. Such transition functions can be specified together with the grammar. The generated parser then controls transition between different levels and accepts only the commands of the actual level. A complete description of those and other features of the parser generator and the generated parsers is given in [3]. This reference contains the description of the scanner generator, too.

Conclusion

Finally, we want to comment on the problems of software construction mentioned in the introduction. In many cases the one who writes a program is also the only one who can comprehend it. There is no widely accepted documentation language except perhaps mathematics. Good tools can be found in the work of those who are occupied with, e.g., the problem of program verification to prove the correctness of an implementation. Program testing is - in principle - unnecessary after a correctness proof. Difficulties with system updating and bad coordination of system modules are phenomena, which can be eliminated on a sheet of paper with the help of good theoretical models. Users' problems in understanding the handling and the working method of a system can be reduced if the system understands more of the users' problems. All those tools could perhaps become generally accessible in the future if programmers become more familiar with the underlying theories and if the theories themselves were further developed because "nothing is more practical than a good theory".

Figures

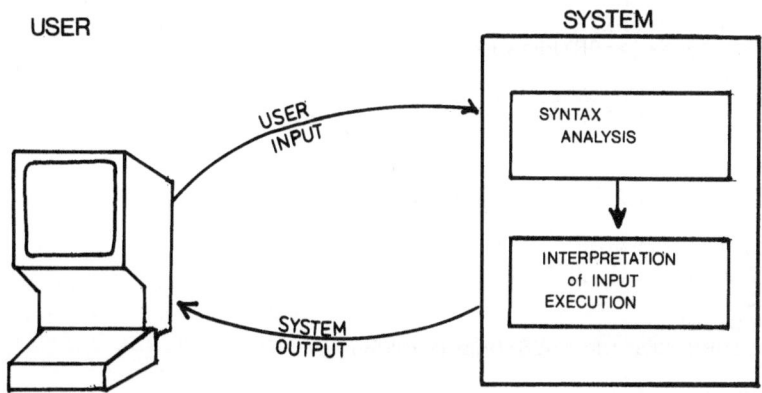

USER

SYSTEM

USER INPUT

SYNTAX ANALYSIS

INTERPRETATION of INPUT EXECUTION

SYSTEM OUTPUT

Fig. 1

```
QUERYP: LL(1) PARSER
 *
 * LEXICAL DEFINITIONS
 *
  QUERYL: SCANNER
    <BLANK>(83)=' '+
    IGNORE(<BLANK>)
    <DESCRIPTOR>(1)=ALPHA(ALPHA|DIGIT)*
    <PRINT>(2)=KEYWORD('PRINT') IN <DESCRIPTOR>
  END
  *
  * GRAMMATICAL RULES
  *
  START=<@START>
  <@START>=<@1><PRINT><@EXPR>
  <@EXPR>=<@2><DESCRIPTOR>
  <@EXPR>=<@3><@EXPR><+><@EXPR>
  <@EXPR>=<@4><@EXPR><-><@EXPR>
  <@EXPR>=<@5><@EXPR><*><@EXPR>
  <@EXPR>=<@6><(><@EXPR><)>
  *
  * ADDITIONAL EXPLANATIONS TO SINGLE FUNCTIONS
  *
  ERKL(1)='PRINT QUERY RESULT'
  ERKL(2)='DESCRIPTOR'
  ERKL(3)='UNION'
  ERKL(4)='DIFFERENCE'
  ERKL(5)='INTERSECTION'
END
```

Fig. 2

```
SYNTACTICAL CONSTRUCTS          MATHEMATICAL SEMANTICS

<@START>=<@1><PRINT><@EXPR>     E(KEY)     →        E(KEY)
<@EXPR>=<@2><DESCRIPTOR>                      →  E(KEY)
<@EXPR>=<@3><@EXPR><+><@EXPR>   E(KEY)XE(KEY) →  E(KEY)
<@EXPR>=<@4><@EXPR><-><@EXPR>   E(KEY)XE(KEY) →  E(KEY)
<@EXPR>=<@5><@EXPR><*><@EXPR>   E(KEY)XE(KEY) →  E(KEY)
<@EXPR>=<@6><(><@EXPR><)>       E(KEY)        →  E(KEY)
```

(Value set for <@EXPR> is E(KEY), the set of all subsets of possible
 keys)

INFORMAL DEFINITION OF CORRESPONDING PROGRAMS

```
    FUNCTION1(X):
     PRINT SET OF KEYS(X);
    END
    FUNCTION2:
     RETURN(SET OF KEYS(DESCRIPTOR));
    END
    FUNCTION3(X,Y):
     RETURN(UNION(X,Y));
    END

    FUNCTION4(X,Y):
     RETURN(DIFFERENCE(X,Y));
    END
    FUNCTION5(X,Y):
     RETURN(INTERSECTION(X,Y));
    END
    FUNCTION6(X):
     RETURN(X);
    END
```

Fig. 3

SYNTACTICAL CONSTRUCTS	MATHEMATICAL SEMANTICS

```
<ƏSTART>=<Ɛ1><PRINT><ƏEXPR>        Z   → Z  (identity mapping)
<ƏEXPR>=<Ə2><INTEGER>                  → Z  (value of the integer)
<ƏEXPR>=<Ə3><ƏEXPR><+><ƏEXPR>     Z X Z → Z  (addition)
<ƏEXPR>=<Ə4><ƏEXPR><-><ƏEXPR>     Z X Z → Z  (subtraction)
<ƏEXPR>=<Ə5><ƏEXPR><*><ƏEXPR>     Z X Z → Z  (multiplication)
<ƏEXPR>=<Ə6><(><ƏEXPR><)>          Z   → Z  (identity mapping)
```

(Value set for <Ə EXPR> is Z, the set of all integers)

DEFINITION OF CORRESPONDING PROGRAMS

```
FUNCTION1(X):
    PUT EDIT (' RESULT IS: ',X) (SKIP,A,F(5));
    RETURN(X);
END
FUNCTION2:
 RETURN(INTEGER);
END
FUNCTION3(X,Y):
 RETURN(X + Y);
END
FUNCTION4(X,Y):
 RETURN(X - Y);
END
FUNCTION5(X,Y):
 RETURN(X * Y);
END
FUNCTION6(X):
 RETURN(X);
END
```

Fig. 4

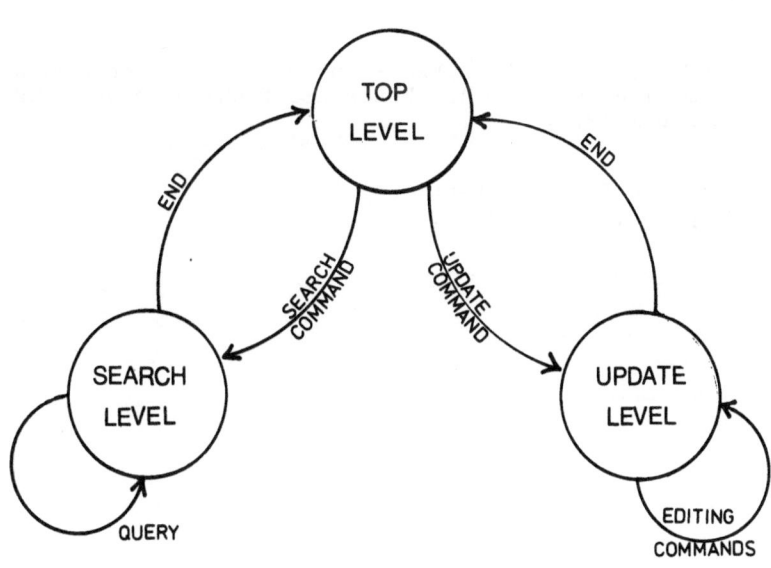

Fig. 5

References

[1]   AHO, A.V., ULLMAN, J.D.: The Theory of Parsing, Translation and
      Compiling, Vol. I. Prentice-Hall, Englewood Cliffs, N. 7, 1973.

[2]   AHO, A.V., ULLMAN, J.D.: The Theory of Parsing, Translation and
      Compiling, Vol. II. Prentice-Hall, Englewood Cliffs, N. 7, 1973.

[3]   BECKER, N., OSTERBURG, G., SCHADEWALDT, K.: PAULA-Generator für
      LL(k)-Parser und lexikalische Analyseprogramme. Tech.Rep. No.10.
      Deutsches Krebsforschungszentrum, ZDV, Heidelberg 1977.

[4]   BECKER, N., OSTERBURG, G.: Generierung interpretativer Systeme.
      Tech.Rep. No.11. Deutsches Krebsforschungszentrum, ZDV,
      Heidelberg 1978.

[5]   GOGUEN, J.A., THATCHER, J.W., WAGNER, F.G., WRIGHT, J.B.:
      Initial Algebra Semantics and Continuous Algebras.
      J. ACM $\underline{24}$ (1977) 68-95.

[6]   GOGUEN, J.A.: Algebraic Specification Techniques.
      Nat.Sci.Foundation Rep., Grant No. MCS72-03633 A04.

[7]   GOGUEN, J.A.: Abstract Errors for Abstract Data Types.
      Nat.Sci.Foundation Rep., Grant No. MCS72-03633 A04.

[8]   OSTERBURG, G.: Zur Semantik formaler Sprachen.
      Submitted for Publication.

[9]   SCHADEWALDT, K., MERX, R.: IDAS - Interaktives Datenbankaus-
      wertesystem. Tech.Rep. No.12, Deutsches Krebsforschungszentrum,
      ZDV, Heidelberg 1978.

[10] SCOTT, D.: Data Types as Lattices.
      SiAM J.Comp. $\underline{5}$ (3) (1977) 522-587.

A DECISION RULE IN PARENTHOOD DIAGNOSIS AND ITS CONSEQUENCES

Cl. CHASTANG, F. GREMY
Groupe de Recherches INSERM U 88
Méthodologie Informatique et Statistique en Médecine
91, bd de l'hôpital, F-75634 PARIS cedex 13

The discovery of the ABO system is at the origin of the study of human polymorphism the latest developments of which have permitted such breakthrough as blood transfusion and organ transplants.

The transmission mode of more than 45 systems of markers is known. So, these data provide an aid to decision in the age-old problems of parenthood diagnosis, for either the purpose of forensic medicine or the validation of data files in genetic studies (nearly 10 % of the families had to be rejected from such studies).

The most frequent of these parenthood problems is to determine if a man is whether or not the biological father of a child. This fatherhood diagnosis can be generalized to a family whatever the number of children is.

The gene, unit of genetic information, presents different forms called alleles. For every characteristics, one receives two of these genes from his parents. These two genes together provide the genotype which determines the observed form, the phenotype.

In the case of a triad $\{$presumed father, mother, child$\}$, the determination of human polymorphism for a sequence of genetic markers leads to 2 situations :
1. the presumed father is definitively rejected as the biological father of the child. For example, an O man cannot be the biological father of an AB child whose mother is A : the child receives allele A from his mother and allele B from his biological father whose phenotype can only be B or AB.
2. the presumed father is not rejected with respect to this child. But it is impossible to ascertain that this man is the biological father of the child.
This decision under uncertainty is particularly important in the forensic framework.

In the absence of rejection, different decisional criteria are used.

In so doing, we wrote a program (1)(2) which performs the following tasks :

a. verification of the parenthood links

b. calculation of parenthood indices

The criticism of these indices led us to propose a new decision strategy which uses an up-to-now neglected index, the percentage of excluded subjects with respect to the set $\{$mother-children$\}$. The application of this decision rule, in the framework of genetic studies, provides important savings in term of financial costs.

I. CLASSICAL DECISION APPROACH

Many decision tools have been elaborated in the case of a triad {presumed father, mother, child}, essentially in order to deal with the most frequent of the forensic problems, the aim of which is to determine if a man is whether or not the father of a child whose mother is known.

In fact, these decisional indices result from a bayesian approach with these two underlying hypotheses :

(H_0) : the presumed father is the biological father.

(H_1) : the biological father is not the presumed father, but according to these authors, he is taken at random from the men population.

The application of Bayes' formula leads to

$$P(H_1/child) = \frac{P(H_1).P(child/H_1)}{\sum\left\{P(H_j).p(child/H_j), j = 0,1\right\}}$$

where $P(H_i)$ is the a priori probability of the hypothesis (H_i). Usually, these two hypotheses are initially taken as equiprobable,

$P(H_1/child)$ is the a posteriori probability of the hypothesis (H_1),

$P(child/H_0)$ is the conditional probability of the child phenotype assuming that the biological father is the presumed father,

$P(child/H_1)$ is the conditional probability of the child phenotype assuming that the biological father is a man taken at random.

In the calculation of these two conditional probabilities, it is usual to assess that every {mother, child} couplet possesses one gene in common, which eventually eliminates some genotypes of the mother and/or the child.

If no genotype of the presumed father is compatible with those of the child, the conditional probability $P(child/H_0)$ is equal to zero, then , the a posteriori probability of the hypothesis (H_0) is also equal to zero. If we are dealing with a feasible system, we may affirm the rejection of the paternity of the presumed father. In fact, in the framework of forensic problems, the biologists used to determine the polymorphism of a fixed sequence of systems without consideration of rejections.

The authors propose decision rules which are very empirical and not based on bayesian methodology.

Hummel, for example, used Essen-Moller's index W which is nothing but the Bayes' formula with an a priori probability of 0.50 and proposes tables giving "parenthood practically proved" when Essen-Moller's index is greater than 0.9975, "likely parenthood if $0.9 < W < 0.95$ and "uncertain" parenthood if $0.45 < W < 0.55$.

The essential criticism concerns the nature of the existing hypotheses : although the 2 hypotheses are formally acceptable, their biological reality is subject to discussion ; actually, the mathematical procedure is only performed in case of an absence of rejection. Thus the non-rejected presumed father should be "compared" to one of the subjects taken at random from the population of men which are compatible with the {mother, child} couplet.

The 2 following hypotheses are so deduced :

(H'_0) the presumed father is the biological father.

(H'_1) the biological father is not the presumed father, but a man taken at random from the population of non rejected men.

Thus, the subjects rejected with respect to the {mother, child} couplet are not taken into account, as they did for (H_0) and (H_1).

These theoretical notions were confirmed on a sample of 138 trios : the correlation coefficient of the percentage of rejected subjects with the a posteriori probability of (H_0) versus (H_1) is 0.49 $(p < 0.001)$, but it is 0.01 with the a posteriori probability of (H'_0) versus (H'_1).

In addition, the a posteriori probability of (H_0) versus (H_1) has a progressively smaller variance (convergence towards 1) if one is dealing with a sufficiently large number of systems.

<u>Figure 1</u>

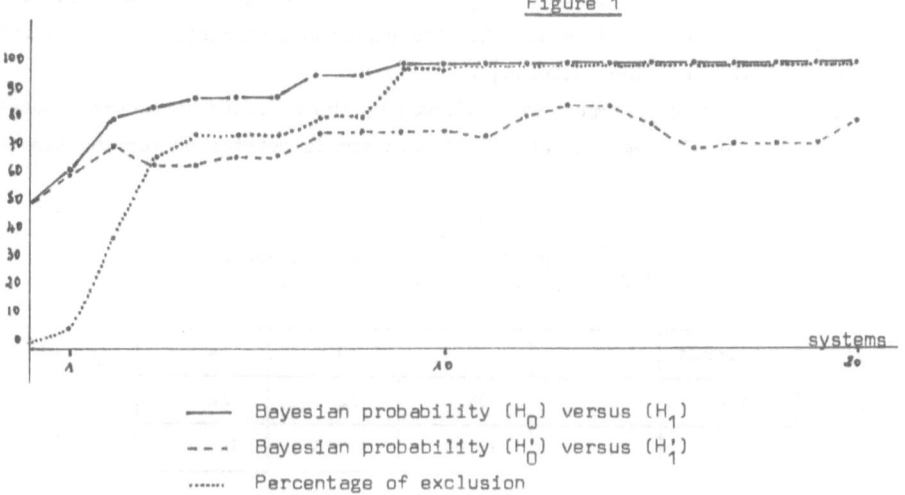

——— Bayesian probability (H_0) versus (H_1)
– – – Bayesian probability (H'_0) versus (H'_1)
……… Percentage of exclusion

Figure 1 shows the evolution of these 3 indices, posterior probabilities of (H_0) and (H'_0) and percentage of rejected men, in a typical case of a triad {presumed father, mother, child}, without rejection of fatherhood after the usual sequence of 20 systems of genetic markers.

In the case of fraternal units not limited to trios, this criticism is the same for the few existing decision tools (forensic medicine rarely tackles such fraternal units).

II. A NEW DECISION APPROACH : THE PERCENTAGE OF REJECTED SUBJECTS

In the classical decision approach, we compare a non excluded man with a stochastic man who is very often excluded. So, in genetic studies, we propose a new decision strategy based on the percentage of men rejected with respect to the set $\{$mother, child$\}$.

In the case of no rejection, we accept the practical null hypothesis which is "the presumed father is the biological father" if the percentage of rejected men exceeds a predetermined threshold p.

If the threshold p is not reached at the end of the sequence, either the family is out of the study, or we establish family polymorphism for unexplored systems.

In so far as the threshold is reached, the Type I error (α) is 0 and the Type II error (β) is equal to 1 - p/100.

In the case of a family with more than one child, we will propose a decision strategy based first on the percentage of men rejected with respect to the $\{$mother, child$\}$ set which must exceed a threshold p, and second, on the percentage of men with respect to each $\{$mother, child$\}$ set which must exceed a threshold p' (p'< p).

With the sequence of 20 genetic markers used in the Tranfusion Department managed by Pr. Ch. SALMON, the expected percentage of excluded men with respect to the set $\{$mother, one child$\}$ is 94.4 %. This expected percentage rises to 98.53 % if we have a set $\{$mother, two children$\}$.

These expected percentages are confirmed by the observed percentages obtained from a sample of 150 families whose polymorphism is determined for the same 20 genetic markers (Table I).

Table I

Observed percentage of excluded men
150 families, 20 genetic markers

Children	1	2	3	4
Number	55	35	32	28
%	94.17	99.01	99.75	99.84

In the serious case of forensic applications, we do not think that it is ethically possible to stop the determination of human polymorphism as soon as a predetermined threshold is reached. But, at the end of a sequence which does not bring to light any rejection, the percentage of rejected subjects with respect to the set $\{$mother, children$\}$ seems to us an excellent index of information. A magistrate will accord a greater likelihood to a triad $\{$man, mother, child$\}$ for which the couplet $\{$mother, child $\}$ excludes 99 % of the men population as incompatible man rather than to a triad for which the percentage of excluded men is 50 %.

III. LEAST COST SEQUENCE

Two reasons make indispensable the research of criteria allowing us to define a subsequence of markers systems which would provide the maximum information for the minimum cost : first, the rapid discovery of new systems, often more than 20 systems are tested today, second, in genetic studies, the validation of the family relationship depends on its cost : a prohibitive cost makes it impossible.

3.1. The notion of cost is taken in a strictly financial sense : the determination of the polymorphism of an individual cost 544 FF. (110 US $) for a sequence of 20 markers systems (ABO, Rhesus, MNSs, P, Kell, Duffy, Kidd, Lutheran, Gm, Inv, Gc, Hp, C_3'-Tf, PAc, PGM_1, AK, ADA, 6-PGD, SGPT, Esterase-D).

3.2. The notion of information

We proposed the use of the percentage of rejected subjects with respect to the {mother, children} set as a decision tool. In the same framework, we may estimate the information associated with a system by the mathematical expectancy of the percentage of rejected subjects or the probability of rejection.

This probability also depends on the size of the fraternal units. However, the correlation coefficients between the probabilities of rejection concerning different sized fraternal units are very high (greater than 0.9). Thus, by finding this optimal sequence, it appeared possible to define a unique decision tool independent of the size of the fraternal unit.

3.3. Determination of the optimal sequence

The assumption of independence between the systems makes this determination particularly simple : all sequences which are permutations of another have the same probability of rejection.

Thus, we have to order this sequence in such a way that the cost is minimized under the condition that fatherhood exclusion should stop the polymorphism determination. This condition is acceptable in the genetic framework.

In the case of a sequence of two systems s_1 and s_2 , the cost of the sequence (s_1, s_2) is :

$$C(s_1, s_2) = C(s_1) + (1 - p(s_1))C(s_2)$$

where :

$C(s_i)$ is the cost of the system s_i and

$p(s_i)$ is the probability of rejection of the system s_i

and the cost of the sequence (s_2, s_1) is :

$$C(s_2, s_1) = C(s_2) + (1 - p(s_2)) C(s_1)$$

We will select the sequence (s_1, s_2)

if $C(s_1, s_2) \leq C(s_2, s_1)$,

i.e. $\dfrac{p(s_1)}{C(s_1)} \geqslant \dfrac{p(s_2)}{C(s_2)}$

The generalization of this rule leads us to order the sequence in descending information/cost ratio.

The application of this criterion to the rejection probabilities calculated for different sized fraternal units leads us to optimal similar sequences composed of 20 systems. This stability allows us to use as the optimal sequence, the one which is determined from the probability of rejection with respect to the $\{$mother, child$\}$ couplet, that is the sequence PAc, MNSs, Rhesus, Hp, Esterase D, Kidd, C_3'-Tf, PGM_1, ABO, SGPT, Gm, ADA, Duffy, Inv, Gc, AK, Kell-Cellano, 6-PGD, P, Lutheran.

IV. EVALUATION OF THE DECISION RULE

In genetic studies, the percentage of rejected subjects with respect to the set $\{$mother, children$\}$ is not only a decision rule, but also a stopping rule according to our strategy.

Giving a threshold, one single error is possible : wrong acceptation of the null hypothesis (β error) (table II). In the case of no rejection, it is impossible to know the right hypothesis and consequently we have to make a decision under uncertainty.

Table II
Decision rule error

Nature / Conclusion	H_0	H_1
H_0	Right	False
H_1		Right

So, in order to evaluate our decision rule and to compare it with the classical approach, we performed it on a sample of 150 families whose polymorphism is determined on the same sequence of 20 genetic markers.

Four cases can be distinguished (table III) :

1. the threshold is reached without rejection and the systems not taken into account do not show any rejection.

2. the threshold is reached without rejection but one or more systems not taken into account lead to the rejection of the family. The null hypothesis is wrongly accepted.

3. rejection is emphasized.

4. the threshold is not reached with the last genetic markers of the sequence.

Table III

Logical outcomes using the decision rule

Whole sequence / Decision rule	No rejection	Rejection
H_0	1	2
H_1		3
No conclusion	4	

Figure II summarizes results obtained for 7 increasing thresholds on the sample of 150 families. For example, given a threshold of 0.95, it is not possible to conclude for 21 families and the conclusion is not right for at least 2 families (further examination may bring an exclusion on the 109 families not rejected with the entire sequence).

Figure II

EVALUATION OF THE DECISION RULE USING THE OPTIMAL SEQUENCE OF MARKERS

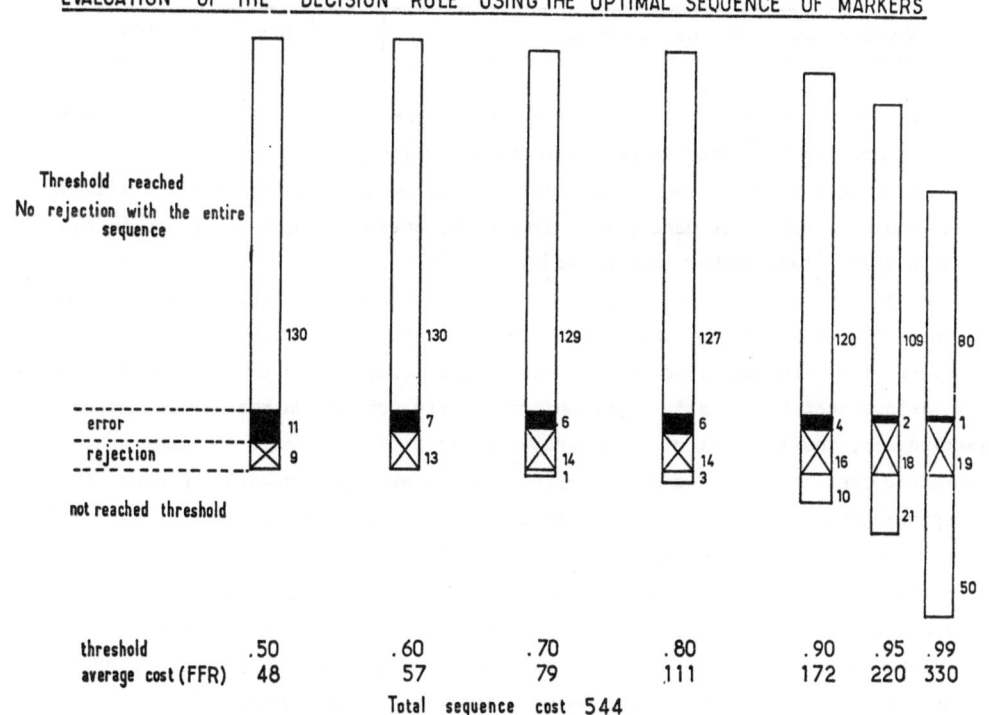

threshold	.50	.60	.70	.80	.90	.95	.99
average cost (FFR)	48	57	79	111	172	220	330

Total sequence cost 544

The computation of the average cost per subject according to this decision rule shows that the cost is an exponential function of the threshold.

The reasonable threshold of 0.95 leads us to an average cost of 220 FF. (44 US $), instead ot 544 FF. (110 US $) if the polymorphism is determined for the entire sequence.

Nevertheless, we must say that these results are really dependent on the size of the family.

Table IV gives, for the same threshold of 0.95, the results for each case according to the family size.

Table IV

Evaluation of the decision rule
according to the family size with a 0.95 threshold

Number of children	1	2	3	4
Number of families	55	35	32	28
THRESHOLD reached No rejection with the entire sequence	28	27	27	27
ERROR	1	0	0	1
REJECTION	7	6	5	0
NOT REACHED THRESHOLD	19	2	0	0
Average cost (FF.) per subject	352	188	127	106

The important result is that 19 of the 21 families for which the threshold is not reached are set {presumed father, mother, one child}.

It is exactly the same to say that we must measure the information brought at the end of a marker sequence. This problem is obviously most important in the case of a triad {Man, Mother, one Child}.

Table V shows for the fixed threshold, the number of families reaching the threshold without rejection, the mean of the percentage of rejection and the mean of the a posteriori probability of (H_0) versus (H_1), according to the size of the family. It is obvious that the classic bayesian probability depends on the percentage of rejection, so, the interest of this percentage in either forensic problems or in genetic studies. Moreover, we may observe that the average percentage exceeds the corresponding threshold, specially if this value is low. Thus, the β risk is, in fact smaller than $1 - p/100$, p being the threshold value.

In addition, table VI shows the interest of our decision rule in terms of number of markers systems ; for each threshold and for different family sizes, we calculated the average number of systems to reach the threshold. This number increases with the threshold value and decreases with the size of the family.

Moreover, the number of markers systems necessary to reach the threshold is surprisingly low. This result confirms the fact that the exclusion can be considered as a Dirac function and also that the percentage of exclusion is without any reason a neglected decision tool.

V. CONCLUSION

We propose in parenthood diagnosis a new decision strategy using the percentage of excluded subjects with respect to the set $\{$mother-child$\}$.

This decision rule points out three main interests :

(i) it is really a decision rule allowing the calculation of the α and β risks

(ii) this rule leads to important savings in the determination of human polymorphism

(iii) it enables us to determine an optimal marker sequence in terms of extracted information and financial cost.

REFERENCES

(1) CHASTANG, Cl. (1977) Parenthood diagnosis aid within a family . MEDINFO 77, Aug. 8-12, 1977. Proceedings p. 219-222

(2) CHASTANG, Cl. (1978) A computer program for parenthood diagnosis within a family Comp. Prog. Biom. (to be published)

<u>Table V</u>

Decision indices according to the threshold and the family size

Threshold / Children	0.50	0.60	0.70	0.80	0.90	0.95	0.99
1 (55)	52/0* 62.95** 74.80***	51/0 68.46 79.25	50/1 76.66 84.45	48/3 84.94 88.80	39/10 93.62 95.70	29/19 97.43 97.34	10/37 99.42 99.77
2 (35)	33/0 66.62 80.21	30/0 72.01 82.14	29/0 80.62 88.83	29/0 89.41 94.11	29/0 93.83 95.58	27/2 97.42 98.41	21/8 99.51 99.66
3 (32)	28/0 77.85 87.26	28/0 80.59 88.12	28/0 85.74 92.35	28/0 90.37 95.22	28/0 93.96 96.90	27/0 97.10 98.16	24/3 99.37 99.82
4 and more (28)	28/0 75.90 89.68	28/0 79.37 90.81	28/0 84.83 95.32	28/0 88.31 96.03	28/0 93.47 96.67	28/0 96.94 98.66	26/2 99.45 99.82

In the (1, 1) cell entry of this table, the interpretation of the numbers is the following :

* among 55 families with one child, 52 reach the 0.50 threshold, 0 do not reach it and 3 (55-52) families are rejected

** 62.95 is the average percentage of exclusion for the 52 families once the threshold is reached

*** 74.80 is the average bayesian probability of (H_0) versus (H_1) in the same conditions

Threshold / Children	0.50	0.60	0.70	0.80	0.90	0.95	0.99
1	3.1 (1-10)	3.8 (1-11)	5.1 (1-15)	7.1 (1-12)	10.2 (2-19)	11.0 (3-17)	13.1 (5-20)
2	2.0 (1- 5)	2.3 (1- 8)	3.2 (1-11)	4.6 (1-17)	6.2 (1-17)	7.5 (1-17)	11.4 (3-20)
3	2.0 (1- 4)	2.1 (1- 5)	2.5 (1- 6)	3.2 (1-10)	4.3 (1-15)	6.3 (1-17)	9.0 (2-18)
4 and more	1.6 (1- 3)	1.8 (1- 4)	2.0 (1- 4)	2.4 (1- 5)	3.4 (1- 9)	4.8 (1-11)	8.2 (2-15)

<u>Table VI</u>

Average number of systems needed to reach the threshold

(the numbers in parentheses represented the extrema values)

INTERACTIVE PROGRAMMING LANGUAGE FOR VALIDATION
AND INTERROGATION OF EVOLUTIVE DATA

J.P.   CHANTALOU

Groupe de Recherches INSERM U 88
Méthodologie Informatique et Statistique en Médecine
91, bd de l'hôpital, F-75634 Paris cedex 13

INTRODUCTION

        Generally the medical data are different from others in the sense that they
contain a notion of evolution. In clinical trials the following situation arises
fairly frequently : for each patient there exist one basic report, several intermediate reports, one final report. The number of reports is generally varying,
because the duration of stationary or ambulant treatment differs from patient to
patient. So a particular development of a data base adapted to such data must be
considered with a query language providing a great number of facilities for the
user. In addition to query and data manipulation facilities, a complete data
sub-language needs facilities for data definition and data analysis.

        Now, the number of interactive programs that require access to a data base
are developped more and more by users not specialized in computer programming which
is the case for most physicians. This fact is certainly contributing to the growing
development of the mini-computer and their sophisticated software (1).

        Therefore, as a high level language, this language must present a number of
particular characteristics (2) :

(i) the nature of the interaction must be simple so that the user has not to
      perform complex statements according to a rigid syntax

(ii) the language must be easy to learn and any program using this language must
      be easy to reread

(iii) it is necessary to supply the user with an online assistance : meaningful
      error messages and possibility to continue the operation sequence. In fact,
      most of high level language such as FORTRAN, ALGOL, PASCAL do not allow the
      efficient control of errors during the execution of the program, which involve
      loss of the totality or a part of the result. It is why a certain number of
      decisions must be included in the system and not at the responsability of the
      user.

(iv) the language must be easily available for both novice and sophisticated
      user

(v) the underlying computer and operating system characteristics must be hidden
      from the user and the size of the software should be limited so that it can be
      implemented on a mini-computer

(vi) the system must be relatively <u>inexpensive</u> from the standpoint of machine costs
   and human resources.

      The purpose of this paper is to describe the language PLD (Programming
Language for Data). Of course, it is not possible to describe a software system
and demonstrate its abilities in a few pages. Nevertheless, it will be tried in
the following sections to show essential features of PLD.

THE OBJECTIVES OF THIS LANGUAGE

      This interactive language aims to reach 4 essential points :
<u>Abstraction</u>. The first characteristic of PLD is to remove the data definition from
the individual application programs, this relieves the application programs from
the burden of physical I/O processing, and keeps the physical data base under central control. Application programs using the data base processor therefore reference
data logically by names assignated to data items instead of physically. These notions
have been reflected in the construction of data base management systems and in the
concept of data independence (CODASYL).
<u>Validation</u>. The main step of data analysis is a good validation of the data handled
by the program.
<u>Interrogation</u>. Consists in :
      (i) restituting on information part according to different criteria
      (ii) giving an one-dimensional description of each data
      (iii) creating other variables
      (iv) converting the variables
      (v) leading to output distribution and n-levels classification
<u>Extraction</u>. To create compatible sub-file with procedures not included in this
system. These sub-files will be directly input by program written in a high level
language like FORTRAN and by the system itself.

DESCRIPTION OF PLD

      Today, this language is essentially composed of 4 types of statements :
- assignment statement
- conditional statement
- unconditional statement
- high level output statement

Assignment statement
      Computations to be performed by PLD are indicated by assignment statements,
which have the general form :
$$V_1 = V_2 = V_3 = \ldots = V_n \; ;$$

where V_1, V_2, V_3 are simple variables, V_n is another simple variable, a number or an arithmetic expression, and = is a replacement operator. The assignment statement causes the object program to evaluate the expression V_n and assign the resultant value to the variables V_1, V_2, V_3, ... Note that the = sign signifies replacement, not equality.

This statement allows the creation of local variable from data base items (global) necessary for statistical analysis. These local variables are created at the time of program entry and are preserved only for the duration of the execution of that program.

The following rules for formation and evaluation apply to arithmetic expressions :

- parentheses specify the order in which elements within an erithmetic expression are to be evaluated. Expressions within parentheses are evaluated first within a nest of parentheses, the evaluation proceeds from the elements within the innermost pair of parentheses to the outermost pair of parentheses.
- when the order of a sequence of operations is not completely specified by use of parentheses, all PLD expressions are evaluated in strict left to right order. There is no precedence among the expression operators except that a unary sign (minus or plus) is evaluated before an arithmetic operator. Additional levels of precedence can be achieved by the nesting of subexpressions. Although there is no logical limit to the depth of nesting, there is a physical limit : size of partition in which program is running.
- an arithmetic expression may begin only with one of following : - + variable and may end only with one of the following :   ) variable
- there must be a one-to-one correspondence between left and right parenthesis in an arithmetic expression ; each left parenthesis must precede its corresponding right parenthesis. But redundant parentheses do not cause a fatal error, they are   unknown : A = (B ✹ (B + C)). The first left parenthesis and the last right parenthesis are not necessary.

Conditional statement. "Data filtering facilities"

One of the key features of PLD is the ease with which conditional statement can be realized.

A conditional statement causes the object program to select between alternate paths (called the TRUE and FALSE paths) of control depending upon the truth value of a test.

Conditional statement has the form : % Query Conditional expression ;

A conditional expression can be only one type : relation condition (greater than, equal to, less than, ...).

A relation condition causes a comparison of two operands, each of which may be a global or local variable, a figurative constant, or an arithmetic expression.

Relational operators specify the type of comparison to be made in the relation condition.

Relational dyadic operators	meaning
<	less than
>	greater than
< =	less than, or equal to
> =	greater than, or equal to
=	equal to
#	not equal to

Relation condition can be combined by either   of two logical operators.

logical dyadic operators	meaning
!	. logical OR. Entire condition is true if either of both of the simple conditions are true
&	. logical AND. Entire condition is true if both of the simple conditions are true

A conditional expression can be composed of either a simple-comdition or a compound-condition. A simple condition is one that performs a single test. A compound condition is one that contains a string of simple conditions connected by the logical operators ! (OR),   & (AND).

The evaluation rules for conditions are analogous to those given   for arithmetic expressions, except that the following hierarchy applies :

- aritmetic expressions
- relational operators
- logical operators

Parentheses may be used either to improve readability or to add levels of precedence.

A conditional expression could contain an assignment statement and   also accept abbreviations in relation conditions.

When a string of consecutive relation conditions appears in a statement, abbreviation can be used, in certain cases, for any relation condition other than the first. The subject, or the subject and relational operator, or the subject, relational operator and logical connective may be omitted.

Example 1 : if the subject is identical in a series of relational conditions, it can
        be omitted in all the relation conditions except the first   :
        In FORTRAN language :
        IF (A.EQ.B.OR. (A.GT.C.AND.A.LE.D).OR.A.EQ.E)

can be abbreviated to PLD :

    8 Q A:B,> C <= D, E ;

Example 2 : in the same way, if   the subjects and relational operators are identical in a series of relational conditions, they can be omitted in all
the relational conditions except the first :
In FORTRAN language :
IF (A.EQ.B.OR.A.EQ.C.OR.A.EQ.D.OR.A.EQ.E)
can be abbreviated to PLD : 8 Q A:B, C, D, E ;

    If the value of the expression is FALSE, control is transferred to the next
conditional statement, when the unconditional statement is not specified. If the
value of the expression is TRUE, control passes to the next sequential statement.

Unconditional statement

    Unconditional statements are of the form : GOTO Label

    A label is a method of marking a place in a program so that control can be
transferred to that point from elsewhere in the program. PLD uses identifiers as
labels. A label is delimited before and after by an exclamation point.
For example : !LAB 1! A = B *C + E ; is an assignment statement labeled by LAB 1.
More than one label can be attached to a statement if required ; thus :
!LND! E2 ! F1 ! A = Ø

    A transfer of control, or "jump", to statement in a program is effected
by a GOTO statement, this statement consists of the character ← followed by the
name of the label attached to the relevant statement.

Example : ! L1 ! A = B * C + E ← L2 ;

            . . .
            . . .

  ! L2 ! 8 Q A:> =   15 ← L1;

High level output statement

    Other key features of PLD are these high level output statements.

    As shown in the previous statements, the data handling features play an
important role in PLD, but they are only means to an end : statistical analysis

    - listing according to different criteria

    - one-dimensional description of each data

    - classification at n-levels

    Missing values or special values are automatically handled correctly.

    Most output statement can be used with one or more options (switches),
which produce different or more ample output.

    Evidently it seems difficult to insert in this system all statistical proce-

dures, because some   procedures are not used frequently. Therefore, a special
output statement allows to create compatible sub-files with procedures not included in this system. These sub-files will be directly input by the library of statistical programs and by the system itself.

TECHNICAL ASPECTS : choice of software interface between the language and the
                    computer

The generation of this language leaves us the choice between various solutions :
- the generation in high level language (FORTRAN, ALGOL) able to be interpreted by
  a compiler and the linking loader
- the generation in primary assembler language able to be interpreted by the assembler and the linking loader
- the generation of relocatable object program, able to be interpreted directly by
  the linking loader
- the generation of an absolute binary code able to be executed directly.

The first three solutions have not been retained which would have been contrary to the objectives that we had decided, to look for, invisibility of the
software with respect to the user, and the impossibility to pass parameters necessary for one task to another one, otherwise than by the intermediairy of the disks.

PLS uses one or more disks devices as the primary data storage medium. Access
to this storage is gained through the use of global variables (data base item).
Unlike local variables, global variables provide permanent storage and can be accessed by more than one user.

To get a clear picture of the situation, the system provides   statistics
of the use of every PLD-statements. This information gives also very useful hints
for optimising the performance of the system.

This language has been developped on a PDP-10 computer with a time-sharing
system. The system is written in Assembler MACRO-10. The current version has about
18,000 MACRO-10 statements. The programs are overlaid and shared and thus take up
minimal space in central core (never more than 4K-words).

CONCLUSION

This language must allow a high scruting of the information contained in
the data base. Little programming language seems to fill this last requirement. The
language PLD is being designed as a language   which provides this possibility and
which is also very easy for learning and use. This language deals items of data
base AIDE (3) as well as those created by a program written in FORTRAN language
or   another data base. It can be used in a satisfactory manner both in iterative

and batch environments. More than 130 schemas have been already analysed with
PLD language.

REFERENCES

(1) RITCHIE, D., THOMRSON, K. The UNIX time sharing system. CACH vol 17, n° 7,
July 1974, 365-375

(2) WASSERMAN, A.I. Reliable interactive software and programming language design
Technical report ≠ 20, April 1976

WASSERMAN, A.I., SHERERTZ, D.D. and ZEARS, R.W. Design of a multiprogramming
system for the MUMPS language. MDC 2/2 5/30/75

(3) de HEAULME, M.,   CHANTALOU, J.P., GARCON, Cl. AIDE : Archivage et Interrogation de Dossiers Evolutifs. Rev. Inform. Méd. vol. 4, 201-208, 1973

A system for computer-aided prognosis
A management function of the medical information system WAMIS

W. Dorda, H. Grabner, H. Neumann

Institute of Medical Computer Science
(Director: Prof. Dr. G. Grabner)
and
The First ENT-Department of the University of Vienna
(Director: Prof. Dr. O. Novotny)

SUMMARY

This article describes a computer-aided system for prognostic decision-making - the system CUMPRO. It has been developed as part of the Viennese General Medical Information System WAMIS.

This system for prognostic decision-making is based on several theoretical models. All relevant symptoms and signs which are stored in the patient's medical record in the central database are used and directly entered into the various algorithms to prognosticate the survival-time or recovery. Several theoretical models for computer-assisted prognosis are described. Their realization in the system CUMPRO and their effectiveness in practical use is demonstrated.

1. Methods for computer-aided prognosis

Several methods for computer-assisted prognosis as aid to medical decision making are shown. Their aim is to present the prognosis of a "new" patient. Thereby it is assumed that the diagnostic findings have been finished and a final diagnosis is known.

All prognostic algorithms try to estimate the survival-time or recovery starting with an array of indicants. The indicants contains all the patient's symptoms and vital signs. Two possible procedures may be applied in computer-assisted prognosis:

1.1 Deterministic Methods

In this case the computer-aided prognosis-system is based on matrices where the medical knowledge about relations of indicants and prognostic indices is stored. These methods may be compared with the deterministic methods in the theory of computer-aided diagnosis (1). In the field of prognosis - on the contrary to computer-aided medical diagnosis - it is nearly impossible to make deterministic statements regarding the relation of indicants and prognosis. Most of these relations are probabilistic and lead to the second group of methods.

1.2 Stochastic Methods

In this case the survival-time of a patient is estimated using statistical methods. There exist two groups of stochastic methods:

1. Estimation of the further course of the disease, based on the previously known facts by the analysis of time-series.

2. Statistical comparison with similar, already closed cases (the control group), whose prognostic indices are known.

This comparison may be done by one of the following methods:

a) regression-analysis
b) density-estimation methods
c) descriptive methods: analysis of factors (3, 15)

Regression analysis has the following two advantages according to Brunk (5).

1. In Regression analysis with continuous variables the total information of the dependent variable "survival-time" is utilized, compared to the density-estimation methods where some information is lost by dichotomizing. There also exist regression models with a dichotomous survival time as dependent variable.

2. Given an array of indicants, a regression method can furnish a probability distribution of the survival-time.

Density estimation methods have two advantanges compared with regression method:

1. Incomplete data can be used, if the "gaps" (missing data) are randomly distributed.

2. Rough estimates of the accuracy of the calculated probability can be made.

1.2.1 Regression estimation methods

1. Multivariate linear regression

This well-known method can only be used in special cases without transformation of the data. The dependent variable survival-time in general decreases exponentially and therefore it is necessary to perform a log-transformation in order to fulfill the assumption of the linear regression.

2. Analysis of covariance

In several application-fields the independet parameters are discrete. Therefore we have qualitative variables which influence the survival-time. In this case the multivariate linear regression-model must be expanded to a general linear model, where the discrete indicants define the design of the model. The continuous indicants are the covariates.A pre-transformation is often necessary in order to linearize the survival-time.

3. Cox-model

Cox has proposed the following model: $F(t/x) = F_o(t)^{\exp(\beta'x)}$

F_o is some arbitrary non-parametric unknown survivor function
t = the survival time
x = the vector, which includes the specified indicants
$F(t/x) = P(T > t / x)$
β = the unknown parameters

The family of the distributions in the Cox model includes the negative exponential model and the Weibul model.

Breslow proposed a parametric approximation of the non-parametric Cox-model. This approximation was used by Brunk (5) in case of breast cancer.

The following models use a dichotomized survival time:

4. Linear Regression Analysis with a dichotomized survival time according to Gehan (8).

This is a special case of multivariate linear regression, with a dichotomous transformation of the survival time. According to Gehan there exists no theoretical foundation for this model, but the procedure has proved successful in some studies (5). Koch modified this method by using weighted least squares for fitting the model.

5. Discriminant Analysis

The survival-time is divided into two (or more) classes which are defined by the physician. A training group is used to calculate the parameters of the discriminant function, by means of which all new patients are classified into one of the given classes of the survival time. As shown in (13) the result of the discriminant analysis is analogous to a multiple variable regression with the following dependent variables:

$$y_i = \frac{- n_1}{n_1 + n_2} \qquad \text{if the patient belongs to group 2}$$

$$y_i = \frac{n_2}{n_1 + n_2} \qquad \text{if the patient belongs to group 1}$$

n_i = size of group i.

Afifi (2) approximated the course of the disease by polynoms and applied the linear discriminant analysis to the coefficients of the polynoms. From the discriminant functions he calculated the prognostic indices in cases of intoxication.

6. Quantal Response Regression (Logistic model) (16)

In this case the survival-time is primarily divided into two intervals. The dependent variable is the logistic transformed pro-

bability of the occurance $t > t_o$ (t = survival time, t_o - constant).
Qualitative or quantitative indicants are allowed in the vector of
the independent variables. The maximum likelihood estimation of the
logistic model was found by Cox.

1.2.2 Density estimation methods

The probability of dying or being cured - given in a special combination of symptoms (danger-situations)- within a definite time-
interval is equal to the incidence rate in similar cases. This leads
directly to the first method:

1. Histogram method (cell-frequency method) (lit. 5)

   The rate of incidence is calculated for all patients with the
   same symptoms. This method requires a very large number of controlled cases, even when only few symptoms are considered. However, it is possible that one or the other cell may have few
   occupants, or may even be empty. In this case the variation of
   the rate of incidence may be rather large and the following methods should be applied.

2. Independence model (lit 5)

   The independence of the parameters is a frequent assumption.
   The survival probability of a special symptom combination then is
   equal to the product of the survival probabilities of single
   symptoms. These survival probabilities may be estimated from
   smaller sample groups. If the parameters are independent good results may be obtained.

3. Logarithmic Linear Models (lit 18)

   Histogram and independent models are the two extremes of the density estimation methods. By the use of the log-linear models one
   tries to find a compromise between these two models. In each log-
   arithmic-linear model, the expected frequencies of the observed
   cases are determined by certain marginal sums. The simplest model
   is the independence model in which only one-dimensional marginal
   sums determine the expected frequency. The histogram-model is the
   most complicated one. In this case no simplifying assumptions are
   made. The whole p-dimensional distribution (where p = number of
   the given parameters) is included into the calculation. The algo-

rithm starts with the most complicated model in order to find the best model and continues with the next simpler one until the end criterium is reached.

4. Orthogonal - Series - Method (lit 5)

Let p (x) be the survival probability according to the histo-gram-model and p_o(x) according to the independence model. The quotient p(x) / p_o(x) is developed in orthonormal series. The orthonormal functions are derived from Helmert-matrices and quoted in Brunk et al (5).

Each of these functions can be developed in linear combinations. Thus, estimates of p(x) which are especially helpful in cases of "nearly independent" parameters are possible.

5. Sequential Maximum Discriminants (lit 8 and 12)

All parameters must be dichotomous. In the first step all para-meters which mostly influence the survival - rate must be found. These dichotomous parameters belong to two groups of patients. The group with the lower survival-rate is taken out of calcula-tion and is not further divided by other parameters. However you must seek among the group with a higher survival-rate for those indicants, which mostly influence the survival-rate; and you carry on in this way. By continuing in this manner you will get a kind of "logical tree" (see diagram) which indicates the pro-gnosis.

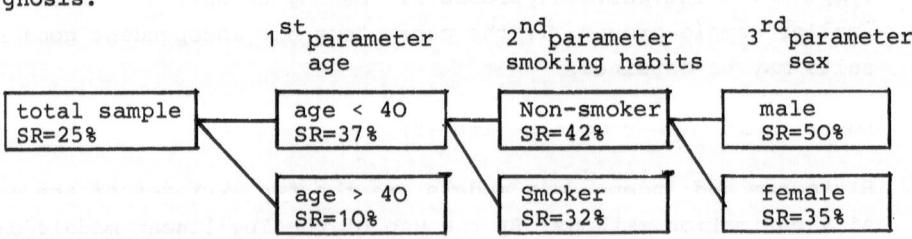

Tree representation of the Sequential Maximum Discriminants-
Method
SR: Survival-rate

6. Ridit-method

If a variable will be Ridit-transformed, it is at first necessary
to choose a random sample in order to identify the distribution
of the variable.

The Ridit-transformation of a discrete variable is defined as
(4, 17)

$$\text{Ridit} (x) = \frac{\sum_{i=1}^{x-1} h_i + \frac{h_x}{2}}{n}$$

where h_i ($i = 1,.., x - 1$) is the frequency of the variable in
class i calculated out of the sample, x is the considered class,
n the total size of the sample.

In analogy to the sequential maximum discriminant-method Neumann
(14), selects the parameters which have the greatest influence
on the survival-time. For that purpose the survival-time is
Ridit-transformed and the Ridits of several groups are compared.
The final result is a series of parameters with decreasing influence on the survival-time. Patients with "as similar as possible" parameters are selected in the following manner. First of
all only one parameter is considered, then the next one of the
series and so on. In every step the number of patients decreases.
This procedure is continued until a point is reached, where not
enough patients remain. So the process stops if a parameter is
developed where it is impossible to start the next iteration step
because of too few similar cases. The last and all following
parameters are declared to be inefficient and are not considered
further on (Compare diagramm). By means of this iteration procedure patients who are "as similar as possible" are found. Their
mean of the Ridits is calculated and retransformed into the original survival-time.

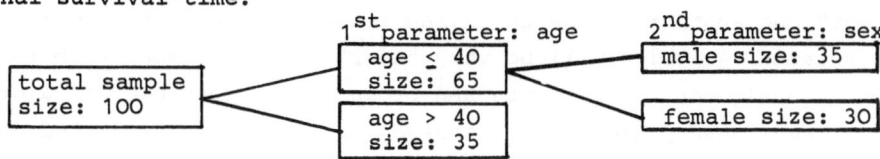

Procedure to find patients who are "as similar as possible" compared with the new patients. For the minimum size of a subgroup
a size of 30 is choosen.

Immich (11) suggested that this mean-difference test statistic
(4) is inadmissible, because of the fact, that mean and standard deviation of the Ridits are dependent. In a Monte-Carlo-study
we examined and verified the idea of Immich. Therefore we restrict the system CUMPRO only to the means themselves. Theoretically this also is inexact, but the positive results seem
to justify the procedure.

7. Modified Histogram Method

As pointed out above the Histogram method requires a very large
number of controlled cases. Therefore we modify this method in the
following way:

The main principle is to find a sequence of the parameters with
decreasing influence on the survival-time. For that reason we
calculate the Kendal-rank-correlation-coefficient between the
parameters and the survival time and sort the parameters according to their coefficients. Then we select the patients who are
"as similar as possible" in analogy to the Ridit-method. The
rate of died or cured patients in this group is calculated and
is used as the prognostic index.

1.2.3 Descriptive methods: analysis of factors (lit 3, 15)

Salmon applies the principal component analysis to

a) the individuals (n points in R^p)

b) the variables (p points in R^n).

This leads to common factorial axes and in consequence to common projections on the planes which are determined by these axes. Thus, if
two individuals are very similar in their indicants, they will be
"near" one another in the Euclidian sense. Similary, two positive
correlated variables will be very "near". In superimposing both planes an assignment of patients and prognosis is possible. If a group
of already dead patients is observed, the variables projected inside
this group lead to an unfavorable prognostic index. Similary, the
variables projected inside a group of patients alive have a good
prognosis.

2. Description of the system CUMPRO and Linkage to the Medical Information System WAMIS

The system CUMPRO is based on several statistical methods and models. In order to prognosticate the survival-time or recovery of new patients it is necessary to use the information of a control group. These control group data are retrieved by means of the evaluation system WAMAS, which is a part of the general medical information system WAMIS. The control group is divided into a training group and a test group, the first one is used to calculate the model parameters, the second one to compare the several models and to choose the best one.

2.1 The General Medical Informationsystem WAMIS

The Viennese General Medical Informationsystem (WAMIS` for german: Wiener Allgemeines Medizinisches Informationssystem) is an approach to an integrated hospital information system (10). This system is destined primarily for medical scientists, in order

1. to provide a source for systematic medical research

2. to obtain an instrument for medical decision making.

Besides these scientific applications WAMIS is built up in order to facilitate the daily work of physicians and nurses. The medical data are collected on-line and stored in the central patient-oriented database. The personal medical record provides the source for systematic medical research, e.g. computer assisted diagnostic decision making (1). The computerized prognosis system CUMPRO is another modul of the information system WAMIS.

2.2 Selection of the control group data by means of the evaluation system WAMAS

The medical evaluation system WAMAS (7) is able to analyze the data stored in the database of the information system in a multiple manner. It is possible

1. to formulate logical expressions in order to select the patient's data

2. to analyze the course of a disease.

All data necessary for the construction of life tables or computerized prognostic algorithms are selected by means of WAMAS and transposed to the system CUMPRO for further handling.

2.3 Calculation of the survival-time

The evaluation system WAMAS provides the date of death or recovery, date of last control, and other significant information in case of special problems concerning survival, recovery or patient's illness. This is necessary for calculating the life tables in the system CUMPRO. If in a special study all patients have died the survival time follows immediately. In case of a study with patients still alive the survival-time must be estimated. The method in use here was elaborated by Chiang (6). Here the estimation of the probability of survival and expectation of life is done according to the maximum likelihood principle. Chiang has shown that the ML-estimator $\hat{p}_{ij}$ of the probability that an individual alive at age x_i will survive to age x_j with $i < j$ is the unique, unbiased, efficient estimator of the corresponding probability p_{ij}. The ML-estimator $\hat{p}_{ij}$ has the minimum variance of all the unbiased estimators p_{ij}, although the Cramér-Rao lower bound for the variance cannot be attained.

2.4 Division of the control group into a training and a test group.

The system for computerized prognosis is based on the data of a control group which constists of completed medical cases. By means of the evaluation system WAMAS all these data are selected out of the database and subsequently divided in a training and a test sample group.

This division is normally done by means of a randomized selection. Another method which is also possible is the following one: The patients in the control group are sorted according to their survival time in ascending order and the training group is composed of e.g. each third case in the sorted sequence, which is advantageous because of a uniform distribution of the patients with long survival-times in the training and test group.

2.5 Data preparation and calculation of the model-parameters

In a special problem it is often necessary to perform a transformation of the data. As above mentioned the dependent variable survival-time in general decreases exponentially. Therefore it is necessary to perform a log-transformation in order to linearize the survival-time if the linear regression model is applied . If necessary the independent variables can also be transformed.

Possible transformations are: power, square-root, exponentiation, logarithms, dichotomizing.

If binary variables are needed and the original data are continuous, the statistical median is used: the value "O" is assigned to all data beyond the median and "1" to the data above.

Depending on the method in use the preparation of the data takes place: patient-oriented, grouped, or cell-oriented corresponding to the factorial design. The physician has the possibility to use several default parameters to specify the model.

The following methods and models are implemented:

1. Multiple linear regression

2. General linear model

3. Logistic model (A program written at the London School of Tropical Medicine was used for the logistic ML-estimation. We use this program with the kind permission of Mr. Scherg (Heidelberg)).

4. Multiple linear regression with dichotomized survival-time

5. Linear discriminant analysis

6. Modified histogram-method

7. Independance model

8. Ridit-method

9. Sequential maximum discrimination (in preparation).

2.6 Model testing and new cases

The test group is used to choose the best model out of the above
mentioned ones. For this purpose the prognosticated survival-time
is calculated for each patient of the test group and each model
and compared with the true survival-time. The percentage of the
correctly estimated patients is used as a quality reference to the
corresponding model.

The survival-time of a new patient is now easily calculated: At
first the relevant symptoms of the new patient are retrieved out
of the database by means of the system WAMAS. In the next step the
best model is selected and the expected survival-time is calculated.

3. Example: Prognosis of the Larynx-tumour

In this example the procedure is briefly demonstrated:

Data-gathering: The basis of all prognosis algorithms of the system
CUMPRO are the patients of the control group who form the training
and the test group. The data of all 718 patients suffering from a
larynxcarcinom, who were first treated at the 1st ENT-department
of the University of Vienna between 1955 and 1969, were documented
and stored in the database. The study was continued for later
check-ups until 1973.

Selection of the control group data:

By means of the evaluation system WAMAS these patients were selected. The following 10 parameters were transmitted to the system
CUMPRO: age, presence of lymphatic metastasis, infiltration, main
symptoms, tumour size, details of location of the tumour, histology,
recidive of tumour, anamnestic duration of illness, smoking-habits.

The definition and selection of these ten significant variables out
of several others is described elsewhere (14).

Calculation of survival. In the case of patients, who died during
the period of investigation the time of survival was calculated as
the difference between the date of death and the date of the first
treatment. A special subprogram was necessary for the patients who

survived the total control interval. In this case the survival time
was calculated by means of a special "cohort-death-table". For further details confer Neumann (14).

The choice of the training - and test sample was done by random.
The proportion of the sample size was 2:1.

For model testing we had to define the admissible deviation between
the calculated and true survival-time. A patient of the test group
is per definitionem correctly estimated, if estimated and actual
survival time are both above or below 5 years. The results of the
model testing are:

Method	rate of correctly estima-ted survival-times in %
General linear model with dichotomized survival time	71,68
Discriminant Analysis	71,24

General linear model:
  transformation of the survival-time:
                Logarithmus
	70,80

Square-root	69,03
without transformations	67,26
Quantal response regression	66,81
Ridit method	66,81
Modified Histogram Method	62,83
Independence model	57,62

Therefore the survival time of the new patient was calculated by
the use of the General linear model with a dichotomous survival-
time.

In addition to these results several statistical parameters are calculated (Mahalanobis-D^2, F-Values, etc.). Thus the physician or the biostatistician has the possibility to determine the quality of the models. Further on he can change the defaults to calculate a modified model.

The system CUMPRO is easy to handle because of the linkage to the medical information system WAMIS together with the selection of a appropriate model. Therefore the user has the possibility to use a typical management-function of the informationsystem.

4. References

(1) Adlassnig K.P., Gergely T., Grabner H., Grabner G.:
    A computer-assisted system for diagnostic decision making -
    On-line usage of the database of the medical information
    system WAMIS
    Medinfo 77, North-Holland Publishing Co., p. 213-218.

(2) Afifi A.A., et al:
    Accumulative Prognostic Index for Patients with Barbiturate,
    Glutethimide and Meprobamate Intoxication.
    New England Journal of Medicine 285 (1971), 1497-1502.

(3) Brdowski I., et al:
    Prognosis of Hodgkin's Disease: A Factor Analysis Approach.
    Medinfo 74, North-Holland Publishing Co., p. 587-592.

(4) Bross I.D.J.:
    How to use ridit analysis.
    Biometrics 14, (1958), 18-38.

(5) Brunk H.D., Thomas D.R., Elashoff R.M., Zippin C.
    Computer-Aided Prognosis.
    In R. Elashoff (Ed.): Perspectives in Biometrices Vol. 1.
    Academic Press 1975, p. 63-80.

(6) Chiang Ch.L.:
    Introduction to Stochastic Processes in Biostatistics.
    J. Wiley 1968.

(7) Dorda W., Kogler W.:
    WAMAS, statistische Auswertung einer patienten-orientierten
    Datenbank.
    Statistical Newsletter 3 (1977) 54-58.

(8) Feinstein A.R., Koss N.:
    Computer-Aided Prognosis.
    Arch.Intern.Med. 127 (1971) 438-447.

(9) Gehan E.A.:
   Use of Medical Measurements to Predict the Course of Disease.
   Nat. Cancer Inst. Monogr. 3 (1960) 53-58.

(10) Grabner H., Grabner G.:
   Aims and Structure of the Vienna General Medical Information
   System WAMIS.
   Medinfo 74, North-Holland Publ. Co. p. 375-379.

(11) Immich personal communication
   Biometrical conference ROES, Krems 1977.

(12) Koss N., Feinstein A.R.:
   Computer-Aided Prognosis: Development of a Prognostic Algorithm.
   Arch.Intern.Med. 127 (1971) 448-459.

(13) Lachenbruch P.A.:
   Discriminant Analysis.
   Hafner Press 1975.

(14) Neumann H.:
   Das Larynxcarcinom. Prognose und Computer.
   Facultas-Verlag, Vienna 1973.

(15) Salmon D., Brdowski I., Michat L., Cabrol C.:
   Computer-aided Prognosis in Early Post-operative Terms for
   139 Cases of Starr-Edwards Prostheses.
   Medinfo 74, North-Holland Publ. Co., P. 501-506.

(16) Scherg H.:
   Quantal Response Regression: Ein Verfahren zur statistischen
   Analyse einer multifaktoriellen Genese.
   Meth.Inform.Med. 15 (1976) 47-51.

(17) Slack N.H., Bross I.D.J.:
   Analysis of Prognostic Factors in Patients with Primary Breast
   Carcinoma.
   J.Med. 2 (1971) 93-111.

(18) Wermuth N.:
   Das Zusammenwirken einiger Risikofaktoren in der Schwanger-
   schaft.
   Meth.Inform.Med. 15 (1976) 251-259.

THEORY OF EVIDENCE AND MEDICAL DIAGNOSTIC.

Ph. SMETS
Department for Scientific Computation
Medical School, Brussels University. (ULB)
Brussels-BELGIUM

1. INTRODUCTION.

Classically the mathematical method used to simulate the medical
diagnostic process is based on the theory of probability. One starts
with a set of well defined diseases (categories), computes the probability that a patient belongs to each category conditionally to the
observations and when a decision has to be taken, the expected utili-
ties are computed.

Such an approach suffers at least from two major criticisms. First,
what is a set of well defined diseases? Disease categories are far
from being so well defined that it is possible to claim without any
ambiguity that a patient belongs to a certain category. These categories are typical exemples of fuzzy sets (Zadeh 1965) and probability theory should at least be adapted to handle fuzzy sets (Smets
and al. 1977a, 1977b). To facilitate the description of the second
criticism let us accept that disease categories are so well defined
that fuzzy sets are unnecessary. Then, does probability theory really
cover the notion of degree of belief as it claims? If my degree of
belief that such patient belongs to the class of infarction is .7,
does it really imply that my degree of belief that the patient does
not belong to the class of infarction is .3, as requested by the
theory of probability? When I have absolutely no evidence about the
fact that the patient belongs or not to a certain class, should I
give a degree of belief of .5 to the proposition "he belongs" and
.5 to the alternate proposition, the same value that I give to the outcome "head" or "tail" after the throw of a piece of money? In one
case I have no evidence at all, in the other, I perfectly know the
pieces of money. Finally, how should I structure the universe of
disease?

Probability theory requests that I describe first all possibilities
as far as some ultimate singleton, that is a possibility which may
not be dissected in subsets. In medical application, it is of course
totally irrealistic to claim that the disease categories are so well
defined that they cannot be splitsed in subcategories.

Shafer(1973, 1976) following ideas of Smith (1961,1965) and Dempster (1968) has introduced a mathematical theory of evidence that avoids all the criticisms presented above and with probability theory as a particular case.

2. THEORY OF EVIDENCE.

2.1 <u>Belief function</u>. Suppose a set of propositions A that belong to a frame of discernement Θ. We define a function of belief Bel that measures our degree of belief that a proposition is true. This function of belief Bel is nul for the empty set (we do not give any degree of belief in "nothing") and is one for Θ the frame of discernement (we are sure at least that the truth is within the frame of discernement). Suppose then two propositions A and B of Θ , we have then

$$Bel(A \lor B) \geqslant Bel(A) + Bel(B) - Bel(A \land B)$$

while in the theory of probability the strict equality is requested. In particular if A and B are mutually exclusive i.e. $A \land B = \emptyset$, we have

$$Bel(A \lor B) \geqslant Bel(A) + Bel(B)$$

As a direct application of this inequality consider the case where a patient comes to the ward with typical clinical symptoms of a myocardial infarction. Then let Bel (infarction) = .9.
Having not yet read the ECG we have no evidence whatsoever that the infarction is anterior or not. So we write Bel(anterior infarction)=0 and Bel (not anterior infarction)=0. As "infarction" is the union of the two disjoint subclasses "anterior infarction" and "not anterior infarction", we would have to give degrees of belief for the two subclasses that add two .9 if probability was to be used to cover our degree of belief.

2.2 <u>Vacuous belief function</u>. A belief function is qualified as vacuous if Bel(A)=0 whenever $A \neq \Theta$, that is no belief is assigned to any strict subset of Θ. This belief function perfectly describes a state of total ignorance.

2.3 <u>Doubt function</u>. We can also define a function that measures our degree of doubt Dou in the truth of a proposition A. Shafer proposes that our doubt in a proposition A is equal to our belief in its negation $\overline{A}$, that is Dou(A)=Bel($\overline{A}$).

2.4 <u>Plausibility function</u>. More usefull is the function Pl(A)=1-Dou(A)
which expresses the extend to which one fails to doubt A, i.e the
extend to which one finds A credible or plausible. We call Pl the
plausibility of A and

$$Pl(A)=1-Bel(\overline{A})$$

2.5 <u>Basic probability numbers</u>. One can also define a non negative
function m(A) on the frame of preference Θ such that for all B $\subseteq$ Θ

$$Bel(B)= \sum_{A\subseteq B} m(A)$$

where the sum is taken over all subsets A of B. Such function m is
uniquely defined by a belief function and uniquely defines such belief
function. The quantity m(A) is called A's basic probability number
and can be understood as that portion of our belief that is committed
exactly to A.

2.6 <u>Bayesian belief function</u>. Classical probability function is a
particular case of belief function where m(A)=0 for all A that is not
a singleton of Θ. In such case for all B$\subseteq\Theta$

$$Bel(B)= \sum_{A\in B} m(A)$$

where the sum is taken on the singletons contained in B. Such belief
function is qualified as Bayesian by Shafer (1977).
The mathematical theory of belief function is fully developped in
Shafer (1973, 1977). Dempster has described a rule to combine belief
functions based on several distinct evidences.

3. <u>EVIDENTIAL GENERALISATION OF BAYES THEOREM</u>.

All mathematical models of medical diagnostic define a set of diagno-
sisses D= {d} and a set of symptoms X= {x}. Let d_i be the singletons
of D, that is "elementary diagnosis" that cannot be splitted in sub-
diagnostic. The symbol $\in$ is strictly reserved for singletons. When
we wrtite x$\in$X or d$\in$D, we mean that x or d are respectively singletons
of X or D. Classically for all elementary diagnostic $d_i\in$D the distri-
bution $P(x|d_i)$ of the symptom x is supposed known. A prior distri-
bution P(d) is formulated on D and the posterior probability of d$\in$D
given a particular symptom x$\subseteq$X is computed by Bayes Theorem

$$P(d|x)=P(x|d)P(d)/ \sum_{d_i\in D} P(x|d_i)P(d_i)$$

This theorem can be generalised within the evidential theory.
Let $Bel_X(x;d_i)$ measure our degree of belief relative to X when
$d_i \in D$ is true. Let $Bel_X(x;d_i)$ be known for all $d_i \in D$. We consider
that $Bel_X(x;d_i)$ is the belief function Bel defined on W=XxD by conditionning on d_i. We have then synthetised such a belief function
on W that contains all and only that information present in the set
of $Bel_X(x;d_i)$. A further conditionning on X provides a belief function $Bel_D(d;x)$ on D analogous to the posterior probability.
The evidential generalisation of Bayes theorem is then

$$Bel_D(d;x) = (\prod_{d_i \in \bar{d}} Bel_X(\bar{x};d_i) - a)/(1-a) \qquad (1)$$

with
$$a = \prod_{d_i \in D} Bel_X(\bar{x};d_i)$$

If one has a prior belief defined on D analogous to the prior probability, both belief functions are combined by the rule of Dempster.
If the prior belief and $Bel_X(x;d)$ are Bayesian, the classical Bayes
theorem is obtained. An important point is that $Bel_D(d;x)$ given
in (1) has been computed with a vacuous prior belief function, that
is the belief function corresponding to total ignorance.

4. APPLICATION.

To show the power of the method we have simulated a realistic exemple
of its application. Real data will be available only when the procedure will have been accepted by clinicians and data accumulated.
Suppose that data are accumulated in three hospitals concerning two
diagnoses; H= Hypertension, D=Diabetes. Let $h_i \in H$ with h_1 = "hypertension absent", h_2 = "renal hypertension" and h_3 = "essential hypertension". Let $d_i \in D$ with d_1 = "diabetes absent", and d_2 = "diabetes present". Let S caractérise the absence (s_1) or the presence (s_2) of
other diseases. We thus have 12 possible diagnostic status (accepting
the proposed diagnosis are exhaustive). Let two symptoms X and Y be
observed where X can be at three levels x_1, x_2, x_3 and Y at two levels
y_1, y_2. In the first hospital, 1000 patients are observed and we
obtain informations relative to the status of their diagnoses and
symptoms. If we had received for all patients the exact status on
H, D, S, X and Y, our theory could be useless. But in practice data

are often only partial, that is some informations are missing. We
could have patients for whom the presence of hypertension is known,
but not its nature (renal or essential) or for whom the data on symptom X are missing. Worse is the case where we find the file of a
patient with two contradictory protocoles and we have no information
to decide which protocole is relevant to the patient. One shows
a renal hypertension and symptom x_1 while the other excludes renal
hypertension and shows symptoms x_2 thus the patient is either
(h_2 and x_1) either ($\bar{h}_2$ and x_2). Classical probability approach is
unable to cope with such "messy data" while the evidential approach
handles them straightforward. To discard such data implies some loss
of information and anybody who has worked with large data base has
often met such embarrassing situation.

Let $f(w)$ be the relative frequency of patients that are classified
in subset w of W, the diagnostic by symptoms universe ($W=HxDxSxXxY$)
and that cannot be classified in a strict subset of w. From the
1000 patients observed we have computed the belief function relative
to the symptoms for the twelve elementary diagnostic classes using
$f(w)$ as basic probability numbers.

In the second hospital, the data obtained from another set of 1000
patients never provided informations on the hypertension status
neither on the Y status (they cannot perform test Y and do not study
the hypertension status).

Finally, in the third hospital, a random sample of 100 patients has
been selected from a population of 1000 patients with their H,D,S
status being respectively h_1, d_1 and s_1. Only symptom Y has been
observed.

The belief function relative to the symptoms obtained from the three
hospitals are then combined by Dempster's rule, providing a belief
function relative to the symptoms for all elementary diagnostic
classes.

By the application of the evidential generalisation of Bayes theorem
one computes the belief function relative to the diagnostic given a
symptom, belief function that describes our belief that a patient
selected randomly from such population belongs to a diagnostic class
when a certain symptom has been observed.

Should we then have some belief on the diagnostic classes obtained
from other evidences, we combine by the rule of Dempster this new
belief function with the one derived from the data collected in the

three hospitals.

5. <u>CONCLUSION</u>.

The theory of evidence has the following advantages relevant for
medical diagnosis:
1. A certain degree of belief in a proposition does not automatically imply our degree of belief in its complement;
2. Total ignorance is perfectly described and avoid all criticisms
   adressed to the proponents of the classical Bayesian probability;
3. An ultimate description of all subsets and elements of the frame
   of discernement is not requested as in the theory of probability
4. Probability theory is just one particular case of the theory
   of evidence.
We consider that the conjonction of the theory of evidence with
fuzzy sets (Smets, 1978) will permit the development of a mathematical model for the medical diagnostic procedure much more acceptable
by the clinicians, much closer to the reality and sufficiently for-
malise that its implementation on computer is possible.

BIBLIOGRAPHY.

DEMPSTER A.P., (1968). A generalisation of Bayesian inference.
J. Roy. Stat. Soc. B-30 : 205-247.

SHAFER G., (1973). Allocations of probability : a theory of partial
belief. Princeton doctoral dissertation, available from
University Microfilms, Ann Arbor. USA.

SHAFER G.,(1976). A mathematical theory of evidence.
Princeton University Press, Princeton, New Jersey. USA.

SMETS Ph., KORNREICH F., BLOCK P., BERNARD R. and VAINSEL H., (1977a)
Fuzzy diagnostic, degree of belief and utility.
In Trends in Computer-processed electrocardiograms.
(Van BemmelJ.H. and Willems J.L. ed.) North Holland,
Amsterdam (pp 257-260).

SMETS Ph., VAINSEL H., BERNARD R. and KORNREICH F., (1977b).
Bayesian probability of fuzzy diagnosis. In Medinfo 77
(Shires D.B. and Wolf H. ed.) North Holland, Amsterdam
(pp 121-122).
SMETS Ph., (1978). Un modèle mathématique simulant le processus
du diagnostic médical. Submitted for publication

SMITH C.A.B. (1960). Consistancy in statistical inference and
decision. J. Roy. Stat. Soc. B-23 : 1-97.

SMITH C.A.B., (1965). Personnal probability and statistical analysis.
J. Roy. Stat. Soc. A-128 : 469-499.

ZADEH L.A., (1965). Fuzzy sets. Inform. Control 8 : 338-353.

BIBLIOGRAPHY

COMPUTER-AIDED CLASSIFICATION OF CHRONIC BRONCHITIS
IN COMPARISON WITH OTHER DIAGNOSTIC TOOLS

THURMAYR, R. - Institut für Medizinische Statistik und
Epidemiologie der TU München, Sternwartstr. 2,
8000 München 80 (BRD)

SCHÜTZ, I. - Werra-Klinik der BfA, Berlinerstr. 3,
3437 Bad Sooden-Allendorf (BRD)

KALIEBE, R., SCHNIEDERS, H., KARL, K., FÜRNTHALER, E. -
Institut für Medizinische Datenverarbeitung der Gesell-
schaft für Strahlen- und Umweltforschung mbH.,
Arabellastr. 4, 8000 München 81 (BRD)

1. PROBLEM

Under the sponsorship and in cooperation with the Bundesversicherungsanstalt für Angestellte (BfA) in Berlin and the Verband Deutscher Rentenversicherungsträger in Frankfurt, a method for computer-aided classification of severity grades for chronic bronchitis was developed.
The purpose of classification into severity grades is to ease the assessment of chronic diseases together with their combinations and to make
comparisons possible. This allows derivation of admission criteria for
rehabilitational therapy which are suited to computerized processing.
Using standardised severity grades permits better evaluation of the
effectivity of in-patient care and monitoring the course and/or result
of the treatment. Computer-aided determination of severity grades is
also feasible in mass-screening programs of out-patient clinics, health
services and health insurances as also in preventive care and epidemiological studies. The objective of this project was to reproduce by
computer the severity grade estimation as made by a physician from
symptoms characterising a clinical picture and to test this method on
routine sample material.

2. METHOD

2.1 Retrospective data acquisition

The diagnostic algorithm for determination of severity grades was developed using 900 case studies of insured patients with chronic bronchitis who
had applied for rehabilitation therapy. For this purpose the symptoms
constituting the clinical picture of 900 anonymous case studies and discharge reports were retrospectively extracted [1]. Simultaneously a team
of 5 physicians determined independently a severity grade from the reports
and agreed on the final severity grade after conferring with one another
when differences occurred. 4 severity grades were used as defined by a
formal decision aid. The final severity grade was used as the external

criterion for discriminant and decision-making procedures which resulted
in a classification algorithm.

2.2 Prospective data acquisition

In developing the classification algorithm the number of variables was
reduced from an original 168 to 70. Selection of the variables depended
beside medical criteria also on the frequency with which they were be
answered in data acquisition. Specifically, frequently missing variables
could not be selected even if they were medically relevant. The frequency
with which these variables were not available from the unstructured verbally composed report seems to indicate that they were difficult to determine in a physicians practice.
Our classification of severity grades is therefore based on material from
insurance practice and on the age group between 15 and 65 years. Extension beyond these limitations is however quite feasible. This reduced variable set was used to construct a formal questionnaire with 70 multiple-
choice questions which was sent to physicians of the BfA together with
directions for application and commentary. The field-test as a prospective
study now provides better data for testing the developed algorithm. 200
completed questionnaires have been returned to date. To check the questionnaire,corresponding medical report is examined and the data corrected
and expanded by our physicians. At this point therefore,two data sets
exist. The uncorrected data from the field-test as it was marked on the
questionnaire and correspondingly,data as it was corrected using the medical report. The severity grade is derived using the same procedure as
the retrospective study by a team of 4 physicians in accordance with the
recieved medical reports.

2.3 Decision-making processes
2.3.1 Boolean equations [+)]

As a first step the severity grades of chronic bronchitis were defined
according to the chronic symptom complexes and their complications
[2,3,4,5]. Then the variable equations of each clinical picture were
combined using boolean algebra which resulted in a severity grade.
To make combinations of the variables transparent, they were developed
stepwise. First the combination defined one of the above general categories of severity-grade (type of bronchitis, asthma, emphysema,
bronchiectases, right ventricular strain, permanent lung and/or thorax
involvement). Each of these 6 derived variables can be subdevided into
doubtful, light and severe cases (Tab. 1).

+) The Boolean equations were practised at advice by Prof.Dr.med.H.-J.Lange

Tab. 1: First stage of logic used (an excerpt)

Derived Variables	Preliminary grade of severity, if found
1. Chronic Bronchitis	
1.1 Simple	1
1.2 Purulent	2
1.3 Slight asthmoid	2
1.4 Severe asthmoid	3
2. Asthma bronchiale	
2.1 With symptom-free interval (s)	2
2.2 Without symptom-free intervals	3
2.3 Severe	4
3. Emphysema	
3.1 Without restriction	2
3.2 With restriction	3
3.3 With severe obstruction	3
4. Bronchiectases	
.	
.	
.	

At least one boolean equation defines each of these severity forms. If the result of an equation is true, a temporary severity grade is given. In the second step the results of the first are combined using boolean equations which result in a final severity grade of chronic bronchitis. Basically the highest temporary grade from the first step is decisive for the final severity grade. Only certain combinations of temporary grades can raise the final severity one step. A further equation gives the possibility of indicating that the diagnosis of chronic bronchitis is false.

The theoretically derived boolean equations are being tested on the collected data. To do this we are using the program system STADAB which was developed by our institute, which allows the use of boolean equations including multiple parentheses [6]. In the first step temporary severity grades are calculated from the derived variables and they again stored. Then the final severity grade for the second step is calculated using an other boolean equation. The identity between the final severity grade and that given by the physicians is used to calculate the rate of correct classifications.

Often missing variables in the equations can be found, when incorrect classifications by the computer are traced. Including new variables into the equation and/or rewriting them permitted the results to be continually improved. Sometimes borderline cases also retrospectively

caused our physicians to change their own assessment of severity grades.
To ease the tracenback the temporary severity grades from the first step
were printed out.

2.3.2 Decision Tables

Since boolean equations are difficult to read when only indexed variables
are used, we have developed a program which takes the variable name from
the data description and prints the equation in a legible form (Fig. 1).

$$
\begin{aligned}
Y(02) := \ &\text{IF ((UPRIGHT-POSITION-V069.EQ.2).AND.AGE-V105.GE40).}\\
&\text{OR.RIGHT-AXIS-DEVIATION-V070.EQ.2).OR.COMPLETE-}\\
&\text{RIGHT-BUNDLE-BRANCH-BLOCK-V073.EQ.2)).OR.}\\
&\text{DYSPNOEA-AFTER-LIGHT-WORK-V032.EQ.2.}\\
&\text{AND.CYANOSIS-V041.EQ.2)) THEN 3 ELSE 0,}
\end{aligned}
$$

Fig. 1: Boolean Equation

> The manifestations of the features are combined in a
> Boolean equation. The logical variables are capable
> of having the values 2: = true and 1: = false.

Translation of the boolean equation into a decision table has been found
to be a further aid. To do this all multiple parentheses are reduced.
Each variable of the boolean equation is placed into one rule of the
decision table, as long as or-conjuncted with the following variable.
Variables with 'and' or 'and-not' combinations are taken into the rule
together. The equation of the first step is then incorporated into
the second step so that a finalized decision table results.

Reducing boolean equations to the form of a decision table has the
advantage that redundancies and logical errors can automatically be
checked [7,8]. This formal error check can be extended in our problem
since severity grades can be sorted ascendingly. If a variable is used
for one severity grade it can be used again in a higher severity
grade only in combination with further variables. Furthermore the
decision table clearly shows which rules have not yet been incorporated.
A program prints them out in legible form and our physicians can then
include them in the severity grade decision or recognize them as contextual contradictions. Those rules which indicate contradictions are
finally combined using or-conjunctes into a boolean equation which
permits detection of erroneous data.

The importance of a variable in the boolean equation can be easily tested. The variable in question is removed from all equations and then the rate of correct classification is determined using the reduced formula for the same data set. If variables are sequentially removed an ascending or descending system such as used in discriminant analysis [9] can be made whereby the importance of the variable may be directly inferred from the increase or decrease in the rate of correct classification.

2.4 Results

When the boolean equations were first defined using 900 retrospective cases we achieved a rate of correct classification of 60 percentage using 120 variables. The equations could finally be improved using corrected data to 75%.

Tab. 2: Acurracy rate of algorithmic Diagnosis

Method / Sample	Boolean equations	Linear discriminant Analysis
Training sample (n=900)		
with missing data	58	75 ⎫
with supplied data	63	81 ⎭ Crossvalidation
Test sample (n = 150)		
uncorrected data	83	29
corrected data	98	56

Direct reuse of the algorithm from the retrospective study to the prospective field-test was impossible since categorical variables been formulated as multiple-choice in the questionnaire and their number reduced from 120 to 40. Therefore the data of the retrospective study was brought into the form of the field-test. This changed data was called the pseudo-field-test. The algorithms were reoriented using this data before they were first tried on the field test. Because of the missing data 120 variables had to be incorporated into the boolean equations of the retrospective study. The field-test only comprised 40. The final decision process now consists of a first step of 17 equations including 40 variables. Each equation combines approximately 5 variables.

The reorientation of the equations in the pseudo field-test (900 cases)
with corrected data yielded a rate of correct classification of between
59% and 63%. When the corrected data from the field test was run with
these equations an initial rate of correct classification of 76% was
achieved which finally was improved to 98%. The incorrect classifications
differed by only one grade of severity from the expected. Using uncorrected data in comparison we registered a rate of correct classification
of only between 61% and 83% respectively (Tab. 2).

3. COMPARISON OF THE METHOD WITH OTHER POSSIBILITIES

Originallly we had begun by developing a discriminant process and had
hoped to avoid the construction of a decision making procedure. When
we recognized that we could not determine the grade of severity without
this, the development and testing of boolean equations and the discriminant process using linear analysis were developed parallel to one
another. The 900 retrospective cases were used as a training sample
and the 150 prospective cases as a test sample [10]. Originally the discriminant analyses achieved a rate of correct classification of 53%
which could be improved to 81% by incorporating missing data and
scaling. The cross-validation using field-test data achieved 83%. This
discriminant formula arrived at a rate of correct classification of 56% when
corrected data was used for new classification. Uncorrected data
allowed only 29% of the patients to be correctly identified (Tab. 2).
The use of discriminant analysis showed an improvement of results after
missing data had been removed. New classification however showed a
strongly overoptimistic assessment of the rate of correct classification
by cross-validation. This was mainly the result of the fact that the selection
of variables had been made using the same material from which the cross-
validation was calculated [11]. The discriminant results of new classification incorporating missing data such as from the field test resulted
in a deterioration bordering on a random destribution for 4 groups.

At first the boolean equations achieved poorer results using the missing
data of the retrospective study than the discriminant analysis had
showed. Restructuring the field test data proved to be much easier with
the boolean equations since the formulae could easily be changed. The
discriminant analysis was more difficult to improve because a large enough
new sample had to be collected to be of any use.
When a boolean equation is reduced in a mathematical sense using times
for "and" and plus for "or" it is possible to recognize the existence
of mixed sections. Therefore, parts of our boolean equations are non
linear. It is thus not surprising that the rate of correct classification

of the linear discriminant analyses is poorer than that of the
boolean equations. The existence of mixed sections also implies that
non-linear discriminant analysis would be the method of choice.
Unfortunately inversion of the covariance matrix results in singularity,
since the type of some of variables is the same for all elements of one
severity grade. Singular matrices prevent calculation of a non-linear
discriminant ananlysis. Using quantitative data from another project,
a marked improvement of results as compared to the linear discriminant,
analysis was detected [12].

4. NEXT STEPS

Great importance must be placed on the question of how the derived
formulas which achieved a high rate of correct classification using
boolean equations can be used in practice. Three possibilities exist:
One lies in the acquisition of the symptomatology utilizing questionaries
which are marked by the examining physician and are amendable to computer
evaluation via boolean equations. This would however result in changes
for the physicians practice and in increased costs which seems excessive
for classification of severity grades of one illness alone.
Another possibility is formulation of the boolean equations as guidelines
for physicians. This is done by writing the equations such that variables
and variable combinations which result in certain severity grades are
listed whereby the most important and characteristic variables can be
accentuated. Only when these are difficult to derive, further variables
on the list can be used as alternatives.
Finally the boolean equations can be represented as a decision table.
Such a table using combination-logic is very compact if "or" combinations
are allowed within one rule. The "and" combinations can then be represented by vertical lines from cross to cross (Fig. 2).
The user of such a decision table first marks the existence of a variable
and then draws a horizontal line to the outermost rule. When all prerequisites of an and-rule reached by such a horizontal the corresponding
action is marked. This results in a temporary severity grade. When more
than one temporary severity grade exists the highest severity grade is
definitive, except in cases where combination of similiar severity grades
causes a rise in the final severity grade. For this purpose those rules
which in combination with others result in a higher severity grade in
the second step are combined in the action part of the decision table.

In summary, the use of boolean equations in routine with questionnaires
and computer evaluation still requires organizational restructuring.
Purely verbal descriptions are not conducive to controls which check
whether or not the rule has been adhered to.

Fig. 2: Decision table with extended logic
(an excerpt)

SYMPTOMS \ SEVERITY	1	2	3
COUGH	X		
EXPECTORATION	X		
MUCOUS EXPECTORATION	X		
BREATH - SOUND PUERILE	X	X	
INFILTRATES	X	X X X	
RALES	X	X	
PURULENT EXPECTORATION		X	
ANTIBIOTICS		X	
RALES MOIST		X	
DYSPNOEA BY HEAVY CHARGE		X	
DYSPNOEA BY SMALL CHARGE		X X	
EXSPIRATION EXTENDED		X	
SONOROUS OR WHISTLING RALES		X	
SLIGHT OBSTRUCTION		X X	
DYSPNOEA BY FITS		X X	X X
NO DISORDERS OF BREATHING		X	
HYPOSONOROUS PERCUSSION SOUND		X	X
NO RESTRICTION		X X X	
SIGNES OF EMPHYSEMA		X	X
BARREL - CHEST		X	
INCOMPLETE RIGHT BUNDLE BRANCH BLOCK ...		X X	
CYANOSIS		X X	
OEDEMA		X	

Using the compressed decision table a physician can make the decision
himself guided by the rule, especially since he can logically review it
at any time. This final form therefore seems to be the method of choice
until symptom complexes can be measured in a form adeptable to data
processing. This becomes increasingly interesting as more illness are
incorporated into the classification of severity grades. We are currently enlarging severity grade classification to encompass coronary heart
disease and chronic illness of the locomotorium.
We have learned from this project that changes in data acquisition
cause difficulties with already existent diagnostic aids, especially as
these changes at times caused by expansion of personal knowledge and
method. The logical decision table proved to be more adaptible since
it is constructed according to medical knowledge and not from a mathematical training sample. We had originally hoped to reach our goal
more quickly by discriminant analysis and thus avoid development of a
decision making process. We were however forced to recognize that a
decision process is already inherent in unified classification by our
team of physicians.

The formulation of boolean equations proved to be the most adequate method for developing a decision making procedure because physicians quickly learned its use. Representation of the decision process in the form of decision tables was also adventageous for automatic error detection.

ACKNOWLEDGEMENT

This work was done under the sponsorship and in cooperation with the Bundesversicherungsanstalt für Angestellte (BfA) in Berlin and the Verband Deutscher Rentenversicherungsträger in Frankfurt.
We are glad to acknowledge our indebtedness to Prof.Dr.med.G.Mäurer, Dr. F.W. Kaufmann (VDR) and Dipl.Ing. H. Dinkloh (BfA) for their encouragement, Dr. B. Dissmann, Dr. E. Kühler (BfA) and Dr. U. Hertig (Werra-Klinik) for their help in estimating the severity grade from records and to R. Kamstieß, M. Müller, Dr.K.Schulz, Dr. G.Wille (BfA) for their continuous collaboration during these studies.
Thanks to C.F-J Götz (IMD) for translation.

REFERENCES

1. Thurmayr, R., Schütz, I., Kaliebe, R., et alii:
    Computerunterstützte Bestimmung des Schweregrades bei der
    chronischen Bronchitis.
    in: Informationsverarbeitung in der Medizin - Wege und Irrwege.
    Bericht über die 22. Jahrestagung der GMDS EV. Göttingen.
    Ed.: Ehlers, C.Th., F.K. Schattauer-Verlag, Stuttgart-New York
    1977 (in Press).

2. Kuntz, E.:
    Chronische Bronchitis. MMW Taschenbuch.
    J.F. Lehmanns-Verlag, München 1975

3. Jelke, G., Möller, R., Schmidt, K.:
    Obstruktuve Atemwegserkrankungen (Teil 2: Stadieneinteilung der
    chronischen Bronchitis und Therapie).
    Med.Klin. 70, 1883-1887 (1975)

4. Lende, R. van der, Hansen-Koster, E.J., Knijpstra, S., Meinesz, A.F.,
    Wever, A.M.J., Orie, N.G.M.:
    Definition of CNSLD: Use in epidemiology and preventive medicine.
    Selected Papers 17, 83 (1977)

5. Lange, H.-J. and R. Reiter:
    DFG-Forschungsbericht "Chronische Bronchitis".
    Deutsche Forschungsgemeinschaft, Bonn-Bad Godesberg (1975)

6. Wolf, H.H.:
    STADAB, Statistisches Datenbank-Auswertungssystem.
    Statistical Software Newsletter 1, 63-66 (1975)

7. Fischbach, F, Groß, J., Ott, W.:
    Entscheidungstabellen.
    Verlagsgesellschaft Rudolf Müller, Köln-Braunsfeld, 1975,
    ISBN 3-481-32711-0

8. Veinott, G.C.:
    Programming Decision Tables in Fortran, Cobol or Algol.
    in: Communications of the ACM, Vol. 9

9. Victor, N., Hörmann, A., Eder, L.:
    STATSYS-Beschreibung und Benutzeranleitung.
    GSF Bericht, MD 24, München (1973)

10. Thurmayr, R., Kaliebe, R., Schnieders, H. et alii:
    Computer-aided classification of chronic bronchitis.
    AWAMI Annals of Wami Quarterly Journal 1978 (in press)

11. Lachenbruch, P.A.:
    Some Misuses of Discriminant Analysis.
    Meth.Inform.Med. 16, 255-258 (1977)

12. Thurmayr, R., Blomer, R.J. et alii:
    Computer aided diagnosis of pancreatic function tests in the
    routine situation.
    in: Decision making and medical care (Eds. by de Dombal and
    Gremy), North-Holland Publishing Company Amsterdam - New York -
    Oxford, 175-182 (1976)

REVIEW OF THE MUMPS LANGUAGE AND ITS APPLICATIONS TO MEDICINE

Joan ZIMMERMAN, Biomedical Computer Laboratory,
Washington University, 700 South Euclid Avenue,
St. Louis, MO 63110, USA.

Frits SCHUTTE, Free University Amsterdam/Department of Medical Informatics,
van der Boechorststraat 7, 1007 MC Amsterdam, The Netherlands.

ABSTRACT

Almost a thousand medical institutions worldwide use the MUMPS concept for medical applications, particularly for hospital and for ambulatory-care medical-record
systems. The number of MUMPS-using institutions grows at about 70% per year, with
the adoption by more groups of MUMPS for such applications as patient identification,
clinical laboratory management, pharmacy, radiology, patient interviewing, physician
consultation, computer-aided instruction, and inventory.

In order to facilitate the transfer of MUMPS applications, the American Department of Health, Education, and Welfare (HEW) and the National Bureau of Standards
sponsored the development of the Standard MUMPS language, and HEW took the initiative in supporting the MUMPS Users' Group. The Standard was defined by the MUMPS
Development Committee during 1973 to 1975. By 1976 several implementations of the
Standard had become available. In 1977 the Standard was approved by ANSI under
standard number X11.1-1977. At that time, the Users' Group started a library of
MUMPS applications that included a questionnaire driver, a series of interactive
lessons teaching people how to program in the Standard MUMPS language, and a package
for documenting applications in Standard MUMPS. In this paper a brief overview is
given of the MUMPS language and the standardization project, existing medical MUMPS
applications are summarized, the application transfers that have been accomplished
by the MUMPS Users' Group Application Library are reviewed, and some plans for future expansions are discussed.

1. INTRODUCTION TO MUMPS

MUMPS (an acronym for Massachusetts General Hospital Utility Multi-Programming
System) is both a computer language and an operating system. Its development began
at the Massachusetts General Hospital (MGH) in Boston during 1965, guided by Dr.
G. Octo Barnett and Mr. A. Neil Pappalardo, and it was first used for application
programming in 1966 (Barnett, 1976). MUMPS' original characteristics and its use
for clinical data management systems were described by Greenes et al. (1969), who
emphasized the speed of application development and modification in MUMPS, and the
strengths of MUMPS in manipulating both text and hierarchically organized data.

Many different institutions became interested in MUMPS soon after 1965.
By 1969, several independent implementations of MUMPS were being developed.

Unfortunately, each implementor had his own preferences for features to be included in and added to MUMPS, so that a variety of different MUMPS dialects appeared. A major disadvantage of this proliferation of dialects was to inhibit application transfer, leading to the parallel development of many similar applications in different dialects (Johnson, 1974). Such concerns led, three years later, to the start of the standardization of MUMPS and the rapid reconvergence of the dialects into Standard MUMPS. The Standard was defined by the MUMPS Development Committee in 1975 (O'Neill, 1976) and approved by the American National Standards Institute in 1977 (ANSI, 1977).

The MUMPS language is a relatively simple procedural language. A novice may learn to write simple MUMPS code in under an hour, although he requires several months of experience in order to be able to write optimal code. The low threshold to writing MUMPS means that people such as physicians, with negligible programming background, can and do learn to develop applications in MUMPS.

MUMPS was designed originally to capture, analyze, store, and retrieve medical data. To this end, MUMPS is able to:
- Handle data input and output easily at video terminals, printers, teletypes, analog-digital channels, and so on.
- Analyze the captured data by such techniques as the comparison of one piece of data or one segment of that data with another, and by verification of its syntax. Data checking is particularly valuable at the time of entry, when wrong data may be corrected immediately.
- Store the data easily in dynamic and readily changeable files. Such files are structured as sparse, multi-level (tree-like) files, just as medical records are organized with increasing levels of complexity. They are easily created and are simultaneously accessible and changeable by multiple users.

The classic implementation of MUMPS is as an interpreter on a dedicated small or medium computer. An interpreter allows a programmer to write and debug his applications interactively and therefore quickly. The application programs are readily tested, modified, and retested in the high-level interpreter environment. In practice, time savings of an order of magnitude have often been observed for programming in MUMPS compared with the use of assembled and compiled languages.

Traditional implementations of MUMPS have included not only the MUMPS language itself but also a time-sharing executive to allocate processing time to MUMPS tasks. Other components are an input/output system for the entry and display of data, and a hierarchical data-base system for the storage of data on long-term storage media. Zimmerman (1977a) listed implementations of Standard MUMPS on 15 different types of computer. For a summary of MUMPS and its classic implementation, see Bowie and Barnett (1976), and for a more detailed description see Wasserman et al. (1975) and ANSI (1977).

2. STANDARDIZATION OF MUMPS

The MUMPS Development Committee (MDC) was formed in March 1973 under the terms of an interagency agreement between the American National Center for Health Services Research and the National Bureau of Standards. The primary purpose of the MDC was to assimilate the many MUMPS dialects into a complete, coherent MUMPS Standard. The main reason for this standardization effort was seen by its HEW sponsors to be the fostering of the "widespread replication of existing MUMPS programs and their assembly into health-care systems" (Glenn, 1974). Mr. David A. Bridger, when he was Chairman of the MDC Standard Specifications and Language Development Subcommittee, saw five major benefits that might result from the MUMPS Standard (Bridger, 1974):

1. Facilitation of the transfer of MUMPS programs and packages between MUMPS users and MUMPS systems.
2. Encouragement of the development of an independent body of MUMPS literature and techniques.
3. Provision of the foundation for the orderly development of MUMPS in the future.
4. Facilitation of the training and transferability of MUMPS programmers.
5. Help in the validation of MUMPS as a legitimate approach to computer utilization in the larger computing community.

For all these reasons, but especially for the first, the MUMPS community has standardized MUMPS. The early acceptance of the Standard MUMPS specification by the MDC on 12 March 1975 illustrated the MUMPS community's commitment to standardization. The approval of the Standard by the American National Standards Institute in September 1977 demonstrated national recognition of MUMPS. Activities of the MDC in further support of MUMPS included investigation of MUMPS implementation, under the chairmanship of Dr. Anthony I. Wasserman (Wasserman et al., 1975a, 1975b, and 1975c), and the establishment under Dr. Jeffrey Rothmeier of guidelines for MUMPS code and data documentation (Peck, 1976).

3. MEDICAL MUMPS APPLICATIONS

MUMPS is used primarily for medical applications, although it is useful in many nonmedical areas such as finance, shipping, television, and library cataloging. An applications list drawn up in mid-1977 contained 230 applications (Zimmerman, 1977a). About 1000 institutions use MUMPS, with roughly two-thirds of the users in the United States and most of the remainder in Europe and Japan; for Europe an overview of medical MUMPS application has been compiled by Schutte (1978a). Workers such as Dr. G. Octo Barnett (1974), Dr. Warner V. Slack (1976), and Dr. Howard L. Bleich (1974), have been concerned with improving the quality of health care delivered to patients, and making the interactions with computers by both patients and providers as friendly and civilized as possible. To these ends, the flexible and responsive characteristics of MUMPS have been emphasized and developed. Some of the most important MUMPS applications are now summarized.

The first MUMPS application was for laboratory management, and this remains one of the most popular applications as seen from Zimmerman (p. 14, 1977a). Justifications for laboratory systems include savings of personnel time, faster reporting of results, more reliable results, availability of better medical and administrative reports, and availability of laboratory statistics. Systems can be purchased for $100,000 to $300,000 for a hospital of approximately 500 beds or 700,000 tests per years. The value of MUMPS as a tool in the clinical laboratory has been described by Barnett (1974), Grossman et al. (1974), and Minckler and McMahan (1973). These authors emphasized automated data acquisition, the conversion of entered data into meaningful results, and the production of cumulative patient summaries. Generally laboratory systems exclude microbiology and emphasize chemistry, but a MUMPS microbiology system for work-card generation, result entry, and report generation has been developed (Lewis and Marr, 1975). The ability of MUMPS to absorb a constant stream of new application developments while maintaining its functional activities is highly valued here.

MUMPS is well suited to handle medical-record systems. It manipulates files readily and also handles text information. A record system can consist of an individual data base on specific kinds of patient. Some examples are cancer patients, thus providing a tumor registry (Milan, 1977); various surgical patients (Merier et al., 1976); pregnant patients (Schutte et al., 1977; Warford, 1978); cardiac patients (Glaser et al., 1975 and 1976; Moore et al., 1976); renal patients (Wakai, 1976); diabetic patients (Achtenberg, 1977); and hypertensive patients. Record systems can also maintain selected important information from all records. This could include a diagnostic code, demographic data, and selected additional information for service, health-care, administrative, research, and PSRO requirements. Small-scale record systems may be established quickly using miniature general-purpose record systems such as MISAR (Karpinski and Bleich, 1971) and MEDINFO.

Ambulatory-care medical records are being developed at the Harvard Community Health Plan and Massachusetts General Hospital (Barnett et al., 1976; Justice, 1974; Lurie, 1974), George Washington University (Baillieul et al., 1976; Waxman, 1976), the Arizona Health Plan (Boyd, 1974), and the Cardiovascular Clinic of Oklahoma City (Wilson and Robbins, 1976). The data manipulated in such record systems include patient identification information and the description of the provider/patient encounter. The encounter description summarizes who interacted with the patient, where, and how, and includes vital signs, test made, problems identified, prescribed therapy (e.g., drugs ordered), and follow-up plans. Major benefits of these systems are improved continuity of patient care and the facilitation of peer review, leading to the enhancement of quality of medical care (Geiss, 1978; Rector, 1977).

Hospital information systems are under development at Hospital Data Center of Virginia in Norfolk, VA, Institute of Living in Hartford, CT, George Washington University in Washington, DC, Kirchliche Gemeinschaftsstelle fuer EDV in Frankfort, Germany (Haase, 1978), Law Hospital in Glasgow, Scotland, and University College Hospital in London, England (Hall, 1978). These complex systems are designed and developed with substantial advice from the future users, in order to maximize their eventual acceptability. They are also designed in a modular fashion, so that the development of one area (say laboratory) may proceed as independently as possible of another area (say pharmacy).

Computer-aided instruction (CAI) is being developed for training medical students (Brigham et al., 1976) and for the advanced training of physicians (Bleich, 1974). The flexibility inherent in the computer-based applications allows a student to work on individualized cases, applying and learning facts and concepts, making decisions, and seeing the simulated results of his actions. A special advantage of CAI is that it provides each student with realistic experiences in health care while avoiding the possibility that the student endangers a real patient in learning the effects of prescribed therapies. Furthermore, it compresses into a few minutes actions that normally last for many weeks or months, thereby giving the student a much clearer perception of the effects of actions than obtainable in real life. Furthermore the MUMPS concept is used to educate medical students in the principal aspects of medical information processing (Schutte, 1978b and 1978c).

MUMPS is proving a valuable tool for pharmacy systems. Braunstein and James (1976) noted the importance of a computer-based outpatient pharmacy system in tracking and monitoring the medications that outpatients use, together with the prescription behavior of various physicians. MUMPS is used for inpatient pharmacy systems such as that at Stanford University School of Medicine (Briggs et al., 1973). There, emphasis is placed upon not only keeping track of what drugs are administered, but also flagging potentially hazardous drug interactions.

Another area in which MUMPS is finding widespread application is radiology information systems, in particular by workers at Columbia, Missouri (Lodwick, 1975). Their system includes a physician-reporting capability that has been shown to halve the time taken for a radiologist's consultation report to get back to the referring physician. Other work on radiology information systems is carried out at the Beth Israel Hospital (Simon et al., 1974), the Tufts New England Medical Center, and the Mallinckrodt Institute of Radiology (Domke and Ragan, 1974).

Patient admitting and census is another most valuable function, providing a hospital with a valid on-line patient data base, reducing clerical errors, and increasing efficiency of in-hospital information and order transfer (Peth et al., 1974).

4. APPLICATIONS FOR THE MUMPS COMMUNITY

The MUMPS Users' Group (MUG) began informally with the first issue of the MUMPS News as a means of developing communication and exchange between MUMPS users (Barnett, 1971). Formal federal sponsorship of MUG began in 1973, allowing the group to provide information to over 5000 requesters during the next 4 years. Meanwhile companion MUG's were started in Japan by Dr. Ichiro Wakai and in Europe by Dr. Boy Glaser.

The MUMPS Users' Group Application Library (MUGAL) is being designed by MUG as a repository for MUMPS applications contributed by the MUMPS community (Forrey, 1977; Zimmerman and Forrey, 1976). The applications are to be primarily small and made available to users at minimal cost. MUGAL's goal is to increase the frequency of successful MUMPS application transfer between users. To facilitate such success, MUGAL requires that submitted applications meet minimal criteria as specified by Forrey (1977).

Three Standard-MUMPS applications were developed under federal funding to the Biomedical Computer Laboratory, St. Louis, for MUGAL. These are the QUEST questionnaire driver (Brigham et al., 1976; Zimmerman and Brigham, 1977), the Standard MUMPS teaching program (Zimmerman, 1977b), and the DOC documentation package (Malamud et al., 1978).

QUEST, developed by Chris Brigham and Joan Zimmerman, allows the authoring and editing of computer-based tutorials, and the teaching and testing of students by means of those tutorials. The lessons are divided into questions or frames, each of which contains text, a question, and logic to check the answer and branch to a more advanced or to a remedial frame, depending upon the student's answer. QUEST differs from other drivers developed in MUMPS by not requiring the user to have knowledge of MUMPS itself to utilize all of the driver's power. No user, whether a student, author, or supervisor, is required to have MUMPS skills.

The Standard MUMPS Teaching Program is a computer-based tutorial developed using QUEST. The teaching program contains 12 lessons that provide guidance on how to use the questionnaire, an overview of MUMPS, and a detailed description of MUMPS' capabilities. The performance of each student that uses the teaching program is evaluated on the basis of whether or not he is re-asked frames (indicating that incorrect answers were given) and how long he takes to respond to the frames. Results for people new to MUMPS and people already familiar with it differ as discussed by Zimmerman and Stimac (1977).

The third application is DOC, which facilitates the documentation of MUMPS routines, programs, and packages. As far as possible, DOC performs the documentation automatically. Where human interaction is necessary, DOC guides the user through a logical sequence of questions to specify the necessary data. The extent and style of the documentation provided by DOC is tailored to the documentation requirements of MUGAL as summarized by Forrey (1977).

By early 1978, QUEST and the Standard MUMPS teaching program had been transferred to 23 institutions and DOC had been transferred to 11. Some of the recipients of QUEST were using it as the basis of their own computer-aided instruction (CAI) programs in diverse application areas, particularly for instruction in surgery to medical students and instructions to paramedical personnel on the care of diabetic patients.

DOC has been used on itself, on QUEST, and on the COSTAR package for the automated ambulatory-care medical-record (Barnett et al., 1976; Justice, 1974). DOC's ability to detect syntax errors facilitated its own development, as did its ability to list local and global variables used and their locations. The use of DOC on CO-STAR was particularly useful in helping us begin to understand this large (900-routine) and complex package. Of particular value were the table of routines listed alphabetically with the routines they invoke and that invoke them, as well as the lists of local and global variables, and the static routine trace. It would be naive to attempt a technical understanding of such a package without use of capabilities like those provided by DOC.

5. HOW MUG CAN FACILITATE APPLICATION TRANSFER

The initial set of applications in MUGAL are basic to disseminating information about MUMPS programming and facilitating the automated documentation of MUMPS applications. In addition the questionnaire driver is a tool for the development of CAI material. Following its successful transfer of these applications, MUG should expand the scope of its library by adding medical applications, preferably those developed under government funding and therefore in the public domain. MUG should be careful to address the technical, administrative, and other problems in application transfer identified by Zimmerman and Forrey (1976). In particular, DOC will help to minimize problems of sparse and inconsistent documentation for the applications MUG makes available.

6. ACKNOWLEDGEMENTS

The development of the three applications described was supported by Grant HS-01540 from the National Center for Health Services Research, HRA, USDHEW. The original development of the MUMPS (Massachusetts General Hospital Utility Multi-Programming System) language was supported by Grant HS-00240 from the National Center for Health Services Research, HRA, DHEW.

REFERENCES

Achtenberg, J., et al., "Data 3 - A Forms-Oriented Data Management System", in Rothmeier (1976), pp. 1-8, 1976.

ANSI X11.1-1977, MUMPS Language Standard, 1977.

Baillieul, P. P., et al., "COSTAR V - Experiment in Transportability", in Rothmeier (1976), pp. 12-15, 1976.

Barnett, G. O., MUMPS News, No. 1, December 1971.

....., "The Use of a Computer-Based System to Teach Clinical Problem Solving", in Stacey and Waxman (1974), pp. 301-319, 1974.

....., personal communication, 1976.

....., et al., "MUMPS: A Support for Medical Information Systems", Medical Informatics, 1, pp. 183-189, 1976.

Bleich, H. L., "Automated Instructional Programs for Advanced Medical Education", in Stacey and Waxman (1974), pp. 289-300, 1974.

Bowie, J., and G. O. Barnett, "MUMPS - An Economical and Efficient Time-Sharing System for Information Management", Comput. Programs in Biomed., 6, pp. 11-22, 1976.

Boyd, J. A., "New 'Handle' on Patient Care", in Zimmerman (1974), pp. 135-139, 1974.

Braunstein, M. L., and J. D. James, "A Computer-Based System for Screening Outpatient Drug Utilization", JAPA, NS16, 2, pp. 82-85, 1976.

Bridger, D. A., "MUMPS Standardization Issues", MUMPS News, #8, pp. 7-10, 1974.

Briggs, R. L., et al., "The Stanford MEDIPHOR System", in Zimmerman (1973), pp. 58-60, 1973.

Brigham, C. R., J. D. Halverson, and J. Zimmerman, "QUEST: A Teaching Program Driver", Journal of Computer-Based Instruction, 3, 2, pp. 42-50, 1976.

Domke, F., and D. P. Ragan, "Diversified Applications Package for Radiation Therapy", in Zimmerman (1974), pp. 74-81, 1974.

Forrey, A. W., "The MUG Application Library", in Zimmerman (1977a), pp. 2-3, 1977.

Geiss, E., "MUMPS Application in Doctor's Office Systems", to be published in Medical Informatics, Editors F. Bagon and J. Anderson, 1978.

Glaser, B., et al., "Thoraxcenter Utility System", in Zimmerman (1975), pp. 60-77, 1975.

....., et al., "Thoraxcenter Utility System (TUS): Level 1 Available", in Rothmeier (1976), pp. 61-68, 1976.

Glenn, W., in MDC/12, "Minutes of the MUMPS Development Committee", No. 2, p. 2, 1974.

Greenes, R. A., A. N. Pappalardo, C. W. Marble, and G. O. Barnett, "Design and Implementation of a Clinical Data Management System", Comput. Biomed. Research, 2, pp. 469-485, 1969.

Grossman, J. H., A. N. Pappalardo, and M. E. Ruderman, "A Commercially Shared Computer Utility for Medicine", in Stacey and Waxman (1974), pp. 267-285, 1974.

Haase, H., Kirchliche Gemeinschaftsstelle fuer EDV, Frankfort, private communication in Schutte (1978a), 1978.

Hall, D. G., "Experience of Transferring an Integrated Hospital Administration System from a Codasyl Database to a Standard MUMPS File Structure", to be published in Annals of the World Association for Medical Informatics (AWAMI), 1978.

Johnson, M. E., "The MUMPS Dialects", MUMPS News, #8, pp. 4-6, 1974.

Justice, N., "The Harvard Community Health Plan's Automated Medical Record System", in Zimmerman (1974), pp. 36-39, 1974.

Karpinski, H. S., and H. L. Bleich, "MISAR: A Miniature Storage and Retrieval System", Comput. Biomed. Research, 4, 6, pp. 655-660, 1971.

Lewis, J. W. and J. J. Marr, "A Low-Cost Clinical Microbiology Computer System", in Zimmerman (1975), pp. 97-100, 1975.

Lodwick, G. S. "The Application of Computers in Diagnostic Radiology", Current Problems in Radiology, 5, 1, 1975.

Lurie, R. S., "COSTAR - Costs and Benefits", in Zimmerman (1974), pp. 140-145, 1974.

Malamud, R. S., R. K. Stimac, and J. Zimmerman, "MUMPS Application Design Manual for DOC, A Documentation Package", Monograph #301, published by the Biomedical Computer Laboratory, Washington University, St. Louis, MO, 1978.

Merier, G., B. Glaser, and R. Brower, "An Interactive Computer System for Assessment of Coronary Bypass Surgery", in Rothmeier (1976), pp. 80-84, 1976.

Milan, J., Royal Marsden Hospital, Sutton, U.K., private communications in Schutte (1978a), 1977.

Minckler, T. M., and J. McMahan, "Our Lab has MUMPS", in Zimmerman (1973), pp. 55-56, 1973.

Moore, P., et al., "A Management Information System Designed to Oversee a Clinical Study", in Rothmeier (1976), pp. 85-95, 1976.

MUMPS Development Committee. For publications, contact Chairman Dr. Richard F. Walters; University of California at Davis, Medical Learning Resources, Davis, California 95616.

MUMPS Users' Group. For publications, contact Executive Director Mr. Richard E. Zapolin, The MITRE Corporation, P.O. Box 208, Bedford, MA 01730. In Europe, contact Executive Secretary Dr. Frits Schutte, Free University of Amsterdam, Dept. Med. Info., NL-1011, van der Boechorststraat 7, Amsterdam, The Netherlands. In Japan, contact Executive Secretary Dr. Ichiro Wakai, MUG-Japan, 5th Fl. Enryu Bldg., 6-25 Shinsakae-Cho Naka-ku, Nagoya, Japan 460.

O'Neill, J. T., Editor, "MUMPS Language Standard", NBS Handbook 118, available from the Superintendent of Documents, US Government Printing Office, Washington DC, 1976.

Peck, L. J., "MUMPS Documentation Manual", MDC 3/6, available from the MUMPS Users' Group, St. Louis, MO, 1976.

Peth, C. F., G. G. Edick and N. W. Hickman, "CGH Admitting System", in Zimmerman (1974), pp. 40-44, 1974.

Rector, A. L., University of Nottingham, U.K., private communications in Schutte (1978a), 1977.

Rothmeier, J., Editor, Proceedings of the 1976 MUMPS Users' Group Meeting, published by the MUMPS Users' Group, Bedford, MA, 1976.

Schutte, F., et al., A Peripheral Data Base in MUMPS", in MEDINFO 77, Editors D. B. Shires and H. Wolff, North-Holland Publ. Comp., pp. 619-623, 1977.

....., An overview of (bio) medical MUMPS applications in Europe", in Medical Informatics, Editors F. Begon and J. Anderson, 1978a.

....., et al., "MUMPS as an Educational Tool", to be published in Medical Informatics, 1978b.

....., et al., "Educational Aspects of Medical Informatics", these proceedings, 1978c.

Sias, F. R., Jr., Compiler, Proceedings of the First Southeastern Region MUMPS Users' Group Meeting, published by the MUMPS Users' Group, Bedford, MA, 1976.

Simon, M., et al., "Computerized Radiology Reporting Using Coded Language", Radiology, 113, pp. 343-349, 1974.

Slack, W., et al., "Dietary Interviewing by Computer", Journal of the American Medical Association, 69, pp. 514-517, 1976.

Stacey, R. W., and B. D. Waxman, Editors, Computers in Biomedical Research IV, Academic Press, 1974.

Wakai, I., "Registry of Renal Failure Patients for Kidney Centers", in Rothmeier (1976), pp. 141-149, 1976.

Warford, H., and E. Jennett, "A Computerized Peripheral Data System", to be published in Annals of the World Association for Medical Informatics (AWAMI), 1978.

Wasserman, A. I., D. D. Sherertz, and R. W. Zears, "Design of a Multiprogramming System for the MUMPS Language", MDC 2/2, available from Medical Information Science, University of California, San Francisco, 1975a.

....., D. D. Sherertz, and C. L. Rogerson, "MUMPS Globals and Their Implementation", MDC 2/1, available from Medical Information Science, University of California, San Francisco, 1975b.

....., D. D. Sherertz, and R. W. Zears, "Implementation of the MUMPS Language Standard", MDC 2/3, available from Medical Information Science, University of California, San Francisco, 1975c.

Waxman, B. D., "COSTAR V - An Exportable Ambulatory Record and Management System", presentation at the Sixth Annual Conference of the Society for Computer Medicine, Boston, MA, 12 November 1976.

Wilson, D. H., and G. P. Robbins, "Introduction of a Computer into Private Physician Practice", in Sias (1976), pp. 14-20, 1976.

Zapolin, R. E., Editor, Proceedings of the 1977 MUMPS Users' Group Meeting, published by the MUMPS Users' Group, Bedford, MA, 1977.

Zimmerman, J., Editor, <u>Proceedings of the 1973 MUMPS Users' Group Meeting</u>, published by the MUMPS Users' Group, Bedford, MA, 1973.

....., Editor, <u>Proceedings of the 1974 MUMPS Users' Group Meeting</u>, published by the MUMPS Users' Group, Bedford, MA, 1974.

....., Editor, <u>Proceedings of the 1975 MUMPS Users' Group Meeting</u>, published by the MUMPS Users' Group, Bedford, MA, 1975.

....., Compiler, <u>Book of MUMPS</u>, available from the MUMPS Users' Group, c/o Mr. Richard Zapolin, the MITRE Corporation, Bedford, MA 01730, 1977a.

....., "MUMPS Application Design Manual for a Standard MUMPS Teaching and Testing Program", Monograph <u>#335</u>, published by the Biomedical Computer Laboratory, Washington University, St. Louis, MO, 1977b.

....., and C. R. Brigham, "MUMPS Application Design Manual for QUEST, a Simple Questionnaire Driver for Teaching and Testing Students", Monograph <u>#300</u>, published by the Biomedical Computer Laboratory, Washington University, St. Louis, MO, 1977.

....., and A. W. Forrey, "MUMPS Application Transfer and the MUG Application Library, in Rothmeier (1976), pp. 150-165, 1976.

....., and R. K. Stimac, "Applications for MUGAL", in Zapolin (1977), pp. 157-163, 1977.

THE COMMUNICATIONAL STRUCTURE OF MEDICAL INFORMATION SYSTEMS AND ITS EDUCATIONAL CONSEQUENCES

by

O. Rienhoff and P.L. Reichertz

Dept. of Biometrics and Medical Informatics
Hannover Medical School

- Abstract -

The paper briefly reviews the state of the art of educational efforts in the field of Medical Informatics. More detailed it analyzes the question of project accompanying education. It is outlined, that not only technical matters have to be taught, but also psychological aspects of system design. As easily performable measurements of communicational and psychological problems are still not available, some guidelines for the setup of educational procedures are formulated. All examples mentioned and the theses derived are based on the experiences of several years of educational activities in connection with the Hannover Medical School hospital information system.

1. INTRODUCTION

During the last years it has been generally accepted, that education and training is one of the key questions of progress within the field of Medical Informatics (1). Several curricula within all subfields have been developed (7). They can be separated into different categories due to the preeducational status, the occupational field and national specialities. It is neither possible to discuss here the analysis and definition of educational needs for all the different curricula (e.g.2), nor is it possible to discuss standards and effectiveness control (e.g.3). Thus only a brief general review will be presented. Less attention has been directed to the main theme of this paper, the detailed description of the educational needs prior, during and after implementation of a concrete information system within a medical environment and its organization. Our experiences, the examples mentioned, and the environment we refer to correspond to the activities of the Division of Medical Informatics at Hannover Medical School and a four years cooperation with the Technical University at Braunschweig. (The Medical School at this moment has nearly 5ooo employees with 14oo beds and 104 clinical and/or theoretical units).

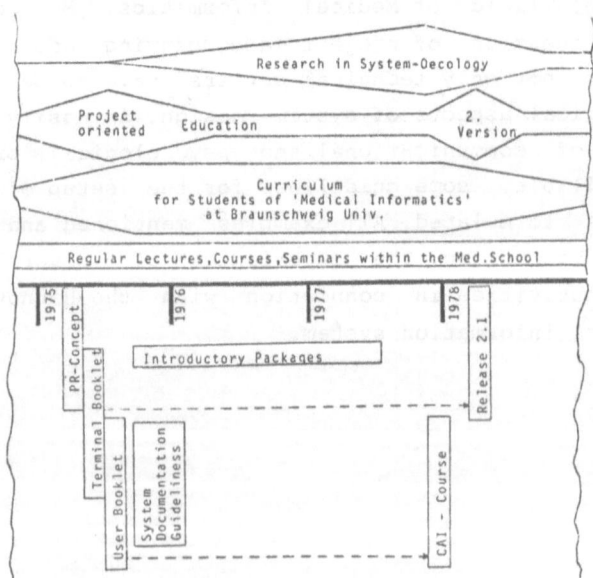

Fig.1: Milestones within the development of curricula by the Division of Medical Informatics in Hannover. In 1978, nearly all different curricula are in the process of final consolidation.

2. OVERVIEW OF THE EDUCATIONAL FIELD IN MEDICAL INFORMATICS

The educational efforts can be divided into those being affiliated with a defined environment or project and those without being oriented towards actual targets. In both cases the education or the training can be realized by universities and schools, by on-the-job training and by special courses offered by system vendors or private spezialized companies. Roughly separating you may distinguish between the academic and non-academic levels and especially in the prior case between pre- and postgraduate training. Further it has to be discriminated between training as acquisition of specific skills and education as acquisition of general principles and skills.

Another order of the various activities is given in Fig.2, stressing the connections between general education by an university hospital (A), the educational programs in the hospital itself (B) and finally the project-supporting education (C). Fig.3 describes the situation in the concrete environment of the Hannover Medical School.

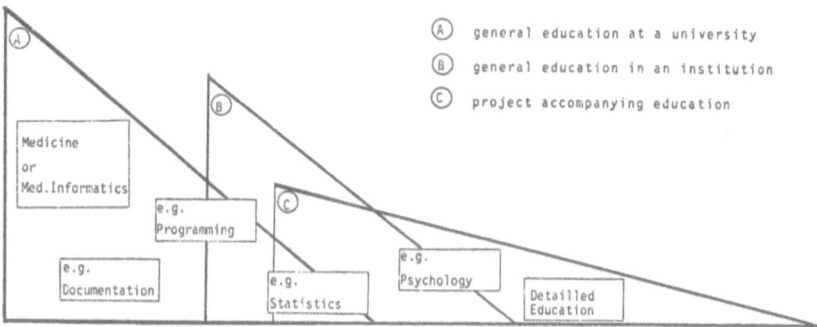

Fig.2: Schematical description of the structure of the educational field in Medical Informatics and the connection of different levels as mentioned in the paper.

Last year, Koeppe (6) described in detail the situation in West Germany and gave first estimates for the number of specialists to be educated in Medical Informatics on an academic level per year. During the Second World Conference on Medical Informatics in Toronto (MEDINFO'77) it became apparent, that the western countries of Europe have developed educational concepts with a higher

318

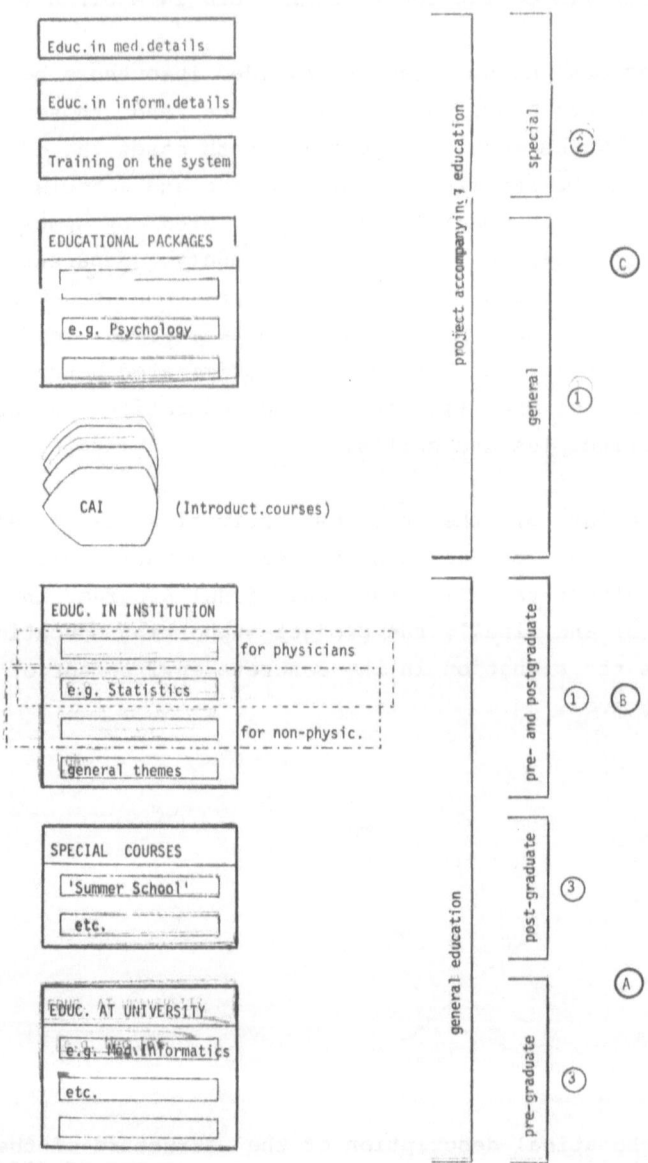

Fig.3: The educational activities of the Division of Medical Informatics at Hannover Medical School as an example for the differentiated educational duties of large scale institutions in the field. The numbers herein correspond to the three levels discussed in the literature (1,2) of courses and the characters to the relating partitions of fig. 2. The computer aided instructions are introductory courses which mainly are supposed to make the use of terminals easier. They are based on the updated versions of a user-booklet from 1975 (8).

priority than the US. As medical computing was exported from the States to Europe twenty years ago, concepts of Medical Informatics now find their way back to the US. In the case of education this is especially true for the academic level, while the education of so-called health engineers is still ahead in the States. Some of the European countries as the Fed. Rep. of Germany still even do not know this profession. Those working in the field of medical documentation, the medical documentation clerks or medical record librarians, have similar basic education concepts in the different countries.

As far as we know, up to now people educated in the field do not have difficulties to find adequate jobs. As specially educated people are yet available, the main institutions in the field tend to employ only those, because they do need less time to become productive than e.g. a general statistician or an economist. However, Koeppe (6) is somehow critical in regard to the increase in production and predicted future demand. One might, however, also foresee an increase of this demand.

Independent from the kind and level of education it can generally be stated in respect to the theme of this paper that in most of the realized curricula the technical aspects are sufficiently taken into consideration. But in all countries the problem arises, how to explain to doctors and nurses the different way of thinking and time priorities of systems analysts -and, the other way round- how to enable the people on the systemside to accept the live characteristics and priorities in a medical environment. We consider the consequences of these differences to be the root of many 'not understandable' difficulties during the implementation of projects, because the differing backgrounds may cause communicational problems, which often are never discussed freely. Therefore it is necessary to make people on both sides conscious of these traps. We are trying to derive a test for the quantification of these difficulties (9). It is difficult to set up curricula containing interdisciplinary aspects instead of teaching the 'others' detailed parts of ones own knowledge for this requires the recognition of new aspects and the development of new teaching concepts. This was mainly the reason why it took several years to create a set of lectures and courses for the students of Medical Informatics at the University of Braunschweig. Even the preparation of a lecture 'medicine in its principles' caused considerable work, in spite of the wave of 'popular' medical books, because those are structured bottom-up (from example to general) instead of the top-down approach needed (principles illustrated by examples). Analytical description of principles in concept, struture and decision making must have priority over knowledge of detail which is necessary in the practice of medicine.

3. EDUCATION AS PROJECT SUPPORT

3.1 Ignoring Psychological and Communicational Aspects

Since early days of system analysis matters mostly have been approached from a technical standpoint. Alternatives have been decided without considering possible educational, psychological or political barriers (5). With 'SAGE', the early US air defense system, these parameters were first systematically introduced into the history of a complex system. But the message of the consequent success reached only 'bitwise' the field of Medical Informatics - mostly too late to save the struggeling medical information systems in the early seventies. Consequently we do not have to focus on the technological questions of systems analysis and its educational consequences, but rather we have to concentrate on the psychological and communicational questions.

The establishment of curricula is time consuming and therefore educational programs have rather been oriented towards the classic solutions than towards new concepts. At teaching hospitals, traditionally courses in programming or statistics are offered or system oriented training courses are sponsored by the software vendors. But -again- this educational approach alone is not any more adequate to our knowledge of the problems which usually arise during the implementation of an information system as results of research in user psychology have shown (10) and as published by IFIP already in 1974 (2). Information systems tend to change the environment into which they are introduced. Therefore not only technically operational matters have to be taught and discussed, but also psychological reactions which will occur during the system implementation phase. This proved to be particularly true the complexer the systems are or the more they perform medical audit analyses.

The lack of consciousness about the influence of psychological and communicational aspects of information systems was extremely reflected in the aggressive advertisement of hard- and software system vendors who successfully sold products to at that point of time innocent users. The confusion and emotionality of the 'used' users was lateron further promoted by those scientific investigators, who presented their work either in the golden shine of success or in dry words decorated with the cream of self-criticism. Only recently the will to inform as objectively as possible about medical information systems starts to prevail.

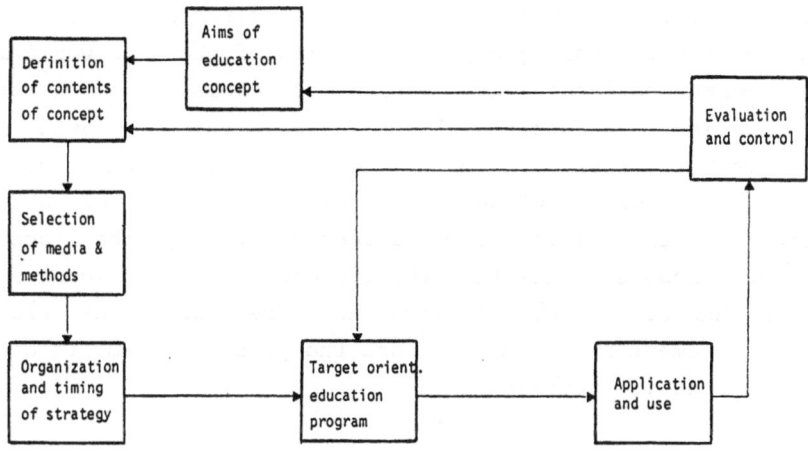

Fig.4: The feedback circuit in the establishment of curricula in any area. It is oriented towards the 'instructional system approach to training' as published by Kaufman (4), and as such a closed loop system which is never considered to be completed. According to our experiences one cycle for programs as described in fig.3 takes at least two years. To realize the five characteristics of the instructional system approach (1. Identification of total training requirements in performance terms, 2. Identification of training subsystems that will interact in accomplishing total instructional system objectives, 3. Provision of a decision making model and of criteria for achieving the system requirements, 4. Provision of methodology for conducting training and 5. Provision of empirical means for the determination whether the system is valid) considerable efforts have to be undertaken. The Hannover concept of fig.3 aims into that direction.

3.2 Formalization of Psychological and Communicational Factors

The first step described above has to be an analysis of the communication structure of medical information systems. After first narrative descriptions of the communicational field reproducible further investigations have to try to structure the problem area. In this case it has to be checked, whether adequate models have already been defined for the field of medical information systems. A review of models of user types and user dimensions was presented by Wersig (12). There are approaches out of social-psychology (e.g.by Paisly, Bock, Allen) and others derived from communication theory. Most of the models reported are rather vague and if integrated end up in so many dimensions of user characteristics that it is difficult to project a given user environment into these dimensions. Nevertheless, all of them identify aspects of user populations which may also be used in more pragmatic models. As the contents of the curricula have to be directed towards the composition of the target group, the mapping of the user world into a formal communicational model is the prerequisite for a target oriented design of educational strategies. This is even more pertinent when the strategy aims at the change of attitudes besides the transferral of knowledge and the development of skills. Formulated in the terms of communication theory the lack of suitable user models means that the elements of the communication system are undefined and therefore the transmission of signals between the element system-manager and the possible elements of the user environment is unstructured.

A rather pragmatic view at a user environment was presented by Virts (11) in connection with the evaluation of the El Camino Project. He defined matrices for participation in decision. These have the function of structuring the decision making process during the design and implementation phases of a hospital-wide information system. The imperative of maximazing participation stands behind this approach. Its pragmatical definition of the user environment (e.g. chief executive, assistants, house staff etc.) may also be used for the educational purposes. The categories may be modified by some of the deductive dimensions reviewed by Wersig and thus lead to a manageable communicational model of the real world of a planned information system. Unfortunately, the use of this concept is limited to rather big projects with enough users to fill all matrix fields. For smaller information systems (e.g. for a department) the description of users may be sufficient, but it will be impossible to set up related sophisticated educational strategies with only few people in single courses. Here only a vertical separation may be tried (e.g. top- and middle management, staff) or a simple occupational (e.g. physicians, nurses, paramedical personnel).

Prior to the setup of a specific education strategy an analysis of the occupational directions and the psychological status of the later user group is further necessary. As stated above, even the formalistic description of the elements of the communication system is basic. A similar situation is true for the aimed psychological measurements (9). The estimation of acceptance in a given communicational network is consequently still a research effort, but not an everyday routine. Therefore the composition of educational strategies that accompany projects in most cases still needs an experienced project manager with careful evaluation of technical as well as psychological and communicational factors influencing the project's history.

Regarding technical questions there exists experience almost everywhere. Regarding system ecology, experiences are still limited. Therefore, it is helpfull to supportthe decision, whether or not special courses have to be integrated in the accompanying education which are oriented towards the solution of possible psychological or communicational conflicts. As decision support we defined seven dimensions, which in our experience describe the possible threats to an information system (fig.5). Within these dimensions we set a rough scale according to which a given system environment can be rated.

The scales are results of experience - they are not validated. Therefore it would be misleading to report profile characteristics and derive special strategy requirements from them. But, it is save to say, that when more than two of the ratings are negative or just one gets into the negative extreme general or specific educational efforts have to be initialized to keep the psychological problems small.

In regard to the attempts to structure the user environment the rating can be accomplished not only for an environment as a whole, but it can be done for different defined user groups separately. In this case, the scaling instrument is already used in a more sophisticated way and it has to be analyzed, whether the dimensions are equally relevant within the different groups. Further sophistication leads to decision tables which are more precise t h a n details are measurable or users can be grouped. It should not be forgotten that this pragmatical procedure intends to optimize the concrete setting up of a project accompanying education and not to yield research results. It is a simple means to structure the non-technological parts of the education supporting the project.

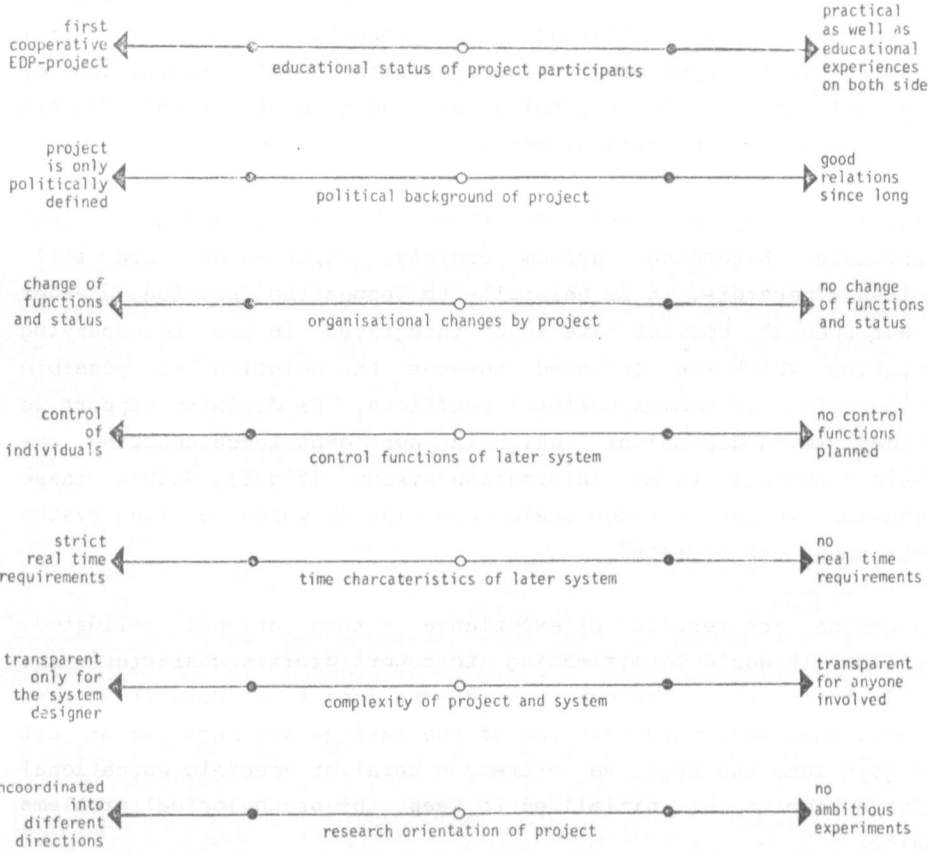

Fig.5: The seven dimensions of 'psychological threat' to an information system in a medical environment projected on a scaling system. The rating scales contain possible roots of psychological problems on the user side as well as on the system-designer side.

3.3 Introduction of Educational Packages into Project Management

The decision to conceptualize the educational needs for a given environment in general and to formulate special needs due to the communicational structure and the psychological characteristics of a project directly leads to the question of feasibility of establishment and maintenance. The answer has to be standardization of procedures. Since a 'structuring' of the 'art of programming' has shown considerable progress in software management, those colleagues believing in the 'art of education' have to be integrated with their know-how into a more formalized solution. At least most parts of the educational concept should be realized in package form. The packages have to contain the logical structure of a defined educational step and necessary material for the preparation of the education. Standardization saves time and allows to concentrate on a didactically good presentation rather than on defining educational targets, gathering contents, and choosing education media. But 'package form' does not only mean standardization in this sense, it also means defining time needs. For example, one way which has proven to be successful, is the installation of crash courses instead of lectures spread over several months.

In this context we have to check which kind of media can be used. The possibilities of computer aided instruction have been discussed extensively. We only use them in project supporting education in a rather simple form as mentioned in fig.3. The use of audiovisual techniques in general has been tried probably everywhere. But the necessary amount of work and money stands in contrast to the difficult updating procedures. Therefore we expect the future trend towards so-called 'question-mark-films' which in few minutes build up a problem oriented motivation within an audience. This consciousness consequently is utilized in analysis and teaching.

The final step is the introduction of these packages and the preceding decision procedures into the regular course of project management (both into system analysis and system implementation). For example equivalent procedures were incorporated into the second version of the "Projektdurchfuehrungsrichtlinien" (project-implementation rules) of the Medical System Hannover in May 1978.

At the end of this paper one point should be clarified to avoid misunderstandings. All educational concepts should neither be abused to educate or train defenseless users in matters they do not want and they do not need, nor shall education substitute inefficient technological solutions. The educational tools have to be optimized to be used within a cooperative approach during the analysis, design and implemetation phases of medical information systems. The set up of an educational project supporting strategy has to be done by the system people and the users - only the tools (as described in the paper) have to be prepared before sufficiently.

5. ACKNOWLEDGEMENT

This presentation is based on the efforts of our coworkers namely I. Moehr, Ch. Moog, H. Haut, V, Hausmann and F. Strauch.

6. REFERENCES

1. Anderson,J. :
   Education of Health Staff in Information Processing Techniques, in
   Shires,D.B.,Wolf,H. (eds.); MEDINFO 77, (North Holland Publ. Comp.,
   Amsterdam,New-York,Oxford: 1977) 975-978

2. Anderson,J., Gremy,F., Pages,J.C. :
   Education in Informatics of Health Personnel,
   IFIP Medical Informatics Monograph Series, vol.1
   (North Holland Publ. Comp., Amsterdam,New-York,Oxford: 1974)

3. Anonymous :
   Comments submitted to the EEC on "A Four Years Programme
   for the Development of Informatics in the Community",
   British Computer Society, March 1977

4. Kaufman,R.A., Corrigan,R.E., Nunnelly,Ch.L. :
   The Instructional System Approach to Training,
   Human Factors, 8 (1966) 157-162

5. Keen,P.G.W., Gerson,E.M. :
   The Politics of Software System Design,
   Datamation (1977) 80-84

6. Koeppe,P. :
   Education in Medical Informatics in the F.R.G.,
   Methods of Information in Medicine, 16 (1977) 160-167

7. Reichertz,P.L.:
   Education,
   Computer Programs in Biomedicine, 5 (1976) 206-14

8. Rienhoff,O. :
    Vorschlag zur Neuordnung der PR-Arbeit innerhalb der MHH,
    Div.of Medical Informatics, Hannover Med.School, June 1975

9. Rienhoff,O. :
    Ein Ansatz zur Optimierung des benutzerseitigen Systemdesigns
    mittels des Semantischen Differentials,
    GMDS Jahrestagung 1977, Goettingen

10. Rienhoff,O., Reichertz,P.L. :
    User Psychology - Or Who is Using Whom in Medical Informatics, in
    Shires,D.B.,Wolf,H. (eds.): MEDINFO 77, (North Holland Publ. Comp.,
    Amsterdam,New-York,Oxford: 1977) 983-987

11. Virts,S.S. :
    Introducing the Hospital-wide Information System to Hospital and
    Medical Staffs, in Shires,D.B.,Wolf,H. (eds.): MEDINFO 77, (North
    Holland Publ. Comp., Amsterdam,New-York,Oxford: 1977) 993-997

12. Wersig,G. :
    Zur Systematik der Benutzerforschung,
    Nachrichten fuer Dokumentation, 24, 1 (1973) 10-14

Address of authors:

Dr. med. O. Rienhoff, Department of Biometrics and Medical Informatics,

P.O.Box 610180, Medical School Hannover, D-3000 Hannover 61,

EDUCATIONAL ASPECTS IN MEDICAL INFORMATICS

F. Schutte, J.H. van Bemmel, A.F.L. Veth and H. van der Woord
Free University
Dept. Medical Informatics
Amsterdam
The Netherlands

1 INTRODUCTION

Besides much older disciplines like physics, chemistry, biology and
statistics, informatics is one of the new sciences recently introduced
into medicine. The use of computers and information processing for
medical research is quite clear; it is also obvious that computers
have a stead fastly growing impact on routine in medicine and health
care, i.e. on clinical management, diagnosis making and so on. The
reason why it is necessary to introduce informatics in the medical
curriculum is for these same reasons clear as well: no doctor - whether
he will practice as General Practitioner, as specialist in advanced
medical care or in social medicine - will be able to escape the confron-
tation with some form of information processing. He will be the supplier
or user of computer data: he will use advanced information processing
systems for his data handling and interpretation; he will store and
retrieve data to or from large medical data bases or he will use the
computer as his clinical research tool, etc.
The main objective and final goal of our educational activities is to acquaint the medical student with our discipline at different
stages during his education and to show him some theoretical backgrounds,
but above all to let him have hands-on experience with some representative small systems for medical information processing. The latter is
only possible if we perform the research in our department in such a
way that spin-off's can be used for teaching and training.
At present we have set up the following educational activities:
- in the 2nd year of the medical curriculum an appreciation course of
  12-24 hrs in medical information processing is given, follwed by a
  mandatory test;
- during the 5th year will be introduced next semester a so-called
  'block course' of one week duration after the internship Internal
  Medicine. During the mornings the student will be taught some aspects
  of medical information processing, whereas the afternoons will be
  available for practical exercises;
- since 1974 almost on an annual basis have been given post-graduate
  courses in medical information processing. These lectures comprise

a total of 12 hrs; also, the above mentioned block course has
incidentally been given for post-graduate training;
- finally, a number of introductory or extensive training courses in
  FORTRAN, RSX and graphics are given. These are being extended by a
  Standard MUMPS course.

It should be emphasized that we do not have the intention to train the
student in whatever programming language; our aim is to give them some
insight in the (im)possibilities of (medical) information processing,
and to give the students some experience in interactive communication
with a computer.

For our real-time applications a Digital PDP 11/70 is available, whereas
a PDP 11/60 is running under the DSM-11 (Standard MUMPS) operating
system. The former is used mainly for research purposes, whereas the
principal task of the latter computer is training.

In this contribution we will restrict ourselves to the description of
a set of software packages for interactive use by the student, which
have been developed in MUMPS and cover several areas of medical information processing and clinical applications. A more extensive review
of our educational activities can be found in material to be published
at the IFIP-TC4 Working Conference on Education in Medical Informatics,
to be held in Munich, November 1978.

2 CLINICALLY ORIENTED PACKAGES

Although we are still in the process of further expanding the set of
training packages for medical informatics, we have already at our
disposal some representative packages which will be briefly discussed.
First of all we will point to the underlying philosophy why such programs have been developed or are being adapted to the training environment. The basic idea is that we will show the student some examples of
information processing in those application fields that he will most
probably be confronted with. We have listed these fields of applications
from 'commonly used by ALL' to 'possibly used by SOME' in table 1.
The scheme of table 1 indicates clearly which fields have to be emphasized heavily and which fields can just be briefly touched. Table 2,
along the same lines as table 1, gives a non-exhaustive summing-up of
practical examples belonging to these fields of applications, although
at the same time one must be aware that several examples belong to more
than one field. For that reason, the most prominent field has been
indicated by a black dot.

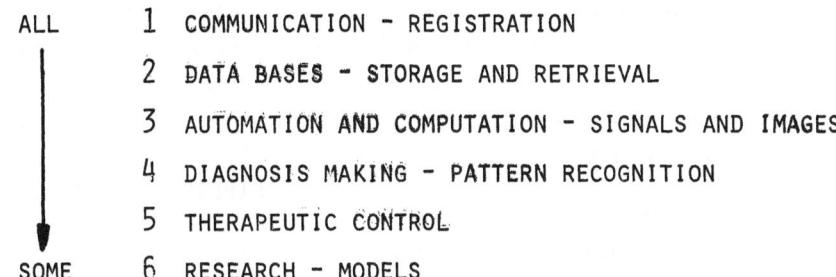

ALL	1	COMMUNICATION - REGISTRATION
	2	DATA BASES - STORAGE AND RETRIEVAL
	3	AUTOMATION AND COMPUTATION - SIGNALS AND IMAGES
	4	DIAGNOSIS MAKING - PATTERN RECOGNITION
	5	THERAPEUTIC CONTROL
SOME	6	RESEARCH - MODELS

Table 1 Fields of applications in Medicine and Health Care, listed from
ALL (commonly used by most physicians) to SOME (possibly used by
a much smaller group)

EXAMPLES	FIELDS OF APPLICATIONS					
	1	2	3	4	5	6
	C&R	DB	A&C,S&I	DM,PR	TH,C	R,M
* MEDICAL REGISTRATION BY TERMINALS	●	O				
* VISUALISATION OF ICU DATA ON CRT	●		O			
* MEDICAL RECORDS	O	●				
* INVENTORY CONTROL		●				
* CLINICAL CHEMICAL LAB		O	●			
* NUCLEAR MEDICINE			●			
* COMPUTER-ASSISTED INTENSIVE CARE		O	●	O	O	
* ECG COMPUTER ANALYSIS			O	●		
* CELL RECOGNITION				●		
* COMPUTER-ASSISTED ANTI-HYPERTENSION				O	●	
* RADIOTHERAPY PLANNING					●	
* THORACIC SURFACE MAPPING						●
* MULTI-COMPARTMENT ANALYSIS						●

Table 2 Practical examples belonging to the fields of applications
listed in table 1

In the demonstration packages for medical education using MUMPS we have attempted to obtain operational examples in all fields, although the fields that will be met by ALL yield most of the attention.
Table 3 shows the examples which have (almost) been made operational indicated by a black dot.

		FIELDS	STATUS
1 HIS	* REGISTRATION - ALLOCATION	1,2	●
	* MEDICAL QUESTIONNAIRES	2,3	O
	* CLINICAL CHEMICAL LAB	2,3	O
	* CODING OF DISCHARGE DIAGNOSES	2(4)	●
	* STATISTICAL REVIEWS	3	O (● in FORTRAN)
	* GRAPHICAL REPRESENTATION OF DATA	1	●
2 DB	* DENTISTRY DATA	1,2,3(4)	●
	* OBSTETRIC DATA	2,3	●
	* PEDIATRIC DATA	2,3(4)	●
3	* SIGNAL ANALYSIS	3,6	O (● in FORTRAN)
4	* DIFF. DIAGNOSIS OF HEPATITIS	4	●

Table 3 Educational packages in different fields of applications operational under MUMPS

(1) *hospital information system*
   a patient census module, modified to the situation and nomenclature of the Academic Hospital of the Free University, with admission, discharge, bed transfer, search, reports etc.; a questionnaire module and a laboratory module are being developed; a package to retrieve coded discharge diagnoses is available.
   For more general use, a statistical package will be converted to Standard MUMPS, whereas means have been developed to allow graphical representations of data.
(2) *data bases*
   a dental data base package, with input of the actual status of a set of teeth, short and long list possibilities, a retrieval module with criteria to be matched, and, in future, a link to statistics; an obstetric/pediatric data base package, which comprises interactive input, storage of obstetric history, trend data during pregnancy, parturition data, data from neurological examinations of the newborn and at later ages, and pediatric data. Retrieval programs are being developed.

(3) *signal processing techniques*

In FORTRAN, a software package has been developed to illustrate a number of signal processing techniques as are in common use in medicine: (i) a library of physiological signals, such as the EEG, the ECG and VCG, the IUP (intra-uterine pressure), the FHR (fetal heart rate), etc., and test signals, and (ii) a set of signal processing techniques to be applied, such as filtering, computation of amplitude distribution, scatter diagrams, power spectra and auto- or cross correlations, and sampling.

(4) *differential diagnosis*

a package to perform a differential diagnosis of neonatal hepatitis and biliary atresia, with patient data input, patient's lists, diagnostic criteria, diagnostic tree, diagnosis and decision table routines.

3 REQUIREMENTS

All packages should embody a common philosophy with respect to the student/user, covering the following items:

- the packages as much as possible should have a relation with or be deduced from research activities with respect to clinical applications
- all packages/modules should be usable in an interactive way
- obviously, the packages to be used should be thoroughly tested on syntactical and dynamical errors
- the generated output should match as close as possible a for the student known and recognizable clinical situation
- the user/student should only be able to access the programs via a security procedure, comprising at least user code, user identification and correct program calling; the user/student should have access to data bases only via the programs; this implies:
o the PRGM INTRPT / CNTRL C / BREAK facility should be disabled
- at any stage in the programs the input of the command HELP or a question mark (<?>) should give access to help routines, by means of which a further explanation of the question involved or a list of possible answers is generated
- in case of non-response, question generation should be repeated and after a number of times consecutive non-response the program should EXIT automatically.

The packages (1) patient census, (2) dental data base, and (4) differential diagnosis have been briefly described in Schutte et al. (1978). The design of (2) an obstetric data base for research purposes is given in Schutte et al. (1977). As an example of our educational packages, in the following section an outline will be given of (3) the package for signal processing techniques.

4 SIGNAL PROCESSING TECHNIQUES

In FORTRAN, a package has been developed to illustrate a number of signal processing techniques as are in common use in medicine. It comprises (i) a library of physiological signals, such as the EEG, the ECG and VCG, the IUP and FHR, etc., and test signals, and (ii) a set of signal processing techniques to be applied. The student may define in an interactive way the signal he wants to process, the technique to be used, the fields on the screen of a Tektronix 4012 on which the signal(s) and the result(s) are to be displayed, and, depending on the type of processing technique, some additional input, such as signal parts, sample points, sample interval, detection level etc.
The general form of the command string is as follows:

<operation>/<input signal>/<output buffer>/<display location>/{<secondary input>}

The <operations> implemented are listed in table 4. Two buffers of each 512 words are available to store any signal or output. The use of this package as an educational tool may be illustrated by a few examples:

4.1 signal_processing (cf. fig. 2)
The first command reads anECG into buffer X and displays it in field 00 (cf. fig. 1). Then the signal is filtered with a moving average filter (MA1), the result is stored into buffer Y, and displayed in field 01. The filter characteristics are automatically displayed in adjacent blocks: the impulse response (left) and the frequency domain (right). The final command calls the level detector to operate on buffer Y (the filtered signal). After indicating interactively a detection level, the result is displayed in field 02.

4.2 Fourier_analysis (cf. fig. 3)
The first command reads an EEG into buffer X and displays the result in field 00. Then a low-pass filter (LP2) is applied. The result is stored into Y and displayed in field 01, together with the filter characteristics, as discussed above. Fourier analysis is applied on the original signal, the result being displayed in field 03 (bottom left), and on the filtered signal, with the result in field 05 (bottom middle). The filtered output is filtered once more, now using a high-pass filter (DI1). The result is stored in X and displayed in field 02. Again, Fourier analysis is performed on this output, and the result is displayed in field 09 (bottom right).

OPERATION		INPUT SIGNAL	OUTPUT BUFFER	DISPLAY FIELD	SEC. INPUT	INTERACTIVE INPUT
REA	read a signal	EXT	X,Y	00-03	-	
FIL	filter a signal digital filters avail.	X,Y	X,Y	00-03	EXT	
PX.	amplitude distribution	X,Y	-	02-13	-	signal part
PXY	scatter diagram 1 or 2 signals	-	-	02-13	*	signal part sample points
FOU	power spectrum	X,Y	-	02-13	-	signal part
LEV	level detection	X,Y	00-03	00-03	-	pos./neg. level
SAM	sample signal	X,Y	-	00-03	-	sample interval
COR	auto or cross correlation	XY,YY	X,Y	00-03	-	signal parts
DET	detection performance of level detector	-	-	02-13	-	detection level
COPY	copy screen on plotter	-	-	-	-	
CLR	clear screen	-	-	-	-	
EXIT	exit from program	-	-	-	-	

Table 4 Command strings for signal processing techniques package

The three power spectra, as displayed in fig. 3, fields 03, 05 and
09, clearly show the effect of filtering on the original signal and
on its frequency contents.

4.3 detection characteristics (cf. fig. 4)

The user specifies the distribution functions to be input in buffers
X and Y and the field(s) where they have to be displayed. Then the
detection characteristics module is called via DET and some levels
are indicated interactively. The results, viz. % Correct Positives
and % Correct Negatives, resp. the Receiver Operating Characteristics,
are given as squares (◻) in the most right displays. Finally, the
continous characteristics are displayed.

All commands may be prepared in advance by creating a command file.
In this way a demonstration can be prepared easily. The user only
hits a key (e.g. the RETURN) in order to proceed with the next command,
and supplies the interaction, as required by several modules.

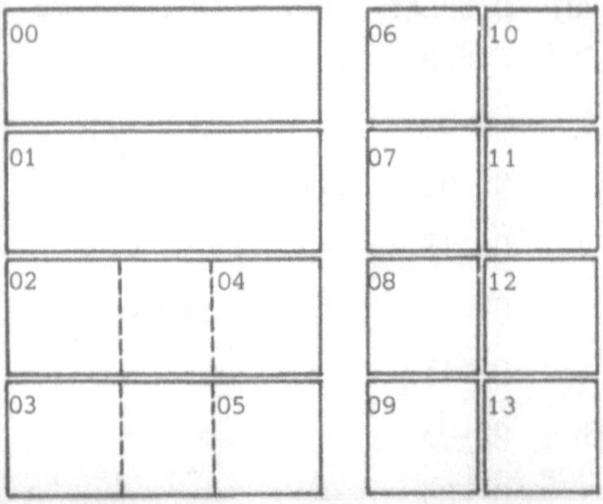

336

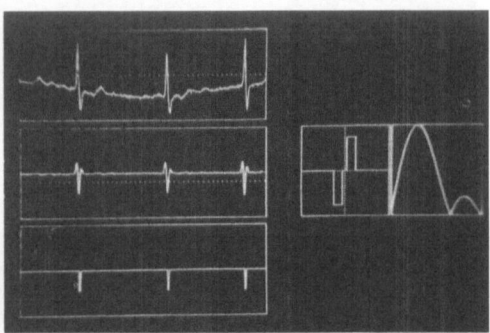

Command strings: REA/ECG/X/00
                 FIL/X/Y/01/MA1
                 LEV/Y/01/02

Fig. 2 Signal processing
        left: ECG, filtered ECG and level
              detector output
        right: filter characteristics:
              impulse and frequency domain

Command strings: REA/EEG/X/00
                 FIL/X/Y/01/LP2
                 FOU/X/03
                 FIL/Y/X/02/DI1
                 FOU/Y/05
                 FOU/X/09

Fig. 3 Fourier analysis
        left: EEG, once and double filtered EE
        right: filter characteristics:
              impulse and frequency domain
        bottom: power spectrum of the three
              signals

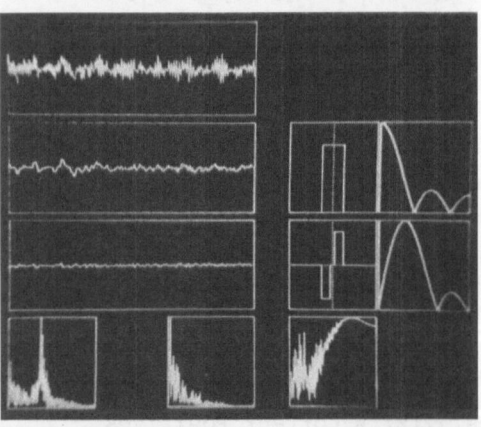

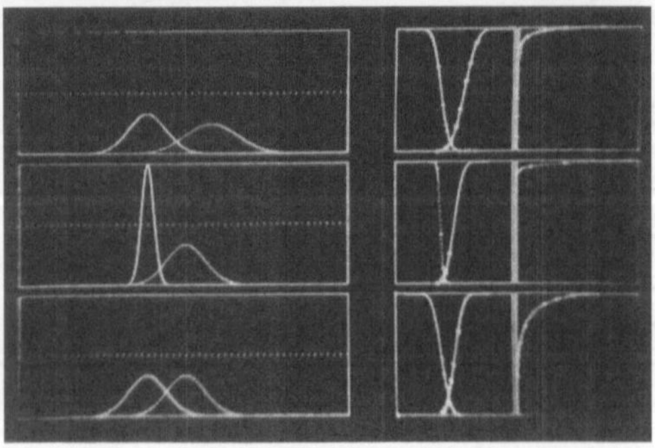

Command strings: REA/GA1/X/01
                 REA/GA2/Y/01
                 DET/07/
                 REA/GA3/X/02
                 REA/GA4/Y/02
                 DET/08/
                 REA/GA1/X/03
                 REA/GA4/Y/03
                 DET/09/

Fig. 4 Detection characteristics
        left: three times
              two distribution functions
        right: the corresponding
              detection characteristics
              and R.O.C.'s

Fig. 1 Definition of fields
        on T4012 screen

CONCLUSION

We have about one year and a half experience with the packages
mentioned, especially in post-graduate courses. The about 50 users
showed a good interest in this set-up and were content with the
facilities offered. This encourages us to continue in this line and
to expand the packages to be used in an environment of educating
medical information processing.

REFERENCES

F. Schutte et al. (1978): MUMPS as an educational tool,
        to be published in Medical Informatics

F. Schutte et al. (1977): A peri-natal data base in MUMPS,
        Medinfo 1977, eds. Shires and Wolf,
        North-Holland Publ. Comp. pp. 619-623

A.F.L. Veth (1978): Signal processing techniques
        Technical note, Free University, Dept. Medical Informatics,
        Amsterdam

COMPADOS : HOW TO CONVINCE A PHYSICIAN TO USE

A COMPUTERIZED MEDICAL RECORD SYSTEM

J. van Egmond, R.J. Wieme

Department for Medical Informatics M.I.G.

University of Gent

De Pintelaan 135

B—9000   GENT

Belgium

ABSTRACT

One of the objectives of the computerized medical record system
COMPADOS, developed at the University Hospital of Gent, is to convince the individual physician of its advantages for patient care,
medical research, medical education and health care management.

Several approaches have been experimented in order to smooth   the
implementation of the system :

- reduction, as far as possible, of the burden caused by the
  daily use of a computerized system
- increase of the advantages e.g. continuous availability of
  user selected information for direct patient care, introduction of some computer aided patient care techniques, care
  for high quality data in the computer record, elaboration
  of facilities for tne scientific use of the registered data.

Distribution of the workload of registration and validation, adaptation of the computerized procedures to the specific structure of a
function a person performs, registration of the medical reality in
all its complexity and consideration of immediate rewards for the
user, are the main characteristics of COMPADOS. In addition, a
sophisticated data protection system meets the ethical criteria one
uses for a medical record system.

Although objective criteria for the evaluation of a medical record
system are not available, it is attempted to evaluate the different
aspects of the system, which is now in routine use in the University
Hospital in Gent.

I. INTRODUCTION

The success of a computerized medical record system (CMRS) depends on the active and "enthusiastic" collaboration of the clinicians. It therefore is of utmost importance to convince the physicians : the advantages of the CMRS for their patient care and for their research must outweigh the burden of its use.

At the University Hospital of Gent, Belgium, the CMRS COMPADOS had to be implemented in competition with the traditional medical record system. The basic goal of the implementation of COMPADOS is the realization of a voluntary participation of the physicians : COMPADOS should demonstrate to the physicians the superiority of the use of informatics to solve the physicians' needs in patient care, medical research and management.

The evaluation of the usefulness of a medical record system is, however, very difficult as no objective and accepted criteria exist for this evaluation.

II. SOME IMPORTANT PROBLEMS FOR THE IMPLEMENTATION OF A CMRS

In addition to financial and organizational difficulties, many problems arise when implementing a CMRS. Most implementors of CMRS's will confirm at least some of the following problems :

1. It is not possible to define one single record system which is usable by all physicians. The debate in the literature between the adepts of the traditional chronological record, of the source oriented record, of the problem oriented record, ... (1) already demonstrates that modern health care struggles with the structure of this basic tool for patient care.

   The computerized medical record must integrate itself into the daily work procedures of an individual physician, who is a member of a team taking care for the patient ! The fact that not all data may be stored in a computer, e.g. analog data and pictures, increases the problem of the use of a CMRS in the daily medical practice.

   It is essential to consider very carefully the philosophy and reality of the local medical environment when implementing a

CMRS. Indicators for the evaluation of the success of the record system may facilitate a stepwise and user (physician) interactive implementation (2) of the CMRS, which is essential for the adaptation of the system to the practice of the physicians.

2. By tradition and, unfortunately also by education - the situation only very recently is changing -, the dedication to a correct medical record is not considered to be important for patient care : the work associated with registration of patient information is a part of the "paperwork" which is always considered excessive by a busy physician. A computerized system increases this workload !

3. Computertechnology is not flexible :
   - the computer terminals are laborious and difficult to integrate into the daily practice of a physician (are physicians good typists ?)
   - computer registration requires a formalization of medical practice

   One should not overestimate the state of art of computer technology neither the existing experience and knowledge concerning medical methodology !

4. Many psychological problems are related to a CMRS, e.g.
   - the collaboration with high level non-physicians, having their own language, own education and own approach to decision problems, may cause conflicts All partners must accept mutual education
   - medical ethics must be respected. Privacy and confidentiality are basic characteristics of medicine. The importance of the ownership of registered data must not be underestimated in a research oriented environment
   - the argument that the CMRS may contribute to realize a better patient care, can incite negative feelings, as this argument suggests that the actual patient care may not be the best possible care
   - everybody is aware of the enormous possibilities of a computer : it can be considered that many uses of a CMRS are per-

haps even not yet conceived. This feeling of starting a venture with an open, perhaps dangerous, future may induce hesi-
tation, ...

The mentioned examples show that the most important problems of a
CMRS are not the hard- and software aspects, but the interaction
of informatics with medical practice. One should realize that a
CMRS is always in an implementation phase, as medical reality is
evolving continuously, particularly when a computer system is introduced.

III. THE CMRS AND THE CLINICIAN : "REDUCE BURDEN, INCREASE ADVANTAGES"

1. Reduce burden :
   the clinician encounters the CMRS while using laborious computer-
   terminals, reading - most often not nice looking - computerprint
   outs, and during the registration and control of data

2. Increase of advantages :
   - it is very difficult to provide direct help in patient care :
     the on-line availability of patient data, selectively aggre-
     gated in accordance with the physician's desire, may be of
     importance. The judicious introduction of computer aided
     decision making techniques may stimulate the use of a CMRS.
     One should also consider literature retrieval systems.

   - a research oriented physician will be convinced by the proces-
     sing appeal of the computer stored data : the possibility of
     processing the computer stored data for scientific purposes
     is a new dimension for the medical record.

   Note : a CMRS without an accepted data protection system should
          not be proposed to physicians.

IV. COMPADOS : AN ON-LINE CMRS, IMPLANTED UPON A HOSPITAL COMPUTER NETWORK

Having realized an item specific data protection system[*], which satisfies the medical faculty as well on privacy and confidentiality
aspects as well on research protection, the main concern of COMPADOS

[*]For each item is registerd : the person responsible for the item and
the level of secrecy assigned by him to the item.

is oriented towards :

1. <u>A not burdening registration of the complex medical reality</u>
   a. principles :
      - for the use in patient care and in medical research the
        computer stored information should reflect in a complete
        and correct way medical reality : the data must be as spe-
        cific and detailed as the physicians sense reality (the
        use of "statistical" codes will certainly not attract the
        clinician - he is not an epidemiologist, neither a public
        health administrator -)
      - the physicians shouldn't feel the registration and valida-
        tion of the data as a burden
   b. a terminology system for medical practice :
      - in order to avoid the problems of definitions of terms, the
        responsible physician, for each item, is stored in the com-
        puter
      - a diagnosis (3) is defined as being the statement summa-
        rizing a clinical situation which induces a specific the-
        rapeutic or diagnostic action
          -- complex medical diagnostic statements are split up
             into "working diagnoses", interrelated by "secondary
             to" (4)
          -- for the registration of a diagnosis two sets of terms
             are used : "disturbance" (actually 2.613 terms) and
             "localization" (actually 9.355 terms)
      - for surgical interventions also a multi-axial system is
        applied : the operation is split up into surgical actions,
        registered as "action", "mode of action", "used foreign
        body" (e.g. heart valve), "localization". The same model
        applies to other diagnostic and therapeutic procedures
      - for clinical laboratory results, the laboratory method is
        also registered in order to increase the value of the result
      N.B. In addition to this "kernel", data about the responsible
           physician, the level of secrecy, the date of the fact,
           ... are stored in COMPADOS.
   c. registration and validation procedures :
      the registration and validation of the data is as much as

possible distributed to those persons who are in daily routine responsible for the data collection. The physicians
only note in full text diagnoses and treatments which are
new in the medical record due to their personal care of the
patient. This information is translated into mnemonic codes
in the Department for Medical Informatics for the on-line
input into the computer system. The computer print-out (fig.1)
being as nice as possible, is sent back to the responsible
physician for control and insertion into the medical record.

  d. evaluation :

- an evaluation of the data base (fig. 2) shows that the number of patients with diagnostic/surgical information is
  growing progressively
- the physicians of the participating departments (50% of
  all departments of the hospital) register correctly
  for 80% of the discharged patients
- the success of the system may also be evaluated by the fact
  that the system is spreading progressively all over the
  hospital.

2. On-line availability of useful information

  a. principle :

- a network of computer system (fig. 3) based on a central
  communication processor (5) ensures the data transmission
  from the laboratories to the medical wards.
- the use of special programs enables the clinician to choose
  selectively the information he needs.

  b. examples :

- clinical laboratory results may be retrieved on-line by
  date of the sample (fig. 3a) or by test (fig. 3b)
- diagnostic information, surgical data, can selectively be
  displayed on the video-terminals.

  c. evaluation :

- some 10 video-terminals are in use on the medical wards
  for the purpose of COMPADOS
- the telephone calls to the clinical laboratory dropped dras-
  tically since the computerized data transmission was installed.

3. Introduction of some computer aided decision making techniques

as COMPADOS is intended for routine clinical use, no attempt
is made to use sophisticated programs : in COMPADOS the calculation of the body surface is one, rather often used
example of computer help for patient care (the computer is
more appealing than the traditional tables).

Note : some other computer aided patient care techniques are
now in routine use at the University Hospital e.g.
the automatic interpretation of the vectocardiograms
(the Veterans Administrations program of Pipberger),
a heart cathetarization program, the monitoring of
patients in the intensive care.

4. Careful consideration of rewards for the clinician

In addition to the on-line availability of patient data, the
computer-printed summary of the patient's history in the medical
record is of concrete help for patient care.

All other rewards are of the long-term type. The statistics
concerning the admitted and discharged patients in the wards
are considered with some interest. The use of the data base
for research purposes is now more and more rewarding, as the
number of stored cases is rapidly growing.

CONCLUSION

The implementation of a computerized medical record system in clinical practice is possible, but very difficult. Each health care
environment needs its own approach. One must also be aware of
the fact that patient care is dynamically changing, adapting itself to medical progress and to the changes induced by the use of
computers.

The collaboration on a voluntary basis of the clinician is the
most important factor for success !

REFERENCES

(1) E. Casiraghi and S. Gorini : "The medical record and the computer : some considerations concerning the implementation of
a computerized medical record system", International School on
foundations of medical informatics, Monte-Carlo, Monaco,
October 9-15, 1977, Foundazione internazionale Menarini,
Piazza del Carmini, Milano, Italy 1977

(2) J. van Egmond, L. Decoussemaker, R.J. Wieme and W. Bossaert :
"Implementation of an Information System for Patient Care in
the University Hospital of Gent", in "Information Systems for
Patient Care" (1976)191-203, ed. J. van Egmond, P. de Vries-
Robbé, A. Levy, Publ. North-Holland Publishing Company, Amster-
dam, New York, Oxford (1976)

(3) J. van Egmond and R.J. Wieme : "Systematized Codification of
Medical Diagnostic Statements" in "Medinfo 74", pp. 931-933,
ed. J. Anderson, M. Forsythe, Publ. North-Holland Publishing
Company, Amsterdam (1974)

(4) J. van Egmond, L. Decoussemaker and R.J. Wieme : "Systematiza-
tion in the registration of medical diagnostic statements", in
"Computational Linguistics in Medicine", ed. W. Schneider and
A.-L. Sagvall Hein, Publ. North-Holland Publishing Company,
Amsterdam, New York, Oxford (1977)119-127

(5) J. van Egmond : "Experience of linking a clinical laboratory
mini-computer to a (418-III) information system", in Proceedings
of the Spring 1975 Univac meeting on Data Networks, Salzburg,
Austria

347

Fig. 1 : Diagnoses of a patient

INTENSIEVE ZORGEN(INTERNE)   DATUM : 28 04 1977

MARTENS.JANUS..............   DOSSIERNR : 76/512......   ARTS : MUSSCHE,MONIQUE   BLZ : 1

PATIENTNR : 101121 019A26

D I A G N O S E N

ONTSTEKING / APPENDIX /
DATUM : .. .. 1915 : ?   DOOR: ZENNER,ROBERT   AZ

ONGEVAL: AUTO / /
DATUM : .. .. 1941 :   DOOR: ZENNER,ROBERT   AZ

FRAKTUUR / FEMUR:DISTALE 1/3(RE) /
GEVOLG VAN NR 2 (DIAGNOSE)
DATUM : .. .. 1941 :
Z.   DOOR: ZENNER,ROBERT   AZ 0

OSTEOSYNTHESE-MATERIAAL / FEMUR(RE) /
GEVOLG VAN NR 3 (OPERATIE)
DATUM : .. .. 1942 :
Z.   DOOR: ZENNER,ROBERT   AZ 0

ACUTE BUIK-SYNDROOM / /
DATUM : 22 03 1948 :
OPMERKING : GRAVE................
Z.   DOOR: ZENNER,ROBERT   RO

GEVOLG VAN NR 6 (DIAGNOSE)
DATUM : 22 03 1948 :
Z.

PERFORATIE / MAAG(N.S.) /
GEVOLG VAN NR 7 (DIAGNOSE)
DATUM : 22 03 1948 :
Z.   DOOR: ZENNER,ROBERT   MZ

ULCUS / MAAGBOVENPOOL /
DATUM : 22 03 1948 :
Z.   DOOR: ZENNER,ROBERT   MZ

ONTSTEKING / LONG(LI) / STAPHYLOCOCCUS SPECIES
GEVOLG VAN NR 7 (OPERATIE)
DATUM : 24 03 1948 :
Z.   DOOR: ZENNER,ROBERT   7. 0

ALLERGIE / / PENICILLINE *
GEVOLG VAN NR 8 (MEDIKATIE)
DATUM : 26 03 1948 :
Z.   DOOR: ZENNER,ROBERT   7. K 0

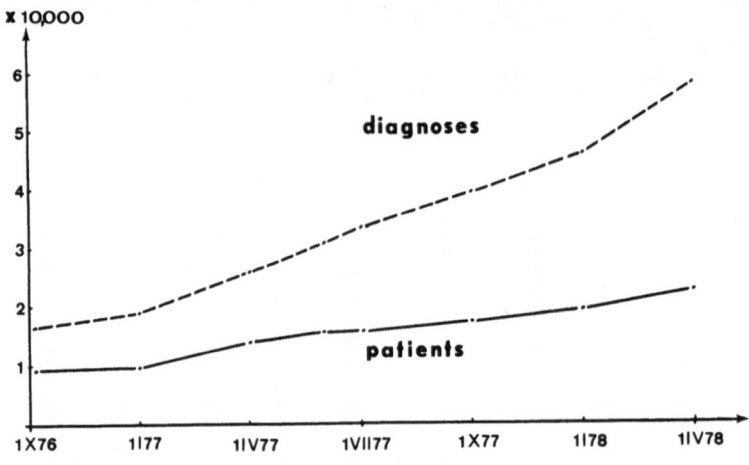

Fig. 2 : The data base of COMPADOS
——— number of patients
---- number of diagnoses

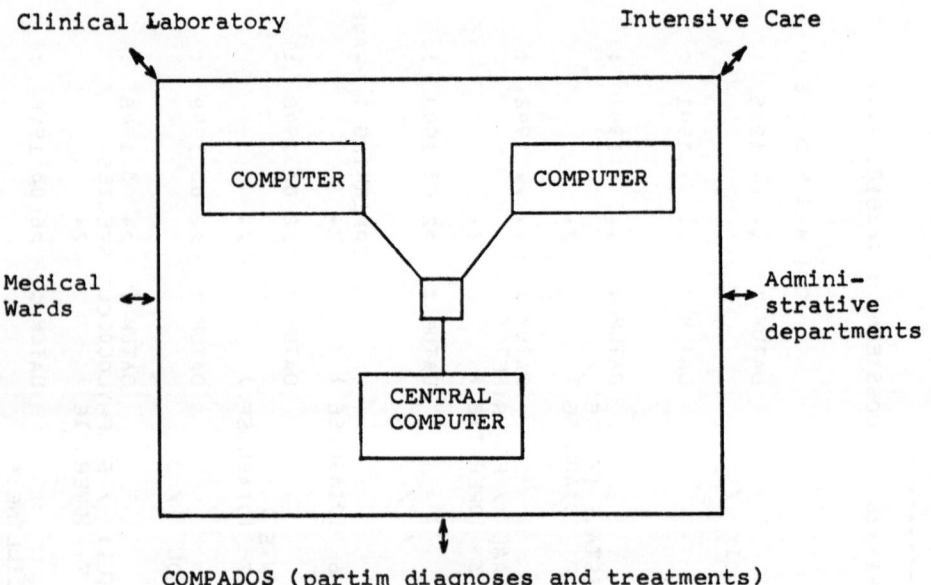

Fig. 3 : The computer network system at the
University Hospital in Gent

```
HLR 101121 019A26                              **FIKTIEF!**
AFDELING: CARDIO  ARTS: ......    MARTENS.JANUS.....................
------------------------------------           21 11 1910 S< .
DATUM: 12 8. 76 1600  AANVR.AFDELING: ......  AANVR.ARTS: ......
LOK: BL  BEPALING: GLUC..
    DATUM        RESULT. EENH.   BIJZ.  METH.   RESP.  GU GA  SP.
12 8. 76 1600   0.9.... G/L...  .....   BKBOGL  RWIEME  .  .  ...
20 8. 76 0745   0.8.... G/L...  .....   GLKAAA  RWIEME  .  .  ...
20 8. 76 1000   1.2...*G/L...   .....   ACACAC  JVE...  .  .  ...
20 8. 76 1400   2.1...*G/L...   .....   ACACAC  JVE...  .  .  ...
20 8. 76 2030   1.8...*G/L...   .....   ACACAC  JVE...  .  .  ...
21 8. 76 0800   1.1... G/L...   .....   ACACAC  JVE...  .  .  ...
22 8. 76 0830   1.2...*G/L...   .....   ACACAC  JVE...  .  .  ...
30 9. 76 0900   1..... G/L...   .....   ACACAC  JVE...  .  .  ...
.. .. .. ....  .......  .....   .....   .....   .....   .  .  ...
WDT/OPM: ..............................  .        TRC: ......
```

Fig. 4a : The retrieval of laboratory results
          by date of sample

```
RBL 101121 019A26
AFDELING: CARDIO  ARTS: ......    MARTENS.JANUS.................
-------------------------------            21 11 1910 S< .
DATUM: 12 8. 76 1600  AANVR.AFDELING: IZE5..  AANVR.ARTS: MMUSS.
                                          T: . SD: . SB: .
BEPAL.     RESULT. EENH.    BIJZ.   METH.   RESP.   GU GA T SP
GLUC..     0.9.... G/L...  ......   BKBOGL  RWIEME   .  . . ...
UREUM.  *  0.6.... G/L...  ......   BEBOEP  RWIEME   .  . . ...
SGOT..  *  120.... MU/ML.  ......   KIBOEP  RWIEME   .  . . ...
SGPT..  *  65..... MU/ML.  ......   KIBOEP  RWIEME   .  . . ...
LDH...     150.... MU/ML.  ......   KIBOEP  RWIEME   .  . . ...
CPK...  *  250.... MU/ML.  ......   KIBOCL  RWIEME   .  . . ...
NA....     145.... MEQ/L.  ......   VLZECO  RWIEME   .  . . ...
K.....  *  3.6.... MEQ/L.  ......   VLZECO  RWIEME   .  . . ...
......   ......  .....   .....   .....   ......   .  . . ...
WDT/OPM: ..............................   ->      TRC: ......
```

Fig. 4b : The retrieval of laboratory results
          by test

THE INFLUENCE OF PRIVACY ACTS ON MEDICAL INFORMATICS

K Boehm

German Cancer Research Center, Heidelberg

Institute of Documentation, Information and Statistics

(Director: Prof.Dr.med.G.Wagner)

In some countries, laws on data protection are under discussion or
have already come into force which are also going to affect medical
data processing. This paper investigates which regulations are of
relevance for medical data, their effect and the costs incurred when
they are carried out.

1. INTRODUCTION

In order to show clearly the relevancy of the problem of data protection, I want to begin by reporting on two experiments which I deem to
be typical for the present situation concerning the protection of
medical data. The first experiment was carried out in a conventional
medical record archive of a university hospital, the second one in
the institution processing these patients' data on an EDP system.

Experiment 1: Upon previous telephonic announcement of their visit,
it was possible for two persons not known to the staff
of the archive to look through any patient records in
the conventionally kept patient registry of the hospital,
to photograph them or to take them away.

Experiment 2: The data processing department was requested by telephone to make up and hand out a printout of part of
patient data with particularly "discriminating" diagnoses. The experiment failed, the main reason, however,
being that the data base to be searched had not been
precisely defined.

Both experiments show that data protection, i.e. the protection of
personal data against unauthorized use, is at present insufficiently
realized in praxi [1]. They show moreover that the problem of data
protection is not limited to electronic data processing but is a problem that occurs equally in conventional archives. Where data is processed conventionally, storage media, access and readability are famil-

iar to any layman; the documents, such as medical records, can,
therefore, be easily interpreted or abused. On the other hand, the
use of data stored in the computer requires specialized knowledge
and access to costly hardware. The basic problem of the protection
of personal data is aggravated by the use of EDP, because the computer permits storage of and access to considerably larger numbers
of data and the linkage of separately stored data which is hardly
feasible with conventional archives on account of the excessive a-
mount of work involved [7,8].

However, the conclusion to be drawn for medical data processing cannot be that we should forego the advantages of progressive technologies and cease to process medical data in computers. We must demand
that in electronic storage and processing medical data be protected
in such a manner as to satisfy the legal requirement of professional
medical secrecy, thus safeguarding the confidential relationship between physician and patient. Persons engaged in medical data processing are themselves as much interested in the regulation of data protection as are the patient and the citizen concerned.

2. REQUIREMENTS OF LEGAL REGULATIONS

The following requirements concerned with the regulation of data
protection are generally recognized:

The person concerned has a right to know

  a) who possesses data concerning him or her;
  b) which data is stored;
  c) to whom his data is passed on;

and he must be sure that

  d) the data is correct;
  e) storage is admissible and predetermined for specific purposes;
  f) the data is safeguarded against abuse.

These relatively extensive rights of the persons concerned are, to a
large extent, taken into account internationally in drafts and laws
already passed on data protection. While the Privacy Act of the United
States is restricted to the regulation of data protection in electronic data processing by public authorities, the corresponding laws in

Sweden and the Federal Republic of Germany extend to the processing of personal data by private institutions. There is no special regulation governing medical data processing. The above mentioned requirements are fundamentally covered by the following principles:

a) Any institutions storing personal data are obliged to announce this or notify the person concerned (duty to announce or notify).

b) Every person concerned is entitled to obtain information on data stored on his or her person (duty to inform).

c) Every person concerned may demand information as to where his or her data is regularly transmitted (duty to keep log records).

d) Inaccurate data must be corrected (duty to correct).

e) Access to any data no longer required or stored without authorization must be barred or else such data must be eliminated (duty to bar access or eliminate data).

f) Any institution storing personal data is obliged to protect such data against abuse (duty to secure data).

Discussion about data protection has so far been largely characterized by manner, scope and technical execution of protective measures, data processing by public authorities being in the foreground. Since such regulations are beginning to extend to private commercial data processing everywhere, the financial implications of data protection are becoming more and more important [5]. Estimates of the costs of data protection known so far are characterized by extreme uncertainty and fluctuation. They vary between 1 and 30 per cent of the present costs of data processing.

In the following, regulations relevant to medical data processing, their effects and their cost will be analyzed.

3. EFFECTS AND COSTS OF REGULATIONS

Medical data related to individual persons is stored and processed by institutions

(i) in the public sector (e.g. hospitals, health offices and places of research),

(ii) in the non-public sector for purposes of these institutions
(e.g. medical practices, places of research, pharmaceutical
industry, insurance companies),

(iii) in the non-public sector for alien purposes (e.g. health
insurance clearing offices and chemical laboratory services).

In the following considerations concerning costs, the law on data
protection of the Federal Republic of Germany is taken as a basis;
it contains different data protection regulations for these sectors.

3.1. Duty to announce or notify

The right of the person concerned to know who stored his or her
personal data is to be safeguarded by the duty to announce or notify.
Different regulations apply to the above mentioned sectors. Public
authorities storing personal data are forced to announce this fact
in an official gazette. No appreciable costs accrew to a public hospital, since it is a case of a one-time publication merely generally
stating the group of persons concerned (patients) and the purpose of
storage. Accordingly, the informative value of this measure is small,
since even an interested person will find it hard to gain a rough
insight into those authorities storing his or her medical data, e.g.
health offices, public research institutes etc.

Non-public agencies processing data for their own purposes, such as
private hospitals, are subject to the duty to notify on the first
occasion personal data is stored. The patient concerned must be personally notified, unless he or she has already learnt about the storage
from some other source of information. As a rule, such notification
will not be required in the case of a new patient, if the patient,
on his first visit to the physician or the hospital, has consented in
writing to having his or her data stored in the computer. Private
agencies to whom patient data may be transmitted, such as research
institutions, other private hospitals or the pharmaceutic industry,
are also obliged to notify the person concerned about the first storage of his or her data in their computer, unless he or she has been
informed about the fact that his or her data has been passed on. Similar regulations apply to non-public agencies whose business it is
to process data for alien purposes, such as service laboratories or
clearing offices. They have to notify the person concerned about the

fact of storage the first time they transmit his or her data, unless he or she has obtained this knowledge from his or her physician.

This way of informing the person concerned is efficient but causes additional expenses by way of administration, computer time, material and postage amounting to about 40 pence. This becomes relevant when patient data are to be stored in the computer retrospectively by non-public agencies. If, for instance, patient records of the past five years are to be stored in the computer of a private hospital with 4,000 admissions per year, the expenditure involved in the duty to notify would in itself amount to £ 6,000. A public hospital proceeding in the same manner is merely subject to the duty to announce, involving costs of about £ 150.-. This represents an enormous inequality between institutions with basically the same purpose, caused solely by the different legal status of these institutions.

3.2. Duty to inform

The right of those concerned to know which of their personal data is stored is to be safeguarded by the duty to inform. Upon request, the data processing agency is obliged to proffer information on the personal data stored. It is obvious that this measure involves considerable expense. Therefore, any laws on data protection provide for a charge for inquiries in order to protect data processing agencies against querulous persons or actual information campaigns which might disturb or even paralyse their work.

However, there appears to be uncertainty as to the nature of this charge for information. While, according to the Privacy Act of the United States, the inquirer merely has to pay the costs incurred by copying his data, but not by the retrieval itself, the law on data protection of the Federal Republic of Germany speaks about a reimbursement of the costs directly connected with the inquiry. The question arises: what are the costs directly connected with the inquiry? Undoubtedly, these are the costs of handling the inquiry and the postage which may be directly attributed as variable costs. However, any data processing agency.is in a position to prove, with the aid of accounting routines, how much CPU-time, connection time, main storage allocation and load of peripheral equipment has been required by the inquiry. These costs can also be declared to be variable and the charge for information will be fixed accordingly.

This manner of calculating costs is, as a rule, questionable from an economic point of view, since costs are not allocated according to the principle of causation. The computer costs, being load-independent fixed costs, are not increased by the inquiry. The additional depreciation caused by increased load on the computer is covered eigther by rental or service agreements and is thus part of the fixed costs and not directly attributable. Exceptions are made only if the increase of load through inquiries exceeds the capacity of the system installed, that is to say if it becomes necessary to run an additional shift.

The problem of information charges also involves a software-technical aspect. If the data base accessed in the retrieval for the inquiry is organized in a person-, i.e. patient-oriented manner, the expenditure caused by the inquiry is relatively small. However, this form of data organization need not in the interest of the storing agency for whom a storage related to facts would often be much more efficient. If, for instance, the typical inquiry in a medical data bank reads: "Which therapy was applied for which diagnosis?" then it can be immensely time-concuming to identify the patients to whom the inquiry refers. For this reason, the data-storing agency can, by freely choosing the form of data organization, manipulate the costs of an inquiry arbitrarily, thus reducing to absurdity the right to information of the person concerned. On the one hand, therefore, it would appear to be imperative to fix a top charge of about £ 3.-; on the other hand, however, it must be anticipated that this charge would not cover the costs of small computer systems where special software and hardware must be made available.

From a medical point of view it is worth considering that, on account of the right to be informed, every patient will be in a position to gain insight into any medical data stored about his person. Thus, the patient will obtain information, e.g. certain diagnoses, which the physician might not wish him to have for medical reasons, or knowledge on therapy plans which might be made use of in litigation.

3.3. Duty to keep log records

The right of the person concerned to know to whom his or her data is
passed on is to be safeguarded by the duty to keep a log record. This
measure, which is handled differently in the American Privacy Act and
the law on data protection of the Federal Republic of Germany, clearly shows the borderline between what is basically desirable and actually workable. The Privacy Act provides for governmental authorities in the USA that, where data is passed on to certain authorities,
a log record has to be kept and, upon request, made accessible to
the person concerned. This makes it possible to communicate necessary
corrections of the data to the recipient. An analysis by Goldstein
[3] of the costs arising by transferring this regulation to the private sector shows that costs amounting to 10 pence per person and
year must be anticipated. The German law on data protection does not
contain the duty to keep a log record, after corresponding investigation [6] had shown the immense expenditure to industry and banks
which would be the consequence of the logging and the subsequent retrieval of such records.

Under these circumstances, the individual concerned will no longer
be able to know where his or her data is stored. Problems are likely
to arise if the information given by an EDP-agency leads him or her
to discover false data. While a correction is possible by this particular agency, it will hardly be feasible in the case of any other a-
gencies who received or transmitted such false data. In this case,
the person concerned must resign himself or herself to the fact that
false data on his or her person is stored somewhere. Alternatively,
he or she will have to instigate a process of clarification by a series of requests for information.

3.4. Regulations on data transfer

In the German law on data protection, regulations on data transfer are
in themselves problematic inasmuch as they specify different procedures for medical data processing on the public and non-public sector.
Data which is subject to professional medical secrecy may be passed
on among public authorities without the patient's consent, provided
the recipient needs the data for the same purpose for which it was
originally obtained by the transmittor, for instance in the information chain: hospital - health office - public research institute. It

is permissible to transfer medical data to agencies outside the public sector if the transmittor can be certain that the recipient would
also be entitled to obtain such data directly from the data-collecting
agency, for instance in the information chain: hospital - hospital -
general practitioner.

A basically different regulation applies to the non-public sector.
Data which is subject to professional medical secrecy and has been
transmitted by a non-public agency, e.g. a general practitioner or
a private hospital, may not be passed on by the recipient. The information chain: general practitioner - specialist - research institution is thereby interrupted. Here, too, as already mentioned in the
case of the duty to notify, there is inequality concerning data processing agencies in medicine depending upon the legal status of such
institutions, with practical consequences for their activities. Medical research relying on personal data is considerably impeded and
thus made more expensive, for instance in keeping a cancer registry,
by the fact that - at least in the case of the non-public sector -
it is by far more difficult to procure data and that it can hardly be
procured at all for necessary retrospective documentation.

3.5. Duty of accuracy

The duty of EDP agencies to correct inaccurate data constitutes the
logical continuation of the duty to inform and is an elementary right
of the person concerned. For this reason, an inquiry leading to the
detection of false data and to their correction is free of charge.
In such a case, the storing agency has to bear the entire costs of
processing the inquiry, retrieval, checking and correction, more than
half the costs being caused by general office work. According to
Goldstein [4], it must be anticipated that about one per cent of the
persons on whom data is stored will make use of their right to information and that 50 per cent of the inquiries will necessitate corrections. This must be regarded as one of the most significant causes of
the costs of data protection. They are, however, inevitable, since
all concerned are interested in the storage of correct data.

3.6. Duty to bar access

If the correctness or incorrectness of data stored cannot be unequi-
ocally clarified, the EDP agency has the duty to bar access to such
data. According to the German law, the right to access to contested
data is to be denied. According to American law, it has to be amended
by a rectifying account of the person concerned. Agencies processing
data for alien purposes are obliged to bar access to any data which
had been stored in their system for five years.

This makes it necessary to keep aging logs as well as to check and
adjust the data bases at regular intervals. The costs incurred largely depend on the fluctuation, the time the data remains in the data
bases and the mode of storage and can only be quantified from case
to case.

3.7. Duty to eliminate data

The duty to eliminate stored data becomes relevant if storage was
inadmissible or if the person concerned demands that data no longer
required be eliminated. The costs incurred are negligeable.

A further financial aspect which concerns data processing agencies
in the non-public sector follows from the obligation to appoint a
person who is responsible for data protection. According to the German law on data protection, private institutions, such as private
hospitals and research institutions employing at least five persons
on processing personal data, have to appoint a person who is responsible for data protection. The tasks of this person are exactly defined by law and it can be estimated that the expenditure for EDP
personnel is thereby increased by about one per cent.

3.8. Duty to secure

Finally, we have to discuss the right of the person concerned to
have his or her data protected against abuse. This is to be realized
by the duty to secure. The comparatively perfectionistic German law
on data protection gives a detailed catalog of 10 demands which have
to be fulfilled by technical and organizational controls. Let me
merely mention two demands which may possibly lead to high costs and

are of particular relevance for medical data processing.

By means of access control unauthorized persons are to be prevented
from gaining access to personal data. If this demand does not only
apply to the computer room itself but also to the rooms where data
is processed on terminals, reorganization or structural changes will
become necessary in many places, such as hospitals or research institutions.

Input control is to safeguard that it is possible to check and ascertain who fed personal data into the computer at what time. It is
at present not yet clear whether the generally available printouts
will satisfy this demand. In case this demand should refer to every
individual record which is fed in or is subject to update, this measure would imply a colossal increase of data bases and, particularly
with small computer systems, would lead to considerable costs.

4. CONCLUSIONS

When measures are taken in the interest of data security, the problem
of drawing a borderline between the costs of data protection and the
costs already incurred by regular data processing becomes particularly
clear [2].

The question arises inhowfar technical and organizational measures
for data security are actually required in the interest of data protection. For, after all, any medical installation is interested in
keeping their patient data confidential within the framework of professional medical secrecy. The demanded measures are, for the greater
part, indispensable for a normal EDP organization anyhow and are already being carried through. For this reason, the costs incurred
should be attributed to the law on data protection to a limited exent
only.

To summarize, I would state that, while the costs of data protection
by the German law are considerable, they are still lower than those
envisaged for corresponding regulations in the USA. However, the
probable costs must be related to the advantages of medical data
processing for the community and the individual patient who can claim
that his or her medical data be treated confidentially.

REFERENCES

[1] Boehm, K.: Datenschutz und Datensicherheit in der medizinischen
    Datenverarbeitung, APIS Newsletter, no. 4, July 1976, 31-38.

[2] Boehm, K.: Kostenimplikationen von Datenschutzregelungen, in:
    Dierstein, R., Fiedler, H., Schulz, A. (Ed.): Datenschutz und
    Datensicherung, Bachem Köln, 1976, 216-226.

[3] Goldstein, R.C.: The cost of privacy, Honeywell Information
    Systems Brighton (Mass.), 1975.

[4] Goldstein, R.C.: The costs of privacy, Datamation, vol. 21,
    October 1975, 65-69.

[5] Lobel, J.: The cost of computer privacy, AFIPS Conf.Proc.,
    vol. 44, 1975, 935-940.

[6] Steinbuch, K., Wacker, H.: Überlegungen zu technischen Möglich-
    keiten des Datenschutzes in Hinblick auf ein Bundesdatenschutz-
    gesetz, in: Drucksache des Deutschen Bundestags VI/3826, 1972,
    213-224.

[7] Wagner, G., Boehm, K.: Data Protection concerning a Cancer
    Registry, in: Griesser, G. (Ed.): Realization of Data
    Protection in Health Information Services. North-Holland,
    Amsterdam, New York, 55-61 (1977).

[8] Wagner, G.: Medizinische Datenbank-Informationssysteme,
    Voraussetzungen und Probleme.
    Z.Datenverarb., vol. 10, 1972, 94-96.

<u>RULES FOR CONFIDENTIALITY</u> -

<u>PRACTICAL EXPERIENCE IN A COMMUNITY BASED REAL-TIME SYSTEM</u>

R H Fisher

The Exeter Community Health Services Computer Project
UK.

<u>INTRODUCTION</u>

It is a time honoured principle that "whatsoever a doctor shall learn about his patient shall remain a secret between them". The practice of modern medicine undermines
this principle; no longer is a patient treated by a single doctor but is cared for by
many professions, each one collecting data and needing to use data from other sources.
The principle of confidentiality is still maintained, however, by the professional
ethics of each of the disciplines working together for the patient's care.

Current BMA policy is agreed in the following terms (ref. BMJ 6.8.77)

Data protection

That in all medical records, information should be regarded as held for the
specific purposes of the continuing care of the patient, and should not be used,
without appropriate authorisation by the responsible clinician or the consent of
the patient for any other purposes.

Because of the community based nature of health care the Exeter Community Health
Services Computer Project was established to investigate the use of a single patient
record contributed to and used by these community services. Thus the problems, now
being considered by the Data Protection Committee in connection with medical records,
have always received consideration in the design of the Project's systems.

The objective of the single record is that data collected during all episodes, whether
dealt with by General Practitioners, outpatient department or inpatient departments of
hospitals, together with results of tests such as X-Rays, blood samples etc. shall be
available from a single source by those who require the data for a specific purpose.

Thus it has been necessary to consider such points as:
- who is responsible for the accuracy of the data
- who can authorise the release of data
- who is authorised to use specific areas of the record;
- what data must be restricted to a single person, and
- how can data be released for research purposes.

These have not been theoretical considerations as the Project has at present the complete General Practice medical records for all patients registered at two Health

Centres. The General Practitioners use visual display units to manipulate these records on a day-to-day basis in their surgeries. In addition there are nursing, service department and administrative records from the hospital accessed via terminals in the wards and departments of two hospitals.

COMPUTER USERS ETHICAL SUB-COMMITTEE (CUE)

To aid the Project and the involved users to determine the rules and to ensure that
the confidentiality of records is being maintained a Computer Users' Ethical Sub-
Committee has been set up. The members are drawn from all branches of the Health
Service with the computer project personnel acting as technical advisers.

The committee is a sub-committee of the Project Committee set up by the Regional
Health Authority to oversee the project, and its terms of reference are:-

> "To formulate rules of procedures for users of the Exeter Computer Systems,
> having regard to the particular areas of need for action and protection, and
> to advise the Project Committee appropriately."

The original members of the committee were drawn from administrators at what was then
Group and Hospital level, Nurses at Group and Hospital level, Consultants, General
Practitioners and the Secretary of the Executive Council. It was discussed at early
meetings whether there should not also be representatives from the Social Services
and the general public. With regard to the former it was thought that as the project
is not actually linking with the Social Services, membership of the committee by
Social Service workers was inappropriate. With regard to the second, at that stage
the only way to have had a representative of the general public would have been to
co-opt a member of the League of Friends or a lay member of the Hospital Management
Committee. It was felt that neither of these was appropriate. The only alternatives
being members of political or quasi-political organisations it was decided for the
time being to drop the matter of public participation in the committee. Since
1 April 1974 however the committee has had two members of the Community Health Council
attending its meetings so since that date the general public might consider themselves
to be represented. The remainder of the committee was reconstructed to represent the
reorganised service.

It was also agreed that to ensure continuity each member should nominate a deputy who
would receive copies of all minutes and papers. The present membership is as follows:

Membership of the Sub-Committee

Group	Representation
1. Nurses	a) District Nursing Officer
	b) Senior Nursing Officer at R D & E Hospital(Wonford)
2. General Practitioners	a) Health Centre at Ottery St. Mary
	b) Second Health Centre
	c) Nominees of District Medical Committee

Group	Representation
3. Hospital Doctors	a) Two from R D & E Hospital (Wonford)
	b) One from Princess Elizabeth Orthopaedic Hospital
4. Administrators	a) Area Administrator
	b) District Administrator
	c) Sector Administrator
5. Community Health Council	Two members
6. Community Physician	District Community Physician
7. Family Practitioner Services Committee	Administrator
8. Project staff as appropriate	

The committee work started with a considerable amount of self-education in the overall problems of confidentiality within the Health Service, the law relating to confidentiality in the Health Service, the nature of the systems that the Project were implementing and the proposals that the project had already to try to ensure confidentiality. The committee met once a month for many months when it first started, and went through a phase of becoming very worried about the whole question of computers and confidentiality and beginning to think about requiring more and more complex technical solutions. After a while, pragmatism set in so that the conclusions that the committee has now reached and the guidelines which it has given the project provide a system which is certainly more confidential than the manual systems without being so difficult that it has become unwieldly.

The committee had its first meeting in July 1972. The following paragraphs illustrate the sort of subjects that have been discussed.

Passwords

Access to the Exeter system is through a system of individual passwords. Should signing on be made easy, that is should instructions about how to use the sign on system be displayed on the screens which might make it easier to break into the system; or should we rely on training users to use a sign on screen without instructions thereby preserving a slightly higher degree of confidentiality. The final solution was a compromise.

Training

The Project felt that there would be a benefit if there was the facility to show any member of Hospital or Health Centre staff any other aspect of the system. This again would increase the individual's ability to break into parts of the system that they were not authorised to use. On the other hand it would give the opportunity to demonstrate the consequences in one part of the system of in-putting inaccurate data in another part. Therefore it was felt that the philosophy that all people should be able to train on all parts of the system was correct.

Access to Waiting Lists

The initial discussions about which Consultants should have access to which Waiting Lists led to fairly restrictive views in that individual consultants wanted the ability to restrict access to their waiting lists to their firm, and the waiting list clerk. This resulted in the situation where some registrars and house officers who were shared between firms had more access to the system than the consultants. In the end the project published a statement of intent (see appendix 1) concerning access to Waiting Lists which was approved by the Ethical Committee then sent to the Medical Executive Committee in the hospital and approved by them.

Protection of Data Base

The Ethical Committee had explained to them the reasons for certain batch programs, that the project runs on a daily or weekly basis, to ensure the continued logical structure of the files. The committee had explained to them that if there were breaks in the logic some parts of the data base might need to be printed out. The project has rules regarding the handling of confidential printout and the eventual disposal of it. These were also explained and as a result of the discussions special forms requiring signatures from project senior management are used when data is required to be printed out from live files. A register of these printouts is kept and is available for inspection by members of the Ethical Committee.

Data for Research

One of the project's secondary aims is to provide data for research. Such data can however only be released by permission of the owner; the project itself will release no such data without such permission. So far there have been no problems about who owns which data but as the systems in the hospital begin to interact much more with the systems in the Health Centres then the problems of ownership will become more acute but will have to be decided on an individual basis. To be absolutely safe in end it may be necessary to decide that all people who have the right to change an item of data can become its owner and that each owner has the right of veto when it comes to releasing that data for research purposes to a non-owner. This last point has not yet been fully resolved by the Ethical Committee.

Data to ICL

Certain software problems result in printout being made available to ICL for their software programmers to examine. The Regional Health Authority tried for a long time to get an indemnity from ICL should any member of ICL accidentally or otherwise reveal data about patients. In the end the Region failed to get this indemnity but the legal view was that having tried to get the indemnity, if it could be shown that ICL were at fault where that data had been revealed, then the Courts would probably rule in the Authority's favour.

Use of Badge Readers

Access to the system is through passwords only. The possibility of using badge readers either in conjunction with passwords or on their own was discussed by the project but it was felt that in systems where the users are changing clothes, i.e. changing from outdoor clothes into uniform of some sort or other to do their work, that badges would either be left in the pocket of the uniform and become a security risk or would be left in the outdoor clothes and not be available when required. It was therefore felt that badge readers would provide more aggravation than security and it was decided not to use them.

Medical Records of Staff

Much discussion was held on whether records of NHS staff should be held on the computer. The final recommendation was that the records of NHS staff should be held on the computer and treated in the same way as the records of other patients. An exception to this has however been made for those members of staff who work on the computer site, i.e. the project staff and ICL engineers. If a printout is being run which contains data concerning one of these people then the Health Centre or Hospital number only is printed, with no identity data, with a note to the doctor who has requested the analysis that this patient is a member of the staff. The general practitioner, if he wishes, should therefore access the records through the visual display unit. I attach a list of papers (appendix 2) distributed to our Computer Users' Ethical Committee. Copies of these papers are in the hands of the Department of Health and Social Security from whom, no doubt, further copies could be sought should anyone so desire.

Evidence to Data Protection Committee

In October 1976 the Computer Users' Ethical Committee submitted evidence to the Data Protection Committee based on our experience to date. The following recommendations are from the evidence. Copies of the full document can be obtained from the Project.

Summary of Recommendations

A   Medical records should come within the general provisions of the legislation and be subject to special defined regulations.

B   Medical records should be defined and be subject to standards.

C   The transfer of data from one system to another should be carefully controlled.

D   Medical records held by organisations other than the NHS should be subject to equally stringent regulations as those proposed for the NHS.

E   A "responsible person or body" should be appointed in each registered installation, as suggested in the Younger Report Cmnd 5012 (Chaps 20 and Appendix O).

F   The legislation should extend to all data banks whether computerised or not containing personal information.

Supporting arguments were supplied for each of the above recommendations but let us consider for instance the points which led to recommendation B.

Standards for medical records

- the subject of the information should not have the right to see the complete medical record;

- there should be an agreed minimum set of medical facts to which the subject can have access (e.g. Vaccination & Immunisation Status, Blood Group, Drug Sensitivity etc.);

- only the subject's identity information (e.g. sex, address, age, occupation, religion and family relationship) can be corrected by the subject, but it can only be changed on the record by an authorised user;

- an identifiable author of an item or items of data should be allowed access to and the power to correct or delete such items;

- an identifiable author of an item of data should have the power to restrict access to such items to the author solely or third parties specifically authorised by the author;

- the release of identifiable medical records for research purposes should only be done if:

  - the research has been considered and approved by an independent Medical Research Ethical body;

  - the consent of the various authors of the data has been obtained;

  - the consent of the subject of the information has been obtained (unless either the Medical Research Ethical body or the authors of the data consider it prejudicial to the health care of the subject for the research objectives to be disclosed to the subject).

The general provisions of the Act that would still apply would be:-

a)   all installations which hold medical records on computer readable media will be
     required to be registered/licenced by the Data Protection Authority.

b)   the existence of the records must be "publicly known" together with the fact that
     they are subject to special rules;

c)   the installation as part of its licence will have to maintain records of:
     - type of records;
     - levels of access to items of data within such records;
     - all access other than those made in the normal processing of the records
       (e.g. in our installation details of enquiry runs on the files);
     - the production and disposition of all data produced in a readable form other
       than through the on-line devices in the normal course of processing;

d)   subject to inspection by the Data Protection Authority (if this is the agreed
     method.

If we look at recommendation F it is an almost impossible task in a computer installation to draw the boundary lines as to where the proposed legislation stops. For example, in the Exeter Project records are reproduced, for standby and home-visit
purposes, as microfiche by the South Western Regional Health Authority bureau. Now
if a complaint of misuse of data is received how will it be possible to establish
whether it was due to misuse of the "computer" or misuse of the microfiche? Similarly if a display on a video terminal is left visible when the user is called away, the
data could be read by a third party and once again, would such an action be subject
to any penalties that may be specified within the Data Protection Act? Where a computer installation is producing one type of output, say printing, this can be controlled and a point established where the responsibility of the manager of the
computer ends and the responsibility of the user starts. But then if the user is to
be subject to the terms of the Act any wrong release of data will not be "misuse of
the computer". It seems that with multitude of devices for producing and displaying
information that is originally stored on a computer readable media this dividing line
of responsibility will be very difficult to define.

It is the view of the Computer Users' Ethical Committee that with regard to the
Organisation of the Data Protection Authority the Data Protection Committee should
take a firm stand. The Younger Report (section 664 et seq) examines two Parliamentary
Bills which set out suggested organisations and no soubt the Data Protection Committee
will consider these previous attempts.

In their considerations we have urged the Data Protection Committee to keep in mind that the Data Protection Authority will have two functions:

a) to act as a registration and licencing agency, and

b) to act as a law enforcement body.

We emphasise these points as the White Paper seems to regard them as alternatives. The only alternative to vesting the second function in the Data Protection Authority is to make the legislation punitive so that any breach could be dealt with by the normal process of civil or criminal law.

CONTROLS IN THE EXETER COMMUNITY HEALTH SERVICES COMPUTER PROJECT

The project files are actively used daily by General Practitioners, their reception-
ists, by nurses, hospital doctors, laboratory and administrative staff. All communication is handled by a real time system and the use of video and teletype terminals
as input-output devices.

Not all the individual rules for access have been defined yet but they will all fall
within the general confidentiality framework, subject to approval by the Computer
Users' Ethical Committee.

The most complete data on file at present relates to health centre systems. I will
use this to illustrate the various levels of protection which exist on the data held
within the Integrated Patient Record:

i) The use of a password to ensure that a defined path with specified actions
is started and that an accessibility matrix is provided for processes along
this path. A user may have a second per pro password which he can allocate
to others to make entries on his behalf.

ii) Where there are specific actions requested, such as Update data, Add data,
Delete data, the accessibility matrix is checked to ensure such action is
permissible.

iii) When information is to be displayed the path allowed to the user ensures
that only permitted data can be extracted from the file.

iv) Certain items of data in the record are specifically labelled to allow
only the author, identified from the password, to be able to recall them
for display. Otherwise the data are indicated as "suppressed".

v) In certain cases items of data for a specific patient can be specifically
labelled by the author to allow access to identifiable users who would
normally not have access to such data. The ability to label such data is
controlled through the password and accessibility matrix.

vi) Should misuse of the system ever be suspected then the project's Systems
Measurement log can be analysed to produce details for any given time
period such as:

. Which password was used
. Which record(s) were looked at
. Which terminal was used at which location.

Example of accessibility matrix for health centre personnel

The method is used in health centre processing and refers to data in the Integrated Patient Record collected by the health centre personnel.

All the following can be overridded by - ANTI (= no display of patient record), STAF (= no display to 'pp' users), Suppressed Lines and when a Leaving Print has been produced.

USER / Patient Status* / DISPLAY	G.P.			REC		L.A.				Hospital		NOTES
	Home	Away		Home	Away	Home		Away		MRD	Doctor	
	Ref N/A	No Ref	Ref Set	Ref N/A	Ref N/A	No Ref	Ref Set	No Ref	Ref Set			
DR REGISTRATION DATA	T	R	R	T	R	R	R	R	R			Referral Marker not used here. User cate category & location of patient govern display.
DS MEDICAL SUMMARY	T	N	A	N	N	N	R	N	R			
DE EXTENSION MEDICAL SUMMARY	T	N	R	N	N	N	R	N	R			
DM MEDICATION	T	N	R	A	N	N	R	N	R			Rec. has 'A' to enable requests for repeat prescriptions to be input.
DA HOSPITAL LETTERS TESTS etc.	T	N	R	N	N	N	R	N	R			

* Ref = Referral Marker in SGNLS on Base Record. 'Ref Set' means the referral marker is applicable to this user at this health centre.

KEY	HOME	=	OWN HC	T	=	Total	R	=	Read Only
	AWAY	=	ANOTHER HC	A	=	Add Only	N	=	None

I would now like to illustrate briefly what the rules, as described, mean when translated to the system as seen by the user.

Figure 1 is the screen which the user will get when they press the 'Sign-On' button on a visual display unit. The 'Sign-On button is one of a group of function buttons on the keyboard. These send messages directly to the computer without any input message appearing on the VDU screen. When the user types in his password it is entered between the brackets but is not actually displayed. The Project gave up the use of the flashing 'unprotected' field and had it turned into an undisplayed 'unprotected' field. It is virtually impossible to read a person's password by watching their fingers on the keyboard unless they are typing very deliberately.

```
)

         SIGN-ON REQUESTED.
              Please make sure the CURSOR is in the CORRECT PLACE

         ENTER YOUR PASSWORD HERE >>>>(      )




                        NORMAL PRODUCTION TIMES.
         Monday    Tuesday   Wednesday  Thursday  Friday    Saturday  Sunday
         0815-2000 0815-2000 0815-2000  0815-2000 0815-2000 0815-2000 0815-2130




                                                                    (
```

Fig. 1

An information service called 'Enquire Within' is the only part of the Exeter system which does not require a password for access. Enquire Within contains Drug information, the Nursing Procedure manual, 'How to Use a Visual Display Unit' and other general information systems.

Figure 2 is the first screen which the General Practitioner will get having signed-on. It reminds him of the facilities available on the system. The first one that we shall look at is 'Log Report' and he obtains this screen simply by overtyping the 'HK' and typing 'LR' in the top left hand corner; and then pressing 'Send'.

```
(HK)Home Keys       -doctors                      Qualifier (          )

    Key  Expansion              Qualifiers Available      Current Value
    HK   Home Keys
    DR   Display Registration   Blank/Patient No
    DS   Display Summary        Patient No
    DE   Display Extension      Patient No
    DM   Display Medication     Patient No
    DA   Document-Archives      Patient No
    CH   Control Hypertension   Patient No
    RD   Reassessments Due      Date                      00/00
    RS   Referral Signals       LA/GP                     00/00
    LL   Leaving List           Blank/Date/GP Initials    01/00
    LR   Log Report                                       02/00
    HS   Hospital Summary       Patient No
    PK   Printer Keys
    RK   Reference Keys



 13/04/78    16/34
```

Fig. 2

376

Figure 3 shows the General Practitioner, for the previous 20 signing-ons up to the latest occasion, the time the doctor signed-on, the time he signed-off and his initials. Where his initials are followed by the letters 'pp' that indicates that a special password (per pro) was used which allowed virtually total access to the data. This facility would be used in a situation where a general practitioner rings up the health centre to find out perhaps the latest entry on the patient's record. In this case the receptionist would use the per pro password and this fact is logged by the computer system. The last column shows the number of the visual display unit from which the signing-on was performed.

Date	On at	Off at	User	VDU
(LR)Log Report	—AA		last update 13.04.78 (	)
06.04.78 *	15.25	15.29	AA	55
	16.03	16.04	AA	55
07.04.78	08.33	08.35	AA	55
	14.39	15.28	AA	10
10.04.78	10.48	12.34	AA	55
	12.00	12.11	AA	54
11.04.78	08.53	08.55	AA	54
	08.56	08.56	AAPP	54
	08.58	08.58	AA	54
	08.58	08.59	AA	54
	09.04	09.06	AA	54
	12.14	12.41	AA	54
	13.39	13.40	AA	57
	17.03	17.04	AA	55
	17.04	17.51	AA	55
	17.34	17.42	AA	54
12.04.78	16.18	17.17	AA	55
	16.40	17.17	AA	54
13.04.78	15.44	15.58	AA	34
	16.34	CLOSE *	AA	57
13.04.78	16.35			

Fig. 3

Figure 4 shows the main screen in the system for general practitioners' use. You can see it illustrates the summarised medical history of a fairly ill patient. This shows the uses of the training system as authorised by the Computer Users' Ethical Committee. The password used is for an imaginary General Practitioner and allows access only to dummy records. This is an imaginary but realistic patient and this is shown by the use of ZZ- at the beginning of her name. The data is displayed in a protected mode on the screen and will only be unprotected should the doctor either type a Y into the space marked 'UPDATE?' in the bottom left hand corner of the screen or by changing the DS to US in the top left hand corner.

```
DS)Display Summary                                  Patient HC No(900223    )
                    ZZ-OTHER,Mrs ELIZABETH VERA"DOLL",34,WEST ST-,NEW
      priority  *HYPERTENSION          age 51 dob 05.11.26 gp 1111 status M
                ALLERGY AMPICILLIN
                DIABETES MELLITUS
                (                    )
      summary history       yr notes                              DAref
      APPENDICECTOMY         50 Uncomplicated.       BP 180/100    1
      BRONCHITIS             72 Ampicillin allergy  CXR LV+ ref XA2314  ECG
    $ FEMORAL CONDYLES,RT    52 Comminuted. RTA. HIN               2
      OA KNEE, RT            70 -78. For knee replacement PEOH WL Apr78
      HYPERTENSION           74 BP 220/120   IVP NAD
        GOOD CONTROL         76 BP 150/ 90              Graphical Control  Ch
      DIABETES MELLITUS      04 Insulin needed
        DIABETIC RETINOPATHY 75 New vessel formation ->Eye Hospital
      (                    ( (                                 (      )
      (                    ( (                                 (      )
      medication IZS-LENTE       BETHANIDINE        Hydrosaluric-K

      current episode      -symptoms,signs etc      /treatment etc    -event
      04.10.77 .1111 Epigastric pain, fever 2 days. HIN RDEW ? Cholecystitis  V
      22.02.78 1111 FEELS DEPRESSED AT THOUGHT OF KNEE REPLACEMENT @15.4.78    A

      Update? ( )   Read Document-Archive? No.=( )               1st page
```

Fig. 4

Figure 5 shows one of the other data screens which general practitioners use. If you look at the line marked 'DATA SUPPRESSED', SH means Social History, the number 1111 is the general practitioner's Family Practitioner Committee number and then 'DATA SUPPRESSED' appears. It is possible in the system for a general practitioner to mark any line of the record for his eyes only; thus excluding it even from the eyes of his partners. Equally it is possible for him to mark lines as being for the eyes of any doctor at the health centre but not for it to be displayed to nurses or to holders of 'pp' passwords. Although the doctor who input the original data is currently signed-on even he does not get this data displayed automatically; he has to ask for it. This is done by asking for the screen in 'Update Mode', i.e. typing a 'Y' in the space marked 'UPDATE?' or UE in the top left hand corner and then 'Sending'. What he then gets back is the screen in Figure 6.

```
DE)Display Extension                                    Patient HC No(900223   )
                    ZZ-OTHER,Mrs ELIZABETH VERA"DOLL",34,WEST ST-,NEW
    signals    LAOI GPOI                   age 51 dob 05.11.26 gp IIII status M
    blood grp  O Rh pos                     registered 26.02.76 printed
    vac & imm  Vac 62,69                    NHS No ASKJ 207C
               Tet 70, R 7. 3.75
               (                      )
               (                      )
       extension history        yr notes                           DAref
    SH IIII DATA SUPPRESSED
       (                    ( (                            (        )
       (                    ( (                            (        )
    OH FTND                 50 9lb 8oz          BP 170/100
       PREMATURE LABOUR     52 8lb stillbirth
       (                    ( (                            (        )
       (                    ( (                            (        )
    FH MOTHER DIABETIC
       (                    ( (                            (        )
       (                    ( (                            (        )

    statistics of attendances etc:-
       "A" 1977-45, 1978-08    "V" 1977-07, 1978-02     "C" 1977-03, 1978-00

    Update? ( )   Read Document-Archive? No.=( )
```

Fig. 5

```
DE)Display Extension                              Patient HC No(900223   )
                    ZZ-OTHER,Mrs ELIZABETH VERA"DOLL",34,WEST ST-,NEW
( )signals   (LAOI(GPOI(   (   (   )   age 51 dob 05.11.26 gp IIII status M
( )blood grp (O Rh pos              )   registered 26.02.70 printed
( )vac & imm (Vac 62,69             )   NHS No ASKJ 207C
( )          (Tet 70, R 7. 3.75     )
( )          (                      )
( )          (                      )
     extension history        yr notes                              DAref
( )SH(IIII Husband beat her   (74(Poor housing & considerable despair (   )
( )  (                        (  (                                    (   )
( )  (                        (  (                                    (   )
( )OH(FTND                    (50(91b 8oz          BP 170/100         (   )
( )  (PREMATURE LABOUR        (52(81b stillbirth                      (   )
( )  (                        (  (                                    (   )
( )  (                        (  (                                    (   )
( )FH(MOTHER DIABETIC         (  (                                    (   )
( )  (                        (  (                                    (   )
( )  (                        (  (                                    (   )

     statistics of attendances etc:-
       "A" 1977-45, 1978-08      "V" 1977-07, 1978-02      "C" 1977-03, 1978-00

              Read Document-Archive? No.=(   )
```

Fig. 6

As you can see this screen is unprotected and the data that was previously suppressed is now displayed. This 'unprotected' facility is available on any patient data screen. At the top of the screen on the left hand side you will see the word 'signals' with 5 spaces for the entry of data. The General Practitioner can by use of these signal spaces refer the patient to a district nurse or health visitor. This system could easily be extended so that GPs could allow doctors in the hospital to have access to the record when the patient is referred to hospital. A patient who is so referred will be listed in the computer so that when the health visitor or district nurse signs-on they will be told that a patient's record has been made available to them. Otherwise health visitors and district nurses at Ottery St. Mary do not automatically have free access to the medical records maintained by the general practitioners.

The General Practitioners have in the system several facilities for printing records but data which is 'suppressed' never appears on a print-out nor does it ever appear on the microfiche copies of the records that are produced for home-visits, night calls and stand-by in the case of breakdown.

Finally, Figure 7 shows what you receive if you attempt to access the patient's medical history and you have only a Health Visitor's password and the patient has not been referred to you.

```
DS)Display Summary                          Patient HC No(900943   )
              ZZ-OTHER,Mrs ANN NANCY,19,SMITH STREET,OSM

    YOUR PASSWORD DOES NOT ALLOW YOU TO ACCESS THIS PATIENT'S CLINICAL DETAILS
```

Fig. 7

CONCLUSION

The majority of the demonstration of the system has been based around the system in use by general practitioners. The general practitioners themselves are convinced that the system is more secure than the manual system, (Letter to the British Medical Journal of 24 February 1976) and they are convinced that the system gives them the ability to offer better care to their patients. (See also the British Medical Journal of 5 June 1976.) Similar protections exist for all hospital users both as regards passwords and with some information limited to certain locations. An authorised user can however obtain the relevant data for most activities from any terminal in the system so exploiting the communication facility of the terminal network. We have had through the whole of our existence to combat the fear of GPs, that they will somehow lose control of their data. It is fair to say that General Practitioners using the full system feel they now have more control over their data than they had in the past. Where I think work is needed is to actually gauge public opinion on the subject of medical records. The work of assessing public opinion will be extremely complicated because fundamentally one would have to show the patient the records that currently exist and then ask the patient whether they would mind that sort of data being transferred to other doctors.

Finally you may remember that the General Practitioner medical records held in the computer are copied to microfiche for home visits, night calls and standby purposes. The entire record, plus copies of letters from the hospital for the entire practice of 11,500 patients goes onto about 200 microfiche. These can be carried in an A4 folder so that the general practitioner can have with him the entire records of the practice plus a microfiche pocket viewer and these are carried around with him. The computer system therefore is as secure, we feel, as we can reasonably make it and the doctor has control over the release of the data. The microfiche represent a potential confidentiality hazard; they are also a considerable factor in the provision of better patient care and thus illustrate the dilemma caused by improved medical record systems.

CONFIDENTIALITY OF WAITING LISTS

Statement of Intent

1. Medical Staff

   (a) Inspection of Waiting Lists

   It will be possible for all medical staff at both hospitals to

     (i) Know which waiting lists any patient is on;

    (ii) Look at the waiting list details for a patient on any waiting list;

   (iii) Examine any waiting list as a whole.

   (b) Selection of patients for admission

   It will be possible for any member of the medical staff at either hospital to input to the computer the selection of any patient from any waiting list.

   (c) Prospective admissions

   It will be possible for any member of the medical staff at either hospital to inspect the list of forthcoming admissions of any consultant.

2. Administrative Staff

   The aim is to limit access to waiting list information to that which is necessary and sufficient for each individual to do his job. The degree of access required by each individual will be assessed by the Medical Records Officers, and the appropriate controls will be then built into the System.

   Agreed to date to have been the following:

   (i) Medical Records Clerks at PEOH do not need and should not have access to Waiting List records, or the list of forthcoming admissions, at Wonford and vice versa.

   (ii) Any Medical Records Clerk who normally uses the Waiting List System only when standing-in for the Admissions Clerk should retain the ability to use the Waiting List System at all times and that this should be possible under her usual password (ie. the password which permits the clerk to perform her normal tasks).

LIST OF PAPERS PRESENTED TO THE COMPUTER USERS' ETHICAL COMMITTEE

1. Introduction to Problems of Confidentiality

2. The Integrated Patient Record and its Users

3. Ownership of Data

4. Use of Patient Data for Research

5. Required Access to Data

6. Chapter 10 "Confidentiality" of the Guide for Computer Users in the NHS

7. Comments on the above

8. Copies of Letters - DHSS to Executive Council
                        Regional Officer to Council

9. The Mechanisms of Confidentiality

10. Extract from "Using Computers to Improve Health Services"

11. Medical Information for Research - Medical Research Council

12. The Structure of Passwords

13. Signing-On

14. Use of Training Systems

15. Confidentiality of Waiting Lists

16. Copy of Chapter 20 of Younger Report

17. Access to Medical Records of Health Service Staff

18. Confidentiality of Waiting Lists - Statement of Intent

19.   - do -   Patients on more than one waiting list

20. Extract from Report of World Medical Assembly on computers and confidentiality

21. Security of Files in Batch Processing

22. Access to the Integrated Patient Record - Interim Statement

The Objectives and Design Philosphy

of the real-time computer project at the

Queen Elizabeth Medical Centre

P.M. Hills,

Director of Computing

1.   The computer project at the Queen Elizabeth Medical Centre was set up in
1968 as part of a programme of such installations, sponsored and funded by the
D.H.S.S. At that time the way forward was seen to lie in the concept of the
large District General Hospital, with about 250 such complexes providing the
main secondary care services across the country. The Queen Elizabeth hospital
was ear-marked for such development, the Maternity hospital had already been
built, and plans were at an advanced stage for the creation of an outpatient
department, accident, emergency and burns units, and more laboratories and
operating theatres, as well as the building of geriatric, psychiatric and children's hospitals all on the same site. The computer system was to be at the
heart of this complex, controlling and integrating the flow of information
between the different units.

        These plans were halted in 1974 and are unlikely to be revived. At the
same time NHS re-organisation was aimed to bring together the primary and secondary arms of the Health Service into a single and more co-ordinated system.
At first sight it might appear that the future expansion path for the project
had been removed, but in practise the context had merely been changed. The
need to control and integrate the flows of information is still there, but are
no longer confined to the environment of the District General Hospital. The
challenge now is to provide this service in the wider context of Area-based
services, as envisaged by NHS re-organisation. Thus the future lies with Area-
based computer systems, but for the present the project at the Queen Elizabeth
hospital is still completing the development of applications that primarily
serve the hospital.

2.   Two main uses of information have been identified:-
        - immediate use, requiring real-time access where computers are involved;
          this is where the use of the information forms part of the function of
          a department or the care of the patient on a day-to-day basis
        - delayed use, requiring batch mode operation, providing for the longer
          term planning or management of hospital or health care resources, and
          meeting the needs of teaching and research.

3.   In the same simplistic manner two main categories of <u>user</u> have been identified, though with considerable overlap:-

- in a hospital context, the users requiring real-time access to information include doctors, nurses, ward clerks, laboratory staff, clerical
  staff in the Records office and in service departments etc .
- those concerned with batch systems and their output include administrators,
  medical and nursing management, statistics, heads of departments and
  teaching and research personnel.

The Queen Elizabeth hospital project has been designed to cater for both types
of use and classification of user. However, the problems of batch mode operation are fairly familiar, and the rest of this paper will concentrate on the
real-time aspects of the overall system.

4.   The <u>Objectives</u> of the project may be defined as follows:-

- to create a system that operates reliably in real-time and is acceptable
  to the users
- to speed information flows within the hospital and in particular patient
  information from service department to ward
- to improve the quality of the information in terms of accuracy, legibility, ease of access and interpretation
- to ensure confidentiality of patient records
- to save staff time, thus improving the use of hospital and NHS resources
- to provide a teaching and research facility
- to evaluate the completed system.

These objectives have by-and-large been met, though the last one is the
task of a separately funded team whose task is far from complete. In order to
achieve these objectives certain design principles were established.

4.1   It seems a fundamental point that everyone who requires access
to patient information as part of their job should have direct access
personally to the computer, if that is where patient information is
to be found. Within the Queen Elizabeth Medical Centre this applies
to more than 2000 staff; if you are intending to have that number of
potential users of the system then this dictates a whole series of
further design principles, such as minimum training, therefore the
system must be very simple to use, therefore it cannot depend upon
the learning of mnemonic codes, and so on.

Not only are there over 2000 potential users, but it is a per-
petually moving population. Most housemen stay only 6 months, and
with a school of nursing on site a number of nurses move on once they
have completed their qualifications. There are in practise normally
about 1200 authorised users of the system at any one time, of whom
half may have occasion to use the system in any week.

4.2   <u>Training</u>. This obviously could be an enormous problem if the
system was complex to learn and understand. There are in effect two
types of real-time user, the "professional" and the amateur:-

- the professional users include the clerks in records offices
  and outpatient clinics etc and many of the staff in laboratories and service departments. These users are numbered in
  dozens; their use of the system is often fairly complex, and
  after initial thorough training by the computer department,
  on-going training is the responsibility of their own department. Their job involves use of the system in the same way
  that a secretary's job involves use of a typewriter or a tel-
  phone
- the amateur users are numbered in hundreds, comprising doctors
  at all levels, nurses, students, physiotherapists, pharmacists
  etc. It is for them that the system has primarily been designed, their use is irregular and incidental to their job.
  They have to be motivated, and it is the computer department's
  responsibility to ensure that they know how to use the system.

This necessary training is carried out by one person in the computer
department on a part-time basis, and it is fairly minimal, since the
system is largely self-explanatory. After a new user has made contact
and his or her identity established, the training officer meets the
person on the ward, allocates a user code and demonstrates the available functions for about 20 minutes. Thereafter the use is learnt
by practise on the job. When a new application is introduced, however,
this is normally implemented one ward at a time, and the initial
training is carried out by the team responsible for that application.
A demonstration system has also been provided, which is in the form
of a self-teaching aid.

4.3   <u>The basic principles</u> of operation are the same for all applications. These consist of selecting an item from a numbered list of
options (tree branching), and making use of named Function buttons.
There is a standard way of identifying a patient - for all inpatients
this is simply to select the name from the ward list. If the ward
is not known, or the patient is not an inpatient, his details may be
accessed either by quoting the Registration number, or by quoting
surname, initial and sex. In all cases a more complete identification
is presented to the user for confirmation that it is the right person.

        Every use of the system is designed as a simple conversation
which follows the same pattern. It starts with the use of the Login
button, and finishes with Logout. The function of logging in presents

the user with an appropriate Home display, which lists the options
available to that user. Having selected the required option and
identified the patient, the user proceeds down the tree structure
till he has retrieved the information he requires or is ready to update the record. At this point he has to press the Confirm function
button actually to update the data-base; alternatively he may press
the Cancel button if he does not wish to proceed with the update.
In either casethe system returns him to his Home display. Pressing
the Home function button will have the same effect, while pressing
Backtrack will take him back up the tree one step at a time. Laboratory results are presented by patient in reverse chronological
sequence. Thus the latest result will appear first and earlier results
can be seen by pressing the Page Backwards button; subsequently Page
Forwards will bring you to the most recent result again.

4.4   <u>Design of the VDU</u> itself was seen to be of the greatest importance. When selecting the hardware in 1971 VDUs were evaluated on
their own, and Cossor 401Es were selected. Subsequently short-listed
mainframe manufacturers were instructed to quote for these Cossor
units. The reason for this was that as far as the user is concerned,
the VDU is the computer system - he is not interested in what you
have in the computer room so long as his terminal does what he wants.
    The main features of the 401E were:-
- a 2000 character screen, giving scope for attractive and
  standardised presentation of data
- clarity of characters, including upper and lower case
- instant filling of the screen (transmission rate of 1.2 Mbaud)
- fast response time (no multiplexing, minimum of queueing)
- a keyboard designed by the hospital, featuring specific
  Function buttons, a number block for rapid tree-branching
  and good editing facilities
- protected fields and full screen send
- login code inhibited from appearing on the screen.

These facilities have combined to make the VDU one of the outstanding
features of the Queen Elizabeth hospital project, and one that is
always noticed and commented on by discerning visitors.
    Another feature is the generally fast response time, and this
has been achieved by the selection of the Univac 418/III mainframe
and the use of fast drums (4 msec access time). The 418/III was specifically designed for real-time use; I/O modules have independant
access to core, which itself has a cycle time of 650 nanosecs per
word, and all channels operate at more than 1 megabyte transfer rate.

Unfortunately this machine is obsolete, and we have yet to discover another mainframe capable of achieving a comparable speed of response. This fast speed is again integral to design for the user, since an easy-to-learn multi-layer tree-branching system has proved very acceptable to users when a response of 1 second or less is achieved, but it rapidly becomes frustrating if the response time exceeds 3 seconds.

4.5   Confidentiality of the data was seen from the start as being of the utmost importance within the overall design principles. In a real-time system access must be restricted to authorised users. Two methods were considered:-

- Card badges
- Codes.

Cossor were prepared to incorporate badge readers into the keyboard of the VDU. However, plastic embossed cards were rejected for the following reasons:-

- they can be lost
- they can be left in the wrong coat pocket
- they can be left lying around
- they can be lent to another person.

Codes also have their dis-advantages

- they can be forgotten
- they can be passed on verbally to some-one else.

However, codes were selected as being the superior method, and the system operates as follows:-

- a new user applies for a code number by completing an application form which is then authorised by his/her head of department. N.B. it is the hospital which decides who can have access to patient data, not the computer department
- A six character alpha/numeric code is then given to the user when they are given their initial training. This code points to an entry in a table which includes the person's name and the staff category. Categories range from 1 - 99, and these control which files the user may access and which they may update
- when using the VDU the user presses Login, types their code number (which does not appear on the screen) and presses Send. The computer responds with the appropriate Home display if the code is recognised. If it is not a valid code, a polite message is presented, together with a message on the console in the computer room. After 3 unsuccessful

attempts to log-in the operator will get in touch by
telephone
- The first 3 characters of the code are fixed and are
recorded against every item of data written by that user.
The trailing 3 characters are variable, and may be changed
by the user at any time. Monitoring reveals that about
30 users change their codes each week
- at the end of a conversation, the user presses Logout.
This blanks the screen again and closes the conversation.

4.6   There are many other features that must be considered in designing a system with the user in mind:-
- to be of practical value it must operate 7 days a week, and
as near to 24 hours a day as possible - the QE system is available for about 20 hours every day of the year
- users must have confidence in the reliability of the system
and the professionalism of the computer staff. To ensure the
viability of the database all input to the system is journal-
ised to 2 magnetic tapes for recovery purposes, all files are
dumped every night, and file integrety routines are run every
day in the background to ensure that all record linkages are
correct. No item of data has yet been lost and an up-time of
99.6% is achieved
- when a breakdown occurs, as they inevitably do, the user needs
to know for how long the break-down will last, and if he was
in the middle of a transaction, whether it was completed or
not. Both these requirements are met
- the length of breakdowns must be kept to a minimum. About
half of those occurring at the QE are of a non-critical nature,
and in these cases the system recovers itself automatically,
without operator intervention, and takes about 1 minute. Manual recovery takes about 8 minutes unless a hardware re-con-
figuration or data-base recovery is necessary. There is considerable hardware redundancy built into the system, such that
it is possible to operate in real-time without the drums, and/
or a channel and half the discs, and/or a channel and half the
tape decks, and/or a printer/card-reader sub-system, and/or
32K of core. However, in this situation development and batch
work would be halted.

5.   Perhaps the most important point of all has been left to the end. The total system must be designed not only <u>for</u> the user, but also with active participation <u>by</u> the user. This is not always as easy as it sounds, since users at first are unsophisticated in computer terms, and are uncertain both of what they want and what is feasible. There is at first a large credibility gap where they cannot imagine how the system will work in practise, nor do they have confidence that the computer can achieve what is being proposed. However, once the first applications have become operational, and practical experience in their use has been gained, their ability and willingness to contribute improves very rapidly.

It is important, also, to ensure in the design of applications that:-

- users are not expected to do the same function twice (there are still sites where the patient is registered manually and then entered into the computer system)
- an additional work-load is not imposed on the user, unless this is unavoidable and other significant benefits are achieved
- the sequence of implementation is such that benefits to the user are apparent from the start.

The formal involvement of the users at the Queen Elizabeth Hospital has been as follows:-

- Each application has been designed by a User group, with the support of a design team
- these groups have included doctors, nurses, and laboratory, pharmacy and records office staff, with combinations of professional staff where applications integrate across boundaries
- separate User groups have been formed to monitor the performance of existing systems
- Chairmen of the User groups, together with members of the M.E.C. and D.M.T., form the Computer Executive who direct the project.

THE UTILIZATION AND VALIDATION OF MATHEMATICAL
MODELS IN MEDICINE AND PUBLIC HEALTH

Norman T. J. Bailey
Unit of Health Statistical Methodology
WHO, Geneva, Switzerland

1. INTRODUCTION

Mathematical modelling is used increasingly over the whole area of medicine and public health, from basic clinical science to policy planning. This attempt to apply in the medical field what has long been familiar in the more exact sciences, whether explicitly called 'modelling' or not, holds considerable promise for the future. However, as with all attempts to transfer techniques from one field to another, careful consideration must be given to the special characteristics of the area to which the new applications are made. These techniques may need unforeseen modifications or developments before they are valid.

This is particularly true of medicine because of the range of applications. Investigations of physiological processes, studies of communicable disease dynamics, the prediction of noncommunicable disease incidence, the testing of drugs and treatments in controlled clinical trials, the allocation of scarce resources, the choice of optimal strategies, the improvement of health care systems, the understanding and use of health economics, the formulation of policy etc., all require different kinds of quantitative analysis. And insofar as any well-organized and well-defined account or picture of certain aspects of the real world entails an appropriate framework of concepts, we are automatically involved in some form of modelling. This can be largely qualitative in character. But as soon as we employ serious rational and scientific thinking major quantitative elements emerge, and we are committed to models which are essentially of a mathematical character.

Judgement and commonsense are required in these matters, in addition to purely technical skills. Since medicine is concerned with curing and preventing disease, as well as with the active promotion of health, the ultimate needs and wishes of the human customers are of primary importance. This means that mental, social and ethical aspects cannot be ignored. Any modelling which is set in a purely mathematical or computer context, no matter how logically faultless, may turn out to be simply irrelevant from the point of view of human needs. There is an ever-present danger of modelling being both unrealistic and expensive. This is why many attempts to develop large-scale systems approaches to health care delivery systems and health planning have been rejected (e.g. Hoos, 1969). Many proposals have foundered on an inability to answer the question, "What you say sounds very interesting, but why should I believe in your particular model?"

If models can be seen to be valid, in acceptable scientific and statistical terms, they are worth examining further for possible cost-effective applications. But if, for example, a vast and complicated econometric style of model is propounded to represent a health care system in which there are hundreds of compartments, thousands of interconnections, and innumerable parameters mostly incapable of estimation, then the absence of validation, not to mention credibility, is sure to entail certain failure, sooner or later.

The issue of model validation is crucial in resolving this mass of contradictions. If medical informatics is to provide effective support to medical and public health decision-making, it must be securely grounded at the technical level. Modelling is one of the key activities, along with statistical planning and design, basic data processing, computerisation, information systems, O.R. and systems analysis etc. But the strengths and weaknesses of modelling must be adequately understood in relation to the tasks to be performed. Moreover, we must be able to tell whether individual models are good or bad, whether to believe in them or not, and how to improve their effectiveness.

This paper attempts to review some of the major aspects with a view to facilitating both the utilization and validation of models in applications within the field of medicine and public health.

2. TYPES OF MODELS

Before discussing the central problems of using, testing and validating models, there are certain preliminary matters of definition and classification to be dealt with. I have already given an elementary treatment of the art of modelling in relatively non-technical terms elsewhere (Bailey, 1977, Chapter 5). For present purposes, the rough definition of a model as a "well-organized and well-defined account or picture of certain aspects of the real world," will suffice.

More important is the question of typology. We are not so much concerned with fine distinctions, important though they may be, such as whether a model includes probability aspects or not, thus entitling it to be labelled 'stochastic' rather than 'deterministic'. But we must take account of any major aspects that call for different approaches, attitudes of mind, interpretations or applications.

For example, it is essential to know whether a model is primarily to be seen as part of a deductive or an inductive process, or perhaps both in alternate phases. Take, for example, a standard model in infectious disease theory, the so-called general stochastic epidemic, involving susceptibles, infectious persons and those who are 'removed', i.e. isolated, dead or recovered and immune. Given certain simplifying assumptions, and supposing that initially there are $\underline{a}$ infectious individuals, $\underline{n}$ susceptibles and a removal/infection ratio ρ, there is a simple threshold theorem about the chance of a major epidemic breaking out. The latter is negligible if $\rho > \underline{n}$, but equal to $1 - (\rho/\underline{n})^a$ if $\rho < \underline{n}$. Such results are obtained purely deductively from the assumptions. They do, however, help to clarify ideas, generate further hypotheses, and provide some general insights into the underlying dynamic mechanisms.

However, there comes a point when there are justifiable doubts as to the credibility of such over-simplified models. We want to know how likely they are to be true, if only approximately. This forces us to look for actual data to test the applicability of the model. We now enter an inductive phase, in which the data are accepted as a starting point from which satisfactory explanatory hypotheses are to be derived. We must embark on a process of estimating parameters and testing 'goodness-of-fit' according to the appropriate statistical procedures. Unsatisfactory models must be rejected, or modified and retested.

Most scientific work is essentially of the inductive kind, though employing deductive phases from time to time for speculative purposes.

When, however, some kind of administrative action is required there is, in the short run, no time for inductive research. Assumptions have to be made and acted on. This is frequently done in a purely intuitive way. A ministerial committee may have to decide on whether to continue or discontinue some kind of vaccination (e.g. as in the past for smallpox). Deductive argumentation can be most valuable in clarifying assumptions, resolving disagreements, working out the consequences of different sets of assumptions, undertaking sensitivity analyses on the effect of possible errors or variations in assumptions etc. The purely rational aspects of the committee's deliberations can depend in large measure on forecasting what will happen if certain suppositions are true. If the models underlying these suppositions are untested and possibly false, the implications for the soundness of the resultant decision-making may be far-reaching.

We merely note in passing that most of Forrester's system dynamics (1961, 1969, 1971), and the later world models of the Club of Rome (Meadows et al. 1972; Mesarovic and Pestel, 1974), fall into this class. A more balanced attitude to the purely preliminary and deductive nature of these studies, as a prelude to inductive modelling that could be subsequently tested and validated, would have avoided much fruitless criticism.

Another major distinction worth making is between what has been referred to in the more philosophical literature as 'positivism' versus 'structuralism' (see Gardner,

1973).   Positivism, or functionalism, deals directly with observed facts, while
'structuralism' tries to explain surface phenomena by means of underlying relationships or mechanisms.   The population dynamics of infectious disease is clearly
structural, dealing as it does with underlying biological processes.   Most noncommunicable disease epidemiology, on the other hand, relies on a largely functional
approach.   Vast quantities of purely statistical data are analysed in terms of
associations and correlations in the hopes that causal connections will be revealed,
leading to ultimate control.   As is well-known, 'correlation is not causation', but
it may be useful in suggesting possibilities.   The relationship between smoking and
lung cancer is one of the few strikingly successful examples of this approach.

An appreciation of whether or not we are dealing with a deductive or an inductive situation, and whether we have a model that merely describes surface phenomena
or reflects more certain knowledge of the underlying processes, is of fundamental
relevance to the valid use of models.

3.   LEVELS OF APPLICATION

An essential aspect of effective modelling is the need for clarity about the
level of the application, because this can seriously affect the criteria appropriate
for judging success or failure.   A useful, but by no means unique, classification
is given by distinguishing between technical models, operational models, information
models, and policy models.

Technical models

This is the basic level of fundamental scientific investigation.   It covers
the traditional disciplines dealing with molecular biology, immunology, biochemistry,
physiology, radiology etc., where the focus of attention is the individual;   and
population phenomena involving demography, evolution, ecology, epidemiology etc.
The keynote here is the search for more scientific understanding, partly for its
own sake, partly in the expectation that it will be useful for the control of natural
phenomena.

The quantitative work implicit in such studies has always entailed some form of
mathematical modelling, examples of which can be traced back to at least the 17th
Century.   The mathematical formulations enable hypotheses to be stated more precisely, deductive analyses to be carried out more expeditiously, and critical testing
against empirical data to be made with greater certainty.

Operational models

This is the level of operational research and systems analysis.   It deals with
man-made systems rather than the natural world.   The emphasis is on a scientific
approach to problems facing executive and administrative authorities.   Much of the

subject matter is thus concerned with organization, management and decision-making. Typical examples in the medical field are: hospital design, outpatient appointment systems, ambulance services, mass health screening, the provision of health services, health planning etc. We may be dealing with anything from a small-scale operational study of an operating theatre to a large-scale investigation of the health service delivery system of a whole country.

Quantitative models are needed to facilitate both deductive and inductive investigations. Complex interacting systems of component parts are logically no different from, say, physiological systems at the technical level. However, in practice, the presence of additional factors such as economics, cost-benefit analysis, resource allocation, decision-making, as well as moral, psychological and social aspects, means that we are effectively working in a substantially different field.

Operational models are aimed at elucidating a complex man-made system in which the administrative control of phenomena involves an understanding of both natural processes and social factors. For example, if a health service delivery system is to be run more effectively it must take into account the natural phenomena of disease incidence and prevalence; the availability of drugs, equipment, and medical manpower; a variety of economic constraints; and the wishes and aspirations of the human consumers, i.e. those whose diseases are to be cured or prevented.

Information models

Information models represent a further step away from fundamental natural phenomena in the direction of human administrative management and control. They are primarily concerned with the flow and communication of information needed for decision-making. In some texts this is regarded as a part of O.R. The preliminary flow chart linking together the system components may be called a 'communication model'. This is seen as a prelude to the specification of a full system dynamics representation. On the other hand, the refining of a specialised managerial instrument to make sure that administrative authorities have the information they need, in the right place, and at the right time, implies that a distinction must be made between such an information system, with its implicit information model, and the O.R. model that depicts the dynamic complex of natural phenomena and man-made decision-making.

There is a good deal of variation in the usage of these concepts. With the classification adopted here, we envisage the broad administrative control of records, reports, payroll, staffing, budgeting, programming, scheduling, etc., using whatever forms of flow-charting, PERT, computerised management, and so on, that may be appropriate.

Policy models

This is the top level where administrators have to deal with broad strategic problems in public health, covering medium-term or long-range planning for large geographical areas of regional, national or even international extent.   Although activities on this level can be crucial to the aspirations, happiness and well-being of millions, they are notoriously susceptible to ill-informed impressions, subjective thinking and arbitrary action.   Inevitable constraints are imposed by what is physically or biologically possible and by what is socially, economically and politically feasible.   Given these constraints, there are horrendous problems in choosing between the available strategies.

To make matters worse, decisions often have to be taken at short notice and under severe emotional and psychological pressures.   Opportunities for relaxed, rational and scientific analysis are restricted, but anything that can be done to improve the situation is worthwhile.   The subject of policy analysis is at a very early stage of development.   Much needs to be done to work out appropriate quantitative models for forecasting the likely consequences of alternative strategies, and choosing what is reasonably good (if not best!).

So far, most policy analysis amounts to little more than a necessary, but preliminary, constraint analysis.   If, however, we follow the view of Majone (1975) that "Policies are, in fact, tentative theories", then we have a point of entry for introducing a more scientifically oriented approach.   Questions of testing and validating the "tentative theories" can be handled <u>via</u> appropriately constructed models.

Some progress has been made in other biologically based fields such as ecology, especially in the areas of fishery management and pest control (e.g. Conway, 1977). While involving numerous human and economic elements, these spheres of application are less complex than public health.   Valuable lessons might be learned, however, from a more detailed study of the results achieved, especially in regard to the implications for the control of vector borne diseases.

4.   TESTING AND VALIDATING MODELS

We have seen above in general terms the kind of problems in medicine and public health that can be investigated using mathematical models.   But what guarantees are there that the <u>right</u> models are being used?   And how do we recognise when mistakes are made?

So long as we operate on the technical level, using traditional scientific methods in contexts which are very close to the familiar areas of physics or biology, there are no serious methodological difficulties. The models can then be seen as an intrinsic part of the hypotheses generated. They are judged by the insight they provide, the stimulus given to new research, and, above all, the extent to which they 'fit' observed data and permit the elaboration of verifiable predictions.

The scientific approach relies on 'trial and error', and repeated experimentation allows a store of more or less successful hypotheses to be built up. When these hypotheses, suitably modified, can be made to fit together into an interlocking conceptual structure, we have an emergent theory. This theory then explains a great many otherwise unconnected observations, and can be used either in whole or in part confidently to predict what will happen in the future under specified, sometimes novel, situations. Theories that continue to pass such tests, with adjustments and modifications as required, gain in strength and credibility. Critical experiments may be suggested from time to time to provide crucial tests of the whole theory. Failure to pass such tests may demand serious revisions of the whole theory, though it may still be valid within a more restricted context.

These ideas have for long been generally accepted within the domain of physics and other near-exact sciences. Relatively small errors of observation can be minimised by averaging repeated measurements. In biology, however, with the large intrinsic variability of living matter, the interpretation of uncertain measurements is far more difficult. Experimentation is liable to be confused by unconscious bias in both the choice of subjects and selection of experimental design. And results can easily be misinterpreted owing to the presence of large, natural, chance variations.

Modern statistical techniques have enabled these problems to be largely overcome by the use of randomisation, factorial designs, standard errors, significance tests etc. Models can be tested by seeing whether they 'fit' the data within the limits of natural variation. Special tests, like the chi-squared goodness-of-fit, enable well-defined results to be obtained in probability terms. Mistaken judgements cannot be entirely avoided, but statistical theory shows how to minimise such errors.

A great deal of medical work, especially in pharmacology, the analysis of clinical data, randomised clinical trials, epidemiological surveys etc., makes enormous use nowadays of such statistical methods. These methods are, however, a refinement to the standard principles of scientific investigation. Repeated experimentation, together with more sophisticated methods of model fitting and hypothesis testing, plus the acid test of prediction, has enabled continuous and reliable advances to be maintained.

On the operational level there has been a certain divergence of the ways. In standard small-scale O.R. approaches to, say, hospital ward design, outpatient appointment systems, mass health screening, cost-benefit studies of expensive and specialised equipment etc., the scientific approach has been able to proceed in much the same way. Plenty of data are available, hypotheses and models can be tested, new ideas can be tried out, experiments planned and executed, and so on. The question "Why should I believe your model?" can be answered by reference to the mass of evaluation and validation work actually carried out.

But when it comes to the larger systems, especially those dealing with complex health services, there is liable to be trouble. The a priori, deductive type of system dynamics approach is highly vulnerable to adverse criticism. It is always easy to find errors, or controversial aspects, of detail. While it may be argued that these approaches are designed to handle the 'big picture', sensitivity analyses will often show that small changes in parametric values or in structural form may have large consequences for the results obtained.

When clarifying concepts and thought, and generating hypotheses, such criticisms can be unnecessarily restricting. But if we are expected to believe the models in their unvalidated state, and to take action on the computed implications, it is a very different matter. For a recent review of developmental trends in the health planning field, see Bailey and Thompson (1974). This collection of papers illustrates the range of possible systems applications, but the question of the validity of the modelling is mostly unresolved.

The heart of the problem is that a big public health system is unique. There is no possibility of constructing a number of alternative health delivery systems for one region or country and trying them all out experimentally. A statistically controlled trial of different 'treatments' is thus impossible. This difficulty is often used as an argument against a systems analysis approach to public health. But this is based on a misunderstanding. Systems analysis is precisely aimed at developing the special methodology required for handling complex, and usually not replicate, systems.

A clue to what is needed for validation comes from the perception that a big system is different from a small well-defined component that might be investigated in a statistically valid experiment. It is much more like a whole body of scientific knowledge constituting a theory. The theory of evolution, for example, has not been developed as a single entity, but by the accumulation of a large number of individually validated items all put together into a coherent whole, followed by various testable predictions.

It follows that public health modelling should _not_ simply consist of a large number of econometric equations asserted without proof to be an appropriate basis for computer simulations, the print-outs of which are to be regarded as an immediate guide for decision-makers. On the contrary, a systems model should be built up slowly and deliberately, with full participation of the eventual users. (Even with technical level infectious disease models, months of discussion may be needed between epidemiologists and mathematicians to reach agreement on the first, tentative flow chart!) The component parts, which may consist of sub-models dealing with demographic aspects, disease incidence and prevalence, medical resources, economic factors etc., must each be carefully selected and tested in the usual way at the technical level.

Even to get this far is a major undertaking. The next step of putting together the components in a bigger system is more difficult, because it is now the overall structure of the interconnected subsystems that is at issue. The question immediately arises "Why should we believe any particular way of putting together the overall system?" At this point we must be quite clear as to which aspects of the modelling are deductive and which are inductive. Obviously, one cannot carry out lengthy research on every possible item, otherwise practical applications would be indefinitely postponed. So it is essential to distinguish between what, at least for the time being, is generally agreed and what needs empirical verification.

It may be possible to utilise technical models of disease incidence and spread, demographic changes, health manpower, etc., which are sufficiently well-established to be accepted. There may be problems with the dependence of public demand for treatment on the actual availability of services. The effect of economic and social constraints may also be uncertain, including the roles of drug advertising and health education. Some of these difficulties can be met by looking for further information on the interactions of certain components. Small special investigations may be worthwhile to establish the mechanisms of interaction between specific components. Everything possible should be done to carry out as much validation as possible at the technical level where standard scientific criteria can be used.

In building up the more comprehensive model it is desirable to do so gradually. Two or three major components can be introduced first. Tentative agreement must be reached between investigators and users on a reasonable way to put the items together. Next, some form of partial validation must be devised, based partly on adequately explaining past data and partly on making verifiable predictions in selected circumstances. If sufficient success is obtained the process can be extended until a large, but reasonably credible, systems model emerges. This too must be rigorously tested before it can be offered as a practical instrument to aid real decision-making and policy planning.

What is more, when such an approach is actually made operational, there must be continual surveillance to check performance. Short-term forecasts, as well as longer term forecasts as time proceeds, should be constantly made and checked, at low, intermediate and top levels of the system, in order to increase the credibility of the model through a demonstration of predictive power.

5. CONCLUSIONS AND RECOMMENDATIONS

It has been possible here to deal only with the broad outlines of the central problems of utilizing and validating models in medicine and public health. Validation is, in particular, a major issue in systems modelling. Until improved means are found for handling this issue effectively, a great deal of systems modelling, which is of vital importance to public health decision-making and policy planning, will continue to be regarded as an excessively expensive and academic exercise.

It is recommended that the approaches proposed in this paper should be applied to a small number of actual public health systems and all the steps worked through in a rigorous manner. In this way practical demonstrations could be provided of just how models can be correctly utilized on the different conceptual levels, how they can be combined into a larger interacting system, and how acceptable validation of the whole system can be achieved.

It is, of course, accepted that some kind of pragmatic compromise must be found between the ideal of complete scientific purity and the pressing need for quick, simple and effective applications to the real-life problems of administrative decision-making and policy planning.

REFERENCES

BAILEY, N. T. J. (1977). Mathematics, Statistics and Systems for Health. Wiley, London.
BAILEY, N. T. J. and THOMPSON, M. (Ed.) (1975). Systems Aspects of Health Planning. North-Holland, Amsterdam.
CONWAY, G. R. (1977). Mathematical models in applied ecology, Nature, 269, 291-297.
FORRESTER, J. (1961). Industrial Dynamics. MIT, Cambridge, Mass.
FORRESTER, J. (1969). Urban Dynamics. MIT, Cambridge, Mass.
FORRESTER, J. (1971). World Dynamics. Wright-Allen, Cambridge, Mass.
GARDNER, H. (1973). The Quest for Mind. Knopf, New York.
HOOS, Ida R. (1969). Systems Analysis in Social Policy. Institute of Economic Affairs, London.
MAJONE, G. (1975). The feasibility of social policies, Policy Science, 6, 49-69.
MEADOWS, D. H., MEADOWS, D. L., RANDERS, J. and BEHRENS, W. W. (1972). The Limits to Growth. Universe Books, New York.
MESAROVIC, M. and PESTEL, E. (1974). Mankind at the Turning Point. Hutchinson, London.

TESTING ALTERNATIVE INVENTORY POLICIES
FOR A REGIONAL BLOOD BANK

B. Page

Technische Universität Berlin

Fachbereich Informatik

Federal Republic of Germany

1. The Problem

The collection, storage and allocation of human blood for transfusion patients presents a problem unlike those encountered in
the production, storage and distribution of industrial products.
Blood cannot be produced at will, but has to be donated by
healthy humans on a voluntary basis. In addition blood cannot
be transfused into any patient, but the compatibility between
the patient's and the donor's blood has to be tested beforehand
("crossmatching"). There are eight different main blood groups
(A, B, O, AB with Rh+ or Rh-), which are basically not compatible with each other. This would not be a problem if the distribution of the main blood groups within the population was
not highly unequal with some very rare groups. The inventory
problem is further complicated by the fact that human blood
has a limited life span of 3 to 4 weeks.

In industrial inventory systems only the demand is stochastic
while in blood bankes the supply, i.e. the arrival of blood
donors, is random as well.

Finally and most important, no emergency call for blood units
can be rejected by a blood bank, because human life would be
endangered. There must be a pool of on-call donors to provide
the blood in need, if a shortage occurs.

Due to the special character of the product "blood unit" and
the poor organization in many regional blood supply systems
frequent shortages with the need for high cost special deliveries and excessive outdating are very common in blood banking.

Even with these additional obstacles in blood banks the fundamental ideas of inventory theory as widely used in industrial
environments can be applied to blood banking systems as well,
where the inventory problem and the problem of optimal distribution
of the units within the supply system exists basically in the
same way.

2. The System

The flow in the total blood supply system is represented by
the following simplified diagram:

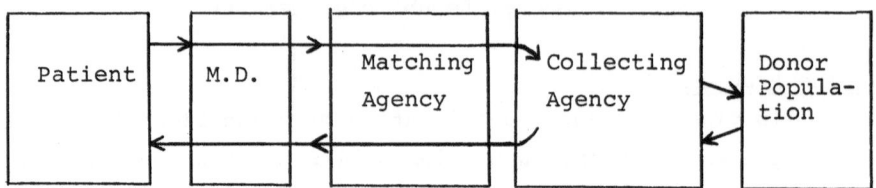

Fig. 1: The total blood supply system

The chain starts with a patient, whose physician decides that
a blood transfusion ist required, supplies the matching agency
with a sample of the patient's blood, and requests a specific
quantity of compatible blood. The matching agency, in turn,
requests blood from the collecting agency which is generally
able to supply it from stocks on hand, but must ocasionally
obtain the required units through a special call to the donor
population. The blood is then delivered to the matching agency
which selects compatible blood and delivers it to the M.D., who
puts it on reserve for this patient, until the transfusion is
performed. The collecting agency is likely to be either a central blood bank or the hospital's blood bank itself, while the
matching agency is, in most cases, the laboratory of the hospital.
Reservation for only one patient means that the blood is normally not available to any other patient until the reservation
is canceled by the M.D.. The need for reservation of blood
units prior to transfusion makes the inventory problem in
blood banking systems more complicated. There are two different
inventories: The unassigned inventory and the reserved inventory.

3. The Model

A simulation model was designed to test alternative inventory
and distribution policies in a regional blood banking system.
At first measures of effectiveness had to be defined to enable
the evaluation of the different inventory policies. The most
commonly used measures in the literature are shortages, wastage,
costs and average age of blood units at transfusion, where only
the first three measures were considered relevant in this research.
In order to avoid the complications of multidimensional objective
functions, inventory cost per transfused unit was taken as the
main measure of effectiveness including waste and shortages
weighted by their costs (cost per outdated blood unit, cost per
emergency shipment).

The model is organized as a centralized system where the regional
blood bank is responsible for all decision on the distribution
of blood units in the total supply system thereby having control
on the hospital's inventory as well.

The structure of the model is shown in Fig. 2, a flow chart of
the events in Fig. 3.

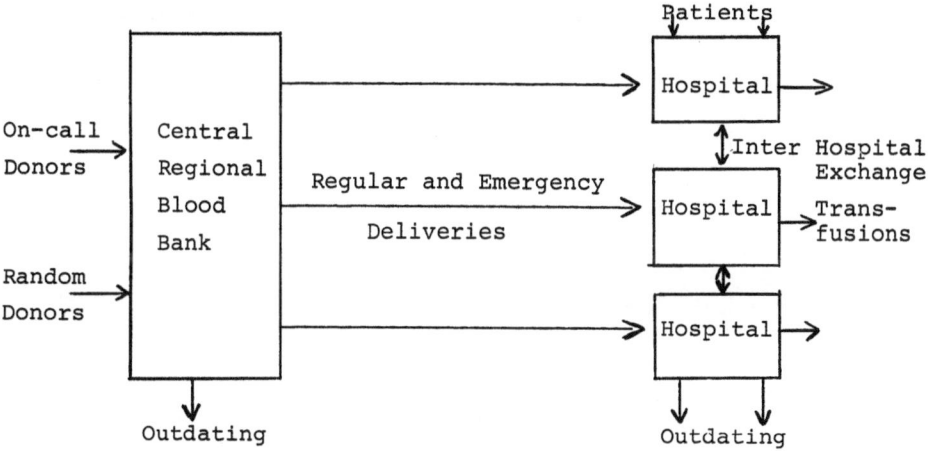

Fig. 2: The structure of the model

Real world data was collected in the regional bank and two hospitals in Berlin (West) on distributions and parameters for the
model, such as patients, donors, blood units per patient, wastage,
shortages, age of units at transfusion, percentage of regular
and emergency deliveries, age of units at delivery, reservation
time, probability for transfusion of reserved units, and cost data.

4. Implementation of the Simulation Model

The complex simulation model was programmed in the discrete system simulation language SIMSCRIPT II.5 on an IBM 370/158 computer with 2 Mbytes of core. All three proposed procedures were implemented in one modular program system. The call up of these modules was controlled by input parameters. The program size is about 2500 lines of code, using 1000 Kbytes of core.

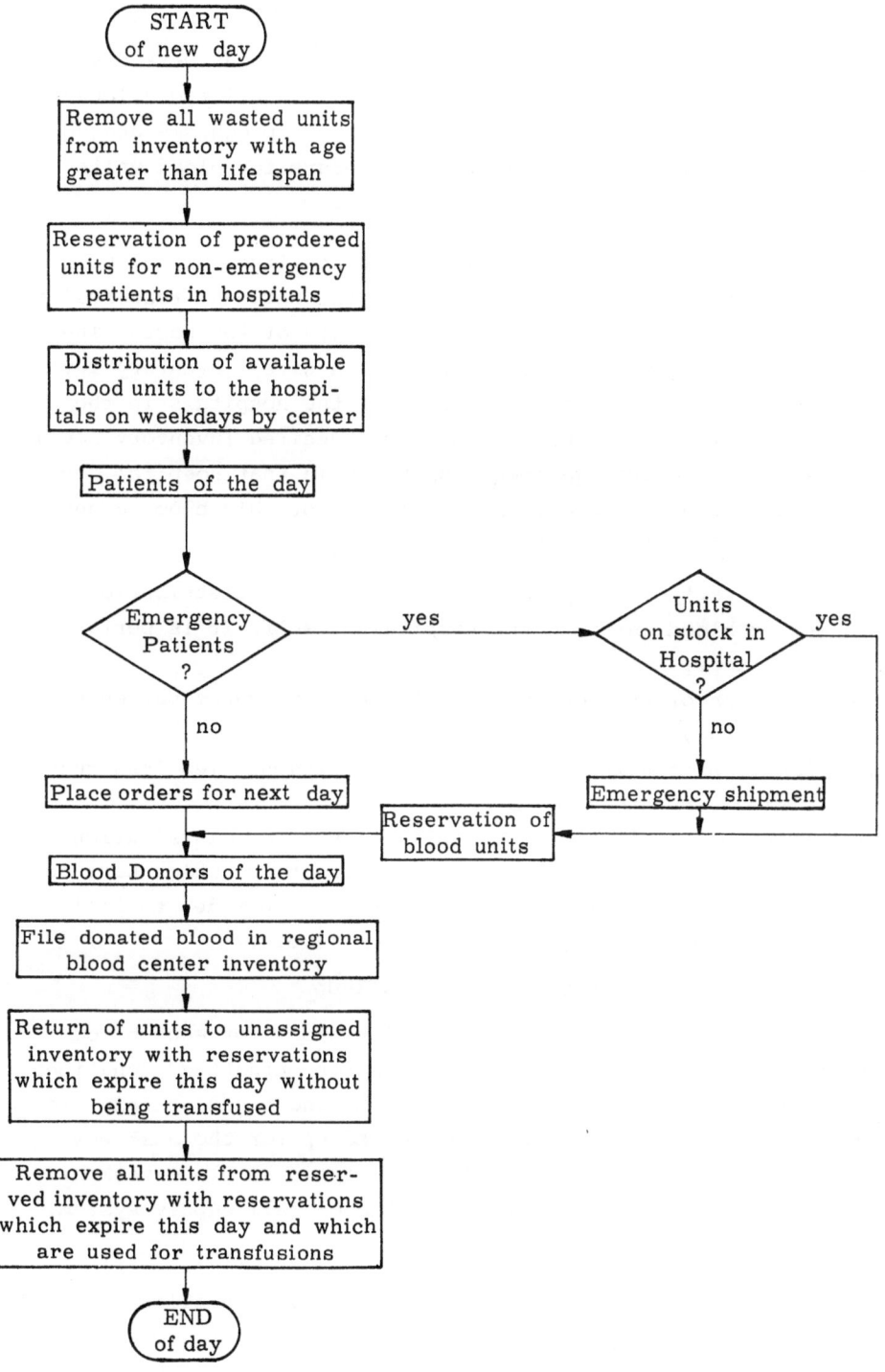

Fig. 3: Flow chart of events in the model

5. Proposed Inventory and Distribution Policies

Three different inventory and distribution methods were developed and tested in the simulation model: A heuristic allocation procedure for blood units, an inventory prognosis and donor
call-up procedure, and a recycling procedure for blood units.

- Heuristic Allocation Procedure

The heuristic allocation procedure concerns itself with the
unequal distribution of blood units in the regional transfusion
blood supply system. The procedure consists of two parts. The
first one deals with the computation of desired inventory levels
for the regional blood bank and each of the hospitals in the
supply system for each blood group. The desired inventory levels
are based on the average demand of blood in that hospital, the
percentage of emergencies, the percentage of this blood group,
and several inventory factors.

The second part of the procedure addresses the distribution
process of blood units to the hospitals itself. It is performed
in three steps:
a) Allocation of preordered units for non-emergency patients
   for that day
b) Allocation of units to hospitals with inventories less than
   a minimum inventory level
c) Allocation of additional units available for distribution
   in the regional blood bank only to hospitals, which have to
   be visited anyway (because of a) or b)), in order to fill
   up their inventories, to the desired levels.

- Prognosis of Inventory and Donor Call-Up

Every week a prognosis of the total inventory for each blood
group is made, composed of estimations for outdating, donations
and transfusions for the following week, and based on this prognosis the number of donors to be called up for the next week
is determined. With this procedure the regional blood bank has
control over the inventory level in the overall supply system.

- Recycling Procedure

Older blood units which are in the inventory of smaller hospitals
are called back to the regional blood center for rallocation to
larger hospitals with a higher probability of transfusion for
these older blood units.

6. Results

Much work was devoted to the validation of the model. Part of the validation procedure was the comparison of model output and real system output, which is shown in Table 1.

Table 1: Output comparison

Results / System	cost per transf. unit	shor-tages	out-dating	age of blood units at transf.	age of blood units at delivery	On-call donors	Reser-vations per unit
Real system	approx. 19 DM	18,8%	18,25%	9,82 days	3,48 days	approx. 5%	1,42
Model of red syst.	19,70 DM	18,76%	18,29%	9,86 days	3,33 days	0,5%	1,44

For the output comparison all 68 hospitals, which receive blood units from the central blood bank in Berlin on a regular basis, where included in the analysis, which led to a CPU-time of approximately one hour for 700 days of simulated blood bank operation. (The length of a simulation run was determined by an acceptable width of the confidence interval for the cost per transfused unit.) Two sets of experiments were run with the validated blood bank simulator. To cut down computer time these experiments were carried out with only nine hospitals (500 sec. CPU-time.)

The first series concerned the stepwise incorporation of the proposed inventory policies to show that they reduce costs. A Multiple Ranking procedure (1) was applied to prove statistically that each of the policies leads to a significant reduction in inventory cost per transfused unit in a regional blood banking system. The results are given in Table 2.

The second set of simulation experiments was directed to the demonstration of setting an optimal inventory level in a regional blood supply system. The results in Figure 4 show that the optimal solution for the real system under investigation is a desired inventory of 1.25 times the weekly demand of blood units for each blood group.

Table 2: Stepwise incorporation of inventory procedures

Results Model	cost per transfu-sed unit (DM)	Shortages (%)	Outdating (%)	Age of blood at transfusion (days)
Model of real system	20,28	18,80	18,33	9,82
Model with Heuristic Allocation Procedure	17,19	4,45	18,27	14,39
Model with aditional Donor Call-Up Procedure	14,90	4,22	15,88	13,24
Model with aditional Recycling Procedure	13,61	4,71	14,3+	13,27

The minimal inventory cost is around 7 DM, which means a reduction to almost a third compared to the real system.

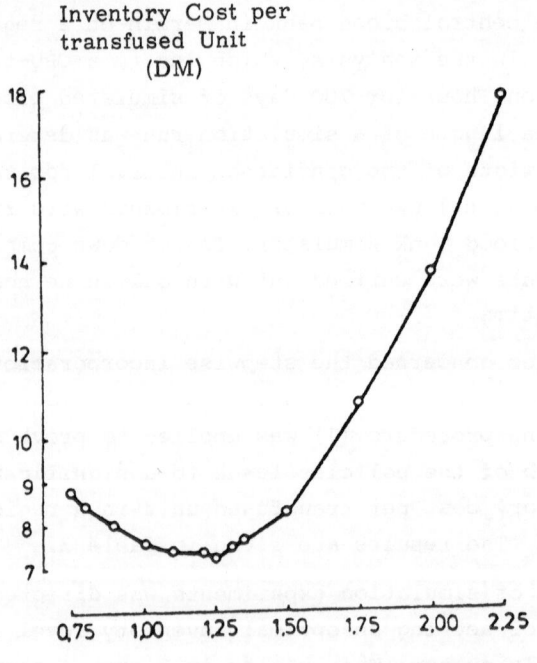

Fig. 4: Inventory level vs cost

7. Literature

BECHHOFER, E.R., DUNNET, C.W. and SOBEL, M.:
"A two sample multiple decision procedure for ranking means
of Normal populations with common unknown variance",
Biometrika 41, 1954

BRILL, E.A. and THOMAS, M.U.:
"Managing a Community Hospital Blood Bank with a Freezer
System", Technical Report Nr. NPS55ZG55TO74011, Naval
Postgraduate School, Monterey, California 1974

BRONDHEIM, E.L. et al:
"Setting Inventory Levels for Hospital Blood Banks",Trans-
fusion 16 (1976)

HULBURT, E.L. and JONES, A.R.:
"Blood Bank Inventory Control", Transfusion 4 (1964)

JENNINGS, J.B.:
"Hospital Blood Bank Whole Blood Inventory Control",
Technical Report Nr. 27, Operations Research Center, M.I.T.,
Cambridge 1967

JENNINGS, J.B.:
"Inventory Control in Regional Blood Banking Systems",
Technical Report, Nr. 53, Operations Research Center, M.I.T.,
Cambridge 1970

MILLARD, D.W.:
"Industrial Inventory Models as Applied to the Problem of
Inventory Whole Blood", in: Industrial Engineering Analy-
sis of a Hospital Blood Laboratory, Engineering Experiment
Station Bulletin 180, Ohio State University, Columbus 1960

PEGELS, C.C. and JELMERT, A.E.:
" An Evaluation of Blood Inventory Policies: A Markov Chain
Application",Operations Research (18), 1970

PAGE, B.:
"Computer Simulation in Health Care Delivery Planning and
Control", in: Bericht Nr. 1 des Arbeitskreises "Medizini-
sche Informatik" an der Technischen Universität Berlin,
Berlin 1976

PAGE, B.:

"Lagerhaltungsmodelle für Blutbanken", Paper on the
"Workshop-Simulationsmethoden in der Medizin und Biolo-
gie" in Hannover, Sept. 1977

PEGELS, C.C. and WALLACE, E.L.:

"Analysis and Design of a Model Regional Blood Management
System", in: Developments in Operations Research, Vol 2

RABINOWITZ, M.:

"Hospital Blood Banking: An Inventory System for distingui-
shable, perishable Items", Dissertation, The City University of New York, 1970

SILVER, A. and Silver, A.M.:

"An Empirical Inventory Control System for Hospital Blood
Banks",Hospitals 38 (1964)

SONNENDECKER, I.P.:

"A Model for Forecasting whole Blood Requirements of a
Hospital Blood Laboratory", in: Industrial Engineering
Analyses of a Hospital Blood Laboratory, Engineering
Experiment Station Bulletin 180, Ohio State University,
Columbus 1960

A MODEL OF THE FOETAL CIRCULATION FOR THE INTERPRETATION OF FOETAL HEART RATE PATTERNS

A.F.L. Veth
Department of Medical Informatics
Free University, Amsterdam
The Netherlands

INTRODUCTION

At present a growing number of obstetricians are making use of the
advances in modern technology to derive information about the condition
of the human foetus during pregnancy and birth. Most commonly the foetal
heart rate (FHR) and the intra-uterine pressure (IUP) are monitored
during labour. The FHR sometimes shows variations, often related to
uterine contractions. One of such variations, called a variable
deceleration, is said to be due to compression of the umbilical cord
during a uterine contraction (1). An example of such patterns is shown
in figure 1.

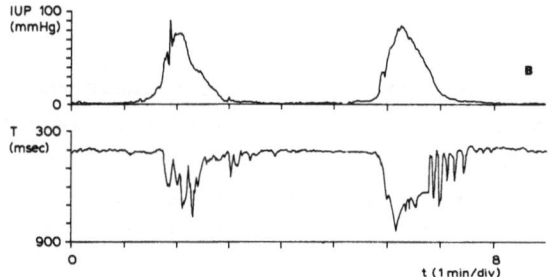

Fig. 1: Registration of the intra-uterine pressure (IUP) and the foetal
RR-interval (T) showing "variable" decelerations.

Several efforts have been made to quantify these patterns, using the
data of a large set of patient material. However, until now such
efforts have had little effect as far as their significance for the
diagnosis of the foetal condition is concerned.
We used a mathematical model in order to select relevant parameters
for the description of these FHR-patterns (2).
The model is based on the results of our experiments on the foetal
sheep and on the data available in the literature (3,4). We restricted
our study to the analysis of the response of the foetal circulation
to temporary occlusion of the umbilical cord, as it also may occur
during birth concurrently with uterine contractions as a result of

414

cord problems. These responses were first studied in experiments on
foetal sheep.
Special attention was paid to the role of the autonomic nervous system
in regulating the foetal circulation, by blocking this system partially
or completely by drugs. The function of the model then was to assist
the development of a mathematical/physiological theory to understand
the mechanisms responsible for the responses during cord occlusion.

ANIMAL EXPERIMENTS

The ewe received epidural anesthesia. After exteriorizing the lamb by
sectio caesarea, the foetal head was covered by a glove, filled with
saline, to prevent spontaneous foetal air breathing. The arterial and
venous bloodpressure, and the electrocardiogram from both mother and
foetus were measured. Since direct measurement of the foetal cardiac
output was considered to be too invasive, this parameter was derived
from the stroke volume, computed from the arterial pressure wave,
using a characteristic impedance method (5).

THE MODEL

A mathematical model has been developed that considers the foetal heart
to act as one single ventricle, while the peripheral vascular bed was
described in a more or less conventional way. The placental vascular
bed was described as a reservoir with an input and an output resistance. An electrical equivalent of the peripheral circulation is given
in figure 2.

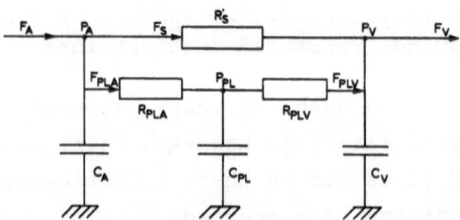

Fig. 2: The electrical equivalent of the foetal peripheral circulation,
including the placental vascular bed.

The parameter values of the model of the foetal heart were estimated
from the scarce data, available in literature. The cardiac output as
a function of the heart rate (HR) and the cardiac compliance (C_H) is
given in figure 3. This characteristic applies for the heart, filled

with a constant pressure of 5 mmHg and pumping against a constant
arterial pressure of 55 mmHg.

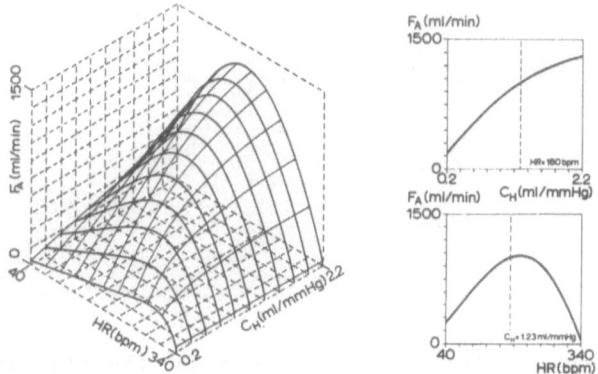

Fig. 3: The cardiac output (F_A) as a function of the heart rate (HR)
and the cardiac compliance (C_H) for the model of the foetal
heart in the steady-state condition. The cross-sections
through the normal operating point are also shown.

The parameter values of the peripheral circulation were partially
derived from literature data, and partially from our experimental
arterial responses to separate occlusion of the umbilical arteries
and veins.
The difference between the two types of responses is mainly determined
by the placental compliance. In case of an arterial occlusion, blood
will flow into the venous reservoir until the pressure into the placental bed (P_{PL}) equals the venous pressure (P_V). The reverse will
take place in case of a venous occlusion. Then blood will flow into
the placenta until P_{PL} equals the arterial pressure P_A.
The steady-state changes in the arterial pressure (ΔP_A) and the
placental blood volume (ΔQ_{PL}) after arterial and venous occlusion
are shown in figure 4.
Since we assumed that a 30-second occlusion of the umbilical cord would
not severely affect the metabolic condition of the foetus, we only
implemented the baroreceptor control of foetal heart rate and peripheral resistance, and the autoregulation of blood flow through the
peripheral vascular bed, into the model.

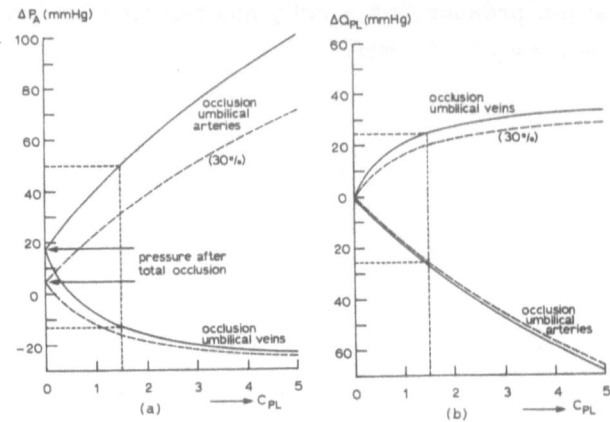

Fig. 4: Change in the arterial pressure (ΔP_A) and the placental blood volume (ΔQ_{PL}) as a function of the placental compliance (C_{PL}) after separate occlusion of the umbilical arteries or veins, predicted by our model. The broken lines represent these changes when deterioration of the foetal heart function occurred.

RESULTS

The responses of the foetal sheep, whose nervous system had been blocked completely, to a complete 30-second cord occlusion can be divided into three types (see figure 5).

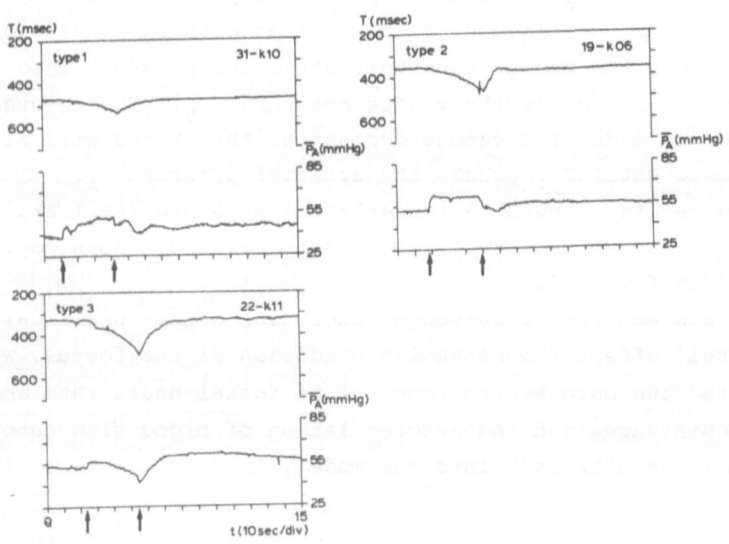

Fig. 5: Some responses of the RR-interval (T) and the mean arterial pressure (P_A) to occlusion of the umbilical cord in foetal lambs with a blocked autonomic nervous system.

The type 1 responses show an increasing P_A during the occlusion, the type 2 a more or less stable P_A, and the type 3 a decreasing P_A during the occlusion. Especially the type 1 responses indicate an increasing resistance as a response to the resistance increase caused by the cord occlusion. This of course cannot be considered to be the result of an overall regulatory system, that may be caused by local autoregulatory systems.

This theory was supported by simulation experiments, showing, dependent on the degree of autoregulation (k_R), the several types of responses (see figure 6).

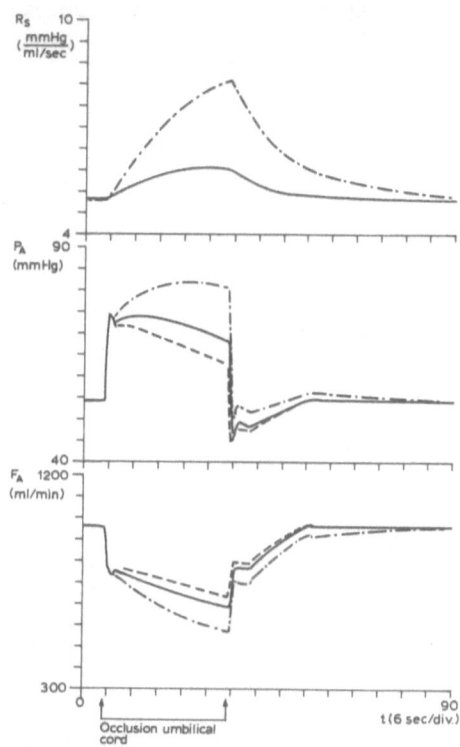

Fig. 6: Model response to occlusion of the umbilical cord, if the RR-interval changes and three different sensitivities of the autoregulation of blood flow: $k_R = 0.06$ sec/ml (—), $k_R = 0$ (---), $k_R = 0.15$ sec/ml (-.-.-).

From top to bottom the systemic resistance (R_S), the mean arterial pressure (P_A) and the cardiac output (F_A) are shown.

The occlusion causes an initial increase of P_A and a decrease of F_A. Thereafter the pattern is determined by the competative effects of a further decreasing F_A, causing a decreasing P_A and a rising R_S, tending to attenuate or even override this effect.

After implementing the regulatory systems we were able to analyse specific FHR-patterns.

As an example we analysed the responses to asynchronous occlusion of the umbilical arteries and veins.

It is often assumed in the literature that the umbilical vein is occluded first during a uterine contraction, since the pressure within this vessel is low (10-15 mmHg) as compared to the pressure within an umbilical artery (50-60 mmHg).

Simulation experiments showed (see figure 7) that, dependent on the time lag between the venous and arterial occlusion, the FHR-pattern may change from a deceleration ($\Delta T=0$) to an acceleration ($\Delta T=5$).

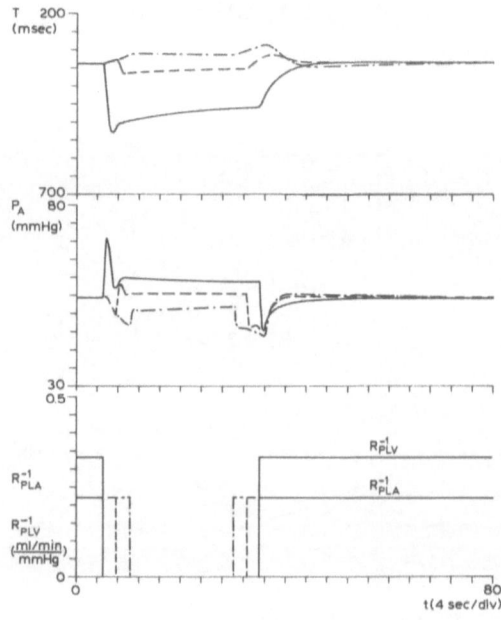

Fig. 7: Model response to asynchronous occlusion of the umbilical arteries and veins for three different time delays between venous and arterial occlusion (ΔT): $\Delta T=0$ (—), $\Delta T=2,5$sec (---) and $\Delta T=5$sec (-·-·-).

DISCUSSION

The ultimate goal of this investigation is, as said earlier, to arrive at a set of parameters that do better describe the foetal condition during birth.

The model approach was therefore selected, since it allows for the selection of physiological relevant parameters, that "contain" the

a priori knowledge about the system.
In order to analyse the relevance and sensitivity of the model
parameters, we are in the process of building a data base of
foetal heart rate patterns. These were selected from well documented
patients from which cord problems have been established at birth.
This data base will be compared with patterns generated by the model,
thus allowing the analysis and refinement of the classification
schemes as well as updating the model.

REFERENCES

1. Hon, E.H.: An atlas of the foetal heart rate patterns
   Hartley Press Inc., New Haven, 1968

2. Veth, A.F.L.: Modelling the foetal circulation: simulation of
   the response to umbilical cord occlusion
   Thesis, Amsterdam, 1976

3. Assali, N.S., Brinkman III, C.R. and Nuwayhid, B.: Comparison of
   maternal and fetal cardiovascular functions in acute and chronic
   experiments in the sheep.
   Am. J. Obstet. Gynecol. 120(3): 411, 1974

4. Rudolph, A.M. and Heymann, M.A.: Circulatory changes during growth
   in the fetal lamb
   Circ. Res. 26: 289, 1970

5. Wesseling, K.H., Nichols, W.W., de Wit, B., and Weber, J.A.P.:
   A beat-to-beat cardiac output computer I and II
   Proc. 3rd Intern. Conf. Med. Phys., incl. medical engineering
   Göteborg, 1972

e patient knowledge about the system.

In Order 5, ... of the underlying equation distillation of fundamental parameters ... are in the product of Bolling's database of ... together with test estimate ... able selected from ... will not be redundant, therefore, but finding how to a solution of ... first. Thus data used ... transparent knowledge and are used by the model. From mixture ... based ... and estimate of the distillation and subsequently ... from the model.

REFERENCES

1. Levin, R.I. and Kirkpatrick C.A. Water based rate control ... Harper Brown 1967, New York, 1965

2. Moore, D.S. and Mabbut ... and distillation test simulation of the ... and later part of column ... Wiley, New York, 1970

3. Spiegel, M.R., Schumann, R.J., C.R. and Bloty ... A comparison of ... extended and total fractionation ... flow line a 13 acute and chronic ... experiments in the sheep.
   Am. J. Physiol. Animal. 440(3) 478, 4914.

4. Hopkins, W.G. and Heywood, K.A. Oscillatory schemes during growth ... in the renal link.
   Circ. Res. Int 244, A479

5. Ossachter, R.A., Nicholls, W.W., O'Lin, R.W. and Wiehl, T.A.R.
   A best fit radiid output computer funct ...
   Proc. ... distribution from data ..., and rmechanical communication ... chamber, 1975.

COMPARTMENTAL ANALYSIS OF THE DISTRIBUTION OF BUFLOMEDIL

P. d'ATHIS[1], E. REY[2], G. OLIVE[2], L. DUSSERRE[1].

(1) Département d'Informatique Médicale (Professeur agrégé L. DUSSERRE) ; hôpital du Bocage, 21034 DIJON CEDEX.

(2) Département de Pharmacologie Clinique (Professeur agrégé G. OLIVE) ; hôpital Saint-Vincent-de-Paul, 75674 PARIS CEDEX 14.

A new vaso-dilator of peripheral blood vessels, Buflomedil, is studied here through compartmental modelling.

EXPERIMENTAL PROCEDURE.

Buflomedil may be administered intravenously or orally.

The intravenous form was studied in 4 women which had been operated (one coelioscopy, one hysterectomy and two Caesarean sections) ; each woman was administered the dose

$$q_o = 100 \text{ mg}$$

The oral form was studied in 3 healthy women : each of them was a physician who accepted to be administered the dose

$$q_o = 450 \text{ mg}$$

Blood and urine samples were collected from each woman just before drug administration in order to check that no other substance than Buflomedil could be taken into account.

Blood time-courses were studied during 12 hours through about fifteen samples.

Urine time-courses were studied during 48 hours through about ten samples.

EXPONENTIAL ANALYSIS OF PLASMA AND URINE DATA.

The date of drug administration is considered as the time-origin ; let Δt the delay for drug to appear in blood : for an intravenous injection

$$(1) \qquad \Delta t = 0$$

whereas for an oral administration

(2) $\qquad \Delta t \geqslant 0$

because drug cannot immediately reach its resorption site.

Now let us suppose that, for any way of administration, the blood level (c) may be related to time (t) by means of a multiexponential function

$$(3) \qquad c = \sum_i a_i e^{b_i (t - \Delta t)}$$

where the b_i's are negative coefficients satisfying the conventional inequalities

$$(4) \qquad b_1 > b_2 \cdots > b_i \cdots$$

By defining

$$(5) \qquad A_i : a_i e^{-b_i \Delta t}$$

the equation (3) may be written

$$(6) \qquad c = \sum_i A_i e^{b_i t}$$

so that, the coefficients A_i and b_i being given, the delay Δt may be computed by solving the equation

$$(7) \qquad \sum_i A_i e^{b_i \Delta t} = 0$$

and the formula (5) allows us to compute the a_i's.

Urine data are used under the hypothesis that renal excretion is a first order process : blood level (c) and urine total amount (u) are related by the linear differential equation

$$(8) \qquad \frac{du}{dt} = f c$$

where f, a time independant parameter, symbolizes the renal clearance of drug.

Now let us imagine a quantity Δu of the first urine sample to be lost : this is not the total amount (u) which is observed but the new function

$$(9) \qquad U : u - \Delta u$$

which, according to (8), satisfies

$$(10) \qquad \frac{dU}{dt} = f c$$

The latter equation, combined with (6), leads us to

$$(11) \qquad U = f \sum_i (\frac{A_i}{b_i}) e^{b_i t} + g$$

(where g is a time independant parameter) then, by expressing that urine contains no drug at time t = Δt, gives us an estimate of the initial urine loss

$$(12) \qquad \Delta u = - g - f \sum_i (\frac{a_i}{b_i})$$

Blood and urine time-courses may therefore be related with time through the endogeneous parameters A_i, b_i, f and g ; the parameters Δt and Δu are then considered as exogeneous.

The endogeneous parameters are estimated with the maximum likelihood method which, because measures done at different times are statistically independant, amounts to the least squares method.

In this case, urine values, being much larger than blood values, tend to attract the fitting towards them : to reduce this size effect, blood data are weighted with the factor

$\|c\|^{-2}$ where $\|c\|$ symbolizes the maximum of blood level according to time, whereas urine data are weighted with the factor

$\|u\|^{-2}$ where $\|u\|$ symbolizes the maximum of urine total amount according to time.

Computations first used one exponential function then two exponential functions : at the first attempt, fitting of theoretical curves to experimental data was not satisfying because of a too low correlation ; at the second attempt, blood and urine fitting were satisfying *simultaneously* in both cases of intravenous injection and oral administration.

Relations (7) and (12) then allowed us to estimate the lag-time Δt and the initial urine loss Δu.

Numerical results are listed in Table I.

EXPONENTIAL ANALYSIS OF PLASMA AND URINE DATA.

Administration	Subject	a mg.l⁻¹	b h⁻¹	f l.h⁻¹	Δt h	Δu mg	r	r'
INTRAVENOUS	1	1.19 / 14.5	− 0.334 / − 9.95	3.02	0.	0.	0.982	0.977
	2	2.61 / 16.5	− 0.321 / − 17.9	1.96	0.	0.	0.997	0.993
	3	3.82 / 80.5	− 0.267 / − 24.0	0.921	0.	4.77	0.988	0.994
	4	2.53 / 34.8	− 0.471 / − 20.5	0.788	0.	0.	0.998	0.970
ORAL	1	− 5.74 / 5.74	− 0.297 / − 2.70	4.27	1.24	0.	0.996	0.966
	2	− 10.6 / 10.6	− 0.295 / − 1.00	4.08	0.571	0.	0.978	0.987
	3	9.58 / − 9.58	− 0.428 / − 0.815	3.00	0.805	0.	0.996	0.998

Table I.

Coefficients a, b, f, Δt and Δu are defined in text.

The letters r and r' symbolize the correlation coefficients between experimental data and theoretical values, for plasma and urine time-courses respectively.

COMPARTMENTAL ANALYSIS OF PLASMA AND URINE DATA.

Exponential analysis proving that every plasma time-course may be broken down into two exponential terms, it is allowed to assume that all processes, besides the renal excretion process, are first-order processes : the smallest compartmental model which may be used is, for intravenous form

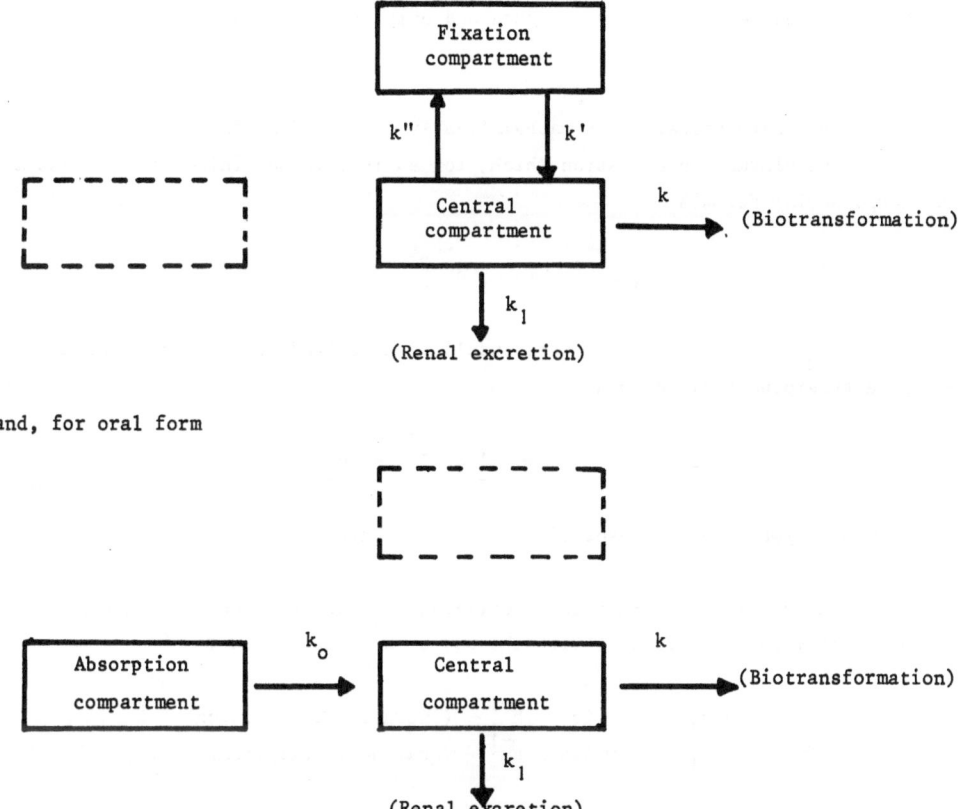

and, for oral form

where dashes mark off compartments which have no or weak influence on plasma concentration.

The intravenous form defines the two-compartment open model whereas the oral form defines the one-compartment open model : the "vanishing" of the fixation compartment, in the latter case, may be explained by the two following laws :

1 : drug gets into the fixation compartment with a velocity proportional to its concentration in the central compartment ;

2 : drug gets out of the fixation compartment with a velocity proportional to its quantity in this compartment.

Orally administered drug slowly arrives into blood where its concentration is much smaller than after an intravenous injection : less drug gets into the fixation compartment (law 1) from where less drug gets out (law 2), which is summarized by an activity reduction of the fixation compartment. Here, activity is reduced down to be undetectable by any measure and only the one-compartment open model may be used.

This interpretation is mathematically expressed as follows.

The plasma concentration which, for an intravenous injection, is defined by a biexponential formula

$$(13) \qquad c = c_1 e^{-K_1 t} + c_2 e^{-K_2 t}$$

where K_1 and K_2 symbolize apparent rates would be described, for an oral administration, by a triexponential formula

$$(14) \qquad c = c_1' e^{-K_1 t} + c_2' e^{-K_2 t} + c_0 e^{-k_0 t}$$

where k_0 would symbolize the resorption rate of the drug.

Our results show that the coefficient b_1, which is present in (6) and (11), does not vary significantly with the way of administration :

$$- 0.471 \leqslant b_1 \leqslant - 0.267 \quad h^{-1} \quad \text{(intravenous injection)}$$
$$- 0.428 \leqslant b_1 \leqslant - 0.295 \quad h^{-1} \quad \text{(oral administration)}$$

whereas the coefficient b_2 strongly varies with the way of administration :

$$-24.0 \leqslant b_2 \leqslant - 9.95 \quad h^{-1} \quad \text{(intravenous injection)}$$
$$- 2.70 \leqslant b_2 \leqslant - 0.815 \quad h^{-1} \quad \text{(oral administration)}$$

These remarks enhance our interpretation if we admit

$K_1 = -b_1$ for both ways of administration

$$0.267 \leqslant K_1 \leqslant 0.471 \quad h^{-1}$$

$K_2 = -b_2$ for intravenous injection

$$9.95 \leqslant K_2 \leqslant 24.0 \quad h^{-1}$$

$k_o = -b_2$ for oral administration

$$0.815 < k_o < 2.70 \quad h^{-1}$$

The great distance between the intervals about the parameters K_2 and k_o suggests the exponential term $e^{-K_2 t}$ to get quickly much smaller than the exponential term $e^{-k_o t}$ then to vanish : so, the plasma concentration quickly gets biexponential

$$(15) \qquad c \simeq c_1' e^{-K_1 t} + c_o e^{-k_o t}$$

We can enhance this phenomenon by choosing, among intravenous injections, the subject who would have the smallest coefficient K_2 (Subject 1, $K_2 = 9.95$ h^{-1}) : the corresponding exponential term would be the most lasting and therefore the most easy to detect. Let us imagine oral administration of a dose of 450 mg to this subject with absorption defined by a rate constant $k_o = 3$ h^{-1} (half-life = 13 minutes) : such a resorption would be nearly as fast as an intravenous injection and, so, the probability to observe a triexponential concentration would be increased.

Computing the theoretical concentration with the exact and approximative formulae yields Table II :

t (minute)	c (μg/ml) Triexponential formula	c (μg/ml) Biexponential approximation
5	10.8	23.2
10	13.8	19.2
15	13.7	16.0
30	9.8	10.0

Table II.

A survey of these results shows that a difference between the exact and approximative formulae would be uneasily detectable at time t = 15 minutes : therefore, our procedure would not allow us to detect the third exponential term, even with a subject being in an optimal state of observability.

A theoretical way to improve our procedure would be to collect blood samples every 5 minutes after administration, during 1.5 hour at least but that would need a large volume of blood, and so cannot be used.

RESULTS.

A full compartmental analysis may be done for the intravenous form of Buflomedil : formulae which give the pharmacokinetic parameters of the two-compartment open model are well-known and are not recalled here.

A partial analysis only is available for the oral form : we can determine, besides the resorption lag-time and renal clearance, the resorption rate and no other parameter can be estimated because of the missing exponential term.

Results are listed in Table III : to make interpretation easier, every process is quantified not with its rate constant k but with its period

$$(16) \qquad T : \frac{\ln(2)}{k}$$

The symbols $\bar{f}$ and $\bar{v}$ respectively designate the renal clearance and volume of the central compartment divided by the subject's weight.

CONCLUSION.

The following properties may be reasonably assumed for Buflomedil :
- its rates of elimination and exchange with the fixation compartment are likely independant of the way of administration (constancy of b_1)
- its renal clearance, divided by subject's weight, is not significantly dependant of the way of administration

$$0.0131 < \bar{f} < 0.0854 \qquad 1.h^{-1}.Kg^{-1}$$

- its fixation is important, which is indicated for intravenous injection by the ratio

$$\frac{k''}{k_1 + k}$$

representing the part of the administered quantity getting into the fixation compartment

$$1.94 < \frac{k''}{k_1 + k} < 6.32$$

PHARMACOKINETIC PARAMETERS OF BUFLOMEDIL

INTRAVENOUS INJECTION

Subject	T_1(h)	T(h)	T'(h)	T''(h)	$\bar{f}$(l.h^{-1}.Kg^{-1})	$\bar{V}$(l.Kg^{-1})
1	1.46	0.260	0.654	0.114	0.0604	0.127
2	1.85	0.400	0.255	0.052	0.0400	0.107
3	0.89	0.174	0.517	0.038	0.0225	0.029
4	2.36	0.139	0.379	0.050	0.0131	0.045

ORAL ADMINISTRATION

Subject	Δt(h)	T_o(h)	$\bar{f}$(l.h^{-1}.Kg^{-1})
1	1.24	0.256	0.0854
2	0.57	0.692	0.0658
3	0.81	0.850	0.0600

Table III.

- its disappearance from the body is rapid, by renal elimination

$$6\% \ \leqslant \ \frac{k''}{k_1 + k} \ \leqslant \ 18\%$$

but mostly by biotransformation

$$82\% \ \leqslant \ \frac{k''}{k_1 + k} \ \leqslant \ 94\%$$

- its oral form is slow to reach its resorption site

$$0.57 \ \leqslant \ \Delta t \ \leqslant \ 1.24 \quad h$$

but is fast enough to pass into blood

$$15 \ \leqslant \ T_o \ \leqslant \ 51 \qquad \text{minutes}$$

REFERENCES.

DRAPER N.R., SMITH H. - Applied regression analysis. New-York, J. Wiley and sons, 1966.

GIBALDI M., PERRIER D. - Pharmacokinetics. New-York, Dekker, 1975.

JONES A. - Spiral. A new algorithm for non-linear parameter estimation using least squares. Computer Journal, 1970, vol.13, p.301,308.

WAGNER J.G. - Model independant linear pharmacokinetics. Drug Intelligence and Clinical Pharmacy, 1976, vol.10, p.179,180.

ACKNOWLEDGEMENTS.

We are grateful to Mrs. D. de LAUTURE, département de Pharmacologie Clinique à l'hôpital Saint-Vincent-de-Paul, for computing assistance.

A LARGE DATABASE ON A MINICOMPUTER

By Bongers, A. and Kouwenberg, J.M.L.
University Hospital Leyden, Rijnsburgerweg 10,
The Netherlands.

INTRODUCTIONS:

An integrated hospital information system (HIS) is being developed at the department of dataprocessing of the Leyden University Hospital (AZL), and is operational since 1974.
Via 120 terminals on a PDP 11/45 users can communicate with a 150-megabyte database holding patient and hospital information concerning 400.000 patients. At the start of the project the decision has been made to develop the operating system in house including teleprocessing part and database handler.

The database software had to meet following requirements:

– highly reliable

– very fast accessable because of a great number of very interactive trans-actions should be handled

– very efficient usage of disk storage because of the size of the patient data

– a strictly formal interface between DB and the application program (written in FORTRAN).

All these aspects will come up for discussion in the next two parts of the paper:

Part 1: the HIS-DB design

Part 2: the HIS-DB use.

PART 1: THE HIS-DATABASE DESIGN   By Ir. J.M.L. Kouwenberg.

CHOSEN STRUCTURE:

After analysing the kind of information which had to be stored in a HIS-DB it seemed very useful to provide for two different storage-methods:

I. a <u>fixed</u> length record structure   – the thesaurus

II. a <u>variable</u> length record structure   – the TVR (Thesaurus Variable Record).

I. Thesaurus: a HIS thesaurus consists of a group sequentially numbered records of _fixed_ length, called elements. These elements are directly addressable by the elementnumber. Besides that, for each thesaurus one or more indexes (derived from the contents of the element) can be defined offering a fast access to all elements that match that index value.

The largest HIS-thesaurus is the PIR (Patient Indentication Record) file at this moment consisting of 400.000 elements used. Every element contains the (compressed) patient information such as: name, address, cityname, general practitioner, insurance ... Direct access to these elements is possible by the elementnumber (= patientnumber) and indirect access takes place via data of birth or name (for women: maiden name or husband's name).

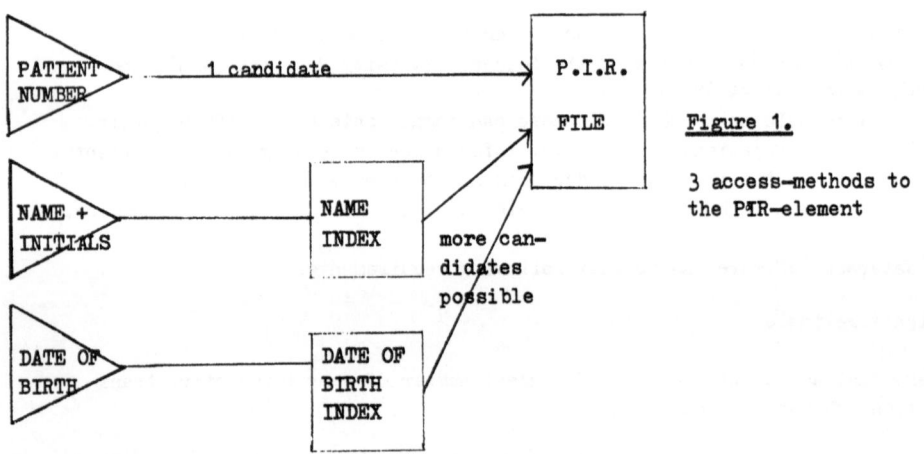

Figure 1.

3 access-methods to the PIR-element

Resuming can be said that a thesaurus consist of:

- mainfile   a group of sequentially numbered unsorted elements of fixed length, all elements having the same logical structure. These elements contain the actual file data.
- index file(s)   comprising a group of logical blocks. The blocks of each index are sorted with respect to a key (see below). Each block consists of a variable number of unsorted records of fixed length containing the sequential number of the mainfile element and additional discriminating information, in the form of an extract from the mainfile element.
- key mechanism   function belonging to each index, which associates for a given item (key information) from the mainfile element the according logical index block. The key mechanism may be in the form of an algorithm or a predefined table.

To illustrate, let us take the city name thesaurus as an example.
- the mainfile consists of elements of 16 words with the following items:

cityname, the post office city code, telephone district number, code
used by the national medical registration office.
- an index has been made for the city name offering a fast access to the elementnumber if the city name (or part of it) is known. For each element in the indexblock the sequential elementnumber and the third, fourth letter of the city
name are stored.
- the key mechanism in this case is a small auxiliary index table, which relates
the first two letters of a city name to the appropriate index block. For
example offering the city name "Dordrecht" the key mechanism gives indexblock
6, being the block in which candidates must be searched. One or more candidates are selected, comparing the third, fourth character "RD" with the
Additional Discriminating Information (A.D.I.) (see fig. 2).

Mind: it is possible to mask the A.D.I. totally or partially by which groups
of elements are selected. In our example all city names are collected
between DE .... and DO ....

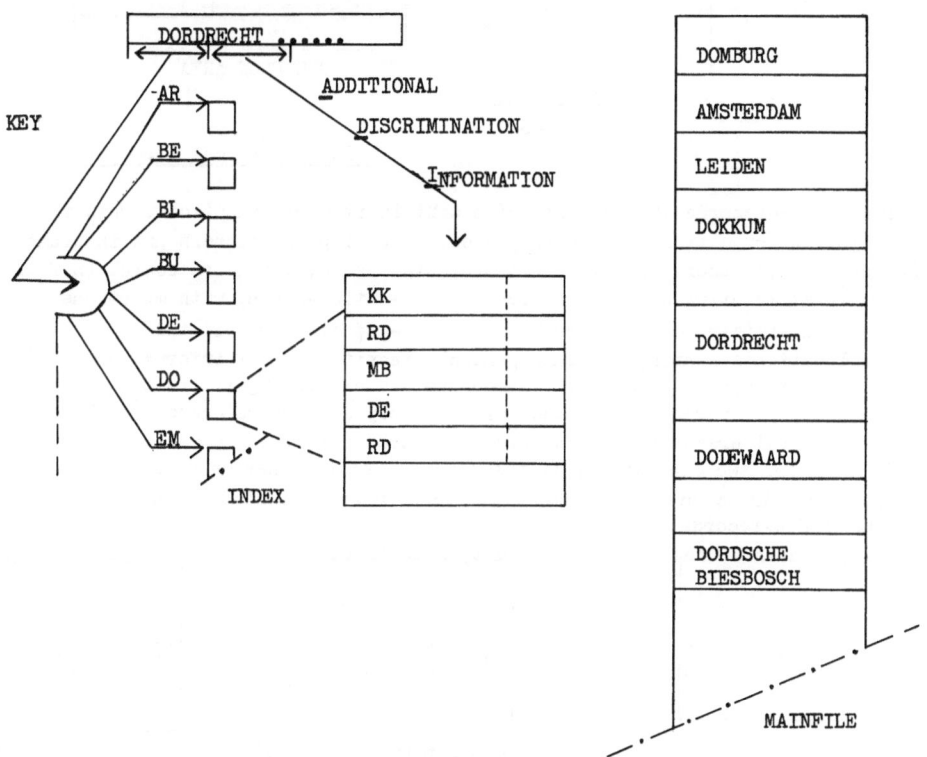

Fig. 2: Thesaurus City Names

The thesaurus of elements with one or more indexes is stored on disc as follows:

434

- the mainfile area resides as one consecutive area on disc. Therefore elements are directly found by their sequential number.
- for each index also, one consecutive discarea is available. To each logical indexblock one disc sector (= 512 bytes) is allocated. If the reserved sector becomes full the system chaines an overflow sector to the full sector (see fig. 3).
- if a small size table excists for the key mechanism it will be core resident. Large tables are stored on disc with only a firts part kept in core.

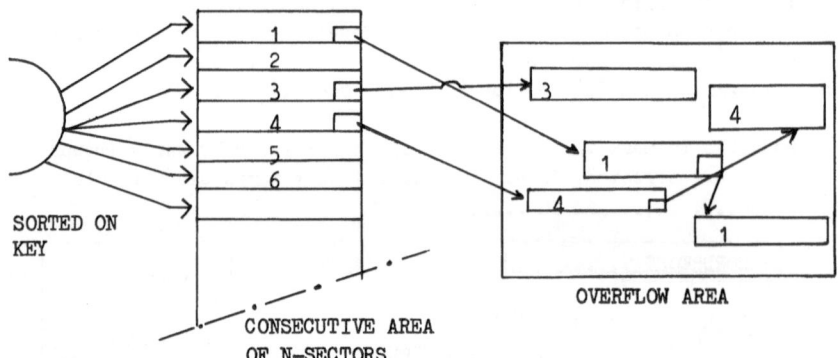

SORTED ON KEY

CONSECUTIVE AREA OF N-SECTORS

OVERFLOW AREA

FIG. 3: Fysical structure.

For many PIR-records the contents of a certain item are identical. This is certainly true for city names, birth places, general practitioners and insurances. For such items, therefore, thesauri are established, which are useful in four ways:
- stimulating standardization
- minimizing data volume
- time-saving with mutations
- fast entry via index.

For all patients sharing the same general practitioner all information about that practitionar is exactly the same. Instead of storing all this information of lets say 50 characters for each patient only a short reference to the element of the general practitionar thesaurus is stored into the PIR-record. This takes only room for two characters. If the general practitioner changes his telephone number or address only one element has to be changed instead of updating thousands of PIR-records.

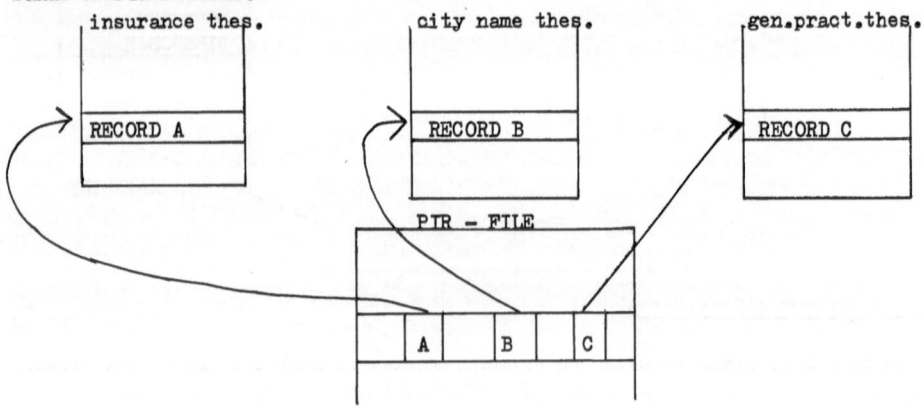

FIG. 4: References to other thesauri.

Resuming can be said that the thesaurus mechanism in the HIS-database is used in two ways:
1) the thesaurus may be used as workfile with one or more indexes to which more users have access to. Contents of this kind of thesauri changes regularly and the protection against "multiple update at the same time" is vital.
2) the thesaurus can be used as reference table, and from other places in the database reference are made to the individual elements. For these thesauri certainly no (essential) changes are made, only enlarging with new elements is permitted.

II) Thesaurus Variable Record (TVR)

The TVR:

To each record of a thesaurus a variable length record can be associated, with a total length of 32767 bytes, the so called thesaurus variable record (TVR). This TVR consists of a chain of subrecords, each identified by a type-number. Every subrecord also contains a length-indication and an indication whether or not the subrecord has been authorized. The TVR-subrecords can consists of a fixed format part (FFP) and a variable format part (VFP). The maximum number of type-numbers is 250. Within one TVR-chain several subrecords of the same type may occur & the subrecords are chained in descending order of type-number. Within a subrecord we distinguish sub-subrecords, that can be identified by a sub-type-number. A thesaurus with a TVR will have a chain-pointerfile, that contains for every thesaurus-recordnumber the startaddress and total length of the TVR. (see figure 5).

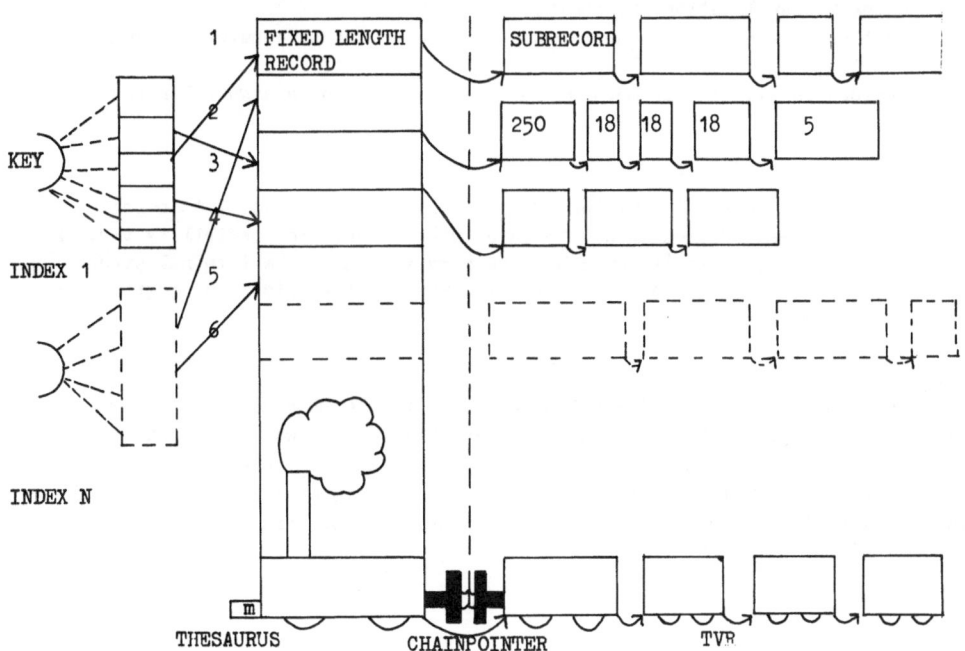

Figure 5: Like a train, the mainfile record is the engine and the subrecords of
the TVR are the waggons coupled to it.

Physical storage on disc:

For reasons of space efficiency, we have introduced in connection with the TVR
a unit of disc space smaller than the sector (= 512 bytes): the miniblock, or
MIB. Six MIB lengths are used, of 16, 32, 64, 256, and 512 bytes. The last four
bytes of a MIB are reserved to contain a pointer to another MIB, so that a
chain of MIBs can be constructed which will accomodate, with very few wasted bits
a record of any given length. Since the TVR is a variable length record, a MIB
chain is an ideal medium for its physical storage. In practice, the required
number of MIBs of each size is calculated by means of an algorithm to give
maximum disctransfers economy, and the TVR is stored on the MIB chain, using
all free bytes consecutively, without reference to its logical structure.

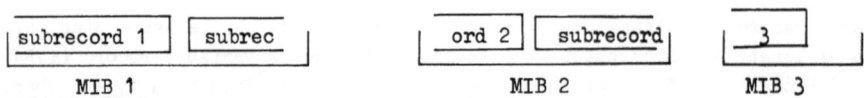

In a MIB chain only 512-byte MIBs are repeated and the tail of the TVR is
stored in a MIB which just

PART 2: THE HIS-DATABASE USE   By Drs. A. Bongers.

INTERFACE:

One of the requirements of our HIS was a strictly formal interface between the
DB and the application programs. The reasons for this were:
1) Modification of the internal organisation of the DB must be possible without
   changing the application programs.
2) Protection of the DB for the user so that the technical consistence remains
   guaranteed.
3) Communication with the DB must be possible by means of a higher language
   (FORTRAN).

Ad 1:

When we started with the definition of the DB-structure (1971), little was
known about the way of use. We had to take into account the possibility that on
the ground of experiences it could be necessary to change the internal structure. Such modifications are impossible if hundreds of application programms
have directly used this internal structure.

Ad 2, 3:

For reasons of security all DB-actions are done by the DB-handler. This DB-
handler has been integrated within the BOS-system. That's why it is also possible to registrate all mutations of the DB on magtape. So this logging is
user-independent. In the seperation between application program and DB the DB-
handler vitually takes care of a number of counters. Only via these counters
the following DB-actions are allowed:

For a thesaurus.

READ function:
A record having a given record number is to be read from the main file. Since the parameters relevant to the indexed files (start address, record length, number of records etc.) are coreresident, the start address of the main file is known, and this operation requires only one discaccess.

WRITE function:
A record is to be added to the main file, and the indexes are to be suitably amended. The record may be added after the record having the highest record number, or may take the place of a deleted record. The handler generates new sequential record numbers as required, and attends to the location and chaining of an overflow sector when an index sector becomes full.

UPDATE function:
A record having a given number is to be changed, new data being stored in place of old data. This may be necessitate corresponding changes in the indexes. To prevent the confusion which would arise if more than one user attempted to update the same record at the same time, a user must offer both the old and the new content of the record; only if the old content offered corresponds with the current content the update will be performed.

DELETE function:
A record having a given record number is to be deleted from the main file, and the indexes are to be amended accordingly. The system maintains a chain of deleted recordnumbers for use in the WRITE operation.

SEARCH function:
A record containing certain given key information is to be located. The function proceeds by means of key mechanism and index as described under Thesaurus to locate any main file record or records which satisfy the given key information. This function returns the recordnumbers of the selected records.

For the TVR.

READ function:
One or more subrecords of a given patient or thesaurus-record are to be read. The user offers the appropriate selection criteria, such as a typenumber, and the TVR is scanned to find all the subrecords which satisfy them. (Since types are stored in descending orders, the read action stops when a lower type is detected)

WRITE function:
A new subrecord is to be inserted in a given TVR at the position appropriate to its typenumber. A new MIB chain is constructed to accomodate the now longer TVR; the TVR in its new form is written on the new chain; the address pointer in the PIR or chainpointerfile is amended and the old MIB chain is released.

UPDATE function:
A specified subrecord of a given patient or thesaurus-record is to be modified.
The entire current content of the subrecord must be offered, and the TVR is
searched until the appropriate subrecord is found. If the new content of the
subrecord has the same length as the old one, it will be exchanged directly;
otherwise, a new MIB chain must be constructed, and the same procedure will be
followed as in WRITE.

DELETE function:
A specified subrecord of a given patient or thesaurus-record is to be deleted.
The entire current content of the subrecord must be offered. The now shorter TVR
is copied to a new MIB chain, and the same procedure followed as before.

AUTHORIZATION function:
A subrecord can be authorized by setting up a bit in the header. When a change
is made in a TVR, the whole chain is reconstructed, and the old chain is
deleted as soon as the requested function has been successfully completed.
This is done to guard against the loss of information (see figure).

EXAMPLE OF TVR : WRITE

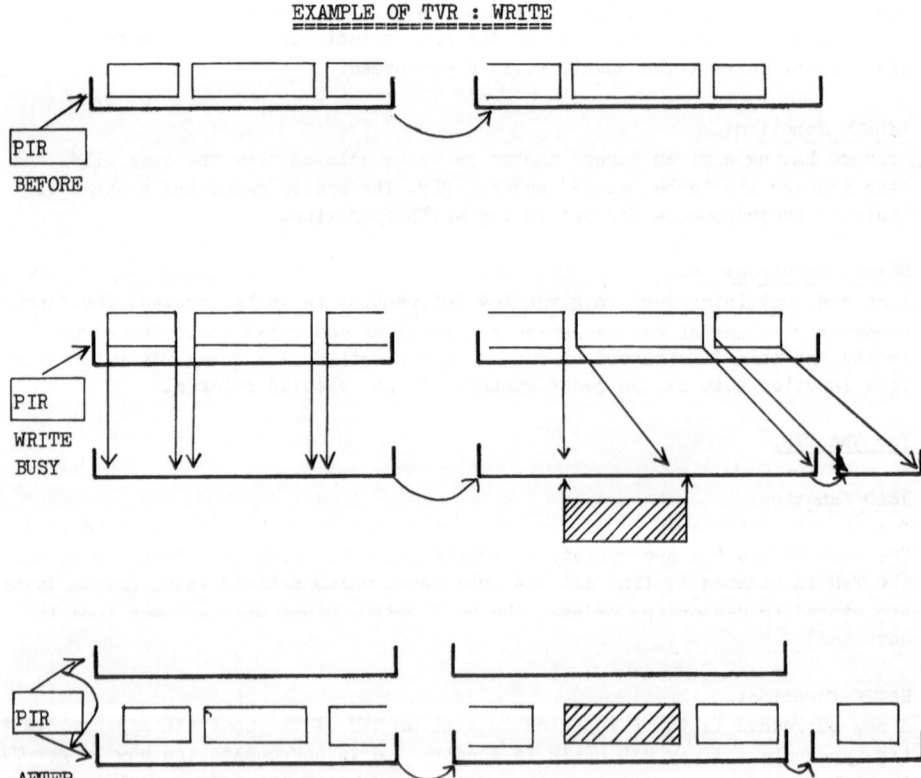

EXTERNAL REPRESENTATION:

With the DB-actions the user only works with the so called external representation
of the thesaurus elements and the TVR-subrecords. The internal storage structure,
the so called internal representation can be quite different and is unknown to
the user. For the PIR a considerable compression takes place. The external representation contains 230 words, while the internal one only has 36 words. Conversion
from internal - to external - representation (and reverse) is done by the DB-
handler. It is clear that in this way, the application programmers need not to
take into account the modifications that take place behind the counters in the
DB-handler or storage structure.

USE OF THE INTERFACE:

Next table shows the number of DB-actions and the number of disctransfers generated by it on a normal day in February 1978.

Actions	Between 07.30 - 17.00		Between 00.00 - 24.00	
	DB actions	disctransfers	DB actions	disctransfers
TVR-read	9317	25489	27972	82503
TVR-write	2832	20469	7084	102139
TVR-delete				
+ update	1342	7625	10018	61796
thes. search	32241	47046	44542	61365
thes. read	128314	127596	244729	243822
thes. delete				
+ update	18192	85814	31506	155463
thes. write	7492	55674	8559	60551

Two periods per day are given while after 17.00 several batchjobs are started
by the operators. So the numbers in the first period represent the interactive
use of the DB.

PRIVACY:

In a Hospital Information System we are very clearly confronted with two basically
contradictory requirements. On one hand, it is important to supply the necessary
data quickly to all who need it (this may sometimes even be of vital importance e.
g. in travel accidents). On the other hand, a part of the medical data are of
a rather confidential nature, in today's health care system even to the patient
himself. The guideline we agreed upon with the clinical staff is that, in
general, all medical data stored in the databank will be available for members
of the medical team concerned with the treatment.
This is worked out in the following steps:
a) access to the system is opened if a valid usernumber is given together
   with the corresponding password. This password can be modified at
   will by the user, and is not shown on paper or display screen. When the
   is accepted to the system, the date and time of the previous usage is

given, together with the number of the terminal used on that occasion. If this unfortunately happens to be an illegal use, the user can change the password and ask the systems amanger to find out from the logtape what was carried out under his usernumber that day. Until now, no such situation has ever been reported.

b) in respect of each application program, the user number of every user who is entitled to execute that program is recorded within the system. Any attempt to run a program on the part of a user not authorized to do so will result in the generation of an error message. This type b protection will shortly be extended to include profiles of authorized users indicated which types of TVR subrecords and thesauri each user is allowed to act upon, and what actions he is permitted to carry out.

c) information is given only if there is sufficient evidence that the user needs this information; for each usernumber, the department the user belongs to is recorded; if the patient has no relation with that department, (under treatment, test requested), the access is refused. However, this level c protection can be overridden by certain users, who have the right to state that the request concerns an emergency case; the information is then supplied, but a message is sent to the head of the medical records office that an overriding because of emergency has occured, together with usernumber and patientnumber.

SOME FIGURES AND MEASUREMENTS

The system started to run in March 1974, when the first programs for patient registration went operational for a few terminals. Nowadays 120 terminals are installed (70 alphanumerical displays; 40 character printers 30 char/sec; 2 remote printers 200 lpm other satellite computers, etc.).

Growth of the patientfile:

From 1968 – 1974 about 205.000 patients were registrated (via batch) with help of the IBM/370 of the Leyden University Computer Centre. Through a magtape the HIS-database has been initialised with these data.

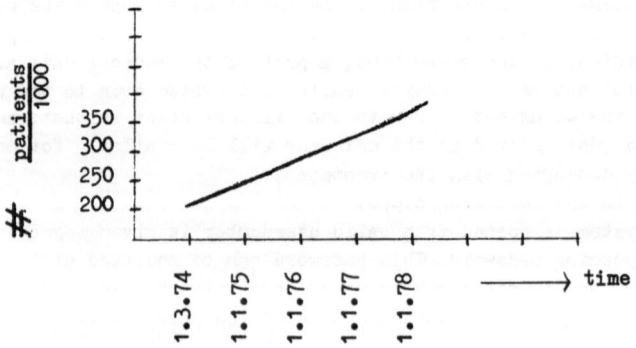

Growth of the number of patients.

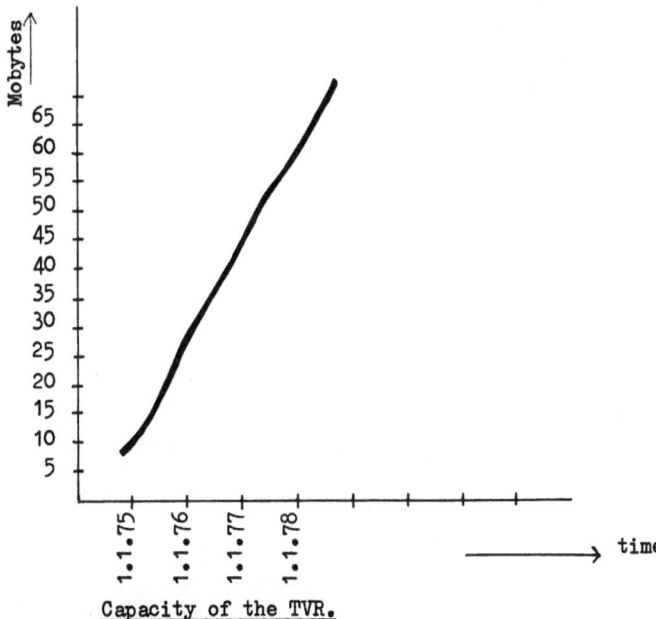

Capacity of the TVR.

Numbers about some subrecords, stored in the DB on 31-12-1977.

Type	Description	$\frac{\#}{1000}$	Mbytes
237	diagnosis	411	7,7
18	lab. results CKCL	308	16,0
1	departments	303	2,6
20	outward-pat.reg.	242	5,1
238	pathology	185	4,1
14	department-data	151	2,1
2	professions	122	1,3
248	anti-coagulant dosage	69	3,1
240	lab. results CKBPL	57	4,5
245	anti-coag. patient data	54	1,5
	rest	940	18

Some characteristic numbers on 31-12-1977.
- number of thesauri   77
- number of reg. patients   400.000
- number of TVR's   390.000
- number of different TVR-types   81
- number of subrecords   3.000.000
- number of messages   160.000

- number of dictransfers   1.100.000
- number of inputchar.   838.000
- number of outputchar.   22.064.000
- number of terminals   120

OP 72 - DATA TECHNICAL ASPECTS
A Hierarchical Data Base Applied to a Complicated Medical Research Project

Fred Bergqvist and Stellan Bengtsson
Uppsala University Data Center and Institute of Clinical Bacteriology,
Uppsala University, Uppsala, Sweden

A medical research project where complex data were analyzed is described. The method chosen used a program system for clinical laboratory data to organize and select data and a general statistics program for statistic analysis. The information
was stored in a hierarchical data base structure independent of the application. The
method was capable of performing most analyses, but the cost was too high and remaining analyses had to be carried out employing conventional programming techniques.
The experience gained from this project has been of value in designing a new data
base system which stores data in a relational way. A short description of this new
system is given.

1.   Introduction

In recent years many general data base systems and data manipulating languages have
been implemented and several more have been proposed. For a particular application
only few users have, however, the opportunity to choose the best tools from the
total list of data storing methods and query languages. They have to use those implemented at the compuer(s) they have access to. This paper discusses the problems
and considerations that often meet the worker who must choose and use a method to
analyse complex medical data.
A research project for the study of postoperative infections was started in an operating department at the University Hospital in Uppsala to investigate the factors
around postoperative infections with the aim of decreasing their frequency. This
work was initiated in 1972 under the name of OPERATION 72 (OP 72). At that time
the data base available was the Medical Data Base (MDB) which had been developed
during 1968-1972 at the Uppsala University Data Center (UDAC). MDB (6) is based upon
IBM's data base management system IMS and is coupled to the statistical program
INTEREST (5). MDB was therefore used for the analysis of the data from OP 72.
The medical research results are presented elsewhere by the medical research
group to which the second author belongs.

2. The medical project OP 72

2.1 Material

The medical project OP 72 comprised all patients operated in four operating rooms during three years. To increase the number of infected patients in the data base, all patients who underwent surgery in the department and developed postoperative infections were also entered into the program. In all, some 4,000 patients were included. The data acquisition process for the approximately 40,000 bacterial samples was based on the principles of the BACTLAB system (a data system for bacteriological routine) (1, 3). The computer technique used for the data acquisition process has been described in more detail earlier (2).

```
          PATIENT HISTORY FOR        SVENSSON KARL
            090313-        P959      PROSP MAN WARD 70C
DATE IN   740915    THEATRE   14     WOUND CLASS    2
DATE OP   740917    OP NO      2     ANAESTH TYPE 6519
DATE OUT  750930    OP TYPE 5351     DRAIN          4
PREDISP FACT:        PREOP              POSTOP
MALIGNANCY    INFECT:   -         WOUND INF SLIGHT,
                        -         PNEUMONIA AFTER 4 DAYS
              ANTIB:  AMPI 1 WEEK AMPI  CEFA
FEVER      INTENSIVE CARE 1 DAY
                                SDG ECA PPM T
                                UOE RLM GVE E
PAT 740917   N-T/ S AUR                2 1 1 RTD/54
    740917   SKIN/ M AUR               1 1 1 RTD/42E/54
    740917   PERIN/ O BETA AUR
    740921   WOUND/ S AUR      211 111 111   RTD/54
                    S ALFA     314 121 122
    740925   WOUND/ M AUR      21  111 111   NT
THEATRE  1   SED/ TOT  95
         2   SED/ TOT 110
                      COL   1
                      AUR   1              1 1 1 RTD/29/42E/81
         3   SED/ TOT  80
                      AUR   1              3 1 1 RTD/29
         4   SED/ TOT  90
STAFF A044   N-T/ ORD
      A046   N-T/ S AUR                2 1 1 53/83A/88
      C122   N-T/ S AUR                1 1 1 29/54
      E116   N-T/ ORD
      F206   N-T/ M AUR                2 1 1 29/54
```

Fig. 1. Example of a patient history.

The collected data were

- results of the bacteriological analysis of samples from patients, staff and environment (air);
- information about any infection, intake of antibiotic drugs, general status before, during and after operation, factors predisposing to infection, etc.;
- information about the operation.

As a result all information about a patient was assembled into a patient history (Fig. 1). These were produced as soon as the patient left the hospital and were used for conventional studies. The same information was stored on magnetic tape for later analysis by computer.

2.2 Requirements of the medical research project

Each patient record consists of a fixed part, with information about the patient and operation in fixed positions, and a variable part with bacteriological findings (Fig. 2). The fixed part is easily analyzed with a standard statistics program after a rather simple formating process to fit the program used. For the variable part this method is, however, not applicable. From the list of queries the following typical examples can be mentioned:

A1. Frequency of wound infection after different operations?

A2. Number of staff present at different operations? Differences between operations followed/not followed by infection?

A3. Total number of bacteria (average) on settle plates at infected and not infected operations?

A4. Number of Staph. aureus on settle plates at operations followed/not followed by staphylococcal infection?

A5. Does a patient who is a carrier of Staph. aureus at the time of operation have a higher incidence of postoperative aureus infection? Is this influenced by the type of carrier site (nose-throat, perineum, forearm)?

A6. Is the number of Staph. aureus colonies on settle plates in the operating room influenced by the carrier state of the patient? by the carrier state of the staff present?

The nature of the project made·it impossible to state all questions beforehand. The results successively gave rise to new questions and relations to analyse. A traditional solution with specially designed programs would therefore have demanded programming work during the whole analysis. The medical researcher, here and in similar situations, accordingly needs a tool with which he can easily specify desired operations, such as selecting, formatting and listing, calculation of frequencies, means and standard deviations, correlation analysis, etc. This should be possible for an arbitrary set of parameters from the material. It should also be easy to modify the questions to include new parameters or exclude others. These needs are commonly recognized and are of course not unique to this project.

3. Computer method

3.1 Choice of method

During 1968-1972 MDB had been developed at UDAC with the aim of realizing the general requirements stated at the end of section 2.2. OP 72 therefore became a test project for MDB. MDB was developed within the MSS project (the Multi Satellite System) for use at the regional level of an integrated information system for health and hospital care. In combination with the statistical program INTEREST, MDB comprises methods to manipulate a data base and select data for editing, listing or statistical calculations. By choosing MDB we hoped to reduce the need of programming considerably. It also gave the researchers the possibility to "get close" to their material and to formulate their questions directly via commands to MDB and INTEREST without the help of an intermediate programmer. Even if the whole analysis was not expected to be realized by MDB, it was still interesting to acquire experience of the method for other similar applications as well as for the further development of data base systems at UDAC. A schematic outline of the principles of MDB and its connection to INTEREST is shown in Fig. 3.

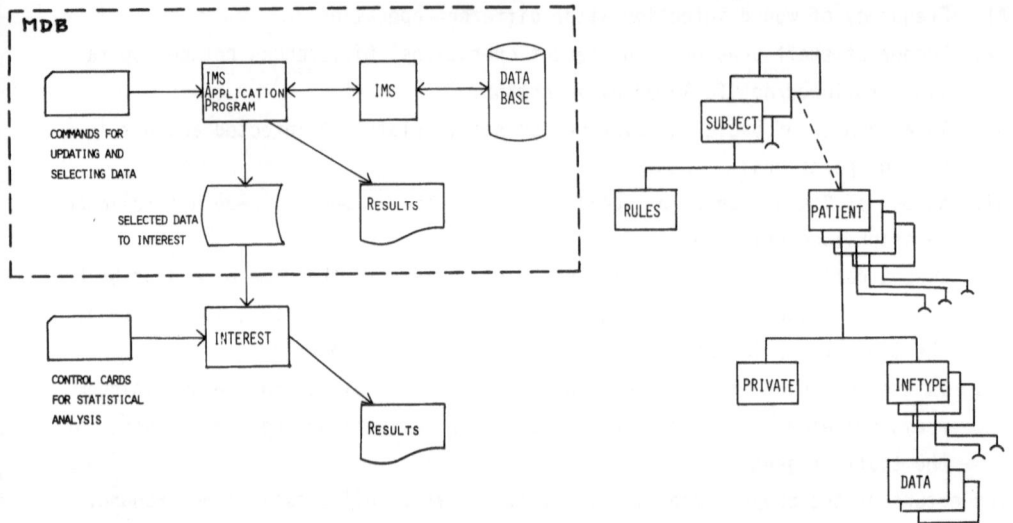

Fig. 3. Main principles for MDB and the connection to INTEREST.

Fig. 5. Logical structure of the subject data base, and the principle for referring to the patient data base.

3.2 MDB - brief description

MDB contains the following data bases
- patient data base: all patient records containing the total medical information about the patient
- text data base: stores all texts for codes in other data bases
- subject data base: defines medical subjects with references to the patient data base.

Data are stored in a fixed hierarchical structure, in our implementation by means of IMS. The general logical structure in the patient data base is shown in Fig. 4. The DATA segment has an inner structure not manipulated with IMS but with the MDB programs (written in PL/1). The reason for this is to unload IMS some work thus getting more rapid searching. The DATA segment is thus a character string with special characters separating the subfields. Fig. 5 shows the logical structure of the subject data base and how it can be combined with the patient data base. MDB runs in batch processing and the user communicates with MDB via transactions. For input and changes

447

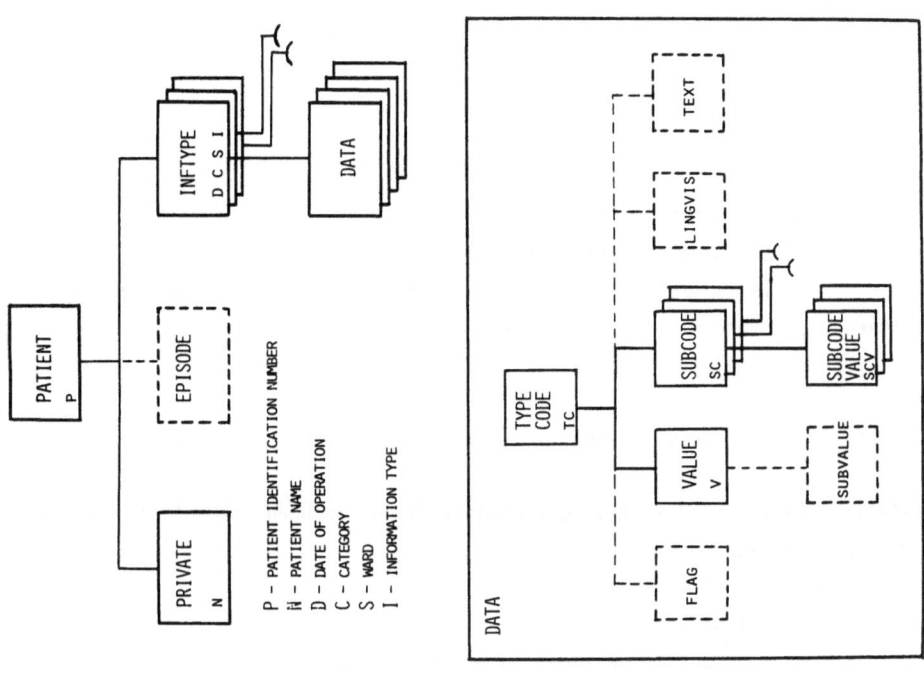

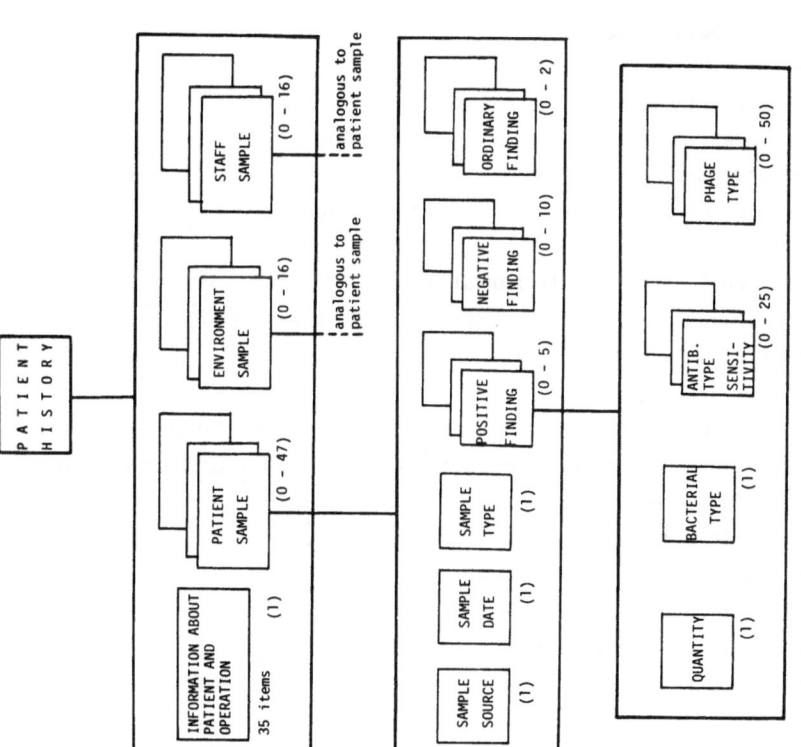

Fig. 2. (above) Data structure of patient records. Numbers within brackets are number of occurrences.

Fig. 4. (right) Logical structure of each patient data base record. Broken lines signify parts not used in the OP72 project.

the following commands are available

    I - insert

    D - delete

    R - replace

    C - change.

For selecting and output there is

    L/V - presentation of patient information in different ways

    T/S - a file is written for INTEREST with or without tabulating the records.

Hence T and S give the important connection to INTEREST. Moreover we have

    G - automatical generation of transactions, e.g., to create subject indices.

3.3 INTEREST - brief description

INTEREST is a well-tested statistical program which has been extensively used outside MDB. Here declaring functions are

    DIMENSION - optimizing of memory

    HEAD   - list headings

    DECIMALS   - number of decimals in presentations

Searching functions

    RECORD   - searching records

    GROUP   - grouping records

Functions for descriptive statistics

    TABLE   - frequency tables

    MEAN   - mean value and standard deviation tables

And functions for analytical statistics

    CORREL   - calculation of correlation coefficients

    REGRES   - regression analysis

A detailed description is given in the manual of INTEREST (5).

4.   Structuring OP 72 data for MDB

For OP 72 the patient data base is utilized as shown in Fig. 4, but parts within
broken lines are not used. The data material has been divided into four information types with the following mnemonics

    1 FX - fixed data

    2 PA - bacteriological samples from the patient

    3 EN - bacteriological samples from the environment

    4 ST - bacteriological samples from staff

The following is a simplified description of the type codes and underlying data.

Information type 1

type code	represents	subcode; subcode value
1	compulsory information	sex, date of admission, operation and discharge, operating room, type of operation, wound class, treatment period, etc (23 items)
2	preoperative infection	type, time
3	preoperative antibiotics	type, time
4	predisposing factors	type (e.g. malignancy, diabetes)
5	postoperative actions	type (e.g. tracheostoma, central venous catheter)
6	postoperative infections	type, time
7	postoperative antibiotics	type, time
8	other	type (e.g. fever, fatal outcome)

Information type 2-4

type code	represents	subcode; subcode value
1-60	sample type	room/category no/normal growth type and quantity of organism
70	ordinary finding	room/category sample type bact type
75	no finding	room/category sample type bact type
100-183	positive bacteriological finding	room/category sample type quantity phage type of Staph. aureus antibiotic sensitivity, etc.

In the preceding table room identifies room and plate in information type EN, and VALUE codes the datum of the sample for all types. Note that type code 1-60 constitutes the inverse to type code 70-183. This permits search via the entry of sample type as well as via bacterial type.

MDB was certainly not designed to utilize the DATA segment with as many subcodes as shown here. This solution was, however, the only one possible which maintained the relation between mutually connected data. Some degree of multiple storing exists, which increases the mass of data to be scanned. This multiple storing is essential for the data to be accessible via different keys, but it is also nesessary in order to make it possible to search for existence of a subcode on the one hand and to pick up its value on the other hand. From considerations of storage space and for loading of data multiple storing is not a serious disadvantage, since the data base is rather static and after loading is used mainly as a data source. The access method HDAM was chosen as being the most effective. A program was constructed to automatically generate transactions for loading the patient data base. This program became a considerable part of the work, mostly dependent on the complex structure of source data. By using the data structure described above all type questions given were solved, and some reserve capacity remained.

5.   Analyzing OP 72 data with MDB

5.1 Selecting from MDB

The most important transactions here are S and REC.
     S   specifies selection from the patient data base
     REC specifies the format of the records for INTEREST. It describes information
           included and how the information should be assembled if several observations
           of the same type exist for one patient.
Syntax:
     S   P=(...),N=(...), I=(...),C=(...),D=(...)
     REC (I(TC:SC,k), ...)
The symbols used here are those shown in Fig. 4.
In the S transaction the operands are optional. They specify values and/or intervals,
e.g.,
     S   I=PA(5,23,36),D=(741001-741321)
which selects data under information type PA and data type 5, 23 or 36 during
October-December 1974.
In REC k is specified as one of
     X esistence   M mean value   U unique (all) values
     H highest value   F first value   G standard deviation
     L lowest value   S last value
Depending on whether :SC is given or not the result is existence of TC or SC
respectively value of V or SCV, which for information type FX is illustrated by
     FX(3,X)   existence of TC=3
     FX(3,F)   first value V under TC=3
     FX(3:7,X)   existence of SC=7 under TC=3
     FX(3:7,H)   highest value SCV under SC=7 and TC=3
     FX(3,U)   all values V under TC 3.

5.2 Practical example

This is question A3 from section 2.2. Two MDB commands are carried out.
     S   C=1,I=(FX(1,6),EN(169)
     REC (FX(1,F),FX(1:5,F),FX(6,F),EN(169:KV,U))

Here the S command specifies the patient category (=1) and the information types (FX and EN). By giving the data types (1,6 respectively 169) the searching is speeded up. The REC command specifies the variables for INTEREST. These are numbered V1, V2, etc. when referred to as values, when referred to in testing for their existence they are called X1, X2, etc. Even if not specified in the REC command V1 and V2 always represent age and sex. Furthermore we have

V3	FX(1,F)	type of operation
V4	FX(1:5,F)	number of operating room
V5	FX(6,F)	type of postoperative infection
V6	EN(169:KV,U)	quantity of total bacteria

As soon as a patient data base record contains any of the requested variables a record is written to the INTEREST file. Since U (unique) is used in V6 one record for each value is created where the other variables are identical. The mean value of total number of bacteria is now obtained by the INTEREST function MEAN, and to put headings we use HEAD

HEAD	(NO INFECT, SLIGHT, SERIOUS, DEEP / OPCL 1)
MEAN	(NOT X5, V5 EQ 2, V5 EQ 3, V5 EQ 4 /
	V3 FROM 1 TO 42 STEP 1 / V6)

The logical operators NOT and EQ (equal to) are used to formulate the conditions. The character / separates arguments for columns and rows. Fig. 6 shows the resulting tables.
By putting

GROUP	(V4 FROM 8 TO 12 STEP 1)

before the HEAD command tables are produced for each operating room. By using the principles illustrated in this example about 50 questions were answered.

6.   Experiences

Data base loading
Generating transactions loading the data base were resource consuming. This is done only once for data bases of the OP 72 type, but it is nevertheless of interest to simplify them. This may be accomplished by using other data base solutions.

Usefulness
MDB is designed to be used by persons without programming knowledge. However, formulating questions in the rigid manner prescribed seems to be inconvenient and is therefore readily left to trained persons. The reason for this is partly that the hierarchical structure influences the syntax of the queries, and that this structure, here as in many other cases, in unnatural.

MEAN VALUE

		NO INFECT	SLIGHT	SERIOUS	DEEP
OPCL	1	99.6	0.0	0.0	0.0
	2	100.8	0.0	0.0	0.0
	3	90.2	92.0	98.8	0.0
	4	89.0	75.0	0.0	79.0
	5	82.2	78.1	0.0	0.0
	6	80.1	88.8	0.0	0.0
	7	122.1	0.0	0.0	0.0

STANDARD DEVIATION

		NO INFECT	SLIGHT	SERIOUS	DEEP
OPCL	1	66.01	0.0	0.0	0.0
	2	32.82	0.0	0.0	0.0
	3	50.59	26.77	11.09	0.0
	4	54.23	38.21	0.0	24.74

STANDARD ERROR OF THE MEAN

		NO INFECT	SLIGHT	SERIOUS	DEEP
OPCL	1	2.39	0.0	0.0	0.0
	2	7.34	0.0	0.0	0.0
	3	2.68	9.47	5.54	0.0

ABSOLUTE FREQUENCY

		NO INFECT	SLIGHT	SERIOUS	DEEP
OPCL	1	764	0	0	0
	2	20	0	0	0
	3	356	8	4	0

FREQUENCY IN PERCENT OF ALL SELECTED CASES

		NO INFECT	SLIGHT	SERIOUS	DEEP
OPCL	1	6.6	0.0	0.0	0.0
	2	0.2	0.0	0.0	0.0
	3	3.1	0.1	0.0	0.0

FREQUENCY IN PERCENT OF COLUMNS SUMS

		NO INFECT	SLIGHT	SERIOUS	DEEP
OPCL	1	7.8	0.0	0.0	0.0
	2	0.2	0.0	0.0	0.0
	3	3.6	1.2	2.4	0.0

FREQUENCY IN PERCENT OF ROWS SUMS

		NO INFECT	SLIGHT	SERIOUS	DEEP
OPCL	1	99.0	0.0	0.0	0.0
	2	100.0	0.0	0.0	0.0
	3	93.7	2.1	1.1	0.0
	4	73.7	7.9	0.0	2.1
	5	97.6	1.6	0.0	0.0
	6	94.0	3.2	0.0	0.0

Fig. 6. List output from INTEREST for the query A3 as solved in section 5.2 of the text.

Query language

Queries of the form

    SELECT (expression) WHERE (logical expression)

are not possible as MDB commands, but would, no doubt, increase the usefulness considerably. Managing <u>all</u> questions is possible only if user-written modules are permitted.

Connection MDB to INTEREST

If the mechanism of selecting was satisfactory for a problem, the automatic generation of the statistic file worked well.

Computer resources

IMS is primarily a general, safe system on a high service level. However, the hierarchical structure with its pointer technique and all the overhead processes used to serve all special features makes IMS far too slow and expensive to use. A comparison of specially designed programs and MDB showed that MDB used 20-100 times more cpu + I/O-time than the special program. Furthermore a fairly great core region is needed to run IMS and its application programs.

To compromise between IMS and own scanning

MDB's own manipulation of the DATA segment in OP 72 makes it lose some of its effectiveness because of the great number of subcodes. In other projects with fewer subcodes this solution has turned out to be successful.

Data base structure

The fixed structure of MDB is not sufficient for OP 72. The DATA segment is overloaded, moreover the hierarchical structure does not fit these data. Another data structure according to the relational model is in our opinion more suitable (see section 7).

Economy

Output involving only the fixed part was economically acceptable. All search involving the variable bacteriological part was too expensive to be acceptable.

Complementary programs

Although the structuring of data was made with great care and attention it became necessary to write far too many special programs.

7. Consequences and further development of data base systems

As appears from the experiences in section 6, the OP 72 data structure is too complex for MDB to be the ideal solution. Since the same assertion could be made about
other similar MDB test projects, UDAC in 1974 decided to take the first steps away
from the hierarchical data base structure and developments based upon it. Some
time-limited projects, among them OP 72, were allowed to proceed to their finish.
These would then give a complete picture of the MDB technique which had not been
possible if they had all been converted to a new technique. Thus, during the later
part of the OP 72 project and after it had been finished, the general data base
system MIMER was developed at UDAC. This system is based on the experiences and
improved knowledge about data base requirements that emanated from earlier data
base projects. A new logical data structure has been adopted and a new mechanism
for physical storing of data has been developed.
The basic software components of MIMER are:
- a data definition facility
- a data manipulating language via a host programming language
- a query language with a relational view of data
- a data dictionary
- a program generation facility, LIDAM

A MIMER data base consists of a number of files. A logical network structure can be
established via the mechanism of file coupling. Any two files can be coupled to-
bether via a common keyfield (primary or secondary). By this coupling mechanism,
queries can be constructed which consist of search criteria from several files.
MIMER is designed around normalized data structures, that is, all data structures
that are not two-dimensional are decomposed into two-dimensional tables. Thus the
concept files means flat files. Any number of fields within a file can be selected
to be a search key (secondary key). For each secondary key an inverted list is created and maintained. The data base may be accessed via the CALL function in the host
programming language. The basic functions are those of OPEN, CLOSE, FIND, COUPLE,
READ, WRITE and DELETE. A high level of data independence between each user application and the manner in which the data are physically organized is maintained by
letting the user retrieve data at the field level rather than at the record level.
The FIND command is introduced to help the user to isolate a record or a set of
records, fulfilling a specified condition. By several FIND commands related to each
other by logical operators, complex logical expressions can be evaluated. MIMER is
now successfully used in several applications, of which SWEDIS (Swedish Drug Information System) can be mentioned (4). The drawbacks of the MDB system described a-
bove have been eliminated. An application for production statistics has shown a
tenfold speed up. A complete query language is under development, which will also
get an interface to a statistical program. Here we have a product that so far is

superior to MDB as regards logical structure and data manipulating. In the few situations where the query language is insufficient the CALL functions in the host programming language are used. The data base system MIMER is now available at the IBM 370, PDP 11 and NORD 10 computers.

References

(1) S. Bengtsson: The Rational Use of Computing in Microbiology. Proc. of First World Conference on Medical Informatics - MEDINFO'74, 1151-1154. Eds: J. Anderson and J.M. Forsythe (North-Holland Publishing Company, Amsterdam), 1974.

(2) S. Bengtsson, F.-O. Bergqvist and W. Schneider: A Data System for Bacteriological Routine and Research. Symposium on Rapid Methods and Automation in Microbiology - 2. New Approaches to the Identifications of Microorganisms, 291-305. Ed. C.G. Heden (John Wiley, New York), 1975.

(3) F. Bergqvist and S. Bengtsson: The BACTLAB system - A Data System for Bacteriological Routine. Computer Programs in Biomedicine 4, 144-157, (North-Holland Publishing Company, Amsterdam), 1975.

(4) B. Dagerus, S.G. Johansson and P. Manell: SWEDIS, A Drug Information System at the Department of Drugs, National Board of Health and Welfare, Sweden. Proc. of the Conference on Computer Aid to Drug Therapy and to Drug Monitoring. (North-Holland Publishing Company, Amsterdam) in press, 1978.

(5) A. Haglund and L. Edblad: INTEREST II Manual (UDAC and IBM Sweden, Stockholm), 1972.

(6) W. Schneider, A. Haglund, K. Vogel, L. Edblad and H. Herrström: IMS, Information Management System, as Data Base for Handling Medical Information (Preliminary technical report). Proc. of 11th IBM Medical Symposium, Heidelberg, Germany. (IBM WT Medical Industry Center, Stockholm), 1972.

Author's address:

F. Bergqvist
Uppsala University Data Center
Box 2103
S-750 02 Uppsala
Sweden

ON THE DESIGN OF A DATABASE SYSTEM FOR CLINICAL RESEARCH

S.C. Chang, A. Hasman and A.B.M.F. Karim
Departments of Medical Informatics and Radiotherapy
Free University
Amsterdam

1. INTRODUCTION

Clinical research is of utmost importance to keep standards of treatment at the highest possible level. This research is often delayed by
the vast amount of time needed to record data on a suitable medium and
then to order these data for analysis purposes. For this reason the
computer is a useful tool for analyzing research data in a fast and
flexible way.
In this paper the design of a database system will be discussed, that
is used for clinical research purposes. The system has been developed
by the Medical Informatics department of the Free University in Amsterdam in cooperation with the department of Radiotherapy, that delivered
the clinical research project. It has been written in FORTRAN IV and
implemented on a PDP 11/70 under the operating system RSX-11D.
In the final draft of the system design the following requirements
were specified:
- non computer-experts should be able to use the system for all kinds
  of applications
- the system should be modularly designed, so that it could be extended
  without much cost and effort
- it should have the possibility of graphical output
- it should pursue data independency
- a simple data manipulation language should be provided to facilitate
  users without any programming experience
- it should contain statistical routines.

On the basis of these requirements the system was divided into the
following modules:
- a data definition module
- a data entry and verification module
- a data manipulation module
- several routines for creating and updating files.

2. THE DATA DEFINITION MODULE

This module generates a user database description. In this description
one must define two types of data:

- General information about the database the user wants to create.
  This information consists of the following data:
  ● the data file name
  ● the name of the file with database item names
  ● user identification
  ● record attributes
  ● user defined keywords.
- Information about items. For example:
  ● itemname
  ● starting position of the value of the item in the record
  ● IO-format
  ● minimum value that can occur
  ● maximum value that can occur
  ● a pointer to the symbolic description of this item.

In figure 1 the general structure is displayed.

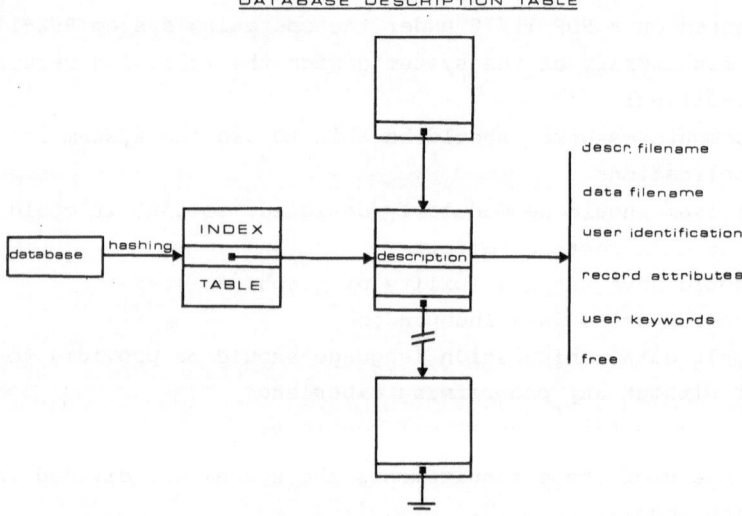

figure 1

In this module the database administrator can either define, change
or delete itemnames and the item attributes.
To give an impression of how an item description is added, the
following example is given:
A/SEX/6,1,1,1,2 (1=MALE, 2=FEMALE)
In this example the literal A is the abbreviation for the command ADD
while the item SEX will be added. The meaning of the attribute list
is the following:

```
6 = starting position of the value of the item in the record
1 = item length
1 = item type  1 = integer; 2 = real; 3 = alphanumeric
1 = minimum value allowed
2 = maximum value allowed
```

The parentheses enclose the symbolic description of the item values
1 and 2. The advantage of defining a symbolic description is clear.
Later on one can use the names MALE and FEMALE instead of the numeric
codes 1 and 2. In this way all the item descriptions are added.
However, for each file this procedure has to be done only once. Later
on it is possible to change an item description, it has no further
consequences for the database software. In figure 2 the way in which
the item description is designed is shown.

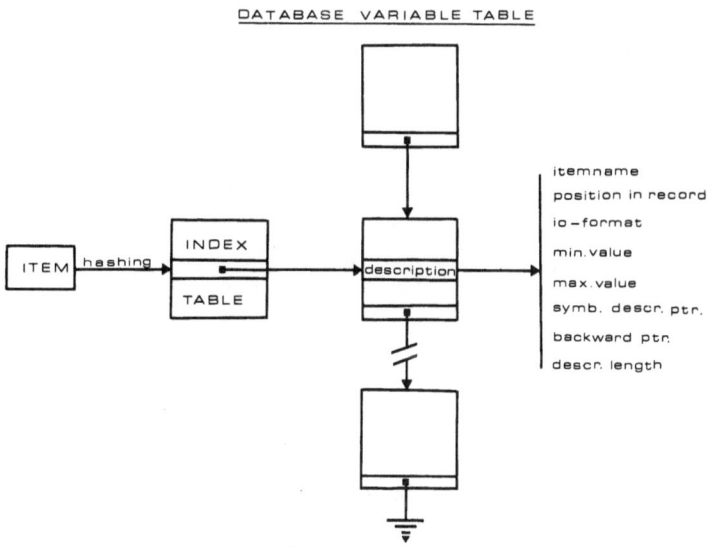

figure 2

. FILE ORGANISATION

In any database system it is important that files can be accessed
very fast. Several file organisations can be compared using certain
criterias as for example:
- the access time
- efficient storage structure
- the difficulty of selecting, changing and adding of records
- the usefulness of an external storage medium.
For each of these criteria one can find a file organization which is
optimal. However, techniques that seem to be better in one respect,
might be less efficient in another way:

- a random file has to be sorted when data must be processed alphabetically or in numeric order
- updating or deleting records in a sequential file takes a long time
- random searching in a linked list is slow.

In this system we have implemented the following techniques:
- hash techniques for the database variable tables
- linked ordered linear lists for the data records
- multiway trees for the inverted files.

To identify a record the user must provide an item as primary key.
This item might be a numeric or an alphanumeric key. The remaining
items are called non-primary keys. The set of primary keys together
with the pointers to their data records are stored in a multiway tree.
Depending of the expected or measured frequencies of non-primary keys
one can also create inverted files for them.

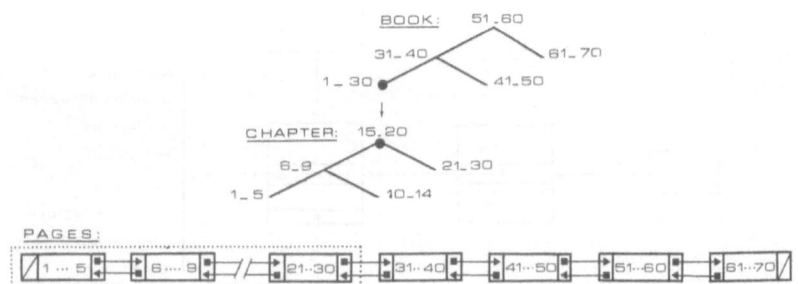

figure 3

In figure 3 an example is given of the logical structure of the inverted
files. The multiway tree consists of three levels. The lowest level is
called a page. The page is a record which consists of the set of
combinations of a primary key and a pointer to a data record.
The next level (chapter) consists of interval data together with pointers
to the corresponding page records. The upper level (book) consists of
interval data with pointers to the corresponding chapter records. The
book level as well as the chapter level are organized internally as
balanced binary trees.

4. THE DATA ENTRY AND VERIFICATION MODULE

The data entry and verification module uses the item description files
for presenting the itemnames and symbolic descriptions on a video display

terminal. The input values are checked and if they are not accepted
the words ILLEGAL ENTRY are flashed on the screen. After the record
has been typed in, the data can be edited in a sequential way (the
values of ten items at a time are presented) or randomly. In the last
case the sequence number of the item has to be specified. The records
are stored in a temporary file and are later on merged with the main
data file by utility programs, that also update the inverted files.

5. THE DATA MANIPULATION MODULE

For the interactive use of the system a keyword oriented data manipulation
language has been developed. We based ours on the presumption that medical
users do not have any programming experience. An example of a keyword
command would be the next expression: SIN (x+y). The keyword is SIN and
its arguments are x and y. Each keyword corresponds with a program
module executing the function. For this reason the system has the
structure as depicted in figure 4.

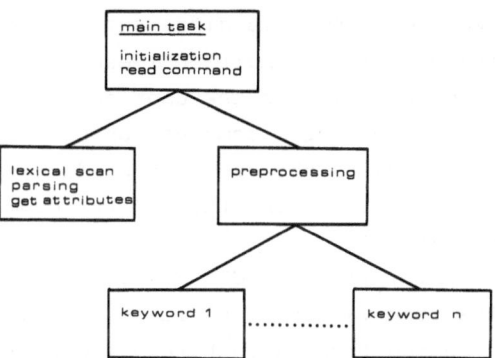

figure 4

Since we allowed conditional expressions, we used a so-called translator
writing system for defining and testing the data manipulation grammar.
For this purpose we used the Langpak system. This system was developed
by Heindel and Roberto (1) of the Bell Telephone Company. The main
advantage of the Langpak system is that a language designer is able to
test his grammar in an interactive way. A disadvantage of this system
is that it is only applicable for simple languages like the one using
keyword oriented commands.
To give the reader an impression of the data manipulation language we
present a few examples of possible commands:

- The first command the user must enter is: LOAD (database name).
  Any other command will be neglected until the LOAD-command has been
  entered. After the LOAD-command the user identification is verified.
- By entering: BYE a query session is ended.
- Unexperienced users frequently enter the TEACH-command. Using this
  command the system will show a list of all keywords. By specifying
  a keyword more information concerning that keyword is given.
- More often than not a research database consists of more than hundred
  items. Few people care to remember all the itemnames. When the
  situation arises that an itemname is imcompletely known, one can enter
  the FIND-command: FIND (beginletter(s) of an itemname)
  e.g. FIND year
  The system will show a list of all the itemnames starting with the
  string: YEAR.
- For some keywords one must know in advance some item attributes like
  the type, the domain or symbolic description of the item. With the
  help of the DESCRIBE-command the system will show these item attributes.
  e.g. DESCRIBE SEX,T,M
- The remaining keyword commands are different from the previous commands
  because they may be used with conditional expressions. A conditional
  expression determines a subset of the user dataset. Arithmetic as
  well as logical expressions or a combination of them are allowed.
  The next example illustrates the use of a conditional expression.
- To display item values one can use the DISPLAY command, e.g.
  DISPLAY PATIENT-NO,SEX,T
  WHERE (SEX=FEMALE .OR. T=TIS).AND.GRADE>=1.
  In this example the item values of PATIENT-NO, SEX and T are displayed
  (T is an itemname coming from radiotherapy and indicating the extent
  of the tumor; grade is a measure of the virulency of the tumor).
- Sometimes one is only interested in the number of records fulfilling
  a number of conditions. In this case the user may enter the COUNT-
  command; e.g. COUNT WHERE T<=T2A .AND. SEX=FEMALE.
- A cross-table is obtained by the TABLE-command, e.g.
  TABLE(2,9) WITH SEX(1,1) AND GRADE(1,1) WHERE T<=T2A .AND. VAR1>2.5
  The system will display a 2 x 9 table with the row variable SEX and
  the column variable GRADE. In this case the variable VAR1 is a
  temporary variable which only exists during the query session. This
  variable is defined with the LET command. The numbers enclosed within
  parentheses indicate the minimum value used and the classwidth.
- In a research environment one often needs histograms of item values.
  This is possible with the FREQUENCY-command, e.g. FREQUENCY SEX(1,1).
  The numbers enclosed between parentheses have the same meaning as the
  ones used in the TABLE-command.

- To display all the item values of a record, one can use the VIEW command, e.g. VIEW WHERE PRIM-KEY = N
  All the item values of the record with primary key N are displayed.
- For several reasons item values can be incorrect. The EDIT-command allows the user to correct these values, e.g. EDIT WHERE PATIENT-NO=53
  Editing is possible in one of two modes: random or sequential.
  This same EDIT function is also built into the data entry module.
- Sometimes one wants to know the value of an item that was not specified in the database but is a function of certain database items. Therefore the user can temporarily (during the query session) define such items with the LET-command, e.g.:
  LET VAR3 = GRADE/2 IF SEX=MALE .AND. T>TIS ELSE VAR3 = GRADE/3.
- To create subfiles of his data set, the COPY-command is available, e.g.
  COPY (FILENAME) WHERE SEX=FEMALE
  It is obvious that a conditional expression is obliged.
- Besides copying of records one can also copy item values. This happens by writing item values into a binary file, e.g.
  WRITE ITEM1,ITEM2,ITEM3 INTO (FILENAME) WHERE SEX=FEMALE
- A statistical package is available with which it is possible to perform statistical tests. Included are graphics routines with which it is possible to obtain scatter plots, histograms, regression curves etc.
- For each application user keywords can be implemented. These keywords are very problem specific. They can be easily introduced into the system.

6. DISCUSSION

A very versatile tool has been presented in this paper. Data entry and retrieval is easily possible for research purposes without the needs for a programmer. The medical researcher can evaluate his data in an interactive way. Several users can work with this system, each on his own research project. The programming effort has to be done only once. The introduction of new keywords is facilitated by the modular setup. Since the beginning of our project, the use of the MUMPS language has become more and more popular. The structure of the database in DEC Standard MUMPS is similar to the structure we used (multiway trees). Therefore the database system will also be implemented in MUMPS, taking advantage of the experience already acquired.

REFERENCES

L.E. Heindel and J.T. Roberto, 1975: Langpak, an interactive language design system. American Elsevier Publishing Company, Inc. New York.

Using CODIL to handle poorly structured clinical information

C.F.Reynolds, Department of Computer Science, Brunel University, Uxbridge, Middx.
and
M.Shackell and G.Sutton, Hillingdon Hospital, Hillingdon, Middlesex.

ABSTRACT

This paper looks at the problems of using computers to handle clinical information
in the context of a small research team where changing requirements and comparatively low volumes can make conventional systems analysis and programming techniques
hopelessly uneconomic. The way in which such difficulties can be overcome are
discussed, and examples are given of an operational system, using CODIL as the
implementation language, which handles clinical information on cardiac patients.
The ease with which such an approach can be extended to other areas is discussed.

1. INTRODUCTION

This paper examines the problems of the medical researcher who wants to
keep case notes, or other information, on a computer. He would like a data base
package tailored to meet his specialist needs at minimal expense. Unfortunately
he will often encounter one or more of the following difficulties:

(a) He is uncertain what his information processing requirements are until he has
had experience of using a suitable system.

(b) His requirements will change with time as a result of medical advances, his
increasing experience of the problem being put onto the computer, etc.

(c) The logical structure of the information may be complex, with different types
of information being collected from different sources at different times.

(d) Some of the information will be incomplete or ambiguous, particularly if it
depends on outsiders to provide data on an ad hoc basis.

(e) The total volume of information involved will often be very small compared
with administrative data processing jobs being run on the same computer.

(f) Existing packages do not fit his requirements without either modifying the
package or his requirements.

(g) He doesn't have a friend in the data processing department who will help him
out for the kicks.

(h) He doesn't have access to unlimited research funds.

As a result the majority of doctors who might like to use automatic
information processing techniques to help in their research activities are unable
to do so.

CODIL is a computer language specifically designed for the class of
user who migh be faced with the difficulties listed above. This paper shows
how the language has been used in the Cardiac Department of Hillingdon Hospital,

assesses the progress made to date and examines the ease with which the findings can be applied to other research groups both inside and outside the medical arena.

2. CODIL as a data base system

CODIL is a computer language (1,2) specifically designed to allow non-computer oriented users to set up and run applications involving ambiguous or poorly defined information with the minimum of help from computer professionals. (3,4,5). In order to provide some degree of familiarity to the user it was decided to build the system around a simplified model of human memory and decision making (5,6,7) which is easy to explain to users and which has proved remarkably efficient to implement. By concentrating on a flexible man-computer interface the package is totally application independent and has been used for tasks as diverse as teaching HNC chemists the basics of information processing through to heuristic problem solving (8). However its chief operational use has been in the field of information storage, processing and retrieval, (9,10) including the application described here.

While CODIL provides the user with powerful "data base" type facilities it is important to realise that there are fundamental differences between it and more conventional data base systems (11). Conventional systems are constructed around a troika of program, data definition and data, with rigid demarcation rules as to the type of information each represents. This approach has proved very successful when the need is to process large volumes of uniformly structured data in routine ways, possibly to meet the needs of some government regulation or administrative edict. On the other hand it is unsuited to comparatively small applications involving poorly structured information. You have only to ask any doctor which parts of his medical knowledge represents program, data definition and data to realise how alien conventional data base software is to the average human being.

Because it is modelled on human information processing CODIL rejects this troika and replaces it with a unified concept of information. All information within CODIL is self-structured and needs no explicit file description. Within the simple syntax of the language the user is free to describe the application in the way he finds most acceptable, and there is no need for him to make arbitrary distinctions between program and data, although if he wishes to think about his problem in this way there are no constraints on him having distinct files of "rules" and "data". In the same way if he wants a file to have a uniform structure there is nothing to stop him, and he is free to vary this as appropriate to cope with missing or extra information should the need arise.

3. Background to the Hillingdon system

In describing the use of CODIL at Hillingdon Hospital it is important to realise that the interests of the various authors are distinct. At the hospital end the aim is to establish a computer file of clinical records of cardiac patients for research purposes. At the University end the aim is to monitor the operational use of the CODIL language.

The work has progressed in a number of stages. Between 1973 and 1975 a pilot study was carried out in conjunction with two undergraduate projects (12,13, 14). This was the first time that CODIL had been used with operational data generated by non-computer oriented users and for technical reasons it had to be carried out in batch mode. The results were generally satisfactory although it was found that the batch punching documents used were over-complicated and tended to give the doctors using the system the impression that they had less flexibility than in fact they had. As a result of this, and trials with different applications, improvements were made in the CODIL interpreter. Unfortunately, it was still impossible to provide a terminal in the hospital, although interactive working was possible within the University. For this reason a far simpler, and more general, punching document was produced and starting early in 1977 clincial information on patients admitted to the cardiac care unit has been recorded. This was extended by the hospital staff to cover a retrospective analysis of patients who had undergone cardiac operations over a period of six years. A range of questions and surveys have been carried out using the data. This is the stage reached by the system described in this paper. Future plans include the provision of a terminal in the hospital, initially to allow file interrogation but eventually to permit direct file update for the cardiac care unit.

4. Description of the Cardiac Information System

In the following paragraphs the various procedures involved in setting up and using the system are summarised. The examples are all artificial to avoid the use of confidential patient data, but have been chosen to illustrate the principle features of interest.

4.1 Direct input procedures.

One of the most obvious differences between CODIL and more conventional data base systems is that there is no need for any prior file definitions before a file is set up. If a user wants to set up a file called HISTORY containing information on a patient's cardiac history all he has to do is to connect with the CODIL interpreter and type:

```
← CREATE = HISTORY.
← PATIENT = SMITH;   YEAR = 1965;   DIAGNOSIS = UNSTABLE ANGINA.
← PATIENT = JONES;   YEAR = 1972;   MONTH = 3;   DIAGNOSIS = MI.
← ............
← END.
```

To list the file in the CODIL default format he types in a simple command and the
system responds immediately:

```
← PRINT ITEM = HISTORY.
  PATIENT = SMITH.
      YEAR = 1965,
          DIAGNOSIS = UNSTABLE ANGINA.
  PATIENT = JONES,
      YEAR = 1972,
          MONTH = 3,
              DIAGNOSIS = MI.

  .......
```

Further statements can be added by using CREATE(APPEND) or the file can be
edited. In the following example the context editor is used to change all
occurrences of DIAGNOSIS = MI to DIAGNOSIS = MYOCARDIAL INFARCT.

```
          ← FILE EDIT.
          FILE NAME = ?
          ← HISTORY.
          TYPE IN AMENDMENT FILE
          ← DIAGNOSIS = MI;   DIAGNOSIS = MYOCARDIAL INFARCT.
          ← END.
```

In practice this degree of flexibility is inappropriate for non-trivial files which
are to be updated over a period of several years and used by more than one
individual. There are also advantages in minimising the volume of batch punching
and interactive input while continuing to use meaningful terminology. For this
reason the hospital files were·initialised as follows:

(a) Abbreviations. To avoid the need to type in long names a number of abbreviations were defined as follows:

```
          ← ADMISSIONS WARD(ABBREV) = AW.
          ← AETIOLOGY(ABBREV) = AET.
          ← ANGIOGRAM(ABBREV) = ANG.
          ← .......
```

New names and/or abbreviations can be defined on any subsequent occasion. However
to prevent the accidental use of an undeclared name it is possible to indicate
that such names are to be reported or rejected.

(b) Semiformatted input. It was agreed at an early stage in the work that all
patient information should be qualified by a serial number unique to the trial and
that no names or hospital identity codes should be used to ensure confidentiality.
In addition all statements were to contain date and time information to an

appropriate degree of detail, together with a "form name" to identify the type of information being input. To handle this a simple routine is created to read in details of the NEXT patient:

```
← CREATE = NEXT.
←  INPUT = SERIAL NO.        )
←  INPUT = YEAR.             )
←  INPUT = MONTH.            )   Reads value of item from
←  INPUT = DAY.             )   terminal or batch stream.
←  INPUT = HOUR.            )
←  INPUT = MINUTE.          )
←  INPUT = FORM.
←  INPUT ALL.                   Reads list of items as required.
←  STORE ALL.                   Stores all items on file.
←  DELETE
← END.
```

This file is used to read data off the form shown in figure 1, which is punched for batch input as follows:

```
NEXT:1234:78:9:4:::REFI:DOB=1913:SEX=M:DI=LV DYSFUNCTION:-
AET=CAD:ORD=INVESTIGATION:REFC=HAREFIELD:E
```

(The ":E" termination is not shown on the form as the actual routine NEXT used in the operation system has been written to minimise punching. The routine can also be used in interactive mode, in which case it will automatically prompt the user for the inputs required.)

(c) Updating the master file. New information is currently made available in batch mode and it would be inappropriate to add it directly to the file of accumulated patient data until there had been an opportunity of removing any data preparation errors, etc. To handle this problem an additional routine READ NEW DATA has been written which copies the input data to a file called NEW DATA, which can be edited, amended, searched for errors, etc. Once this file is free from errors it is merged with the master file. It is worth noting that the biggest part of the initialisation process is the list of abbreviations used by the doctor.

4.2 File listing facilities.

In addition to the default file listing facility - which can be bulky for large files - it is simple for the user to write his own routines for controlling the way in which information is printed. The following example involves the creation and use of the file, LIST PATIENTS, and shows some of the tabulation and other facilities available for controlling the layout of the printed page.

CODIL

HILLINGDON HOSPITAL DATA FORM

		NUMBER	YEAR	MONTH	DAY	HOUR	MIN	FORM
	NEXT	1234	78	9	4			REFI
:DOB	=1913							
:SEX	=M							
:DI	=LV DYSFUNCTION							
:AET	=CAD							
:ORF	=INVESTIGATION							
:REFC	=HAREFIELD							
:	=							

FIGURE 1

```
← CREATE = LIST PATIENTS.
← $TABULATE = 0.                    Start printing at beginning of
← PRINT(4) IS = SERIAL NO.                a new line.
← PRINT(2) IS = YEAR.              )
← PRINT(2) IS = MONTH.             ) Print appropriate item value
← PRINT(2) IS = DAY.               ) (if any) to occupy the given
← PRINT(2) IS = HOUR.              ) number of column positions.
← PRINT(2) IS = MINUTE.            )
← $TABULATE = 21.                  Align on stated print position.
← FORMS.                           Look up full form name in
← PRINT (16) IS = FORM.            "table" of form abbreviations.
← PRINT ITEM > FORM.               Print all items following
← END.                             "FORM" in the list of items.
←
← $STARTLINE = 21.                 )Define default page margins
← $ENDLINE = 60                    )
← HEADING(1) = " NO  Y  M  D  H  M  FORM          DATA.
← LIST PATIENTS = NEW DATA.        Define heading and list file.
.
.
 NO  Y  M  D  H  M  FORM                          DATA

1234 78 9 4        REFERRAL INFO      DATE OF BIRTH = 1913; SEX = -
                                      M; DIAGNOSIS = LV DYSFUNCTION; AETIOLOGY-
                                      = CAD; OBJECT REFERRAL = INVESTIGATION; -
                                      REFERRAL CENTRE = HAREFIELD
```

Although not shown in this example the CODIL interpreter automatically adjusts for undefined or multivalued information with the minimum of user inconvenience.

4.3 File searching facilities.

Files are searched by comparing a pair of files. The first contains the definition of the search and the second the information to be searched. The

following example prints out a list of all the patients who have died according
to the file PATIENT FILE.

```
- CREATE = SEARCH.
- FORM = DEATH; PRINT IS = SERIAL NO.
- END.
-
- SEARCH = PATENT FILE.
3 5 9 19 28 37 41 43 56 69 76 .....
```

Queries can involve several different items of information. For instance the
next example looks at all patients referred for investigation to Brompton or
Harefield hospitals where the diagnosis included the word ANGINA. Information on
the patient's serial no. sex, and age are printed.

```
← CREATE = SEARCH.
← OBJECT REFERRAL = INVESTIGATION,
←     REFERRAL CENTRE = BROMPTON,
←     OR REFERRAL CENTRE = HAREFIELD,
←        DIAGNOSIS CONTAINS ANGINA,
←           PRINT(4) IS = SN.
←           PRINT IS = SEX
←           PRINT IS = 1900 + YEAR - DATE OF BIRTH.
←           PRINT.
← END
←
← SEARCH = PATIENT FILE.
  34 M 51
 104 M 64
 195 M 57
 205 M 53
 ......
```

Questions involving several different events in the patient's history need to be
formulated more carefully as the information is held in patient/date/time order
and there is no limit to the number of statements about any one patient. Sometimes this can be done by using an additional item to indicate that an earlier
event has been noted relevant to the enquiry. In this case the item BROMPTON
PATIENT is used to hold the serial number of the last patient referred to
Brompton in 1973. This is used to select such patients who were seen at a follow
up session in 1977.

```
← CREATE = SEARCH.
←  REFC = BROMPTON; YEAR = 1973; BROMPTON PATIENT IS = SERIAL NO.
←  FORM = FOLLOW UP; YEAR = 1977; BROMPTON PATIENT IS = SN; PT IS=SN.
← END.
←
← BROMPTON PATIENT = 0.
← SEARCH = BROMPTON PATIENT.
197 209 667 905 ........
```

Complex questions are best asked by using files as conditions of indexes. For
instance in the last example the result could have been stored as a list of
serial numbers on a file called BROMPTON F U 77 rather than being printed out.
This file could then be used to identify such patients immediately on any
subsequent occasion. This can be done for any category that the user finds

useful. Given files such as ANGINA PATIENTS, BUGGINS PATIENTS and SURVIVED 5
YRS, and using the experimental indexing facility, it is possible to list out all
clinical information on Buggin's patients who suffer from angina who have
aurvived for a period of 5 years.

```
← CREATE = SEARCH.
←  SURVIVED 5 YEARS; ANGINA PATIENTS; LIST PATIENTS = PATIENT FILE.
← END.
←
←  SEARCH = BUGGINS PATIENTS.
.................
```

The effect of using files in this way is analogous to a user being allowed to set
up indexes on any items, or combinations of items, that he feels would be useful.

4.4 Data vetting.

The flexible nature of CODIL means that there is inherently less control over the
format and structure of the information being stored as compared with a more
conventional data base system. For areas of the application where the user
requires more control over the structure and content of the information being
processed there are a number of optional facilities. In addition the user can
write his own checking routines. This account will restrict itself to two
different approaches.

The first is a CODIL library routine, MAKE CHECK LIST. This scans through a
file and extracts all items with a given name, cross referenced by the key item,
which for this application happens to be the patient number. The result is an
alphabetical list of values, with appropriate references to the patients. By
scanning this list the doctor can quickly see the terms used in the systems,
spot unintended synonyms, etc. He can then use the results to amend the master
file or to chose suitable phrases for use in a search query. MAKE CHECK LIST can
also produce a file containing all the valid values of the given item and this can
be used to check whether a newly input item has a novel value or not.

The second approach can be considered as an extension of the file searching
techniques used earlier, except that the files being used contain valid items or
lists of items. For instance there might be a file called NORMAL REFERRALS that
links the surgeon's name with the appropriate hospital.

```
← CREATE = NORMAL REFERRALS.
←  SURGEON = SMITH,
←  OR SURGEON = JONES,
←       REFERRAL CENTRE = HAREFIELD.
←  SURGEON = BROWN,
←  OR SURGEON = GREEN,
←  OR SURGEON = YELLOW,
←       REFERRAL CENTRE = BROMPTON.
← END.
```

Given a file that contains the data checking appropriate to the input the above file could be used in one of two ways. Embedded in a statement such as:

FORM = REFI; NORMAL REFERRAL NONE; ERROR MESSAGE = ?? REFC/SURGEON.

it will produce an error message whenever a referral form does not contain a valid surgeon/referral centre combination. Alternatively the user might want to do no more than record the name of the surgeon, leaving the CODIL system to add the referral centre. This can be done using a statement as follows:

REFERRAL CENTRE NONE; NORMAL REFERRAL.

This will cause the appropriate referral centre to be added to the statement being examined.

5. Future plans with the Cardiac Information System

Despite the lack of a terminal at the hospital the system is operating in a satisfactory manner and currently holds details of some 500 or so patients. The next stage is to give the hospital staff unsupervised hands on experience by providing a terminal in the hospital. It is hoped to do this later this year and it will be initially used for file interrogation activities, switching to file update a few months later. Associated with the change over will be a switch from sequential to indexed files and the introduction of improved data vetting facilities under the control of the doctors.

In making these plans due note has been taken of other trials using the CODIL language. One of these involves the processing of the weekly job statistics for the University Computer Science Department. This has proved the ability of the language to handle comparatively routine tasks peaking at about 1000 transactions a week. Another application is built round a data base of genealogical information on about 1400 individuals - which contains poorly structured biographical inform-ation with the need to generate family trees, etc. This has proved invaluable in examining the need for file indexing more rigorously than would be possible with the cardiac system.

6. CONCLUSIONS

The system described above has proved valuable to all concerned. The medical staff have computer files of clinical data on their patients and there has been valuable feedback on the design and implementation of the software. The Cardiac Information System could be modified to handle any other clinical area simply by providing a different set of names/abbreviations - and of course changing any data vet facilities to match the requirements of the new system. In this connection it is worth commenting that the CODIL interpreter will run on almost any ICL 1900 computer, has been transferred to a CDC 6600, and should run on most mainframe systems with the minimum of alteration.

The next stage in this research is to examine the use of CODIL in field conditions, both inside and outside the medical environment. Because of the success of the language in artificial intelligence type applications the approach may well have some relevance to diagnostic systems.

7. ACKNOWLEDGEMENTS

The work described here would not have been possible without the earlier pilot trials involving Dr.D.Orton, then of Hillingdon Hospital, and Messrs. Palmer and Marmion, then undergraduates of Brunel University. Christine Godfrey of the University Computing Unit carried out the thankless task of punching the forms and other colleagues, too numerous to mention, have given help and advice. In addition a Science Research Council grant covers certain aspects of the work.

REFERENCES

1. C.F.REYNOLDS, (1971) CODIL Part 1, The importance of flexibility. Computer Journal, Vol 14,p217-220.

2. C.F.REYNOLDS, (1971) CODIL, Part 2, The CODIL language and its interpreter, Computer Journal, Vol 14, p327-332.

3. C.F.REYNOLDS (1974) Designing an interactive language for the pragmatic user, Proc. European Comp.Conf., p991-1006.

4. C.F.REYNOLDS (1977) Matching the computer language to the user, Report CSTR/14, Brunel University.

5. C.F.REYNOLDS, (1978) A new look at the problem of open-ended applications, Pragmatic Programming and Sensible Software, 239-251.

6. C.F.REYNOLDS (1978) A psychological approach to language design, Workshop on Computing Skills and Adaptive Systems.

7. C.F.REYNOLDS (1978) The design and use of a computer language based on production system principles, Report CSTR/15, Brunel University.

8. C.F.REYNOLDS (1975) TANTALIZE, a conversational problem solver written in CODIL Second one day conference on Recent Topics in Cybernetics.

9. C.F.REYNOLDS (1971) Handling cave fauna data on a computer, Trans. Cave Research Group of Great Britain, Vol 13. p160-165.

10. C.F.REYNOLDS (1976) A data base system for the individual research worker, Selective Dissemination of Information, IEEE, p1-7.

11. C.F.REYNOLDS and D.OMRANI (1978) Formalism or flexibility? Int.Conf. on Manafement of Data.

12 L.R.NEAL (1977) The computer handling of medical information for research purposes, Medinfo 77, p651-655.

13. R.J.PALMER (1974) A computer based data retrieval system to aid research into myocardial infarction, B.Tech dissertation, Brunel University.

14. K.MARMION (1976) The study and use of the CODIL language in a patient recording system in Hillingdon Hospital, B.Tech dissertation, Brunel University.

A LABORATORY DATA PROCESSING SYSTEM FOR NON-NUMERIC RESULTS

P.J.L. SEQUEIRA
CENTRAL SEROLOGY LABORATORY
WITHINGTON HOSPITAL
MANCHESTER M20 8LR

History

The Central Serology Laboratory was set up by the Manchester Regional Hospital Board to provide a syphilis Serology Service for the whole region. My particular interest has been the development and assessment of Serological tests, especially for the diagnosis of syphilis. As in that field, one is interested in a few occurrences in ten thousand or more specimens, a data processing system capable of analysing very large numbers of results is required, so to this end, the reports and records of the laboratory were put on a punch card, sorter, tabulator system in 1962. This system was developed over the years and proved a satisfactory if rather laborious method for reporting, recording results of four hundred or so specimens a day and which also provides detailed statistics of the origins, age distributions and other data for analysis, quality control and administrative purposes in the laboratory and hospital.

Reporting was by exception, sort control cards were included along with cards to produce a negative report for every specimen. Where the results were other than negative, the sort control cards lead the cards of the report into an appropriate pocket and the resulting exception reports re-sorted and listed out for checking. A deck of cards containing the postal addresses was added and the resulting composite deck sorted by postal address on a three column field and then listed out on pre-printed report forms. A summary card (to which we will return) with coded results and clinical data was added, the main deck of cards sorted by Laboratory number, and listed to provide internal records. Finally, a sort procedure extracted the summary cards and their associated patient data which were listed to provide entries in a cumulative card file of positive findings. Sorting and tabulation of the patient data and summary cards allowed analysis of the material examined by the Laboratory

About ten years ago, the Central Serology Laboratory and the Virus Laboratory of the Public Health Laboratory collaborated to provide a diagnostic Virology service for Manchester and the surrounding towns.

The Serology was carried out in the Central Serology Laboratory, the Isolations in the Public Health Laboratory. For various reasons including the lack of space, the Virus reports and records were put on the existing punch card system.

The requirements of the two Laboratories were very different. The Syphilis Serology was high volume, but all except a few results were available by the end of the working day after receipt of the specimen, and the total number of tests small - say three to eight.

The Virus work was of low volume, divided into Serology which required the reporting of a dozen to twenty results, ideally on two or more specimens and isolation work in which the specimens might be examined by special techniques for certain viruses in addition to the routine testing for the more common viruses. In both of these groups some results might be delayed for several weeks, but in the virus isolation work, the positive findings generally occur in a few days to a couple of weeks after inoculation, while the negative results are produced in larger blocks after two or more weeks of incubation as batches of unsuccessful tissue culture tubes are examined and discarded.

About seven years ago, it became clear that the life of the system was limited as maintenance services on the equipment were to be discontinued. An available alternative was limited time on an IBM 1130 which my colleague Dr. Gowland was running on-line to a Technicon 12/60 and 6/60. The system had a CPU with 8K core and console typewriter, a single disk drive, a card reader-punch and an 80 line per minute printer. Analysis suggested that the system was just large enough provided every economy of running time and facilities were made. At IBM's suggestion, R.P.G. was selected as the programming language and the system developed, largely based on the well defined requirements derived from our old system. The exception was that our "Summary card" became input datum for results and clinical data and our card files of complete and incomplete results became disk files. This system served us well for two or three years but increasing pressure on prime time by my system and the work of the Chemical Pathology Laboratory made the acquisition of additional computing capacity essential.

About $3\frac{1}{2}$ years ago we obtained a Data General Nova Computer with 32K of core, twin Diablo disk drives, 2 VDU's and a Centronic line printer. A multi-task system was developed based on the additional experiance gained on the IBM 1130, and which provides a data base for the two laboratories, with old data dumped to disk for future analysis.

Discription of System

The system was programmed in FORTRAN IV sublemented by Data General's Commercial and String Handling Subroutines.

Each terminal, when at rest, displays a "menu" of Services available, these include entry of various forms of data, typing a file, editing of input and recovery of data either from a reference number or the use of an alpha-numeric index.

One terminal controls the "house keeping" of the system using an alternative menu from which the appropriate job, e.g. data entry, printing reports or printing out files is selected. When one of these jobs has been initiated, the terminal reverts to its own "menu". The "house keeping" out-put device is the line printer.

One disk carries the main data files, the other the system, programs, library files and temporary files which include those of input data awaiting editing or entry and others associated with the "house keeping" of the day's reports or records. When the data disk is full, old records are dumped to other disks for storage. Current data will also be held on a backup disk or/and cassette, thus data from the inception of the system is available for analysis on the computer or one of the other Novas on the campus. The data from the IBM 1130 records are also available on disk or cards.

The concept of the system is that patients' and other data is entered and stored as it becomes available. If an input datum is a test result, a cumulative report and internal record is prepared, and the resulting data is retained in a machine readable form.

There is provision for storage of clinical data, generally in coded form in addition to patient data and results.   The resulting files provides a data base from which information on any specimen can be recalled, either on a terminal, or as line-printer tabulation, or a releatively simple program can be written to analyse any combination of data required.

Coded data to be printed out "in clear" is converted by use of a Dictionary file containing test names, results and comments.   This file is accessed using a two character key (sorted in a tag file) or by record number and provides an eight character block and a 38 character block of text which is then set up as appropriate for printing or VDU display. Serological results and cell lines are entered and stored in the record files as single character codes which are converted into two character codes for print-out.   Comments are entered and stored as two character codes.   A portion of the comment file is reserved for free narrative which is entered between quotes and is automatically alloted a code which is entered in the record file.   This section of the comment file is periodically over-written.

The system provides seperate files for each type of data, these files are referenced using the six digit laboratory number, the first digit of which indicates the record type.   Each specimen is represented by a 128 character file entry.   In addition, virus specimens have an 85 character file entry in a seperate file for patient data.   The first 84 characters of the non-virus files are identical in lay-out to the first 84 characters of the virus patient file entries.

Record Linkage

Where more than one specimen has been received from a patient, the records are linked using two fields in each record, one recording the laboratory number of the previous specimen (if any), the other the laboratory number of the subsequent specimen (if any).   Thus if any specimen from a patient is found, previous and subsequent results may also be found.   This feature is used in reporting virus serology results where the results of up to four specimens are reported together for comparison of titres, and for VDU display of previous or subsequent results.

Linkage between the serology and isolation files is provided by entering the laboratory number of the last specimen from the patient in the "subsequent specimen" field of the last entry for that patient in the "other file".

When supplied with the laboratory reference number of a previous specimen, the Record Linkage Sub-routine finds this entry, and checks the "subsequent specimen" field.   If this field contains a laboratory number from the same file, the end of the patient's record chain has not been reached, and the latter record or records are checked until the "subsequent specimen" field is blank or contains a laboratory number from another file. This record is then linked to the new record and any cross reference to the "other file" re-established with the new last record.

It would appear possible to link a patient's record in more than two files in this way by forming a ring, thus a record in file 'A' might be linked to a record in file 'B', 'B' to 'C' and 'D' to 'A'.   In this example finding a record in file 'C' from a record in file 'A' would be via the linkage in 'B', but a call in the reverse direction via the linkage in 'D'.

Patient Identification

As the laboratories receive specimens from many centres, we do not have control of the format and content of the patient data. Virology requests also frequently involve the examination of mother and baby and it is sometimes not clear from which the specimen has been collected, we usually edit the requests before data entry. The index feature on the VDU will either display a page of 20 entries starting from the first match of an 8 charactor key or full matches only. Experience with our rather undisciplined data shows that a match of even less than the whole key field plus a match of another field e.g. date of birth, or hospital reference number is adequate in all but exceptional circumstances. Of these fields date of birth was the most satisfactory as it was not invalidated by the transfer of the patient to another centre.

There are no serious programming or operational problems in setting up a full automatic linkage system, giving a print-out of full matches and "near misses" for subsequent monitoring and if necessary editing.

We have been running such a program for over eight months which prints out "matches" and "near misses".

Experience with this program suggests that, with an amendment to differentiate between twins, the "match" criteria are satisfactory and editing these could be abandoned but that the "net" for "new misses" requires widening to include common transcription errors normally guarded against in computer practice, for example 1 for I, and others suggested by experience such as for example H12345 for H/2345, 12668 for 12688, and dropped or additional characters.

Having widened the net, the true "near misses" requiring human editing or clarification by the sender might be separated from the "bad shots" by accepting a limited number of errors in the same way that a human editor uses the redundancy normally present in the data.

Conclusion

The value of such a system as a research tool will depend on the value attached to the data passing through the system as it allows retrospective analysis impossible by other methods. In the field of syphilis serology, the full analysis of results on many thousand specimens require a data processing system. In the virus work, the recording of as much clinical data as can be gathered in a reproducable manner in addition to results provides a data base which can provide insight into problems which no mannual form of analysis would allow.

Recent examples have been the analysis of Influenza A results week by week over the full period that records are available to attempt prediction of Influenza epidemics and the search of records for certain virus infections to allow the assessment of long term prognosis. A major project has been the analysis of over sixty thousand ante-natals patients routinely tested for rubella antibody to assess the variation in results due to age, area, antigen batch and technique, and measure the success of the school vaccination program.

If the data system can provide the equivalent of a "day-book" the labour of data entry of patient data into the system replaces and is generally more efficient than manuscript entry into a book and as the master entry, is consistant throughout the laboratory and records.   The provision of a machine generated index of patients eliminate the need for more complex filing than be accesion number order, and is supplimented by compact printed records.

Analysis of methods of entry of result data and of interpretation of results can, by allowing the most efficient mode of entry for the datum in question, provide considerable saving in time both to the person reporting on the specimens and to the clerical staff especially where one specimen may result in the generation of results in different parts of the laboratory or on different days.   The generation of the laboratories reports ready sorted and addressed for posting reduces misdirection of reports, eliminates hand sorting of reports and duplication of posting to individual addresses.

As described, the system is meeting the needs of two laboratories with very different operating characteristics and is producing reports of three different formats.   Alterations or additions to the Dictionary, and adjustments of the program associated with rational design of the input data would allow reporting of other non-numeric results from Histology, Cytology and Bacteriology Laboratory or of X-Ray reports.

A SURGICAL PATHOLOGY FILE

EXPERIENCES WITH 30,000 RECORDS

M.Härringer and H.Becker
Pathological Institute
University Graz
Graz / Austria

I. Introduction:

The surgical pathology findings collected at the Pathological
Institute in Graz, are conceived completely in free text. Three
reasons have been given for the necessity of a speedy and reliable
retrieval of these data:

a.) Recall of previous findings in the daily routine-work:
   Not only but especially in the case of an intraoperative
   biopsy examination, the possible existence of a previous
   record of the patient in question provides a very good support
   for the examiner. The claims made on the EDP are relatively
   simple to formulate:

   1.) the retrieval of the record in question is based on the
       name of the patient or his identification number. This has
       to be done within a small interval of time and also has to
       contain the complete wording because shades in the formu-
       lation of the report can often be decisive.

   2.) the fast processing of the input, because it is of an
       essential interest to have the data base up to date. This
       necessity becomes obvious in the case of an autopsy
       shortly after a surgical intervention has led to a biopsy.

b.) Scientific interpretation:
   Here, time does not play an important part, moreover a
   convenient retrieval system is needed. Epidemiological studies
   can be based on both relevant findings and age diagrams.
   Epidemiological changes or variations due to regional facts
   can be found only by screening the data according to the
   supplying physician or hospital.

c.) Hospital Information System (HIS):
   A combination of the two points mentioned above is necessary
   to install a HIS. Moreover a structure must be found to
   guarantee the portability of the data.

The necessity to put such a system into practice is obvious.With regard to our institute,the very beginning was in 1969 /1/. The decision was made to build up a processing of the complete free text records by using a thesaurus described later in detail.Starting by using punch cards and paper tapes,the data input was performed off-line and had been processed by means of a UNIVAC 490.

II. Present stage:

a.) Since 1972 our cirumstances have been improved by the installation of a UNIVAC 494 with an adequate peripheral completion.Using the new configuration,we have succeeded in processing a greater data bulk both faster and much more comfortably. Essentially up to a few months ago,we did not have direct access mass storage at our disposal,which were voluminous enough to allow a turn over from a serial retrieval by means of tapes to a direct access storage.Good progress was made by the installation of a terminal of our own in our institute at a distance of about 4 km from the computer in use.

b.) The development of our software for both UNIVAC 490 and UNIVAC 494 was done by utilizing completely the present system.Due to the available hardware,the 30.000 records are stored on magnetic tapes for the sequential retrieval.On the other hand,the thesaurus with its 50.000 entries wasfirst stored on a drum,then on a disc.A special handler respresents the special software for the teleprocessing via an open 4-wire data line.At present,the data input is carried out using the terminal.The records are stored off-line on a digital cassette.The computer asks on-line for them.After being processed,the data are at our disposal for a retrieval without any restriction.To perform the retrieval,we have developed a special meta-language that can be learned by the medical staff within a few minutes.

It has three machine statements:

1) SUCHE (to open the collection of search criteria)
2) GO   (to close the criteria and to start the retrieval)
3) ENDE (to stop the communication)

Five options (ZAHL = sum, ALTER = diagram, KOPF = heading, BEFUND = report, CODE = code) contribute to the specification of the output and seven search terms (NUMMER = number,of the report,EINSENDER = supplier, NAME = name, ALTER = age,

MATERIAL = specimen, MAKRO = gross pathology and HISTO = microscopy)
in Boolean combinations (and,or,not)allow the retrieval.Fig.1 is the
equivalence of a retrieval,based on all non-malignant teratomes of the
testis,with a surgical intervention,not performed in Graz,and with the
patients age not exceeding 20 years.The output has to include both age
diagram and in addition the reports in question with the complete
wordings.

```
SUCHE *ALTER *BEFUND 'ALTER 1-20' AND
'MATER TESTIS' AND NOT 'EINSENDER GRAZ'
AND NOT 'HISTO CARCINOM' AND
'HISTO TERATOM'
GO
```

fig. 1 Retrieval statement

III. Positive experiences:

Because it is simple to learn,the metalanguage does not provide
an obstacle for using the system.To the physician the transformation of his question (which is generally formulated
inaccurately) into the clear metalanguage represents neither a
real nor an emotional problem.After having made a few attempts,
he can formulate his questions in the correct way by himself.
It is clear,without any reservation,that the decision to process
the free text,not on a string comparison but on a thesaurus
basis,was right,retrospectively judged.The 50,000 entries in our
thesaurus are a synthesis of SNOP /3/, an input word list by
Röttger /7/,the CIOMS lists /2/,a diagnostic key /5,6/,
extractions of the WHO-Monographies /8/,and supplements having
their origin in the practical use of the thesaurus through
years.With this,we had the opportunity to solve the synonym
problem in a simple but nevertheless extremely efficacious way.

Moreover,the search was optimized automatically by utilizing fully the
hierarchy,because,by using a thesaurus,a retrieval is done based only
on the codes and not on the free text words.The construction of mask
expressions based on the codes of the search terms leads in a
relatively simple manner to this convenience in retrieval.With regard
to the scientific interpretation of the medical records,this method
produces a level that can only be reached in this way,because the use
of mask expressions brings a high intelligency into the system.
The use of the thesaurus bears even more fruit:
The retrieval based on the codes allows (at least theoretically) the
evaluation of data bases in different languages with the same
convenience if the same codes are used to encode the same facts.
Furthermore,there is another more practical and existing advantage
that can be derived from the use of a single thesaurus by several
hospitals: It is relatively easy to build up a condensation point of
a HIS containing free text with a direct access to all records in the
complete wording that has an easy and efficacious retrieval with a
direct benefit to both physicians and patients /4/.
Differences in nomenclatures can only be eliminated indirectly in
looking for the codes.The data become compatible and other hospitals
have access to them.In this way,they become applicable immediately to
the support of individual therapy.
The same code applies as well to the clinical term M.Waldenström
(macroglobulinemia)" as to the pathological diagnosis "immunocytoma".

IV. Problems:

Due to the changes in the hardware configuration,it was essential
to make an attempt to adapt the software in the best way to the
hardware,one step following the other to make the system as
convenient as possible to the medical user.Therefore it was
necessary to use statements and even routines that were not in
congruence with the international standards.Because of this and
to an even greater extent by using assembler routines,the
change-over from UNIVAC 490 to UNIVAC 494 and now to a UNIVAC
1100/81 was not possible without difficulties originating in the
construction of partly new software.Therefore,this adaptation
had to be done in several stages with a great investment of man
power.Additional difficulties arise when there are changes
concerning the execution system and / or the philosophy of the
hardware configuration. Often we found the necessity to
redevelop greater parts of the software which took up to several

months,because,in addition,no familiarity with the new system
existed.

To search through 1,000 records within 1 min was satisfactory
especially in consideration of the fact that we had the possible to
process up to 9 questions within one search and that we had only
magnetic tapes as large mass storage at our disposal.In opposition
to the UNIVAC 494,the UNIVAC 1100/81 will have only discs as mass
storage and tapes only for data security.Unquestionably ,a direct
access to the records using the data base systems DMS 1100 or
UNIDAS 1100 will be much faster and more comfortable in comparison
to our own system,but it will be necessary to develop new software
with an investment that is not negligible.

Our data base has the character of a pilot project.Therefore the
capacity of both man and machine power was extremely restricted.The
single terminal that was at our disposal had been put to optimal
use.A part-time employee performed the data input of the biopsy
records.For the remainder of the day,it served as a stand alone
unit to support the development of software,to test the system and
to improve the retrieval.This is the explanation for the fact,that
we have only 30,000 records at our disposal,that is a year's class
of biopsy records,written in the conventional way by a six persons-
writing staff in addition to 2,500 autopsy reports.

Another bottleneck is the maintenance and development of the
thesaurus.To do this extremely important work,we have only a student
who has nearly reached the end of his education at our disposal,
because we have always failed to gain a physician to do this work.
A last bottleneck exists in the fact that we have no computer of our
own but must share one with the institutes of two universities.
Whereas the technical institutes only need to process relatively
small databulks with great and intensive software and only need
little mass storage (with exception of scratch files).We,on the
contrary,need an extremely large mass storage,especially considering
the fact that the data base of a pathology institute becomes
interesting, and relevant if it contains at least 6 year's classes
of biopsy records (in our case,this would be some 200,000 records).
Solving this problem of mass storage is not very simple because it
must be taken into account,that we would need a third of all
available mass storage.

V. Conclusions:

It is an open secret,that a complete and rigorous free text
processing is the most convenient way to perform a free text
processing, in which a thesaurus is used to make a hierarchically
oriented multidimensional retrieval but there is,on the other
hand,a great bulk of uninteresting ballast to be processed and
stored. It is obvious that it necessary to construct a good free
text concentrator to optimize the economical aspect of the
problem.Up to now,we have not succeeded in answering the
question,if there will be installed a black and white drawing up
to a certain degree suppressing the grey tones that are often
vital in medicine.We consciously answered the question of
introducing such a concentrator negatively,because if a
concentration of the free text takes place,the information
concentrated away can never be retrieved.Furthermore,information
looked upon today as unimportant,may be brought under a new light
by new knowledge.But having been processed away by using a text
concentrator,the now interesting data can be never retrieved,because
they have been eliminated.We think that we have created a universally
usable software package.Based on its modular conception it is able
to satisfy the special needs of a pathology institute,moreover with
little modification it serves as well in the field of clinical
medicine /4/.
The package qualifies as a free text processing component of a HIS.
Due to the evolution of technology,one can only speak of a
preliminary end to this pilot project,a phenomenon,very familiar to
all who have developed complex software packages.It is necessary to
use all possibilities and chances of new hardware,even if it would
demand greater investments in the area of software.
But we also think we have created a system that proved itself, not
only in an experiment,but in the hard every day routine too,as a free
text component of an information system for a hospital with 3.000 beds.
The preliminary work to reach this goal has been finished.The further
development will show,if our model,which passed a thorough field-trial
stage,will be put into routine work.The main problem that arises must
be seen in the economic situation of our country.

ACKNOWLEDGEMENTS:

This work was supported by Grant No.1944 and No.2677 from the
Austrian Research Fund.

We want to thank the Computing Centre Graz which enabled us to
install test our system.

REFERENCES:

1/ Becker,H;G.Gell, F.Schwarz,H.Enge,W.Muhri:Klartextanalyse mit
    internationaler Klassifikation.Überregionales Pathologie-
    Register für 31 Krankenhäuser.In:G.Fuchs u.G.Wagner(ed):
    Krankenhausinformationssysteme - Erstrebtes und Erreichtes.
    (Stuttgart - New York 1972) 247-259

2/ CIOMS-Projekt,Deutschsprachiges Sekretariat des CIOMS (ed) vol I-III
    (1973-1974)

3/ College of American Pathologists (ed):Sytematized Nomenclature of
    Pathology (SNOP)(Chicago 1965)

4/ Härringer,M;H.Becker,G.Schober,G.Gell,G.Schneider: Computerized
    interclinical cross-check of radiological and pathological
    data.
    Med.Inform. 2 (1977) 141-149.

5/ Immich,H.:Bemerkungen zum Klinischen Diagnosenschlüssel (KDS).
    Meth.Inform. Med. 5 (1966) 140-143

6/ Immich,H:Klinischer Diagnosenschlüssel (KDS) (Stuttgart-New York
    1966)

7/ Röttger,P.:Wingert F.,Feigl W.,Graepel P., Gross W.M. and
    Matakas F.: Structure and development of a thesaurus for
    accomodation of autopsy and biopsy records to automatic
    free text evaluation. 4th Congress of the European
    Society of Pathology,Budapest 1973.

8/ World Health Organization (ed): International Histological
    Classification of Tumors.vol. I-XVI,(Geneva 1967-1977)

DATA STRUCTURES AND DATA BASE PROBLEMS IN CLINICAL CHEMISTRY INFORMATION SYSTEMS

A.J. Porth, I. Mieth
Medizinische Hochschule
Hannover, Germany

1. Introduction

The implementation of data processing in clinical chemistry has led to the development of many different computerized laboratories.

The initial approach to this problem was very pragmatic failing often to make full use of computer's potentials.

Until now there have been more publications an work lists, sample identification, data acquisition and other practical problems of laboratory computing than on the inherent data structures.

On the other hand one of the main goals of clinical chemistry data processing is the development of portable systems. It is therefore imperative to focus on data structures and data base problems.

2. Essential Requirements of Data Structures

It is one of the principals of data processing that "the main objective of the definition of data structures should be the optimization of both: data retrieval and the further processing thereof."

This would seem to be self-evident. However, one of the main errors of EDP-systems is that the structure of data sets is mostly defined by acquisition facilities available. Therefore a lot of data are input to the computer without anybody knowing what their use is. This has led to the creation of large data cemeteries which can never be processed even if such were possible.

Only well defined aims for the processing and the filing of data will lead to the development of suitable structures.

With the regard to their use four different types of data have to be distinguished:
- data for system control and structure description
- fixed user data that must be permanent available
- variable user data for current use
- variable user data for long term filing and archivation.

2.1 System Control and Structure Description Data

The importance of this type of data has grown in the last years. The aim is to extract system and project specific data out of the programs and embed them into structured data sets. This procedure leads to a higher flexibility with the regard to the use of a program (or a program module) within different user systems. This type of data reduces individual adaptation of programs and facilitates service and maintenance of program packages, and last but not least, increases the degree of portability.

Two main functions are controlled by this kind of structured data set: 1. The integration of program segments, modules, subroutines and specific application routines to a "task", that deals with a certain project. 2. The definition of the behaviour of these tasks within real daily routine situations. The actuel behaviour within the context of all situations having to be considered is given in "decision tables".

Type one above will be used mainly during project development and implementation and further for supplementation to and alterations of structures.

Type 2 provides the requisite flexibility for adaptation to new situations, which however, must have been forseen principally upon layout of the program package.

2.2 Fixed User Data that must be permanent available

These are project internal information which have to be codified at the commencement of project installation. These data have never or relativly seldom to be changed, replaced or complemented (e.g. testnames, mnemotechnic abbreviations, measurement units, normal values, reference limits, textelements for validation of results, etc.).

2.3 Variable User Data for current Use

This kind of data has to be available to the system over a well defined period of time and has to be updated continuously (e.g. current requests, measurement values, result output of a work station, patient data and laboratory results accumulated over his stay, quality control data for actual and retrospective survey, etc.).

2.4 Variable User Data for long Term Filing and Archivation

Parts of the data kept for a defined period of data handling are later stored for many purposes, e.g. for statistical use or to be made available when a patient returns to the hospital or the physician. Long term filing and archivation has to solve the problem of large amounts of data. Therefore mass storage media (discs, magnetic tapes etc.) are used, upon which the data are stored blockwise sequentially along with a corresponding index. Structures and codification have to be defined extremely careful since each alteration may influence data which have been previously stored and may affect programs in current use.

In the following are presented some detailed reflections on the structures of fixed user data for permanent use and variable user data for current use.

3. Data that must be available to Clinical Chemistry Laboratory

Within a Clinical Chemistry Laboratory there is a specimen flux and an accompanying information flux. Laboratory data processing organizes this information flux from the registration of the request data to the reporting of the result data.

3.1 Reference Data for Laboratory Data Handling

The main work of a laboratory is the performance of certain tests upon request of a physician and the delivery of the results. The catalogue of tests and the parameters for their description, their function and the checking results have to be communicated to the computer over a reference data set which has to be permanently available. It contains parameters with numeric information (e.g. normal values, measurement limits etc.), others with alphameric information (e.g. the test name, the test code, etc.) and some special codified information (e.g. packed indicators). No standardization has been developed in this field and therefore most systems refer to their individual set of tables and codes.

3.2 Laboratory Results

There are three stages of result handling within the computer:

492

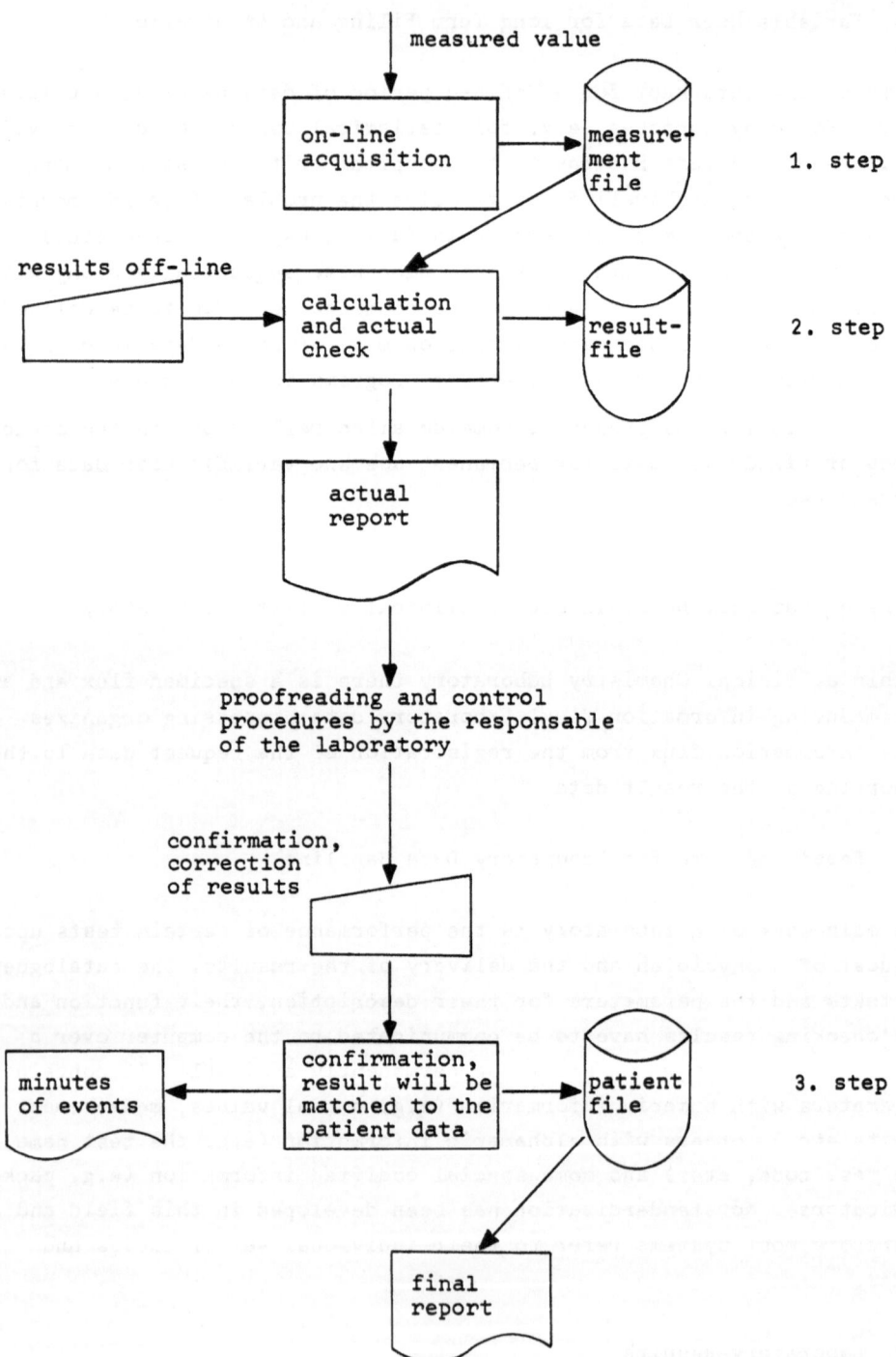

Fig. 1   The three steps of result handling

- acquisition of results
- calculation and check procedures
- storage in the patient report file

Files are required corresponding to these three stages. (Fig. 1)

3.2.1 Control File of Measurement Values Input to the System

Results input to the computer are in random order since multiprogramming serves several sets of technical equipment. It is reasonable to
put these data upon arrival into a common disc pool where they are
available to other programs working under less strict time criteria
than the measurement acquisition procedure. These input minutes are
very useful for trouble shooting.

3.2.2 Work Station related Control Files

The technician orders a report by calling up the measurement evaluation
and check program, which uses parameters from the data handling reference tables presented above. These reports should be stored on disc
in work station related order.

After proofreading the results the technician responsable for the equipment confirms, corrects or cancels the results reported.

3.2.3 Specimen and/or Patient related Control File

After the confirmation of the results they have to be stored in the
patient and/or specimen files. During the storage procedure the program checks whether there are duplicate values, whether results are
present which have not be requested etc.

All results stored in the patient and/or specimen files have undergone
a variety of cross checks and are thus made available for final reporting to the physician.

3.3 Patient Data

Within a Laboratory Information System (LIS) the patient data have
considered variable data for short term filing and current use. They
have to be stored in structured data sets to be in a position to locate
and retrieve all required information. With unstructured patient data
statistical evaluation will be difficult or impossible.

3.4   Administrative Data

Data for administration may be fixed or variable. Data for billing or for insurance purposes are fixed and must be permanently available. Variable data for short term filing and current use are mainly concerned with administrative patient data.

4. Retrieval Problems with Regard to Clinical Laboratory Data

In a Laboratory Information System all relevant data have to be available promptly at any time as information for the physician in order to check failures and for data correction.

4.1   Patient oriented Data

The communication to the user of the data required must not be dependent on any single item of information on the patient such as e.g. the patient ID with or without check number, the name only, the hospital registration number or the sample number (specimen/request number). Independent of the search argument selected the information has to be retrieved and presented to the user.

4.2   Work Station related Data

The laboratory technician needs be in a position to request a list (or display) of all or a subset of the values from a certain work station or from a certain method. It may be for example that there is a need to look for special events, or a particular trend is suspected, etc.. For such purposes the work station specific laboratory results control file suggested in 3.2.2 is very useful.

4.3   Quality Control oriented Files of Data

Current and retrospective quality control data have to be available at any time in the required form. It may be that the user needs the control list for a particular method for the previous month or day. He may, in addition, need e.g. the daily control list for the 12 parameters of a multi-channel analyzer. It may therefore be useful to store the quality control results on special files to facilitate access and organization of data.

5. The Structure of Laboratory Data Files

Having described the data we need for Clinical Chemistry data processing and tasks required to retrieve them within an information system, it remains to reflect upon the structures of the files themselves. Some common criteria define them:

5.1. Space Optimization

It is self-evident that data have to be stored in a way that the space on disc (or other storage media) is used efficiently. The data have therefore to be structured in subsets which are both: small enough to make full use of the space available and large enough to contain all necessary information.

5.2 Optimization of Storage and Retrieval Search Time (access)

The structures have on the other hand not to be too fine and sophisticated in order to avoid an inacceptable increase in access time and number of accesses which thereby lead to inflexibility of the information system.

5.3 Update Facilities

In addition to optimization of space-usage and search/retrieval time it is essential to optimize update facilities.

a) Update of fixed User Data that must be permanent available.

Though it seems to be a contradiction that "fixed" data are to be updated, within a laboratory new methods have to be integrated into the information system, as well as parameters having to be changed such e.g. measurement units, reference limits etc.. Such alterations have to be analyzed and carried out very carefully. It is essential to guarentee complete compatibility of the new tables and structures with the old ones, since the results already produced under former conditions will then be handled under the new ones as of the day these data have been changed.

b) Update of variable User Data that is in current Use

As mentioned above these data need to be updated continuously during the actual daily routine run of the computer.

The update of patient data, result data or quality control data has to be considered from the point-of-view of the laboratory organization as being separate tasks. Therefore data structures should be built up in problem oriented files interfaced with one another for comprehensive use as required by a report system, for instance.

6. Conclusion

All these aspects of clinical chemistry data handling should be considered under the condition that only problem oriented languages as FORTRAN (or perhaps BASIC) should be used since the main goal is to produce portable information systems which are adaptable to computers from different manufactures and to future developments.

Comprehensive data structures have to be created so that the user may select his project specific data sets.
The combination of these two points provides a good basis that enables the development of portable clinical chemistry information systems.

CLINICAL LABORATORY SYSTEMS

S Sargent

Queen Elizabeth Medical Centre

This paper will describe in general terms the Laboratory Service provided by the Univac 418 III Real Time Hospital System at the Queen Elizabeth Medical Centre in Birmingham. It is in two parts; the facilities provided for laboratory management and reporting and the service offered to the wards and other departments of the hospital.

A profile of the hospital functions so far included in the computer system is set out in Appendix 1. Patient Administration services have now been extended to two other hospitals. Four laboratories are included and some details of these are set out in Appendix 1. Each of the laboratories functions as an independent unit with its own Head of Department. Clinical Chemistry has two departments. The Wolfson Laboratory headed by Professor T.P. Whitehead is an experimental and development centre for new forms of automation and has its own laboratory computer. Less automated tests are performed in another laboratory which performs a much wider range of tests. Previous to the Real Time (RT) system Bacteriology, Clinical Chemistry and Haematology were using punch card methods of reporting. Haematology is still being developed but an interim system using punch card input to the RT files has been in use since 1976. It may seem difficult to justify the inclusion of Histopathology due to its low volume of reports. In fact this was developed from a "Free Text" facility in the Bacteriology system using only five man months of programmer/analyst resources and was not included in the original scheme.

At the initial stages of design we considered the three laboratories to be one unit as far as possible so that common procedures could be established. This saved time and also made it relatively easy for VDU operators to change from one laboratory system to another. The list shown in Appendix 2 is the VDU screen common to all laboratories and shows the range of services provided. Also shown in Appendix 2 is an example of one of the standard laboratory request forms which accompanies the specimen. Both the request document and specimen container are identified by labels produced by the Patient Administration system.

It was a design decision not to require ward staff to make requests via the ward VDU. From the laboratory point of view it would have served little purpose since the hospital has no laboratory based specimen collecting service.

At ward level it was considered that doctors should not be required to enter information at the VDU which was not essential. It is doubtful if this reason is valid in the light of experience but seemed a sound reason at the design stage. Two other considerations however are still valid. A standard requesting method is used throughout the hospital whether the service is based on the computer or not and in the event of a computer breakdown there is no need for a requesting back-up method.

The schematic diagram at Appendix 3 is an attempt to show the relationship of the four laboratories, the function of Request Entry, Results Entry and Results Checking and the Computer files.

An important feature of the Laboratory systems is the Pathology Data Unit (PDU). Originally each Department had its own operators and produced its reports independently. The systems analysis identified that peaks of work were occurring in each of the three laboratories at different times of the day. It was also obvious that each Department was vulnerable to periods of sickness, holidays and staff leaving. It was decided to set up the PDU as a data processing service to the three laboratories. Reductions in the number of staff required to maintain a service has been made due to the improved methods of recording data by VDU, the more even spread of work load throughout the day, and the absorption of under utilised time made possible by the merging of three previously independent small units. Staff numbers are now one supervisor and the equivalent of $3\frac{1}{2}$ whole time operators to provide the service for $5\frac{1}{2}$ days, a reduction of $2\frac{1}{2}$ operators.

Request forms and labelled specimens are received at each laboratory and a Laboratory Number is added to the specimen and request form. The forms are then taken to the PDU where the Request Entry is made, and the file record is created in the Laboratory Orientated Files. A linkage is created for Registered Patients so that a search can be made by patient. Work sheets are produced for Clinical Chemistry on teletypes in the PDU and the specimens are associated with them before they are sent to the laboratory.

The next stage is Results Entry from work sheets. Bacteriology is recorded in coded form by the technicians at the bench, Clinical Chemistry is mainly numeric and Histopathology is text. A level of validation is applied where appropriate and the valid results are added to the Laboratory files. At this stage results are not available for the wards.

Request and Results Entry is performed by trained operators in the PDU but the checking is done by authorised senior members of each Department at VDU's located in their laboratories. At this stage the report is presented on the VDU to the person checking, in the same form as it will be presented to the wards. Bacteriology reports have been translated from code to text. When performing the Results Checking sequence previous results for the patient are available at the VDU. At this point the person checking the test results has the option to approve and 'Certify' the report, he may 'Cancel' that test report so that it never appears on the ward or he may 'Hold' for further investigation. At this point a copy of the results are transferred from the Laboratory Orientated files to the Patient files and are then available at the ward VDU. This process is continuous throughout the working day.

The Wolfson Laboratory has its own computer which controls the processes of that laboratory and prepares the data which is fed to the Patient files in the RT system. No further checks are performed by the hospital computer since all necessary levels of validation have been completed by this very sophisticated laboratory computer system.

Appropriate Clinical Chemistry Results are subjected to a further level of validation. Each result is checked to fall within pre-set limits for that test, if it fails it is put onto the "Results Check List of Abnormal Values" file. If it satisfies the limits check, this result is compared with the previous result for this test, if this has occurred within the last seven days. Should more than a pre-set percentage or numeric variance occur the result is also added to the Check List file. The records of this file are inspected at a VDU by a responsible member of the Department who will decide on the action to be taken. This method ensures that every result is checked against a set of predetermined criteria, and the unusual results set aside for further investigation. These criteria are held in table form and are easily adjusted.

Each laboratory has a "Daybook" in Laboratory Number order produced automatically and a program can be called from the VDU to search the Laboratory files for an "Outstanding Work" list to be printed in the PDU. Periodically details of all specimens and reports are moved from the RT Laboratory files to Archive files kept on magnetic tape. These provide the source data for management information and research studies.

Reporting to the wards is on demand at VDU's and a cumulative printed report is produced when an update to a patient's record has been made. These cumulative reports are produced by line printer in the early evening and distributed from the Computer Unit with other reports and lists as a single postal round. It was possible to design the report presentation in such a way that the VDU and printed report are virtually identical. There is an obvious benefit in having achieved this but it is impossible to measure its effect on the doctors use or acceptance of the method of reporting. Examples of the printed form, and therefore the VDU format, of report presentation are shown as Appendices 5, 6 and 7.

The current Laboratory Reporting facilities available are shown as Appendix 4 which is a copy of the screen presented to the user immediately after having indicated the patient required. Choice 8, Progress Report, causes all of the Laboratory Orientated files to be searched for the current state of specimens sent to, all four laboratories. This information is presented in two parts. Firstly results which have been released within the past 48 hours are shown. This is followed by information relating to all unreported specimens currently held in the Laboratories, together with the stage it has reached. e.g. 'Specimen Received', 'Results entered but not Checked'. The process of entry and checking is continuous throughout the day in the PDU so that the Progress Report presented will always indicate the current position in the four laboratories. Telephone calls to the laboratories from the ward have virtually ceased.

The printed reports have two functions. During the patient stay in hospital they provide a back-up function in the event of a computer breakdown and the final cumulative reports produced ensure that a well ordered, complete and chronologically correct report is retained in the patient's notes folder. For the majority of patients one sheet of paper for each test grouping is all that is retained in the notes thus contributing to a saving in filing space.

Little comment is necessary about the features of the reports since these are perhaps mostly self-evident: Two features of the Clinical Chemistry report are worth mentioning. For each test result the 95% Analytical Confidence Limits (ACL) are quoted in the report. These factors have been derived from a long term programme of self assessment and relate to the equipment and techniques used in this hospital. The Standard Deviation Difference (SDD) expresses the deviation from the norm for a person of the same sex and age range. Tables are stored by sex and ten yearly intervals of age, and represent the normal values as derived from tests conducted in these laboratories over many years. Only variations in excess of 2 SDD are printed as a general indication of abnormal results.

In conclusion it is important to restate the point that this is an integrated service whereby both laboratories and wards derive the maximum benefit from improvements achieved in the complete cycle of requesting through to reporting back to the ward. Many of the laboratory based small computers achieve improvements in laboratory performance and report presentation but the service to the wards is not significantly improved in respect of the speed of reporting or current information regarding the status of their specimens in the laboratory. A summary of the Benefits and Improvements is listed in Appendix 8.

QUEEN ELIZABETH HOSPITAL

BIRMINGHAM

DISTRICT GENERAL HOSPITAL (TEACHING)

620 BEDS   50 VDUs IN WARDS AND DEPARTMENTS

COMPUTER APPLICATIONS - LIVE
    PATIENT ADMINISTRATION
    LABORATORY SERVICES
    NURSING ORDERS AND RECORDS
    INFORMATION - DRUGS
            - LABORATORIES

COMPUTER APPLICATIONS - UNDER DEVELOPMENT

    DRUG PRESCRIBING

LABORATORIES

WEEKLY WORK LOADING

LABORATORY	OPERATIONAL	REQUESTS	TEST RESULTS
1. BACTERIOLOGY	JULY 1975	900	2,600
2. CLINICAL CHEMISTRY	NOV. 1975	2,160	13,600
3. HISTOPATHOLOGY	SEPT. 1976	90	170
4. HAEMATOLOGY		1,300	8,100

APPENDIX 2

LABORATORY SERVICES

1   REQUEST ENTRY - REGISTERED PATIENTS

2   REQUEST ENTRY - EXTERNAL PATIENTS

3   PRINT ALL UNPRINTED WORKSHEETS

4   RESULTS ENTRY

5   RESULTS CHECKING

6   REPORTS - REGISTERED PATIENTS

7   REPORTS - EXTERNAL PATIENTS

8   PATIENT ENQUIRY

9   REPORTS DELETE - REGISTERED PATIENTS

10 RESULTS CHECK LIST OF ABNORMAL VALUES

20 INFORMATION

NAME JENKINSON SARAH M	REG No G999061/8		CLINICAL CHEMISTRY			
		DATE OF COLLECTION (START)	TIME OF COLLECTION	PERIOD OF COLLECTION (FOR FLUIDS)		H

AGE 035 SEX F WARD E1A CONSULTANT DR W.T.COOKE

RELIGION CE CIVIL STATE M DATE OF BIRTH 03/04/42

AFFIX LABEL FOR PATIENT IDENTITY

LABORATORY USE ONLY - LAB NO.

DATE OF COLLECTION	TIME	TEST		H
020	10	SODIUM, POTASSIUM, UREA		SERUM OR BLOOD
	30	CALCIUM AND PHOSPHATE (FASTING)		
	40	CREATININE		
	74	THYROXINE		
021	50	GLUCOSE (FLUORIDE BOTTLE)		
011	18	H⁺, PCO_2, STD. BICARB. (CAPILLARY BLOOD)		
013	18	PO_2, H⁺, PCO_2, STD. BICARB. (ARTERIAL BLOOD)		
015	41	CREATININE CLEARANCE		
	80	SODIUM POTASSIUM (INDICATE FLUID)	URINE, FAECAL, FISTULA, GASTRIC, ILEOSTOMY, WOUND ASPIRATE	FLUIDS

CLINICAL DETAILS

LABORATORY USE ONLY
S.   T.

SPECIAL INSTRUCTIONS OR OTHER TEST/ SPECIMEN :

M.O. SIGNATURE

QUEEN ELIZABETH HOSPITAL

QUEEN ELIZABETH HOSPITAL

LABORATORY SYSTEMS

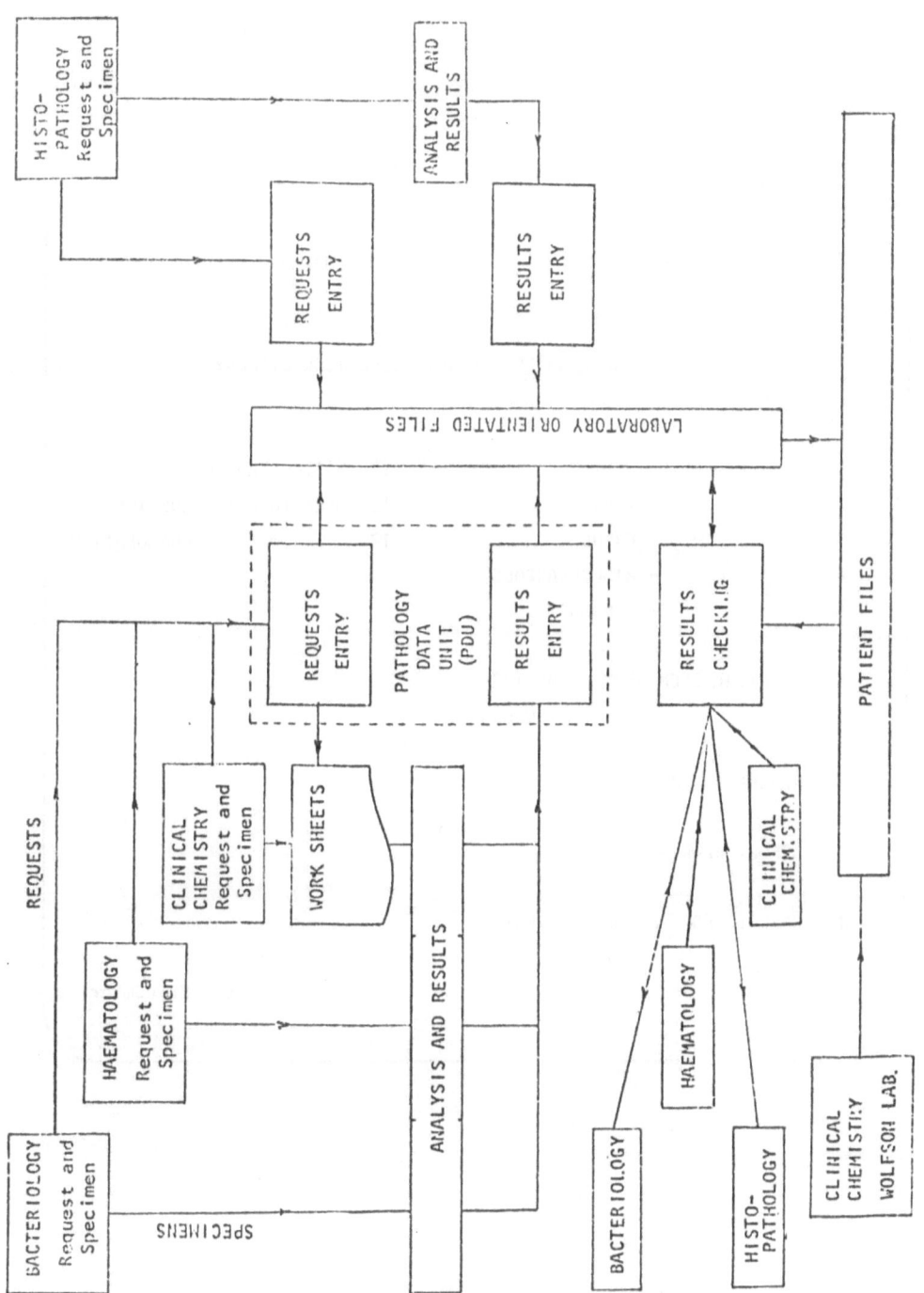

```
WWI JENKINSON SARAH M      G999061/8     FEMALE    age 34  DR W.T. COOKE


                 LABORATORY REPORT  SELECTION DISPLAY


     1    BACTERIOLOGY - SPUTUM          11   HISTOPATHOLOGY
     2                 - SWAB            12   HAEMATOLOGY - ROUTINE
     3                 - URINE           13               - COAGULATION
     4                 - MISCELLANEOUS
     5                 - SEROLOGY


     6    CLINICAL CHEMISTRY - ROUTINE
                             - MISCELLANEOUS


     8    PROGRESS REPORT


     9    REPORT REPRINT


     10   REPORTS FOR ANOTHER PATIENT


                                         Select ONE number ..
```

Appendix 5.

HMR 101a
BACTERIOLOGY   Printed: 24/08/76   Report group: URINE — PAGE 1

Patient's Name	Registration No.	Sex	Age	Admission Date	Ward	Consultant
SMITH ALAN C	G222222/9	M	21	12/08/76	E3A	DR.A.B.JEKYLL

MID-STREAM URINE   LAB NO.   236143
COLLECTION DATE   16/08/76

```
  REACTION - ACID                    * ANTIBIOTIC SENSITIVITY
  PROTEIN - PROFUSE                  * ----------------------
                                     *                    1
  MICROSCOPY                         *
  ----------                         * PENICILLIN         R
  EP.CELLS - OCCASIONAL              * AMPICILLIN         S
  ORGANISMS - OCCASIONAL             * CEPHALEXIN         R
  WBC COUNT - 400 PER C.MM.          * TETRACYCLINE       R
  RBC COUNT - 200 PER C.MM.          * NITROFURANTOIN     S
                                     * CO-TRIMOXAZOLE     S
  CULTURE                            :
  -------                            *
     VIABLE COUNT: 10,000-100,000 PER C.C.  *
  1 STREPTOCOCCUS FAECALIS: LIGHT GROWTH    *
                                     *
*****************************************************************
```

CATHETER SPEC URINE   LAB NO.   26731X
COLLECTION DATE   20/08/76   COLLECTION TIME   0800

```
  REACTION - NEUTRAL                 * ANTIBIOTIC SENSITIVITY
  PROTEIN - NONE DETECTED            * ----------------------
                                     *                    1  2
  MICROSCOPY                         *
  ----------                         * PENICILLIN         M  -
  EP.CELLS - OCCASIONAL              * AMPICILLIN         S  R
  WBC COUNT - 230 PER C.MM.          * CEPHALEXIN         R  R
  RBC COUNT - NIL                    * NITROFURANTOIN     S  R
                                     * CO-TRIMOXAZOLE     S  S
  CULTURE                            * NALIDIXIC ACID     -  S
  -------                            * SULPHONAMIDE       -  S
     VIABLE COUNT:   100,000 PER C.C.  *
  1 STREPTOCOCCUS FAECALIS: MODERATE GROWTH *
  2 ACINETOBACTER ANITRATUS:MODERATE GROWTH *
                                     *
*****************************************************************
```

HMR 101b
CLINICAL CHEMISTRY   TEST DATA EXAMPLE   PRINTED 12/04/76   PAGE   1

Patient's Name	Registration No.	Sex	Age	Admission Date	Ward	Consultant
JENKINSON SARAH M	G999061/8	F	34	29/03/76	WW4	DR W.T. COOKE

COLLECTION: DATE	TIME	Fluid Type	Volume ml	Period h	Sodium mmol total	Potassium mmol total	Urea mmol total	Protein g total	Creatinine Clearance ml/min	Creatinine µmol/l	Sodium mmol/l	Potassium mmol/l	Urea mmol/l
30/03	NG										121	6.8	60.0
30/03													
30/03													
30/03													
31/03	NG										128	7.1	65.4
31/03	1500	UR	1657	24	166	25							
01/04	1440										136	5.6	63.9
01/04													
03/04													
05/04	NG									1255	138	3.6	62.5
08/04	NG									1103	138	3.6	56.0
12/04	NG									1042	135	3.5	49.1
PLEASE DESTROY PREVIOUS VERSION OF PAGE 1													
A.C.L. (95%) ± S.D. Difference										83 / 63	3	0.1 / -2.2	2.5 / 43

COLLECTION: DATE	TIME	Bilirubin µmol/l	Asp. T. U/l	Alk. Phos. U/dl	5'NT U/l	Albumin g/l	Globulin g/l	Calcium mmol/l	Phosphate mmol/l	Urate µmol/l	Cholesterol mmol/l	Glucose mmol/l
30/03												
30/03	0800					27						
30/03	0800							1.54				
30/03	1400							1.50	2.56			
31/03												
31/03												
01/04												
01/04												
03/04												
05/04	NG	9	28	20		24	38	0.89		795	4.1	5.8
08/04	NG	7	25	17		24	37	0.86		740	4.0	7.0
12/04	NG	8	21	16		25	39	0.81		790	4.4	7.4
PLEASE DESTROY PREVIOUS VERSION OF PAGE 1												
A.C.L. (95%) ± S.D. Difference		1	4	2 / 3.3		3 / -4.7	4 / 2.5	0.04 / -13	0.13 / 8.6	47 / 7.1	0.4	1.1 / 2.4

COLLECTION: DATE	TIME	Ala. T. U/l	Amylase units/dl	Iron µmol/l	IBC µmol/l	T4 nmol/l	T3 uptake test	Free T4 Index	H+ nmol/l	Pco2 kPa	Standard Bicarb. mmol/l	Po2 kPa	Insp. O2 %
30/03													
30/03													
30/03	NG												
30/03													
31/03													
31/03													
01/04													
01/04	1440								56	5.3	16.8		

Appendix 7.

HMR 101c
PATHOLOGY   Printed: 18/08/76   T E S T D A T A E X A M P L E   P A G E   1

Patient's Name	Registration No.	Sex	Age	Admission Date	Ward	Consultant
SMITH ALAN C	G222222/9	M	21	12/08/76	E3A	DR.A.B.JEKYLL

```
BIOPSY                                    LAB.NO.   000029
COLLECTION DATE   13/08/76
NATURE OF SPECIMEN - GALL BLADDER
             ***MACROSCOPIC APPEARANCE***
A PARTIALLY OPENED THICK WALLED GALL BLADDER MEASURING 8 CMS IN
LENGTH. AT THE ONE END THERE IS YELLOWISH TISSUE ON THE SURFACE AND
IN THE LUMEN A SINGLE MULTI-FACETED STONE WAS FOUND AT THIS POINT
             ***HISTOLOGY***
THE WALL OF THE GALL BLADDER IS CONSIDERABLY THICKENED BY FIBROSIS
THE MUCOSA IS ULCERATED IN AREAS AND ASCHOFF-ROKITANSKY SINUSES ARE
PRESENT. THERE ARE LARGE COLLECTIONS OF FOAMY HISTIOCYTES WITH
OCCASIONAL GIANT CELLS WITHIN THE WALL TOGETHER WITH FOCAL
COLLECTIONS OF ACUTE AND CHRONIC INFLAMMATORY CELLS REPRESENTING
AREAS OF CHOLEGRANULOMATOUS REACTION
DIAGNOSIS- ACUTE ON CHRONIC CHOLECYSTITIS
---------
                          PATHOLOGIST  E. L. JONES
              3017,B,C,1234,1,2,3,4,5700,4200,0000,0000,**
```

A COMMON APPROACH TO A VARIETY OF CLINICAL LABORATORIES

David R Mace

Senior Systems Designer

The London Hospital

U.K.

1. SUMMARY

This paper describes in outline the Clinical Laboratories computer system operated
as part of the overall integrated hospital system at The London Hospital.
Computer-based requesting services which relate directly to the bedstate and
hence admissions System, are well - established for almost all pathology services.
In the last two years laboratory worksheet and associated results capture
services have been added for the three major laboratories of Microbiology,
Clinical Chemistry and Haematology.

The degree to which the system is basically independent of the laboratory
concerned, while at the same time being varied and flexible enough to meet
laboratory requirements, is the main topic of the paper. It has proved to be the
case that, by the use of two main files into which laboratory and test specific
data have been abstracted, a fundamentally common system is operated in the three
main laboratories. This is true, not only in the more remote requesting aspects
of the system, but also in the laboratory worksheets and associated documentation
services used within the laboratories themselves, and it is this aspect in
particular that the paper explores.

2.   INTRODUCTION

The London Hospital operates a real-time, integrated computer system providing
administrative and information dissemination services throughout the hospital
and, where appropriate, within the district as a whole (1,5)

The Clinical Laboratories system within this project commenced as a requesting
service from wards at the main site, together with necessary services to facilitate collection of specimens and to control their transportation to the relevant
laboratory. This requesting service is operated from ward visual display units
(VDU's), based upon the current patient list for that ward as set up by the
admission services and the related patient index. Requests can be made for
investigations in Microbiology, Clinical Chemistry, Haematology, Blood Transfusion,
Immunology, Virology, Cytology and Histopathology laboratories.

This requesting system uses basically common software throughout, distinctions
between investigations being controlled via the test dictionary file, which
provides all the necessary data specific to a given investigation.

A concurrent development was the provision of a reporting subsystem, whereby
laboratories enter results to the request file using their own terminals, and the
system generates printed cumulative reports overnight for distribution to the
wards. Results are also viewable from the ward terminals as soon as they are
entered.

The transit times between requesting of investigations and specimen delivery and
between performing tests and receipt of results were thus reduced (2,3). The
reporting suite was only used by Microbiology at first, but the programs were of
common applicability, inter-laboratory and inter-test variances being reflected
in the dictionary file.

The latest set of problems to be addressed were within the laboratory itself,
where the processing of specimens had relied on request forms (mainly computer-
printed) which were either returned with results added or used as the basis of
clerical entry of results via a terminal. Two distinct areas of potential
computer assistance were identified namely:

        a)   Aids in documentation and control of specimens within the
              laboratory.

        b)   Capturing results directly, thereby avoiding the potential delays
              and transcription errors associated with entering results.

As developments in these areas progressed it was of interest to assess the
prospects of maintaining the commonality of software which had so far been a
feature of the system. This was appropriate, as the overall project initially
came under the experimental heading applied by The Department of Health and

Social Security.

The system has now been developed to a **po**int where internal laboratory services have been implemented in the three major clinical laboratories of Clinical Chemistry, Microbiology and Haematology. In general, a common system exists for all aspects of the **s**ystem except those relating to the direct capture of results, where non-computer automated equipment in use in the laboratory has a major effect. This paper seeks to show how the general system commonality has been maintained while meeting the varied technical and adminstrative requirements of the three named laboratories.

3. SYSTEM OUTLINE

The processing of laboratory requests follows a route involving the following main steps:-

a) Requesting

As with most services on The London Hospital System, this service involves a series of "menu-selections" from lists on the VDU's. The act of requesting creates a record in the requests file, using the test dictionary file to define test specific items, notably the format of the result block, which includes sub-test names and units of measurement. A request form will be printed, either immediately for urgent requests or as part of the scheduling subsystem for next day collections, whereby the forms are sorted by ward and specimen type to facilitate collection.

b) Check-in

Upon arrival at the laboratory, a specimen is first "checked-in" to the system, i.e. the fact of its arrival is recorded. Where the request is already known to the system, this simply entails transcribing the request reference number from the request form into the VDU. In some cases, specimens are received with manual forms, usually relating to specimens from outpatients or other hospitals. In these cases, an abbreviated form of the requesting suite is used to create a request record as part of the check-in process, or as a clerical function in preparation for check-in.

There are three main effects of check-in:-

i) A date and time are added to the request, so that the progress of the request may be observed from ward VDU's.

ii) An entry is created in the logsheet file, so that the item is included on the appropriate list of specimens received in the laboratory.

iii) One or more entries are created in the worksheet file. This is basically an index file with pointers to the request file, where the index is sorted into work categories so that each laboratory bench or technician receives a list of work. Test items are directed to a given work category depending upon the test dictionary record used. One or more test types may be included on a given worksheet, as the laboratory requires. A laboratory number is also allocated to each specimen, sequentially within work category. This number is used as an identifier of the specimen at the work bench and to direct the sequence of running for chemistry automated categories.

c) Logsheet printing

The logsheet is a form of day book showing specimens received in chronological sequence. In Microbiology and Haematology this is the only function of logsheets, whereas in Clinical Chemistry they are used to specify the sub-division and numbering of plasma samples before the performance of the tests.

d) Worksheet printing

It is not necessary to use a printed worksheet for the direction of technicians, the request form based system being operable within laboratories. However, all three laboratories do, in fact find it advantageous to use worksheets for almost all their work categories. These sheets are printed off in real-time and delivered to the bench along with the associated specimens.

e) Result derivation

In Haematology there is computer assistance in result derivation. Here a small laboratory computer system with handset terminals assists in the calculation of cell counting results. The two Coulter counters are also linked to this local Haematology computer, so that results of some 85% of Haematology work are captured in this way, including differential cell counts, reticulocyte counts etc.

Clinical Chemistry also has an internal laboratory system, capturing results from the SMA-Plus and Technicon Mark II auto-analysers used in the laboratory. The system provides some monitoring information and assists by deriving results from on-line analysis of the analogue signals from the auto-analysers.

f) Result entry

Individual results and associated comments may be entered using the request reference number to give direct access to the request file. However, the majority of results are entered using the worksheet file in its role as index to the results file. In the automated cases in Haematology and Clinical Chemistry, there are data transmission links between the two laboratory computers and the main hospital machine and these account for over 70% of the work of these two laboratories. Safeguards are incorporated into the system to minimise the risk of associating any result with the wrong request.

For the remaining categories of work, and as a fallback mechanism for the auto-mated categories a VDU-based service for entering results sequentially from a printed worksheet is provided, using the allocated specimen number as key.

Results entered in either of these fashions are considered "unapproved", that is to say that the laboratory have not finally released the result. These unapproved results may be seen over the VDU's, but are clearly marked to warn the medical staff that a correction may occur.

g)   Result approval

The act of approval signifies the authorised release of a result by the laboratory. No printed report can be issued by the system until it has been approved.

An individual result may be approved (or initially entered as approved) via the request reference number. Much more usually, the service for approval via the worksheet file is used. In this case, firstly an approval sheet must be printed, this being a copy of the worksheet with the associated results actually printed on it, giving the senior laboratory staff a copy of what the system actually holds for each test. Having checked these results the approver may then indicate their release to the system using the work category identifier and specimen number range. Alternatively, a branching mechanism may be followed to amend any erroneous result or to look up associated results.

h)   Printing and distribution of reports

The result having been approved, the system next takes appropriate action to prepare printed results for delivery. Where the patient is the subject of cumulative reporting (currently, only main site inpatients), the result will be included in the overnight print of cumulative reports, positioned according to the layout rules in the test dictionary. For other results, the act of approval adds an entry to a list per distribution heading, usually an outside hospital or a local clinic. Individual reports are then generated on demand according to delivery location to tie in with the hospital and district transport and mailing systems.

i)   Result viewing

From ward VDU's, progress of requests and any results available may be viewed for patients admitted to that ward, or recently discharged. The progress of requests service allows medical and other ward staff to keep track of what requests have been made and whether the specimen has reached the laboratory and been processed. A separate laboratory service operates via a search of the worksheet file accord-ing to given criteria to assist in query handling. A version of this service, restricted to requests from given sources, is used in another hospital in the district to reduce the main site laboratories' enquiry load.

j) Clinic lists and laboratory copies

A number of result lists are produced to show results approved in a given day or week by a given laboratory or for issue to a given hospital or clinic. For the laboratory, this provides a long-term reference copy of results, since results are removed from the computer system soon after patient discharge or, for individual report cases, soon after distribution of results. The hospital and clinic lists are a security mechanism guarding against the loss or mis-delivery of individual report slips.

4. COMMONALITY OF LABORATORY ASPECTS

Aspects of the system external to the laboratory use a largely common set of programs regardless of laboratory or test details, these being inherent in the data structure of the test dictionary file, and extracted into the request file as required. These aspects of the system are discussed fully by Wills (2).

The advent of the worksheet file and the linkage between work category and test dictionary record provide for an extension of the principle of parameterising test-dependent factors and thereby permit the continuation of the laboratory independent philosophy of the system into the laboratory documentation area. Each aspect of the intra-laboratory processing will now be considered and the degree to which commonality of software is applicable explained. It is also interesting to note that certain test-specific developments have proved to be of use in totally different areas of operation.

a) Check-in

This service operates via totally common software. Where a request record is set up by check-in, large parts of the requesting suite are embedded into the check-in process, making use of the test dictionary as the sole test-dependent aspect. The association of a test with a work category is based on the dictionary record number to preserve integrity. In a number of cases, notably in Microbiology and Haematology, a work category incorporates a number of test types, e.g. the variety of tests performed in the Coagulation Room in Haematology and the various fluid culture tests in Microbiology. Occasionally a duplicate dictionary record has been created, the most important example being the Çoulter work in Haematology. There are two Coulter counters and work has traditionally been divided between them according to the originating hospital of the request. The computer system meets this requirement by using different but equivalent dictionary records in setting up requests.

b) Logsheets

The logsheet is basically a chronological list of specimens arriving and tests required in a given laboratory. The facility exists, currently used in Haematology and Chemistry, for common categories of work to be shown on the log-sheet in a columnar fashion with specimen numbers shown. The name of the test required is shown for non-columnar categories. Items are associated with a given logsheet by means of a worksheet file parameter and columnar items are also directed via this file.

In Microbiology and Haematology, the logsheets are primarily a record of work received, no direct use being made of them in daily operations except for reference purposes. There are two Chemistry logsheets, however, dependent upon whether the specimen is of blood or not. The Blood Chemistry logsheet is used to direct the sub-dividing of the initial specimen to provide samples for each bench involved and for the labelling of these samples with specimen numbers.

c)   Worksheets

The worksheet file contains a set of records for each work category in the system. All category related data is stored in this file as well as it acting as an index to the request file as described earlier. Some of the topics controlled via work-sheet file parameters are:-

i) Worksheet print layout

The main factor here is whether the worksheet follows a basically columnar layout or whether each entry has a dictionary result block printed. Currently, the columnar layout is used for the automated categories in Clinical Chemistry, such as Urea and Electrolytes, and for the E.S.R. category in Haematology. The facility could easily be extended to any category with short (e.g. numeric) results. The number of items per page is also parameterised.

Items of data other than the standard ones of patient identifying information and result area can be printed from the request file or the work area onto a specified point within each specimen entry by use of worksheet file parameters. For example, in categories where more than one test type is performed at the same bench, then the actual test requested may be needed, or the type of specimen or the patient's recent travels. There are many such data items printed on various worksheets according to laboratory needs. Another provision of this nature is to print other results or parts of the same request for reference.

ii)   Parameters for validation of numeric results

These fields are used to control the entry of results across the link from the Clinical Chemistry computer and the entry of results of certain categories over VDU's.

iii)   Positioning of non-specimen entries

Some worksheets require the facility to insert standard specimens at fixed
positions in the sequence for calibration checks, drift control, quality control,
etc., this being controlled via worksheet record parameters. Additionally, an
occasional gap may be set up to receive any urgent specimens or dilutions. The
requirements for such insertions are generally a function of the type of
analytical equipment in use, and there has been no call for such a facility in
Microbiology.

d)   Result entry

The method of entering results by request reference number, i.e. direct to the
request file, is totally independent of laboratory. A VDU "form" is presented
to the user giving the relevant result block extracted from the test dictionary.

Entering results via worksheet generally presents the same "form" for completion,
but automatically skips down the worksheet page to allow easy entry of successive
items from the worksheet. For some categories, the results entry service will
present a set of 5 or 10 specimen numbers for entry on one screen. These
categories are usually, but not necessarily, those where columnar print layout
is used. Two further items associated with results entry are worthy of note:-

i) Interim reports

Some types of laboratory investigation involve an initial report followed by a
further or more detailed investigation and a further report. Sometimes this
process may be reiterated a second time. For this type of work category a
facility has been included in the system whereby the item concerned is transferred
to a new "follow-up" work category following approval of the interim result.
This service was initially provided for the Acid Fast Bacilli work carried out in
Microbiology and was subsequently applied to the Thyroid Function Tests category
attached to Clinical Chemistry.

Where interim reports are less likely or where a second work category is not
desirable for local administrative or technical reasons, interim reports are
nevertheless permissible and are handled in a uniform manner.

ii)   Standard comments

In all three main laboratories there are situations where a selection from a
standard list of comments will frequently be appended to a result. For a variety
of reasons, both technical, historical and organisational, these are handled in
different ways by the system. In Haematology they are incorporated in coded form
within the local laboratory computer system. In Microbiology they are included
within the results entry suite, again coded and in Chemistry, where they are least
common, they are incorporated as an additional numeric code field in the work-

sheet results entry service for the relevant categories. Despite the variations in handling the principle of coding comments for entry is well established as being a general laboratory system requirement.

e) Result approval

The worksheet based approval service is entirely uniform within the system as a whole, requiring the user to specify work category identifier and range of specimen numbers to be approved and have reports released. Equally, resultant individual report slips, which are produced centrally in one of the laboratory offices are sorted according to patient and location and a print batch for a location will therefore include results from all laboratories.

f) Result viewing

The ward-based result viewing services provide for looking up results based on the patient identity and the list presented for selection is in chronological order regardless of laboratory.

The laboratory-based viewing service involves the inclusion of search parameters, such as a code identifying the hospital originating the request, in the index section of the worksheet file. As such, the service is generalised over laboratories, but the result seeker requires to know the correct work category of the test.

The primary operational advantages arising from the commonality of the system as seen in the laboratory lie in the interchangeability of clerical staff and of terminals. Where the system is basically standardised between the user environments, staff sicknesses or failure of terminal equipment can more readily be covered by use of the resources usually involved in another laboratory.

5. CONCLUSION

Despite the variation in work performed, working methods employed and management structure between the three main laboratories, The London Hospital Clinical Laboratories computer system is a fundamentally common system across the laboratories. By abstracting the test-specific aspects of the system into two related reference files, the test dictionary and the worksheet file, it has proved possible to write common programs to provide requesting services in the wards, laboratory management and results entry services in the laboratories and reporting services. In two of the laboratories, local smaller computers are used to assist in the calculation, derivation and transmission of results to the central computer system, thereby acting as a form of intelligent data capture. The links from these local laboratory systems to the mainframe use the worksheet file as an interface, as does the results entry service through the VDU's.

The primary advantage of this commonality lies in the reduction in analyst and programmer time associated with adding services for further laboratories, development work relating largely to the area of result derivation. Although there may be some modifications or additions to the existing system to cater for laboratory-specific requirements, the majority of the services are already available, notably the requesting, reporting and laboratory documentation services. Any additional parts to the system, for example the collection of workload statistics, can be provided for use by all relevant pathology departments and experience so far indicates that even apparently very parochial requirements can prove of great use in other areas.

Experience at The London Hospital has shown that a general common pathology system can be developed for use in a variety of laboratories, accruing benefits in transit times and in laboratory efficiency. This can lead to a relatively economic addition of further laboratories onto the system in terms of development effort. Additional computer hardware needs are limited to terminals and extension of file space.

Operational benefits also accrue in the interchangeability of staff and computer terminals within the laboratory area and reports are returned to requestors in deliveries combining all reports related to a patient. The delivery process itself is also simplified by virtue of the centralisation and pre-sorting associated with report printing.

The only apparent disadvantage associated with centralising the system lies in the need to handle a high volume of transactions through a single system, leading to occasional slight increases in response times over the excellent standard to which users are accustomed.

All in all, the advantages of a common system covering pathology services in a teaching hospital, based upon an underlying admissions system, greatly outweigh any potential difficulties, as has been proven at The London Hospital. Laboratory-specific requirements can be met by suitable parameterisation and data abstraction and laboratory reports can be presented sorted in the fashion most suited to the distribution system and the requestors, all of which is to the ultimate benefit of the hospitals users - its patients.

6.   REFERENCES

1.   Barber B. and Abbott W. 'Computing and Operational Research at the
     London Hospital', Computers in Medicine series, Butterworths, 1972.

2.   Wills A.R. 'A computer requesting and reporting system for a variety
     of clinical laboratories', Proceedings of Medcomp '77, P. 151.

3.   Evaluation Report 47 'Transit Times'. 1975. The London Hospital
     Project Evaluation Team.

4.   File Description - Clinical Laboratories Worksheet File, The London
     Hospital Project Documentation.

5.   Barber B., Cohen R.D., Scholes M. 'A review of The London Hospital
     Computer Project'. 1976. Medical Informatics 1 (1).

A 128-CHANNEL ELECTROCARDIOGRAPHIC DATA ACQUISITION SYSTEM

P Block, J Tiberghien, I Raadschelders, A Lenaers,
Ph Dewilde, E Van Thiel, Ph Smets, F Kornreich, O Steenhaut

For Reprints : P. Block, MD, Department of Cardiology
University Hospital Jette (V.U.B.)
Bosstraat
B-1090 Brussels - Belgium

I. METHODS

1. System layout (fig. 1)

This data acquisition system is composed of two parts : the recorder and the pre-processor.

The recorder is a special purpose hardware equipment, which acquires data on the patients body and writes these data on a digital magnetic tape.

The preprocessor is a general purpose mini-computer which reads the tapes generated by the recorder, eliminates the artefacts introduced by the recording process, selects, with the aid of an operator the best recorded systoles, averages them, locates on the resulting systole the QRS and T points and writes all this information on a new magnetic tape in a convenient format.

This tape is stored and used for diagnostic and research purposes.

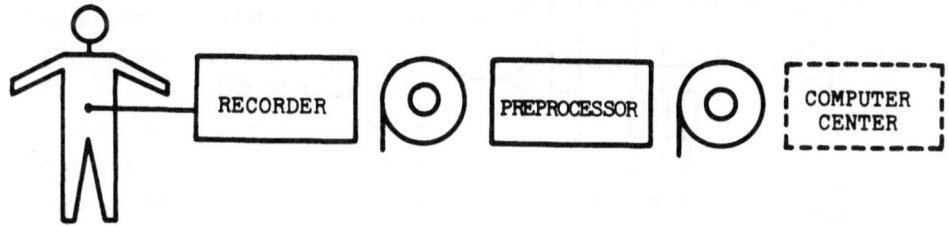

Fig. 1 : System layout

2. The recorder

Five main functional blocs can be distinguished in the recorder : the patient interface, the analog filters and amplifiers, the sample and holds, the multiplexers and analog to digital converter, the mag-tape interface and the mag-tape drive.

2.1 The patient interface

2.1.1 Specifications

- The potential in 117 thoracic locations is to be measured with respect
  to a reference potential similar to the Wilson central terminal, defined
  as the mean value of the potentials on the two shoulders and the left
  limb.

- The impedance of the measurement electrodes has to be sufficiently high
  to avoid any perturbation of the potential distribution.

- Artefacts resulting from movements of the patient during an exercise
  test are to be minimised.

- Since the recorder is to be used in hospital environment, the input
  signals have to be protected against capacitively and inductively
  coupled 50 Hz or 60 Hz artefact sources.

2.1.2 Realisation (fig. 2)

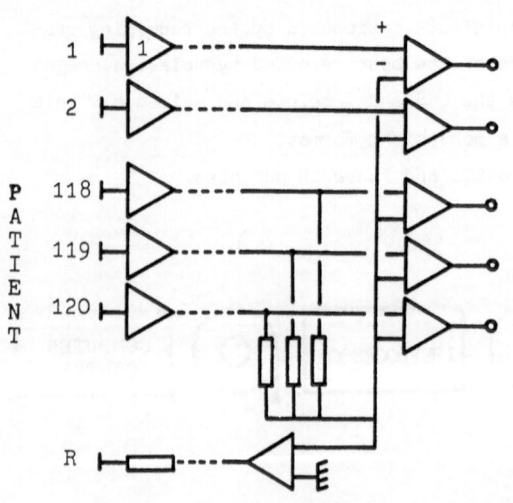

Fig. 2 : The patient interface.

Physically the patient interface can be divided into two parts :
-The first part, directly fixed on the patients body is formed by
classical silver-silver chloride electrodes, on which two transistor
miniature buffers are mounted.
These buffers have a voltage gain very close to 1 and a current gain
of at least 25,000.
By this technique, the input impedance of the measurement system is
at least 25,000 times higher than the impedance seen by any noise
source coupled with the patient cable. This practically eliminates
artefacts caused by capacitive coupling between the AC wiring of
the testroom and the patient cables, and by the tribo-electric effects
arising when the patient cable is moved up and down during an exercise
test.

-The second part, located in the main cabinet, computes the reference voltage and substracts this voltage from all the channel voltages. To reduce
the common mode rejection requirements of the differential amplifiers used
for this substraction, the reference voltage is kept close to the equipment ground potential by driving the (insulated) patient by the inverted
and amplified potential difference between reference signal and equipment
ground.

2.2 The filters and amplifiers

2.2.1 Specifications

- The signals have to be amplified 1,000 times.

- The signals have to be filtered to attenuate as much as possible all
  components out of the 1 to 80 Hz domain.

- The high pass filter design has to be a compromise between two require-
  ments :
  - A sharp cut - off is required to eliminate efficiently respiration and
    movement artefacts.
  - A smooth cut -off is preferable to avoid severe waveforms distorsions
    resulting from important in band phase rotations associated with sharp
    cut -off filters.

- The low pass filter also has to be a compromise.
  To avoid serious alliasing errors associated with the relatively low
  sampling frequency (250 Hz), imposed by the limited mag-tape speed, a
  very sharp cut -off is required, but such a sharp cut -off can be a
  source of severe waveform distorsions (overshoot).

2.2.2 Realisation

Since the distorsions resulting from severe filtering are perfectly known
and linear, and thus recoverable by subsequent filtering, and since at the
other hand, the errors resulting from high amplitude low frequency artefacts (amplifier saturation), and from the alliasing phenomenom are essentially non recoverable, it was decided to opt for severe filtering.
The high pass is a third order Bessel filter and the low pass a fifth
order Butterworth. The Bessel high pass filter was chosen so that if the
filtered waveform is displayed for control purposes, an M.D. should recognise without too much difficulty the familiar ECG waveform.

The resulting amplitude and group delay characteristics are shown in
fig. 3.

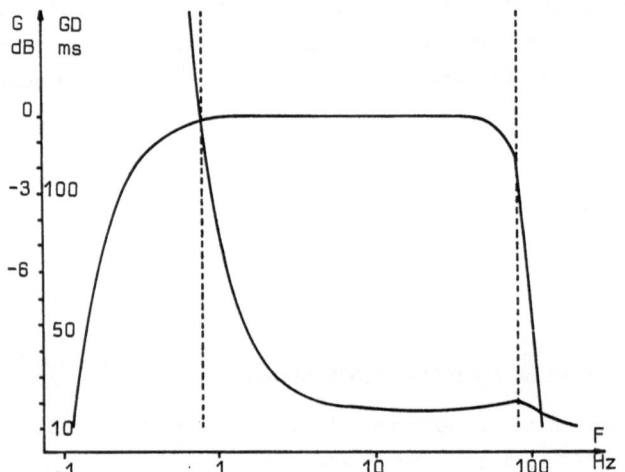

Fig. 3 :
Amplitude and
Group Delay
characteristics.

2.3 The analog to digital converter and associated circuits (fig. 4)

2.3.1 Summation networks

The three components of a vectocardiographic signal are obtained by summing through resistor networks the appropriate ECG signals.

2.3.2 Sample and Holds

All 123 channels (120 body signals + 3 summation signals) are sampled simultaneously, every 4 ms. The aperture time of the sample and holds is
31 μs.

2.3.3 Analog multiplexer

A 128-channel analog multiplexer connects successively all 123 channels to
the input of the analog to digital converter.

2.3.4 Analog to digital converter

The analog to digital converter converts successively all the 123 analog
signals to 9 bit, two's complement numbers.

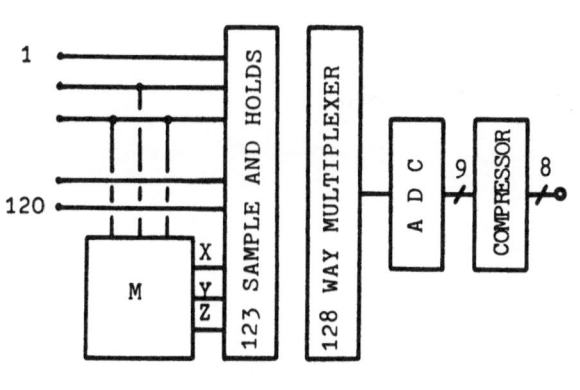

Fig. 4 : Analog to digital conversion
and associated circuits.

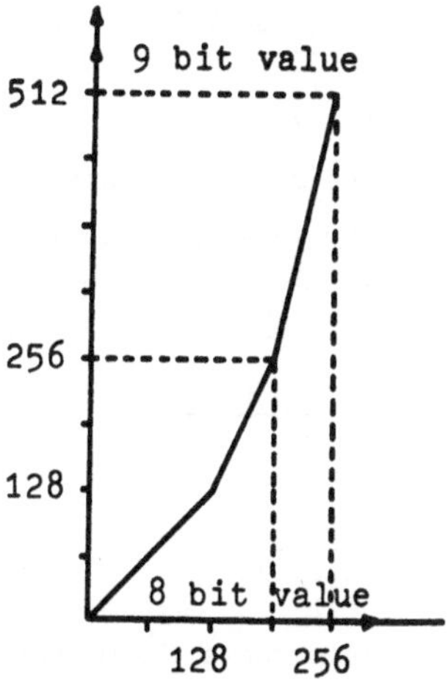

Fig. 5 : Compressor

2.3.5 Digital range compressor

The data words which can be stored on magnetic tape are only 8 bit long.
A pseudo logarithmic range compression scheme is used to reduce the size
of the measurements from 9 to 8 bits.

This conversion scheme, represented in fig. 5 assures a 20 µV resolution
for signals up to 1,2 mV, and a range extending from -5 to +5 mV. The
maximum relative digitalisation error is, with this technique, 3.3 %.

2.4 The Magnetic tape interface

This interface, built around a 4 K x 8 bit Random access memory, provides
the necessary buffer capacity to allow, while acquiring continuously data
from the patient, blocked recording on the mag-tape of those data. The
blocks are 4096 bytes long.

2.5 The Magnetic tape drive

A commercial (HP 7970) magnetic drive is used.
The recording format is NRZI, 800 BPI, 9 track.
The tape speed is 45 IPS.

3. The preprocessor

3.1 Hardware

To process the magnetic tapes written by the recorder an HP, 21 MX computer
with 112 K bytes memory, a 7900 disc, a 7970 mag-tape drive, a Tektronix
4010, graphic terminal and a Tektronix hard copy unit are used.

3.2 Software

The preprocessor programs running under the RTE III operating system have
6 different tasks.

3.2.1 Selection of good systoles

The 3 components of the summation vectocardiogram are plotted on a graphic
display, in 30-sec batches. An operator with a light cursor selects the
"good" systoles, in order to eliminate extra systoles and systoles distorted by movement artefacts.

3.2.2 Averaging (1)

All the selected systoles are averaged. This requires careful alignement
of these systoles. To find the optimal alignement the component of the
vectocardiogram with highest amplitude is used.
The first systole is digitally filtered to eliminate possible 50 Hz hum,
and then each systole is moved along the first. The covariance function,
integrated over the QRS interval is computed for each relative position of
two waveforms and when this function is maximal, the systoles are considered as aligned. This alignement is used to perform the averaging in
all 123 channels.

3.2.3 Equalization of filter characteristics

A software group delay equalizer is used to eliminate the unwanted effects
of the severe analog filters. This equalizer transforms the 123 averaged
waveforms into their complex Fourier spectra, corrects the phase relationships between components at different frequencies, and retransforms the
spectra to the time domain.

3.2.4 Base line correction (1)

When selecting good systoles, the operator is requested to put his light
cursor in the PQ interval. The base line correction routine, determines
in the neighbourhood of that point the 16-ms interval in which the electrical activity is minimal. By definition voltages in the center of this
interval will be equal to zero in all 123 channels.

3.2.5 QRST localisation (1)

The QRS and T waveforms are localized on the vectocardiogram. The results
are extrapolated to all the channels.

3.2.5.1 R onset

This point is defined by threshold crossings of the first and second
derivatives of the amplitude of the vectocardiogram.

3.2.5.2 R offset

This is defined as the point located at least 80 ms after R onset, in
which the second derivative of the amplitude is maximal.

3.2.5.3 T offset

This point is defined by a threshold crossing of the low pass filtered,
first derivative of the amplitude.

3.2.6 Display and storage of results

Finally all 120 waveforms are plotted, in groups of 30 on the graphic
display, and recorded on a new magnetic tape.

---

(1) These algorithms were proposed by H.K. WOLF.

II. MATERIAL

The populations observed consisted of a group of 25 ostensibly normal subjects
(age 28-59, mean : 41) and of 25 male patients diagnosed as having CAD but without
evidence of myocardial infarction (MI) (age : 40-55, mean : 47). The notion of
Normality was based on the assumption that no heart disease or other diseases that
might alter the ECG were detected, neither in the history, the physical and radiological examinations, the resting standard 12-lead ECG or on the myocardial scintigraphy during exercise.
All patients presented abnormalities of the coronary arteries (narrowing of the
lumen > 50 % in one or more of the arteries), while other diseases with possible
ECG alterations were, as already stressed, excluded. None of the subjects, either
normal or with CAD, demonstrated any abnormality during repolarization in the
resting standard 12-lead ECG (whether abnormal downward slope of ST-segment > -.05 mV
or abnormal negative T waves).
In all subjects at least one recording at rest in sitting position, one at the end
of a graded exercise test on a bicycle and one immediately after interruption were
examined. The interruption criteria of the exercise test were those preconized by
the W.H.O.
A myocardial scintigraphy was performed in each subject, after an intravenous injection of 2 mci 201 TL.
The technical aspects of this examination have already been described.

III. RESULTS

As far as the depolarization is concerned and as previously described, we observed
the same features as those described by Taccardi.
No significant differences were observed between the normal subjects and those
with CAD but without a known myocardial infarction, either at rest as during exercise. A slight to moderate increase in the amplitude of the maximum and minimum
of QRS was frequently observed (in 14/25 of the normals and in 18/25 of the patients
with CAD). But 6 out of the 25 patients with CAD demonstrated an increase of the
late positive potentials in the upper mediastinal and right subclavicular areas with
a decrease of the late positive potentials in the left precordium, these features
were not observed in our normal group.
In the normal subjects, during the repolarization, at rest as well as during exercise and in the early recovery period, a region with negative ST forces appeared
only on the right scapular, upper dorsal and right thoracic area, at least during

the major part of the repolarization.

With an exception for the first instants of the repolarization (first 10 to 50 msec), and this mainly at exercise, the precordial and left hemithoracic areas were positive in all but 3 out of the 25 apparently normal subjects. However, the amplitude of these negative potential areas was less than -50 µV.

Although only patients with normal repolarization in the standard 12-lead ECG at rest were selected, 5 out of them nevertheless showed abnormal ST patterns in the body surface maps when recorded at rest. The abnormality was characterized by ST negative potentials > -50 µV beside the normally negative areas in regions not scanned by the 12 standard leads, one example of which is shown in fig. 6.

For the study of the ST mapping images recorded during exercise, our attention was mainly focussed on the instant ST60 (60 msec after the J point), since on the basis of previous studies   and of the inspection of the mapping images, recorded on the 10 msec, this instant provided indeed the best discrimination between normals and subjects with CAD, although ST70 gave approximately identical results. Taking into account the features observed in the normal subjects, we considered as pathologic the presence on the body surface maps of a negative ST60 region > -50 µV beside the normal negative ST region as described before. With this criterion, a sensitivity of 100 % was reached for a specificity of 88 %.

If instead of a level of -50 µV we took -90 µV as critical value for the negative ST60 area, a specificity of 100 % was reached but at the cost of a lower sensitivity (84 %). In both cases, however, the performance was much higher compared to that obtained with the classical criterion consisting of a horizontal or downward ST depression $\geq$ -.1 mV in V_{2-4-6}, with performances which reached respectively 94 % and 92 % instead of 80 % (p < .05) with the classical criteria.

No ST elevation in the left hemithoracic and hence in the precordial leads was observed in any out of the 25 patients with CAD. The modifications at exercise of the T waves were less systematic and their examination did not improve the diagnosis of coronary insufficiency.

The recordings at the early recovery as well as the time-normalized ST criteria (1/8 ST) did not improve the results. This is in concordance with previous findings obtained with the XYZ leads recorded at exercise.

Examples of isopotential mapping images at the instant ST60 recorded at rest and during the end of the exercise in a normal subject and in one patient with CAD are shown in fig. 6.

Despite the excellent separation of subjects with and those without CAD, no relation was observed between the location of the abnormal ST regions (ST60 > -50 µV) and the site of the coronary artery obstructions as visualized by the coronary arteriography. A complete agreement occurred in only 55 % of the cases, a figure which is comparable to that reached by myocardial scintigraphy at exercise (table 1).

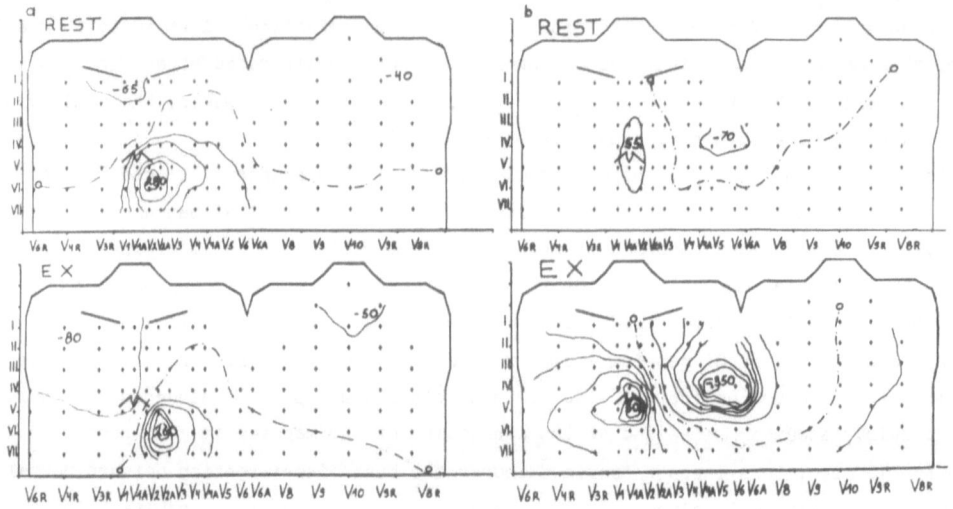

Fig. 6 : Isopotential mapping images of ST60 recorded at rest and at the end of the
exercise test in a normal subject (a) and in a patient with CAD (b). Each
corresponds to the location of one thoracic electrode. The 3 limb electrodes according to the technique of Mason are not indicated.

TABLE 1	Mapping images		Scanning images	
	Correct	Inaccurate	Correct	Inaccurate
Stenoses > 70 %	diagnosis	diagnosis	diagnosis	diagnosis
LMCA or LAD + Cx	3	0	1	1
LAD	5	1	4	2
RCA or Cx	2	1	1	0
LCA + RCA	4	9	2	5
Total	14/25 (56 %)	11/25 (44 %)	8/16 (50 %)	8/16 (50 %)

Correct diagnosis : all the stenosed coronary arteries are correctly diagnosed
without any false positives.
Inaccurate diagnosis : too many or too few stenosed coronary arteries are diagnosed according to coronary arteriography findings.
Remark : only 16 of the 25 patients with CAD underwent myocardial scintigraphy
at exercise.

The discordances were found mainly in the cases with more than one significant
coronary artery stenosis. Indeed, the results appeared better in the small number of cases with single vessel disease, especially for the differential diagnosis
between right coronary (RCA) or circumflex artery (Cx) and left anterior descending
(LAD) or main left coronary artery (MLCA) stenosis.

IV. CONCLUSIONS

The described equipment allowed for the first time the recording of complete potential distribution during an exercise test. Due to the careful design of the equipment an acceptable signal to noise ratio was obtained.
Concerning the results obtained in the small group of 50 subjects, the diagnostical
performance (92 to 94 %) was comparable to this obtained by the scintigraphy images
recorded during exercise (92 %), and much higher than these obtained by the classical ECG criteria determined on the conventional leads, whose diagnostical performance was comprised between 80 and 84 %.
In conclusion, as far as the diagnosis of coronary insufficiency at exercise in
male subjects and with normal rest ECG is concerned, the recording of surface potential mapping images allowed to reach the same very good results as those obtained by the myocardial scanning images. Both were much better in comparison with
the one got by the classical exercise ECG techniques.

FEATURES TO SEGMENTATE EEG RECORDINGS: A COMPARATIVE STUDY

B.H. Jansen, A. Hasman, S.L. Visser
Department of Medical Informatics
and EEG department, Valerius Clinic,
Free University, Amsterdam

INTRODUCTION

At our institution, techniques are developed to parameterize and classify the human, spontaneous EEG. Ongoing changes in an EEG should be detected with the aid of these methods in an early phase.
We learned from a previous study (1) that the intra-individual variability is much smaller than the inter-individual variability of the EEG recorded from normals. This was shown by means of a classification procedure. The nine recordings of each subject (registrated within a three weeks period) were divided in 90 epochs of 10 seconds each. Using half of these epochs to estimate mean vector and dispersion matrix of each subject, 90% of the other intervals were assigned correctly by means of a least-chi-square analysis method. However, the classification was much worse if the EEG was recorded one year later than the other nine registrations. This indicates a relatively large intra-individual variability over 10 sec. epochs due to e.g. fluctuations in level of vigilance. Therefore, it was suggested to develop a segmentation technique in order to cope with this problem (2,3). This technique comprises four steps. Firstly the EEG is subdivided in short intervals of 1 to 2 seconds. Secondly, these segments are parameterized and each segment is compared with every other one in a learning procedure (third step). The learning procedure reduces the EEG to a number of different intervals ("patterns") which can be used to simulate the original EEG by replacing an original interval by the most similar "pattern". Differences between two EEG recordings of the same individual can be expressed e.g. as differences in the number of times a certain pattern occurs in each recording. The outcome of the above outlined strategy depends on the choice of the methods and features used for parameterization. In order to detect the most powerful features for each method used, stepwise discriminant analysis was applied on a number of "stationary" EEG intervals which were selected and classified visually by one of the authors (SLV). This paper reviews the methods used and presents some results.

534

THEORY

1. Feature extraction

As a first step, the EEG is subdivided into segments of fixed length, such that each segment overlaps the preceding one by half. This overlapping makes the procedure of determining the point where the EEG changes more accurate. These segments, preferably 1.28 seconds long, are quantified.

In this study three different methods are applied:
1. autoregressive modelling
2. power spectral analysis
3. texture analysis
From each of these methods parameters are extracted.

1.1 Autoregressive modelling

Several authors (4,5) have reported the application of an autoregressive model to quantify an EEG interval. This model is represented by the equation:

$$y(t) = C_1(t)y(t-1) + C_2(t)y(t-2) + \ldots + C_n(t)y(t-n) + W(t)$$

where $y(t)$ represents the EEG sample amplitude at time t.
The coefficients $C_i(t)$ (i=1,2,...,n) are the model coefficients and $W(t)$ is the white noise term. The order n of the model determines the variance of $W(t)$ and is 10 in this study. Isaksson (6) describes a method, based on a Kalman-filter, to estimate the model coefficients. Once the model is adjusted in such a way that the original signal resembles the model output, the coefficient vector (state vector) can be used to represent the EEG. Here, the averaged state vector is calculated for each segment of 1.28 seconds.

1.2 Power spectral analysis

The most well-known and widely used quantification technique in EEG analysis is probably power spectral analysis. In this study, the EEG segments are transformed by means of a Fast Fourier Transform as described by Cooley and Tukey (7). From this spectrum, 14 features are extracted and listed in table 1.

```
total power:    ptot
relative power delta band ( 0 -  4 Hz): reld
     "        "   theta band ( 4 -  8 Hz): relt
     "        "   alpha band ( 8 - 12 Hz): rela
     "        "   beta  band (12 - 25 Hz): relb

 e
  log of power in the delta band        : logd
     "   "    "   "   "   theta   "      : logt
     "   "    "   "   "   alpha   "      : loga
     "   "    "   "   "   beta    "      : logb


peak frequency                          : pk - f


mean frequency in the delta band        : fm - d
     "       "    "  "   theta   "       : fm - t
     "       "    "  "   alpha   "       : fm - a
     "       "    "  "   beta    "       : fm - b
```

Table 1: listed are the features
extracted from the
power spectra

1.3 Texture analysis

This method builds up a kind of transition matrix called the
texture matrix. Each element (i,j) in this matrix is incremented
by one if the amplitude from one sample to the consecutive one
changes from the value i to the value j. The procedure is visualized in figure 1. A number of features were extracted from these
matrices, containing information about frequency and amplitude of
the EEG segment concerned. Moreover, the number of zerocrossings
and the standard deviation of the signal amplitude were computed
too. Table 2 gives an overview.

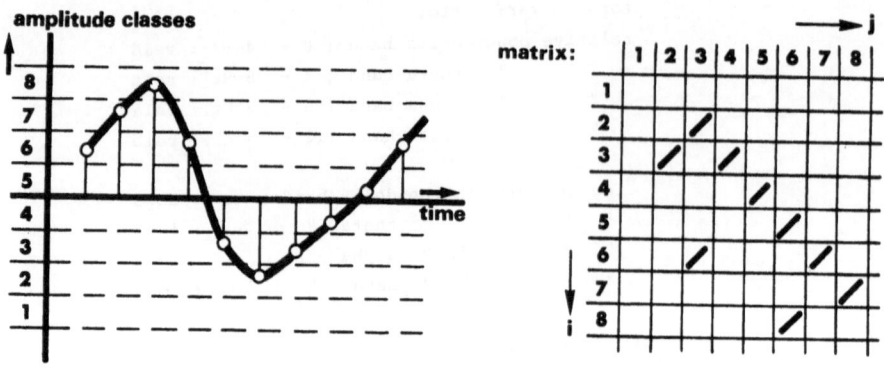

figure 1: composing the texture matrix

hgth : largest, vertical distance between two filled elements

$$\text{eij} : \sum_{i=1, j=1}^{n\ n} (i-j)^2 \qquad , \text{ n = order of matrix}$$

$$\text{eijn} : \sum_{i=1, j=1}^{n\ n} (i-j)^2 \times N(i,j) \qquad N(i,j) = \text{contents of element } i,j \text{ of matrix}$$

$$\text{ampl} : \sum_{j=1}^{n} (\frac{n}{2}-j)^2 \times N(j,j)$$

$$\text{freq} : \sum_{i=1, j=n-i+1}^{n\ 1} (\frac{n}{2}-i)^2 \times N(j,i)$$

$$\text{asym} : \sum_{i=1, j=1}^{n\ n} \{N(i,j) - N(j,i)\}^2$$

dev : standard deviation of amplitude

zero : number of zerocrossings per 1.28 seconds

Table 2: listed are the features extracted
from the texture matrices

2. Feature selection

In this case, the aim of the feature selection is to search for
those variables that characterize the different segments best.
These parameters can be determined by the multiple analysis of
covariance as described by Cooley and Lohnes (8) assuming that
1. the features have a multivariate normal probability distribution
2. and the variance-covariance (dispersion) matrices of all clusters
   are identical.
It was shown earlier (9) that slight deviations from normality do
not affect the outcome of the procedure.

3. Classification

The usefulness of the selected features can be established by means
of a classifier based on similar assumptions as mentioned in paragraph 2. For this purpose the following discriminant function is
suitable:

$$g_i(\vec{x}) = (\vec{x}-\vec{\mu}_i)^t \Sigma^{-1} (\vec{x}-\vec{\mu}_i)$$

where $\vec{x}$ is the feature vector belonging to the segment to be classified, $\vec{\mu}_i$ the mean vector of cluster i and Σ the pooled-dispersion
matrix. The feature vector $\vec{x}$ is assigned to that cluster for which
the discriminant function is at a minimum. Both the feature selection
procedure and the classifier are part of a larger interactive statistical pattern recognition package (ISPAHAN), developed by
Gelsema (10).

RESULTS AND CONCLUSIONS

In this study, two sets of EEG recordings (P_3-O_1) were segmented and
classified visually by an electroencephalographist. One set, consisting
of 6 EEG's recorded from 4 subjects (2 renal patients and 2 healthy
students) served as training set. The second collection was used for
testing purposes and consisted of 7 EEG's recorded from 2 renal patients
(one patient was also part of the training set, but now the EEG's were
recorded immediately before and after a dialysis instead of 24 hours
after dialysis as was done with the EEG of that patient used in the
training set). During the training phase, the best discriminating
features were determined and evaluated by means of a least-chi-square
classifier. The validity of the hierarchy thus obtained was proven in
the testing phase.

1. Training phase

The electroencephalographist distinguished eleven different types
of segments (clusters) each containing about 30 seconds of EEG.
Typical segments of each cluster are shown in figure 2.

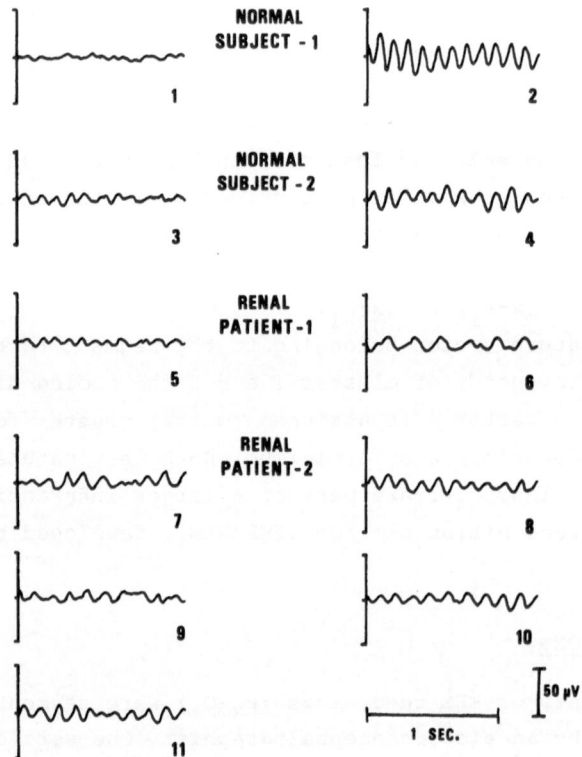

figure 2: Typical members of the eleven clusters as distinguished by
an electroencephalographist

After calculation of the power spectral features, the autoregressive
coefficients and the texture parameters, the feature selection
procedure was applied on half of the data set.

autoregressive coefficients	power spectral features	texture features
c 4	loga	dev
c 1	fm - a	eijn
c 6	relt	zero
c 3	ptot	eij
c10	fm - t	asym
c 8	logb	hgth
c 7	fm - b	ampl
c 5	fm - d	freq
c 9	logd	
c 2	logt	
	pk - f	
	relb	
	rela	
	reld	

Table 3: features hierarchically structured
according to their discriminating power

Table 3 shows the hierarchy of the parameters for the three different feature extraction methods. The higher a feature ranks in the table, the better it discriminates between the clusters. The 10 autoregressive coefficients, together with the five best discriminating features of the other methods were used again as input for the selection method. The resulting hierarchy is depicted in table 4. Note the dominancy of the autoregressive coefficients.

1	c 4		11	relt
2	loga		12	fm - a
3	c 6		13	ptot
4	c 1		14	dev
5	c 3		15	eijn
6	c10		16	zero
7	c 8		17	asym
8	c 7		18	eij
9	c 5		19	c 2
10	fm - t		20	c 9

Table 4: feature hierarchy for the combination
of the parameters of the three extraction
methods

The classification procedure used the same data to compute the mean
vectors of the eleven clusters and the pooled dispersion matrix.
The remaining data were then assigned to that cluster for which the
discriminant function was at a minimum. Extending the number of
features with the next best discriminating one resulted in a classification performance as shown in figure 3.

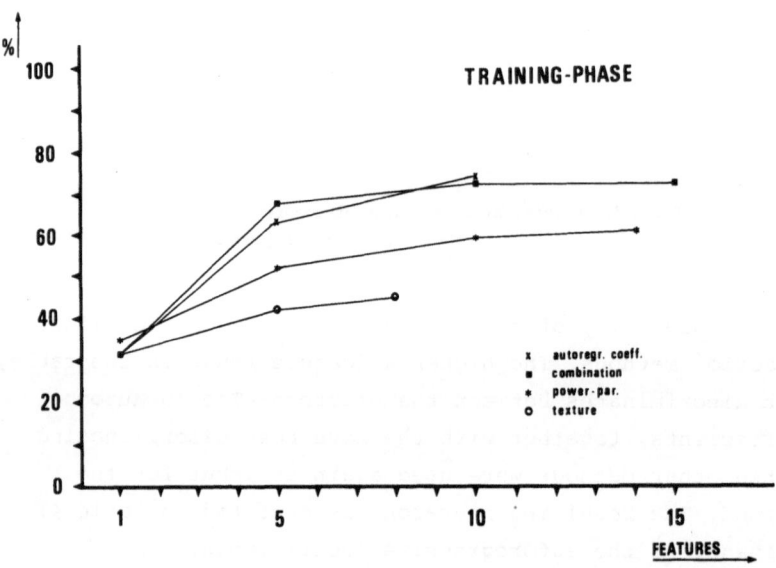

figure 3: Classification results as a function of the number of best
          discriminating features. The numbers along the horizontal
          axis refer to table 4.

Using the 5 best discriminating features, 68% correct classifications
were obtained. It can be seen from figure 3 that the autoregressive
coefficients alone performed almost as well. It appeared that these
10 features in combination with a measure for the signal amplitude
gave the best results: 74% when LOGA was used for that purpose and
78% when DEV was included. As can be seen from the confusion matrix,
shown in figure 4, most of the wrong classified segments are from
the clusters 7 through 11. Although the electroencephalographist
distinguished these clusters visually, the differences are not very
distinct. Therefore, the consistency of the visual classification
was checked. All the data, used thus far, was presented to the
electroencephalographer a second time.

	1	2	3	4	5	6	7	8	9	10	11
1	21										
2		24									
3			24	3							
4			4	7							
5					30	1				4	
6						8					
7							13	1	8	1	
8							3	6		2	1
9							7		17	1	
10							4	4	3	23	10
11							5	3		7	19

figure 4: Confusion matrix, using 10 best features as shown in table 4.
Horizontal: posteriori classification
Vertical : a priori classification
The number of correct classifications is depicted on the
upper-left, lower-right diagonal

Now, he was able to distinguish only seven clusters. This lack of
consistency is probably due to the fact that an electroencephalographer is much more accustomed to classify longer intervals (e.g.
10 sec.) than 1.28 second intervals.
Figure 5 shows the rearrangement of the data in the form of a
confusion matrix. From this matrix, it can be seen that only the
original clusters 1 and 6 were a one to one projection of the
newly formed clusters 2 and 4, respectively. Especially clusters 7
through 11 were mixed up although cluster 8 could be completely
distinguished from cluster 9. These findings are in ful agreement
with the computer-classification results as already shown in figure 4.

	1	2	3	4	5	6	7	8	9	10	11
1			4				25		15	9	
2	52										
3			17		80						6
4						17					
5		52		13							
6			6	10			10	26		56	42
7			38	5			15		42	28	24

figure 5: Consistency of the visual classification:
        horizontal: a posteriori classification
        vertical : a priori classification

2. Testing phase

The seven EEG's used in the testing phase were visually segmented
into 12 clusters by the electroencephalographist. Half of the data
were used to estimate the parameters of the probability density
functions. The other half was used as input for the classification
procedure. Application of the 10 best discriminating features, as
determined during the training phase, resulted in 61% correct
classifications. This classification result is much lower than
obtained with the training set. However, from figure 4 it can be
calculated that the correct assigned segments of the EEG's of the
two renal patients used in the training phase is also 61%.
Moreover, this is comparable to the 63% correctly assigned segments
when the 10 best discriminating features were used that were obtained
by applying the feature selection method on the data of the testing
set. Moreover, this hierarchy was almost the same as the one obtained
during the training phase: again the autoregressive coefficients
were high ranking features in combination with amplitude measures
as LOGA, PTOT and DEV.

Classifying by means of the combination of the 10 autoregressive coefficients and LOGA or DEV gave the best results here too: 62%, respectively 65% correct assignments.

Therefore, it is justified to assume that autoregressive coefficients, estimated by means of Kalman filtering, in combination with some measure for amplitude, are best suited to segmentate EEG-recordings.

LITERATURE

(1) F.M. Grosveld, B.H. Jansen, A. Hasman, S.L. Visser:
La reconaissance des individus à l'interieur d'un groupe de seize
sujets normaux
Rev. EEG Neurol.Physiol., 1976, 6, 2, 295-297

(2) B.H. Jansen, A. Hasman:
Quantification of the EEG variability
Accepted for publication in Int. Journal of Biomedical Computing

(3) A. Hasman, B.H. Jansen, G.H. Landeweerd, A.W. van Blokland-Vogelesang:
Demonstration of segmentation techniques for EEG records
Accepted for publication in Int. Journal of Biomedical Computing

(4) P.B.C. Fenwick, P. Michie, J. Dollimore, G.W. Fenton:
Simulation of the electroencephalogram using an autoregressive series
Biomedical Computing (2), 1971: 281-307

(5) L.H. Zetterberg:
Experience with analysis and simulation of EEG signals with parametric
description of spectra
Automation of clinical electroencephalography (eds. P. Kellaway,
I Petersén), Raven Press, New York, 1973

(6) A. Isaksson:
On time variable properties of EEG signals, examined by means of a
Kalman filter method
Techn. Rep. no. 95, April 1975, Telecom. Theory / Electr. Eng.
Royal Institute of Technology, Stockholm

(7) J.W. Cooley, J.W. Tukey:
An algorithm for the machine calculation of complex fourier series
Math. Comp. 19 April 1965

(8) W.W. Cooley, P.R. Lohnes:
Multivariate Data Analysis - John Wiley & Sons, Inc., New York, 1971

(9) B.H. Jansen:
Quantitative aspects of EEG variability
Internal report, Dept. of Med. Inf., Free University, Amsterdam

(10) E.S. Gelsema:
ISPAHAN Users Manual, 2nd edition, department of Medical Informatics,
Free University, Amsterdam, September 1977

ABSCESS

A SYSTEM FOR THE ANALYSIS BY SMALL COMPUTER
OF EEG SIGNALS IN A CLINICAL SETTING

B.B. MacGillivray, D.G. Wadbrook, P.M. Quilter and J. Douglas
The Royal Free Hospital
London

The clinical electroencephalogram, (EEG), is a recording, customarily of 16 channels of ten to fifteen minutes duration, of the electrical activity of the cerebral cortex carried out for the purpose of establishing the presence and nature of physical or biochemical disorders of the brain. The EEG is to the brain much as the ECG (electrocardiogram) is to the heart, but is far more complex and its generation less well understood. It is primarily used as a screening device, to detect whether the brain is normal or not and in the elucidation of the diagnosis of epilepsy and it shows the presence of structural changes such as occurs with strokes and cerebral tumours and infections of the brain, for example, abscess or encephalitis. It is a sensitive test of function but commonly limited in its ability to precisely locate discrete lesions which are better visualised by x-ray methods.

The EEG is in itself, save for a few particular conditions, non-specific with respect to the pathology of brain disorders, but taken in conjunction with the clinical features of a problem, it can often differentiate between a number of possible causes. Interpretation is largely empirical and based on long experience and although there are some general principles, the theoretical background is poor because of the complex nature of the brain and our present limited understanding of its mechanisms.

The EEG signal itself consists of a complex sequence of wave patterns which vary in time and in location on the surface of the head. The main characteristics taken into account in interpretation are shape, frequency characteristics, amplitude, topographic distributions and variance with time.

A report on an EEG consists of a short description of the main features usually couched in simple jargon, a conclusion which summarises the abnormality and its location, and an interpretive statement which relates the findings to the clinical problem. The last two are frequently combined.

From the early clinical use of the EEG in the middle thirties, various techniques have been used in an attempt to measure and quantify EEG patterns, mostly based on filtering techniques and the frequency domain but also using time domain methods (see recent reviews in Dolce, 1974 and Rémond, 1977).

Computing of course, vastly enhances the power, speed and sophistication of these processes but has up until now largely been used as an ancillary to visual inspection. We have set out to automate the whole process from the recording to the conclusion and interpretation. The primary motivation is practical, to reduce the demands on a limited number of skilled personnel and to improve accuracy and consistency by eliminating the subjective component of EEG interpretation. To date we have been moderately successful in achieving an output which compares with that of a skilled clinical interpreter using eye-balling methods. Quantification and formalisation of the interpretive process also provides the background for heuristic development of new procedures.

The general system requirements from the outset have been as follows:

1) collection and storage of upto 24 channels of analogue EEG and other signals for ten minutes or more.
2) data processing to achieve comparisons between channels and against archival records including normal reference values.
3) interpretation in relation to clinical data.
4) acceptable output.
5) ease of use.

Methodology

We have used Fourier spectral analysis as the primary data processing procedure because it is well understood and produces a frequency domain solution familiar to EEG interpreters using traditional methods. Additionally the availability of low cost Fourier transform hardware allows real time analysis of multichannel signals.

Data acquisition is preceded by an interactive system check routine carried out by the recording technician which includes a calibration procedure. The latter allows the verification of all twenty four channels and the calculation of gain correction factors for each channel, which are automatically implemented during data acquisition. Digitisation is normally at 128Hz, 12 bits, and storage is on disc, for immediate use, and tape. Normally five minutes of routine data are collected from the subject under controlled conditions of alertness and rest.

Patient data, personal details, and clinical information are entered by VDU keyboard at the end of recording and the relevant segments of the record, excluding obvious artefacts, identified for computer processing. The remainder of the process to the production of the final report is automatic. Staff indoctrination is minimal.

Pre-processing of the raw data includes gain correction and removal of unwanted signals generated by the eye fields which are a prominent and unavoidable source of confusing artefact in EEG analysis. (The normal eye is a bio-electric cell generating 7 to 10 mv between cornea and retina. EEG signals are typically to 20 to 100µV). The process, which is of fundamental importance to the success of the system and has been described elsewhere, (Quilter, et al, 1977) uses co-variance products between the recorded EEG signals and signals taken from electrodes place about the eye to calculate correction co-efficients which are applied to all the data. The algorithm allows the calculation of the coefficient K_1 and K_2 in the equation shown below:

$$M(t) = E(t) + K_1 V(t) + K_2 H(t)$$

where $M(t)$ is the signal measured at some position on the scalp, $E(t)$ is the part of the signal of true cortical origin and $V(t)$, $H(t)$ are the vertical and horizontal components of eye movement artefact measured around the eye. It can be shown that K_1 and K_2 can be estimated by:

$$K_1 = \frac{C_V/P_V - (C_H/P_H) \cdot (C_C/P_V)}{1 - C_C^{\,2}/P_H \cdot P_V}$$

$$K_2 = \frac{C_H/P_H - (C_V/P_V) \cdot (C_C/P_H)}{1 - C_C^{\,2}/P_H \cdot P_V}$$

where

C_V is the covariance product of the vertical eye movement signal

C_H is the covariance product of the horizontal eye movement signal

C_C is the covariance product between vertical and horizontal eye movement signal

P_V is the power in the vertical eye movement signal

P_H is the power in the horizontal eye movement signal

Data processing proceeds by computing the frequency spectrum of a sequence of
one second epochs overlapped by 0.5seconds, using a hardwire FFT system, (Wadbrook,
et al, 1977) . The resulting fourier co-efficients are summed to form five filter
bands between 1 and 30Hz and a total energy band.

The entire sequence of data analysed in this way produces a corresponding
time series of filter band values in one second epochs for each filter and for
each channel i.e. 96 time series. The first order statistics of these time
series are used to identify those epochs containing energy levels significantly
differing from the mean level for each filter band. Using this method reliable
estimates of the overall broadband spectral content of the signal can be made.
Epochs containing energy levels exceeding four standard deviations from the mean
in each time series are labelled 'paroxysmal' or 'transient' and treated
separately in the further analysis. These epochs often contain the most
significant information in the record or the only abnormality.

The overall mean broadband activity (96 values) is compared with thresholds
derived from a set of normal values (based on 100 normal subjects) to determine
'abnormality'.

In addition to the short epoch spectral analysis, the entire record is
scanned using an algorithm to detect sharp maxima and minima. These are the
'spikes' of traditional EEG interpretation and relate to epilepsy. A 5 point
moving window is used to find positive or negative maxima with slopes exceeding
a present threshold ($2\mu V/msec$). The crude spike list generated in this way is
subject to validation by eliminating sharp waves associated either with rhythmical
normal alpha activity (which often has sharp wave characteristics) and muscle
contamination. The spectral content of two seconds data centred on the 'spike'
event is examined to detect a dominant 8-12c/s component (alpha) or excess fast
frequencies (muscle). In practice some 1% of 'spikes' as recognised by visual
methods are missed in this process (of no practical significance) but there are
also some errors of commition i.e. not true spikes by visual criteria, and it is
necessary to add some refinements, for example the presence of a spike requires
also coincident maxima in adjacent channels i.e. three in all.

The mean background energy levels derived from the short epoch analysis
are used to produce two derived measures. Firstly, the differences in mean
energy in each filter band taken from recording sites equidistant about the
midline are computed and give rise to an estimate of symmetry between cerebral
hemispheres. Like comparing left and right hands, this is a sensitive and self

justifying measure of normality. Secondly the ratio of mean background energy
in the signal channel by channel measured in the alert and resting situation gives
a measure of responsiveness. We use a simple reaction task to randomly switched
small LED lamps to maintain alertness (neglect of this simple physiological
parameter has prevented other workers from establishing clear cut normal values.
Drowsiness produces EEG changes which might be confused with abnormality.).

In addition to these basic analysis procedures several other variables
are measured to establish for example the dominant frequency of the spectrum,
the actual frequency of the alpha band activity and the voltage range of the
signal.

From these results summarised outputs of the mean background activity, the
percentage deviation from normal and the percentage asymmetry are printed for
each filter band in schematic form in a 4 x 4 matrix which corresponds to the
topographic distribution of activity across the head. Any paroxysmal activity
occuring in the record is printed separately in a similar fashion.

An example of the printout (re-typed for clarity) is given below:

MEAN VALUES

	ALPHA				DELTA				THETA		
46	38	33	40	74	49	36	56	65	44	38	45
62	54	47	57	64	53	49	62	81	54	51	65
76	60	29	34	77	50	38	36	117	71	40	44
70	50	47	61	79	50	47	62	106	68	66	86

% ABOVE NORMAL LIMITS

	ALPHA				DELTA				THETA				SPIKES		
-	-	-	-	-	-	-	-	-	-	-	-	-	-	-	-
-	-	-	-	-	-	-	-	32	-	-	1	-	-	-	-
-	-	-	-	-	-	-	-	35	-	-	-	-	-	-	-
-	-	-	-	-	-	-	-	43	-	-	19	-	-	-	-

% ASYMMETRY

	ALPHA				DELTA				THETA		
14	14	-	-	23	23	-	-	30	14	-	-
7	13	-	-	2	2	-	-	19	5	-	-
54	50	-	-	52	23	-	-	61	44	.	-
13	6	-	-	20	5	-	-	19	2	-	-

A factual report is generated based on this data, the computer producing a text description of the record using the standard EEG reporting terminology. The text includes a description of the alpha band activity together with the location and magnitude of any abnormal delta, theta or beta band activity. Any spikes occuring in the record are reported and finally a description of paroxysmal events is given. The text generation system uses the results of the analysis procedure and a word dictionary currently containing about 300 entries to form the output text. The example below shows the factual report which accompanies the printout already given. The subject had suffered a moderate head injury.

EEG REPORT ON PATIENT NUMBER

NAME ....
AGE 53
DATE OF RECORDING ... 6.10.76

THE RECORD CONTAINS ABNORMAL BACKGROUND ACTIVITY, WITH NO DOMINANT ALPHA ACTIVITY IN POSTERIOR QUADRANTS, POOR BUT SYMMETRICAL ALPHA BLOCKING OCCURRED ON EYES OPENING.

ABNORMAL CONTINUOUS HIGH VOLTAGE THETA ACTIVITY WITH MODERATE LEFT-SIDED ASYMMETRY IN TEMPORAL REGION. ABNORMAL HIGH VOLTAGE SYMMETRICAL ACTIVITY IN THIS BAND IN ANTERIOR TEMPORAL AND TEMPORO-OCCIPITAL REGIONS. RHYTHMICAL 6 HZ ACTIVITY WAS SEEN IN POSTERIOR QUADRANTS.

NO SPIKES WERE DETECTED IN THE BACKGROUND ACTIVITY.

PAROXYSMAL THETA ACTIVITY WAS SEEN IN RIGHT FRONTO-CENTRAL, RIGHT ANTERIOR TEMPORAL AND RIGHT TEMPORAL REGIONS. NO SPIKES WERE DETECTED WITHIN THE PAROXYSMAL ACTIVITY.

CLINICAL DATA; HEAD INJURY 10 DAYS AGO. NO SIGNS.

COMMENT: INTERMEDIATE SLOW ACTIVITY IN LEFT TEMPORAL REGION OF LOCALISING SIGNIFICANCE. CONSISTENT WITH CLINICAL DATA.

To be of full value to the clinician, the EEG findings must be related to the clinical circumstances. In ABSCESS, clinical as well as personal data is entered through a VDU key board from a coded data sheet by the EEG technician at the end of each record. The sheet, which is arranged in six short trees, only two being required for any one patient depending on the condition, is completed by the technician on the basis of the information given on the routine hospital request form supplemented by that obtained from the patient. Understanding the significance of signs and symptoms and medical terms is a normal part of technician training, and is a major factor in job satisfaction, so that the sheets are reliably completed and not regarded as a burden. The reliability is much higher, incidentally, that from busy clinicians for whom form filling is an anathema.

Normally it is not necessary to provide more than six to seven items of information on a data sheet tree e.g. 1) paralysis; 2) left, right, both; 3) duration from onset; 4) suspected cause; 5) epilepsy; 6) drugs.

The clinical data, besides allowing a relevant interpretation of the EEG records prevents simple errors, for example in a grossly asymmetric record with both hemispheres abnormal, the high amplitude side may reflect a significant 'active' disturbance, or the low amplitude side could be significantly depressed. The clinical signs will usually direct interest to the correct side.

The results of data processing are brought together with the clinical data in one or four major decision trees which are symmetrical with normal (1) or abnormal (2) threshold values, or asymmetrical, normal (3) or abnormal (4). Since any of the categories of record may also have additional information in the form of paroxysmal data tests for this are included in the diagnostic decision trees.

It is apparent that possible combinations of the various items of processed data for any one record are very large indeed, but in practice, real combinations are much fewer, perhaps 200-300 (it is not a defined set). For this reason, and because there are advantages to the subject in analysing the requisite decision logic, we have opted for decision tree processing. The final output statement is derived from a dictionary. In the present structure a final decision is reached in not more that 22 nodes in the worst case, often in 3 or 4. Each node may, however, depend on the result of a previous, extra, decision tree processing, or may itself involve additional processing in order reach the yes/no output. This process yields some economies since unnecessary tests are

not applied to all records whether they are relevant or not. An example of
part of the decision tree logic is as follows:

Abnormal   no   yes   yes   yes   yes
symmetrical ----(PD-S)────►(PD-sym) ─────►(PD-alpha) ─────►(loc not 0) ─────►(CCD-MT) ─────►P(14)
tree   ↓y   ↓n   ↓n   ↓n   ↓n

where   PD   =   paroxysmal data

                    S   =   spikes (verified)

                  sym   =   symmetrical

                alpha   =   8-13c/s rhythmical activity

          loc not 0   =   location not in posterior 8 channels

          CCD - MT   =   clinical coded data - metabolic/toxic

                P14   =   print statement number 14: abnormal symmetrical fast
                          activity in (location) with paroxysmal (frequency in c/s)
                          activity in (location) consistent with midline
                          effects consequent on a metabolic/toxic disorder of
                          moderate degree.

    In the above example, CCD-MT is a conclusion from a separate decision tree
which looks at the clinical data to determine that the clinical problem is, or
could be, a metabolic or toxic disorder, and further, that it is not associated
with localising neurological signs or symptoms. The reference to 'midline' in
the print statement is to the presumed mechanism for the abnormal findings, that
is, the involvement of the midline brain systems, and is intended as a reminder
that midline effects may be due to other that metabolic/toxic disorders. It
will be noted that the 'location' is given again (the result of considerable
data processing in itself) because very often it is only the conclusion which is
read and acted upon by non-neurologists. At present there are just over 200
print statements on the type given with more than half of these including a
variable (location) and/or (frequency) component (giving some thousands of
strictly non-identical outputs (!)).

    It might be appropriate to list the particular problems and lessons we
have learned: in general, of course, we underestimated the time and programming
effort involved, but we have had no unforeseen snags of major consequence. We
have had to make some changes in recording procedures and we lost quite a lot of
early achieval material because it did not include eye movement monitoring when
we were not sure that we could resolve that problem except by editing. The
system is undoubtedly very complex and heavily dependent on thresholds at
various points - a relatively small threshold adjustment required for 'tuning'
to make a particular record go the 'right way' can result in other records going

'wrong' and the need to change logical tests to catch errors of this kind.

Of the lessons, we are, glad that we tackled the problem as a 'whole' from the beginning. That is we took the whole of adult EEG practice from recording to conclusion and all possible conditions, as the material on which to work. In this way we have had to arrive at general solutions and maintain economy. In fact there are considerable advantages. We have, for example, been able to resolve problems because we had access to 16 channels of synchronous data, which, if we had been dealing with only a few channels would have required a considerable overhead of complex pattern recognition techniques. The best example is a form of epilepsy, petit mal, which is associated with a characteristic EEG pattern of 3c/s spike and wave activity. Treated as an isolated wave complex, it is almost impossible to recognise by computer methods except of considerable sophistication. In ABSCESS, the diagnosis is easy because this form of epilepsy uniquely occurs as a major paroxysmal event, simultaneously all over the head and has a spike and a slow wave together between 2 and 4 times a second. It is the simultaneous occurrence of a large paroxysmal event in a relatively normal background across all sixteen channels of data which provides the key to recognition of an otherwise complex wave form.

There is no doubt that a sophisticated operating and file management system and the use of high level programming language has been a great advantage.

How do we see the future? When we are satisfied with the system and we can demonstrate the clinical acceptability of the output, it will be possible to produce a turn-key version implemented with micro-processors and incorporated in the primary recording device. A problem remains with the large amounts of sampled EEG signal to be stored during the processing, the capacity of low cost floppy disc or digital cassette system being insufficient. One solution to this problem is to use standard analogue cassettes storage devices. We have constructed a prototype 24 channel cassette storage system which will provide continuous storage of up to sixty minutes of EEG.

It may be possible ultimately to do away with the paper record and therefore the expensive polygraph writing systems, however, these would have to be replaced by some form of soft display device.

References

DOLCE, G., KUNKEL, H, 'CEAN - Computerised EEG Analysis'. Fisher Verlag, 1974.

RÉMOND, A. 'EEG Informatics', Elsevier Scientific Publishing Co. 1977.

QUILTER, P., MACGILLIVRAY, B.B., WADBROOK, D.G. 'The removal of eye movement artefact from EEG signals using correlation techniques'. IEE conference on Random Signal Analysis, Publication No. 159. 1977. pp 93-100.

WADBROOK, D.G., MACGILLIVRAY, B.B., QUILTER, P. 'Analysis of EEG using short epoch Fourier transfroms'. IEE conference on Random Signals Analysis, Publication No. 159. 1977. pp 53-64.

COMPUTER ANALYSIS OF MOTOR UNIT
DISCHARGE PATTERNS

Lars Philipson
Dept of Clinical Neurophysiology
Lund University Hospital, Sweden

INTRODUCTION

Motor unit analysis in the clinical EMG laboratory usually is based
on recordings of EMG activity, in which individual motor unit potentials are considered to belong to the same motor unit if they have
similar shape. Each motor unit then can be characterized by the amplitude, duration and number of phases of its potential. By examining
several potentials from the same unit and calculating the mean values
of these variables, the quantitative characterization can be made more
reliable. Even with more sophisticated EMG equipment the procedure is,
in principle, the same.

In this kind of analysis the properties of the discharge pattern of
the motor units are left out. The only information of that kind that
may be available is the rattling from a loudspeaker connected to the
recording equipment. The main reason why the discharge pattern characteristics are not taken into account is not that they are less interesting, but that they are hard to obtain with conventional recording
technique. The ordinary motor unit recording contains potentials from
several units. The problem of studying the discharge pattern of one
of these therefore implies the problem of distinguishing its potentials
from the others. Even when this has been accomplished, e.g. by using
special recording technique, the practical problems of making quantitative analysis from recordings consisting of graphs on paper are
substantial (Hannerz 1974).

By using modern computer technique it is possible to make such an
analysis automatically, to make all desired computations on the data
and to produce the result in a comprehensive graphical form. That may
be the first step in order to evaluate the clinical significance of
different discharge pattern properties. In a second phase it is then
necessary to interpret different results in physiological terms and
adapt the technique to the clinical needs.

METHOD

Recording

The recording of motor unit potentials was done using a commercial
EMG recording device (DISA 1500) and needle electrodes. An analog
data tape recorder (HP 3960A) was used to store the signals for later
reexamination.

After filtering and amplification, the signals were fed into an A/D
converter (12 bits) connected to a minicomputer (Varian V73). Data
sampling was made at a rate of 10 kHz, corresponding to 100 micro-
seconds per datapoint. The resulting digital data was stored on disc
memory. Using direct memory access and double buffer system, this
was done without any data loss.

Analysis

All analysis was done off-line after finishing recording of a suitable
data sequence, when all the data was available in digital form on disc.
Programming was made in Fortran, which made it easy to introduce all
desired modifications during the period of clinical tests. The actual
analysis consists of two parts, motor unit separation and discharge
pattern analysis.

The program for motor unit separation was developed as part of a
masters thesis at Lund Institute of Technology (Mandersson 1973).
Each time the signal reaches a preset triggering level, the peak of
the corresponding potential is detected and used as time reference.
The potential first detected is kept as a temporary reference. Shape
comparison between new potentials and current references is made
according to two different criteria, absolute difference in single
points and relative square sum difference over a preset interval.
If both these values are within preset limits, the new potential is
considered to belong to the same class as the reference in case. Then
the mean value of the two for each sample-point wull be computed and
the result will be kept as a refined refernce. Six such classes may
exist at the time, and there are certain rules to eliminate false
references. Similar methods for separation of motor units have been
used elsewhere (Bergmans 1971, Prochazka et al 1973). The result of
this procedure is a considerable noise reduction.

Reliable values of the amplitude and duration of the potentials in each class then can be determined just by examining the reference potentials. The duration was computed according to a combined level-derivative criterion (Lee and White 1973). The whole procedure is controlled by a number of parameters that can be set and changed by the user, which has made it possible to find out the optimal setup for clinical use.

During motor unit separation the time references for all accepted potentials were kept for the <u>discharge pattern analysis</u>, which is then based on the sequence of time references for each class separately. An interval histogram and a sliding mean interval curve for five

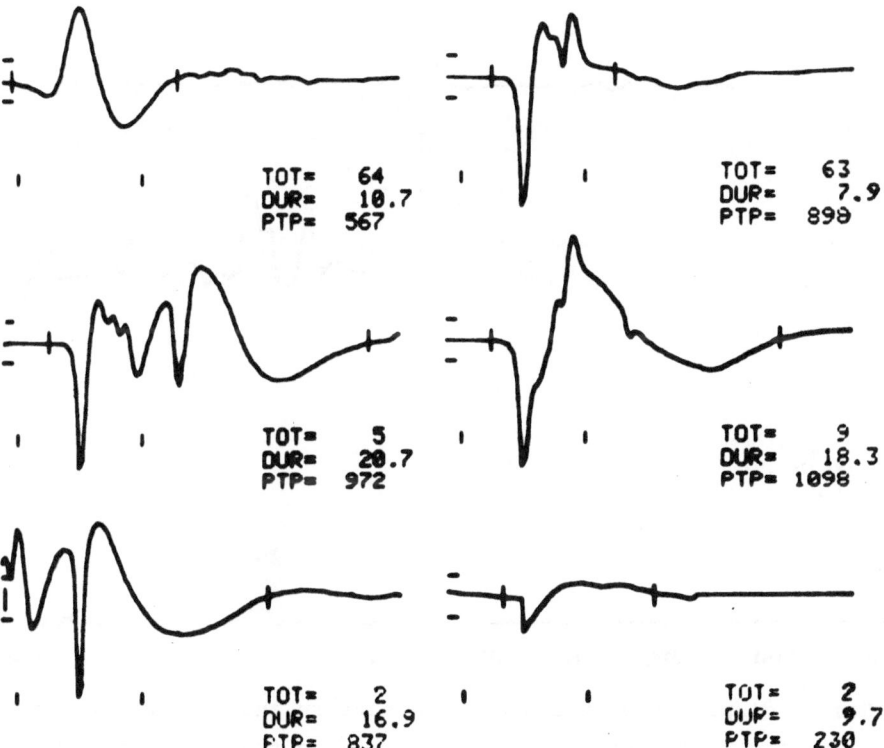

TOT=   64
DUR=   10.7
PTP=   567

TOT=   63
DUR=   7.9
PTP=   898

TOT=   5
DUR=   20.7
PTP=   972

TOT=   9
DUR=   18.3
PTP=   1098

TOT=   2
DUR=   16.9
PTP=   837

TOT=   2
DUR=   9.7
PTP=   230

<u>Fig 1</u>. A typical example of the result dispaly from the motor unit separation. Each of the six possible references is shown (25 ms sweep) together with the number of included potentials (TOT), the duration in ms (DUR) and the peak-to-peak amplitude in microvolts (PTP). The triggering level, the computed duration interval boundaries, and the interval for the square sum difference criterion are also indicated.

successive intervals are computed. As descibed below, certain calculations on histogram data may also be done.

Result displays

Data recording and analysis was controlled from the keyboard of a
graphical terminal (Tektronix 4010), which was also used for the
result displays. All the results from the analysis was presented in
two types of displays, cf fig 1 and 2. The forward/backward interval
diagram has shown to be useful to detect certain pathological firing
patterns, e.g. from fibrillation potentials (Prochazka et al 1973).

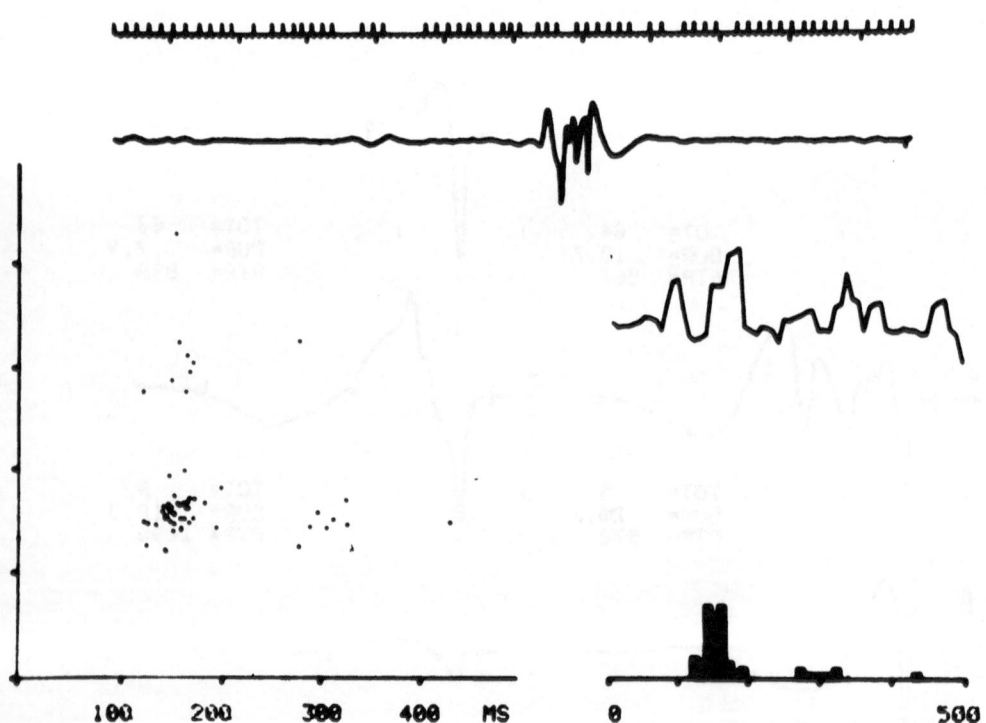

Fig 2. Result display from the discharge pattern analysis of the first
potential in fig 1 (TOT=64). On the time axis on top with the time inter
val marks downwards, each potential in this class is indicated by an
upward spike. The sequence of time intervals is shown in three other
ways in the same display. Bottom right is the time interval histogram
and above is a sliding mean interval curve. The two-dimensional diagram at bottom left shows each potential as a dot, with the x- and y-
coordinates corresponding to the forward and backward interval.

In fig 2 the discharge pattern looks very regular, except for a few
gaps in the sequence. There are two possible explanations to such
gaps, either they reflect actual gaps in the motor unit discharge
behaviour, or they reflect unsuccessful recognition of that particular
unit during the separation procedure. The most reliable way of finding
out if the last alternative is applicable, is to look at the actual
signal in the gap interval. This possibility is included in the system,
and in fig 2, below the time axis, a 250 ms part of the original data
is shown, corresponding to the first gap in the sequence. It can easily
be seen that two different potentials have been mixed and therefore
become unrecognizable for the separation algorithm.

In other cases the separation may become too detailed, so that potentials from one motor unit will be split into two or more classes. The
system contains the possibility of merging several such classes in the
discharge pattern analysis, in order to compensate such class splitting.

RESULTS

The following examples of results are based on analysis of tape recordings made during clinical routine examinations on patients with suspected neuromuscular disorders. All motor units studied belonged to
m. tibialis anterior.

Fig 1 shows a typical example of the result from an analysis of a 12
second sequence, where 145 motor unit potentials have been separated
into six different classes. The two types in the top row seem to correspond to the two different motor units that dominate the sequence, the
two in the bottom row are too few and too different from the others to
be considered, and the two in the middle row may be mixed potentials.
The discharge pattern analysis (fig 2) confirms this for the first
potential. The time sequence, completed by checking the actual signal
in some of the gaps, shows a motor unit with a fairly regular behaviour.
From the histogram we can read off that the mean interval is 150 ms
corresponding to 6.7 Hz firing frequency, and from the sliding mean
curve we can see that this mean frequency has no particular trend.

In fig 3 and 4 differnt types of irregularities in the detected discharge pattern are shown. Fig 3 shows a synchonized discharge pattern,

which has the characteristic regular 'square' type of forward/backward interval diagram and an interval histogram with 'harmonics'. These are typical artifacts caused by unsuccessful recognition during the separation procedure due to interference between potentials from different motor units. Most often this can be clearly distinguished from actual arythmia of the unit itself, which is the case in fig 4. The histogram shows that even if the pattern is fairly iregular, the unit seem to keep a well defined characteristic frequency of approximately 10 Hz whenever it fires.

Observations of this kind have led to the conclusion that the most useful part of the discharge pattern analysis display for routine purposes is the time interval histogram. From that the characteristic frequency can be computed as the mean frequency of the main peak. The standard deviation of the intervals in the main peak is a measure

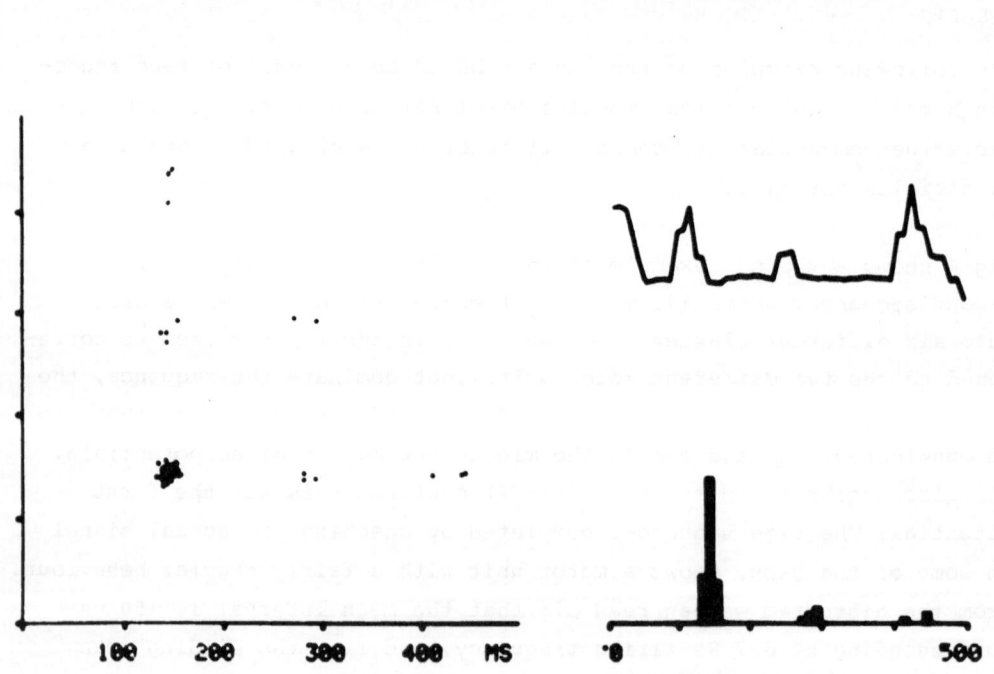

Fig 3. Example of a highly regular discharge pattern in which there are some gaps due to unsuccessful recognition during the motor unit separation.

of the regularity of the characteristic frequency, and the relative
amount of potentials in the main peak compared to the whole histogram may be an indication on the overall regularity of the unit.
These values can easily be computed and displayed together with the
histogram. Fig 5 shows how the interval histogram together with these
three computed values may be used clinically.

In order to find out if the whole analysis may be done in real time,
which is necessary in order to be useful in the clinical routine,
the critical parts have been implemented on a microcomputer system.
Using the microprocessor Z80A with 4 MHz clock, the data aquisition
in a ring buffer with 5 kHz sampling frequency will take 11% of the
CPU capacity. With a simplified algorithm for pattern recognition it
seems to be possible to handle four classes of potentials if the total
number exceeding the triggering level does not reach 60 per second.

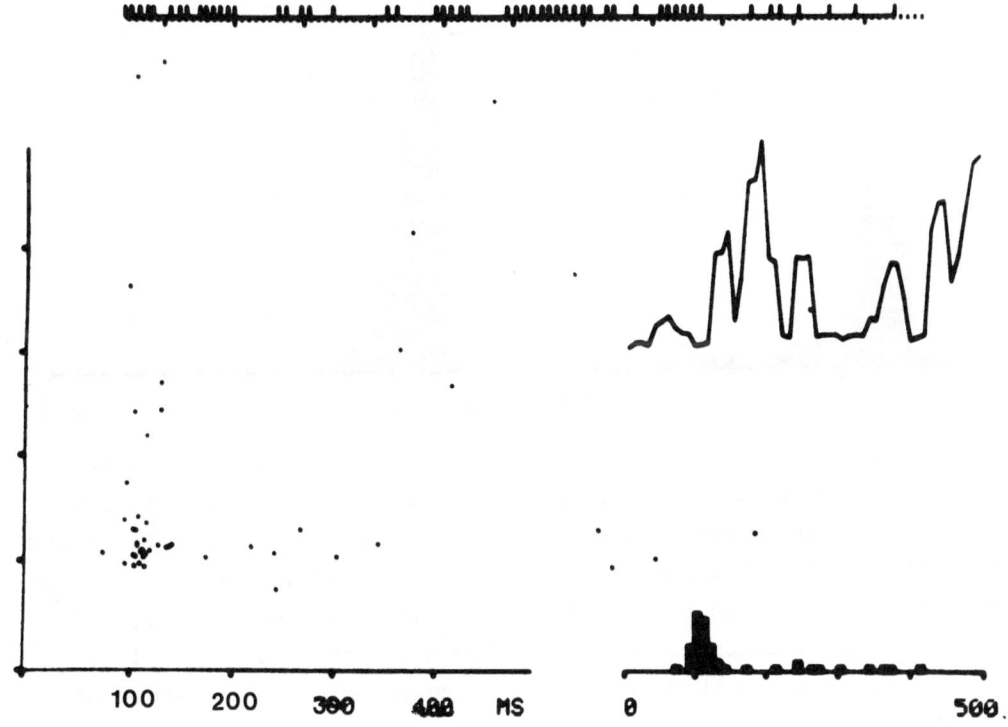

Fig 4. Example of a motor unit with irregular discharge pattern.
Note however that it seems to keep the frequency very well when
it eventually fires.

562

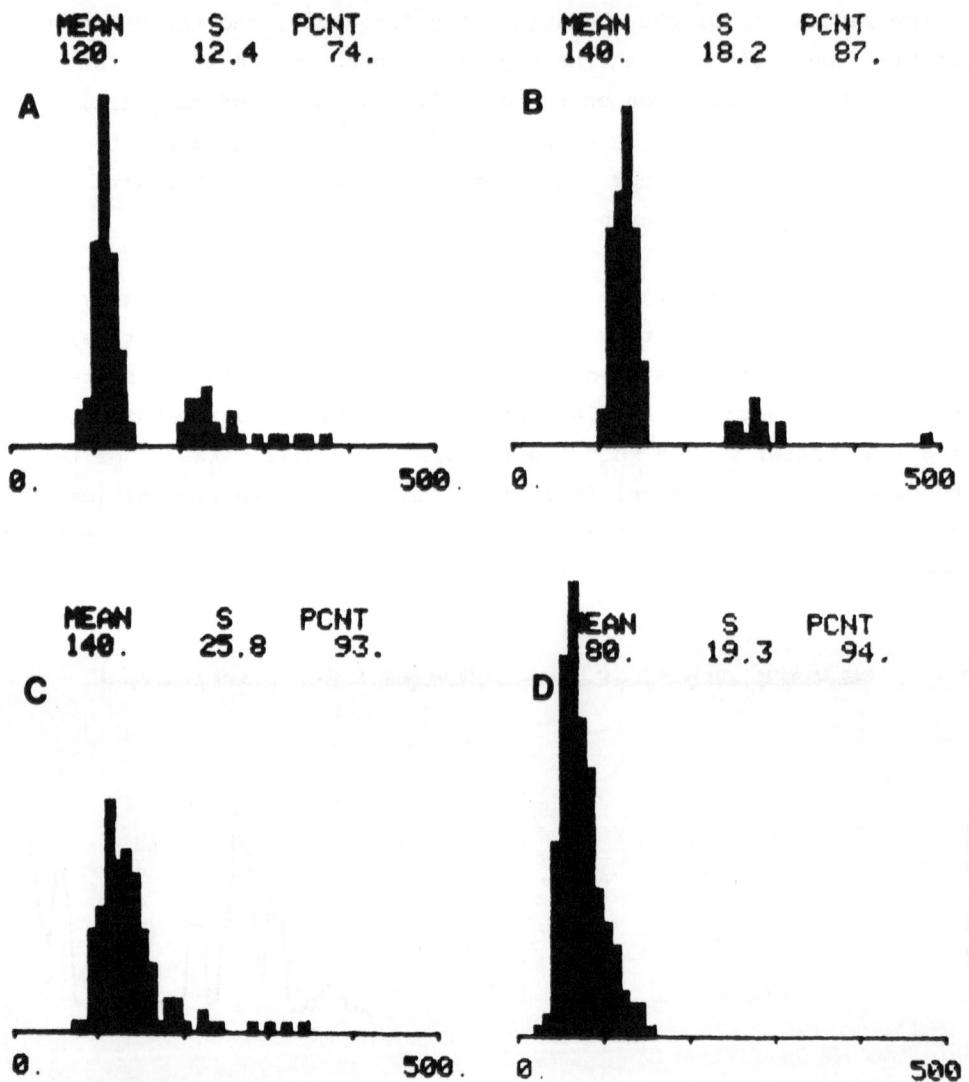

Fig 5.Example of the clinical use of the interval histogram alone.
The figures above the histograms show mean frequency, standard deviation and relative content, all referring to the main peak. Fig 5 A-C
show four different units from a patient with partial central paresis
in the right leg. Fig 5 A-B show motor units from the left leg with
normal, regular discharge patterns. The units from the right leg,
fig 5 C-D, show a marked irregularity indicated by a broadening of
the main peak. When pain stimulation of the foot was given during
voluntary contraction, the caharacteristic frequency increased due
to facilitation through the pathways of the pain reflex, fig 5 D.

REFERENCES

Bergmans J: Computer assisted on line measurement of motor unit
    potential parameters in human electromyography. In: Computers
    in the neurophysiology laboratory Vol 1, Digital Equipment,
    Munard, Mass, pp 9-19, 1971.

Hannerz J: Discharge properties of motor units in relation to recruit-
    ment order in voluntary contraction. Acta physiol Scand, 91,
    374-384, 1974.

Lee R G and White D G: Computer analysis of motor unit action poten-
    tials in routine clinical electromyography. In: Desmedt J E (ed):
    New developments in electromyography and clinical neurophysiology,
    Vol 2, Karger, Basel, 1973.

Mandersson B: Automatic computer analysis of motor unit potentials
    (in Swedish), Dept of Telecommunication, Lund Institute of
    Technology, Lund 1973.

Prochazka V J, Conrad B and Sindermann F: Computerized single-unit
    interval analysis and its clinical application.
    In: Desmedt J E (ed): New developments in electromyography and
    clinical neurophysiology, Vol 2, Karger, Basel, 1973.

NEUROPHYSIOLOGICAL SIGNALS AVERAGING STIMULI MINIMIZATION.

Drs. J. Villalobos and X. Majem

Depart. of Clinical Neurophysiology

Clinica Corachan

Barcelona. Spain

INTRODUCTION.

The purpose of this work is to surmount medical and mathematical problems that implies convencional averaging process in Neurophysiological domain.

From the medical point of view a large number of stimuli are needed to obtain a valid response in conventional averaging process, so to that system is inherent: Patient habituation to stimuli, dificulty to remain patient in the same state (EEG trace, retinal conditions, audition threshold) and a lot of problems to get a reliable response in some special patients (Children, mental disorder etc...).

From the mathematical point of view conventional averaging process assumes hypothesis of stationarity of background noise (Donchin 1969, Basar 1975). This hypothesis is rather hard to reach in long records used in the above mentioned process (Praetorius 1967, Isakson and Wennberg 1975).

Furthermore to surmount Medical and Mathematical problems previously discussed, this method allows make some test in Clinical routine that would have never been carried out due to long duration recording.

MATHEMATICAL APROACH.

Number stimuli minimization is achieved by Wiener Filter. This filtering method seeks to minimize the mean square estimation error.

The hypothesis to apply this filtering are:

= Stationarity of signal and noise.

= Additive relationship and statistical independence between signal and noise.

The general formulation of the coefficient of Wiener filter is:

$$H_m = \frac{S_{ss}(m)}{S_{ss}(m) + S_{nn}(m)}$$

Where: m is the mth coefficient of the filter.

S_{ss} is the Power Spectrum of the real signal.

S_{nn} is the Power Spectrum of the noise.

In averaging process we want to emphasize signal against noise.

The formulation to use in this case is:

$$H_m = \frac{\frac{N}{N-1} S_{\overline{xx}}(m) - \frac{1}{N-1} \overline{S}_{xx}(m)}{S_{\overline{xx}}(m) + \frac{1}{N(N-1)} \overline{S}_{xx'}(m)}$$

Where: $S_{\overline{xx}}$ is the Power Spectrum of the averaged process.

$\overline{S}_{xx}$ is the averaged Power Spectrum of individual processes.

N is the number of averaged stimuli.

The output signal would be:

$$\overline{X}_m = H_m \cdot X_m$$

wrere: X_m is the Power Spectrum density of averaged signal.

$\overline{X}_m$ is the Power Spectrum density of filtered signal.

INFORMATIC DEVELOPMENT.

The practical realization of this research is running on a PDP II/40
32Kwords memory core under a Real time operative system(RT-11).
The system uses as peripherals 2 disks of 1.2Mwords each,an
analogical signal acquisition module(LPS-11) and a graphical display.
The programming languages used are Basic and Fortran IV.

The first version of this work was made in three steps:
The first one included acquisition,A/D conversion and data storage.
It was supported by a Basic program.

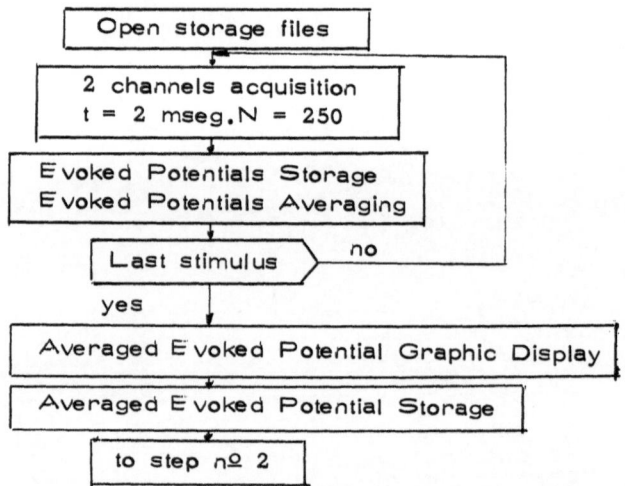

We adquired 500 mseg.of recording in real time from the patient,with
a sample interval of 2 msec.
In this step is important to point out the fact that long time
acquisition implies good frequency resolution but the ratio between
signal and noise(Power Spectra) disminished(Basar 1975).

The second step implied calculus of Wiener Filter coefficients and the stimated output signal. This step was supported by a Fortran IV program, using the F.F.T. (Fast Fourier Transform) algorithm, that allowed the calculus of two sets df real data at the same time.

We modified the input signal by a Turkey window to overrun "Leakage" effect. The inverse F.F.T. will transform the filtered averaged response to the temporal domain for the usual graphic display.

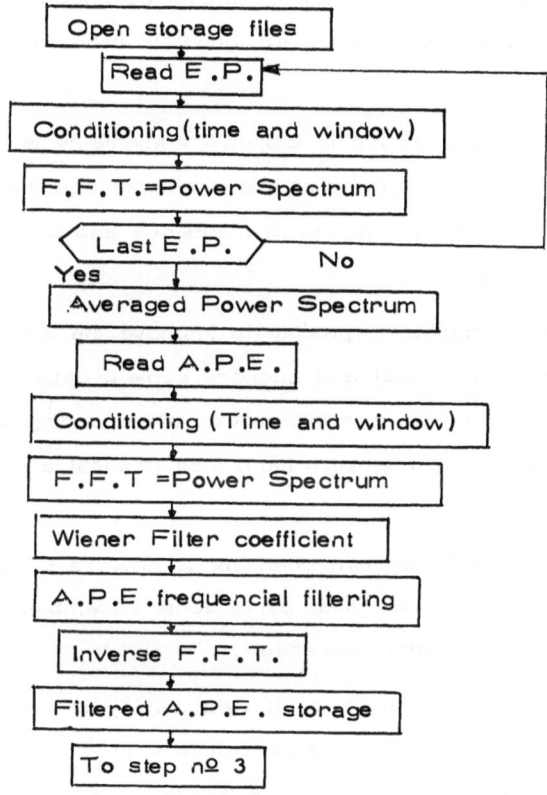

Last step implied smoothing, interpolation, when required, of averaged filtered response and graphic display.

RESULTS.

The system previously described is being used in our laboratory of Clinical Neurophysiology to obtain Evoked responses in some kind of patients (Children, behavior disorder etc...) and long duration tests (Objetive audiometry).

The number of stimuli used in conventional averaging is close to 60. With this new method we use only 6 stimuli over a "clean" E.E. G. trace. The Evoked response pattern obtained is usually satisfactory if the input averaged signal is reasonable clean of artefacts.

The use of Wiener Filter in Objetive audiometry is especially interesting due to simplicity of this response and the need to repeat the same test a lot of time (each frequency and a few energy tones as stimulation).

In the Clinical routine is posible to improve the acquisition characteristics. In visual and auditory evoked potentials a sampling frequency of 100 Hz. and 400 msec. of recording is sufficent (previous low-pass filtering) from mathematical and clinical requirements.

The computer time for two channels is now 13 sec. although is possible to improve this time using some assembler program and hardware floating point processor.

In the two following pages is showed, display of the program for evoked responses (comparing conventional averaging, N =60 and the new method, N = 6) and an example of audiometry test.

In a near future we intend to apply tis method to processes with low signal to noise ratio, as Cochlear Potentials, that imply a large number of stimuli in the conventional averaging.

Patient   nº 1

Patient nº 2

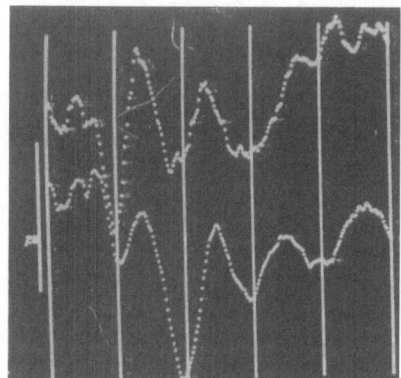

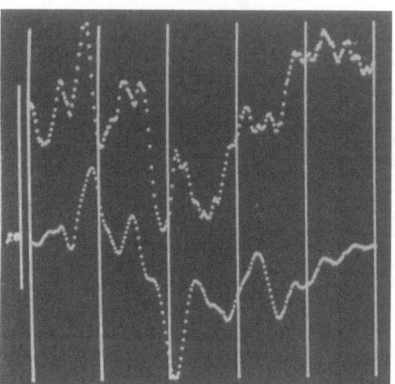

Conventional Evoked Potentials.
Upper line 6 stimuli
Lower line 80 stimuli

Conventional Evoked Potentials
Upper line 6 stimuli
Lower line 80 stimuli

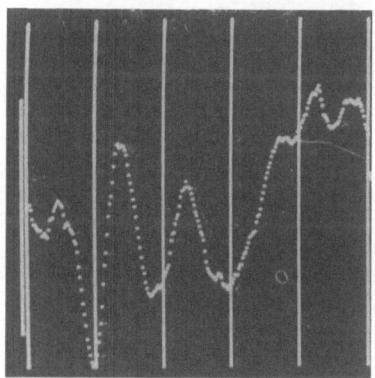

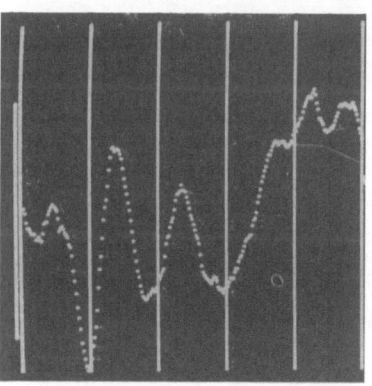

Filtered Evoked Potentials
6 stimuli

Filtered Evoked Potentials
6 stimuli

Two case of filtered Evoked Potentials comparing conventional
averaging(upward) and filtered Potentials(downward).

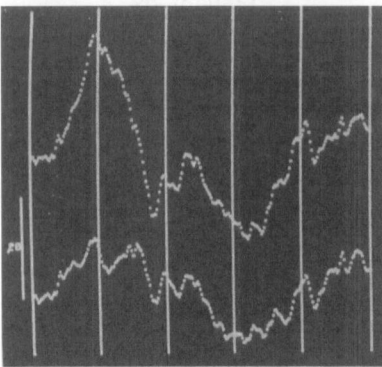 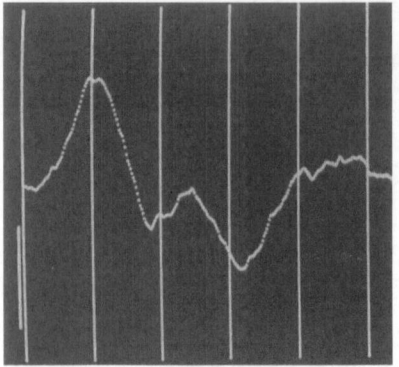

Bilareral auditory stimulation

Averaging(conventional).500 Hz   80 dB   Filtered averaging.500 Hz.

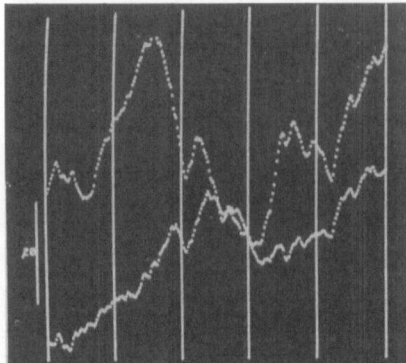 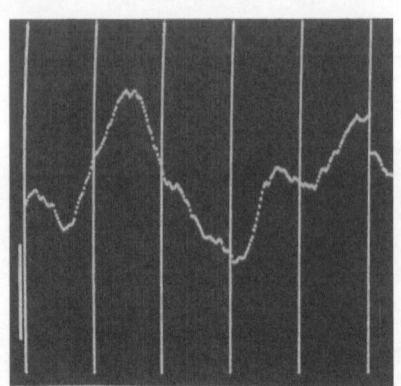

Conv.Aver. 2000 Hz.   Bilateral auditory stimulation.Filter.Aver.

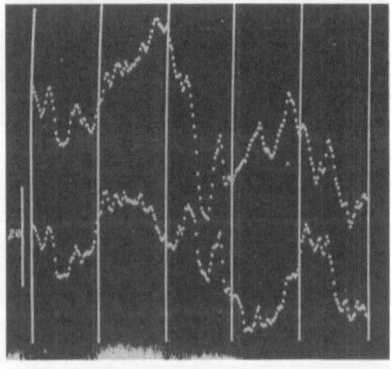 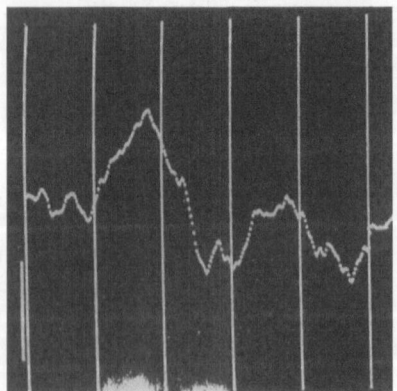

Conv.Aver.4000 Hz. Bilater.audit.stimul. Filtered averaging

Bibliography

Albretcht.Some comments on the derivation of the Wiener filter for average evoked potentials.Bio-Cybernetics 1976

Basar   .Comparation of Wiener filtering and selective averaging of evoked potentials.Clinical Neurpph.1976.

Doyle   .Some comments on the use of Wiener filtering for the estimation of evoked potentials.EEG and Clin.Neuroph.1976

Isaksson .Spectral parameter analysis of EEG and evaluation of stationarity by means of Kalman filtering.

Radix   .Introduction au filtrage numerique.Ed.Eyrolles 1970

COMPUTERIZED DETERMINATION OF LUNGFUNCTION PARAMETERS

L.H. van Montfort and L. de Pater
Lab. for Medical Physics, State University of Groningen
R. Peset Reig and K. de Vries
Internal Clinic, University Hospital Groningen

Introduction

In the Departments Allergology and Lungfunction of the Internal Clinic of the
Groningen University Hospital the routine spirometric measurements to determine lungfunction parameters have been computerized. These routine measurements
consist of the determination of the inspiratory Vital Capacity (VC) and the one
second Forced Expiratory Volume (FEV or FEV_1). The measurements are performed
by means of a Spirometer connected to a dedicated, on line, real time minicom-
putersystem (PDP-8/E). Both departments run their own program at the same time
in the same computer. The Lungfunction program can only service one spirometer
and assists the lungfunction technician by a heavy graphical feedback from the
computer and consequently has the highest priority. The Allergology program can
service up to five spirometers simultaneously. This multiple of spirometers is
necessary because of the time dependency of the lungfunction parameters is determined during and/or after the administration of an increasing amount of a
drug which gives a long occupation of each spirometer.

Objectives and Requirements

The main objectives of our computerization were
1. to obtain fast, accurate and standardly determined lungfunction parameters
   to be presented to the lungfunction technician as soon as available, to
   assist in the decision making to conduct and/or to prolong a measurement.
2. to reduce the vast amount of clerical work performed by the technician by
   generating an automatic, standard and more elaborated final result report.
3. to obtain a database for statistical evaluation in the future.
4. to include, in the final result report, for the Lungfunction department,
   the spirometer curves leading to the final results of the VC and FEV_1 values
   as well as all results obtained in their proper time sequence.

The main requirement we stated for the computerization was to retain, as much as
possible, the procedures used to perform all necessary measurements. Especially
to maintain the responsibility of the technician for the quality of the results,
because the technician has to decide on the sequence and the total number of
blowing manoeuvres performed by the patients. This requirement excluded definitely
tape recordings, *Shonfeld et al.,(1964)*, *Rosner et al.,(1969)*, *Derret and Brown
(1975)* and prescribed predefined manoeuvres, *Bouhuys (1970)*.

The ability to enter patient data into the computer from a position located near
the spirometer was another requirement. An additional strong requirement we
posed for the Allergology program was the ability to include easily on line, all
kind of new (unique) time/drug dependent measurements and to add comments to the
final reports on a per measurement base and to the complete report.

The signal analysis

The spirometer signals are sampled with 200 Hz, which is reduced to 50 Hz by
averaging four consecutive samples. In addition to the spirometer signal, the analog
differentiated signal (flow signal) is sampled, because numerical differentiation can be too inaccurate. The spirogram analysis is based upon the detection
of flow commutations to determine the end of an inspiration and the end of an
expiration. After noise elimination in the spirometer signal the inspiratory
volume of a respiration is a tentative VC value and each expiration is used to
calculate, by an extrapolation scheme, a tentative FEV_1 value. Each of both
values is compared with, and eventually substitutes, the stored largest previously
obtained (initially zero) corresponding value. At the end of an analysis the determined final lungfunction parameters will be the largest values of VC and FEV_1
encountered during that analysis. The lungfunction program additionally retains,
to obtain a history of the patients performance, all values no more than 15%
smaller than the largest value at the moment that the new value is determined,
but restarts collecting when the new value is more than 15% larger than the largest
value, to discard non-optimal performances.

Equipment

Both departments use 10 liter water-sealed Spirometers modified to provide for
an analog electrical output. The computer is a 16 K PDP-8/E with a 16 channel
10 bit unipolar Analog to Digital converter, a digital magnetic tape (DEC tape)
as external mass storage, Programmable Clock and a special time-of-day clock.
All special devices are built to speed-up program execution.
The Lungfunction program can run in 4 K memory as a stand alone program. The
Allergology program needs 8 K of memory and uses the interrupt routine of the
Lungfunction program, and synchronizes the A/D sampling with that program because both use the same A/D converter. The program input and output devices are
quite different for both departments.
The Lungfunction department has a special multi purpose input device PP(see fig.1)
i) to enter patient data and directing commands to the program, ii) to filter,
differentiate and send analog signals to the computer along permanent cables
($\pm$ 300 meter), iii) to perform initially each day (at power up) a simple calibration of the analog hardware. The output device is a memory oscilloscope

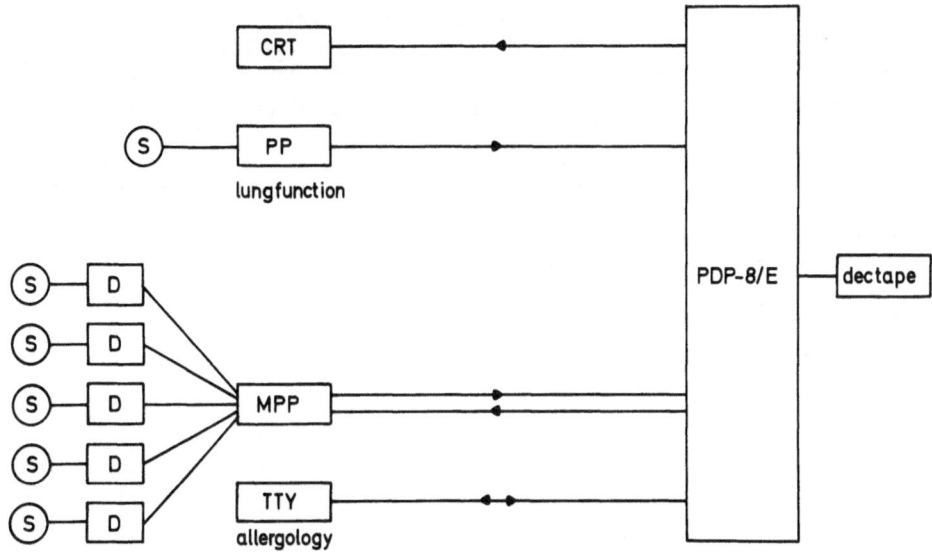

Fig. 1. Simplified diagram of the equipment for the computerized determination of lungfunction parameters. *S*, spirometer; *PP*, preprocessor; *MPP*, multi-preprocessor; *D*, display; *CRT*, oscilloscope; *TTY*, teletype.

Tektronix 611 with a special computer interface, to present all intermediate computer results and to generate the final result report. This report can be copied by a Hard Copy Unit. On the oscilloscope a constantly updated 20 second history of the spirogram is displayed in a non store (refresh) mode to deminish the repeated switching of the technician's attention between the patient, the spirometer and the oscilloscope, by eliminating the need to look at the spiro-meter where normally the spirogram is written.

The Allergology department has, located in the same room as the five spirometers, a teletype for data input, for program directing and as an intermediate and final report generator. All Allergology final reports are stored on digital magnetic tape. The analog preprocessing and calibration hardware as well as a digital input/output distribution has been build into a special device MPP (see fig.1). The computer is extended by a special digital input/output interface, connected to the distributor. The distance to the computer is $\pm$ 150 meter. On a small box connected to each spirometer all temporarily numerical computer results are presented to the technician and start/stop commands for the signal analysis can be send to the computer. The results are presented in four 3 digit LED displays. Start/stop commands are given with a button provided with a signal light.

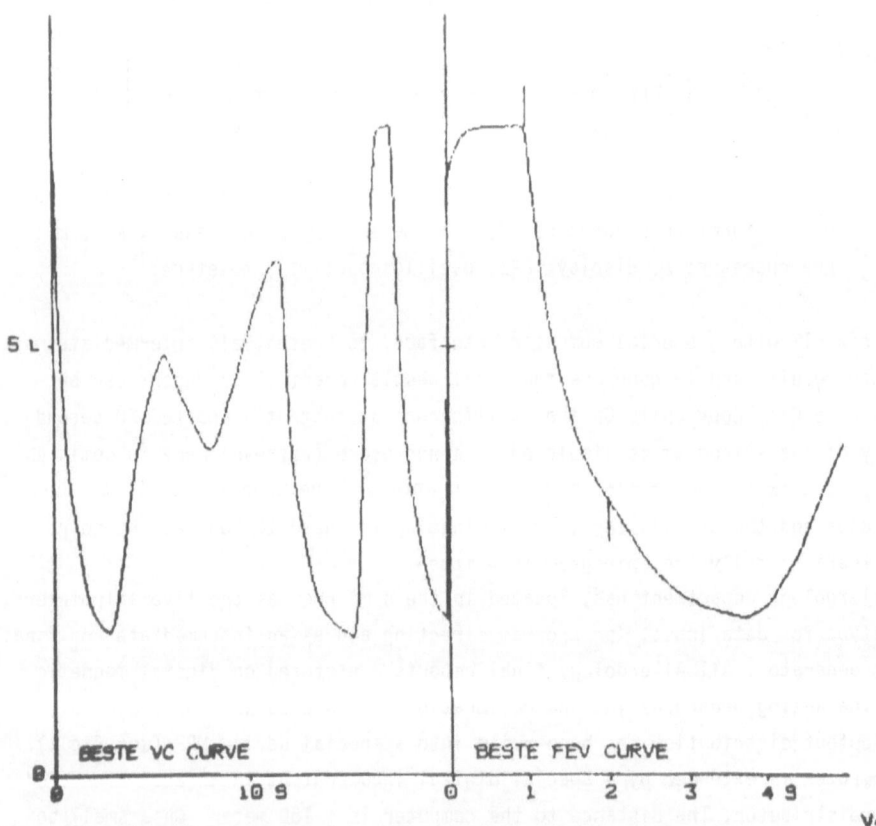

Fig. 2. Example of the final report of the Lungfunction program.

Results

In fig.2 an example of the final report of the Lungfunction program is given.
In fig.3 an example of the final report of the Allergology program is given.
The computerized lungfunction parameter determination at the Lungfunction department is in permanent use since November 1975. Twice the computer results
have been extensively compared with the results obtained from the usual method.
Each time all patient results have been calculated during a week by Lungfunction
technicians. The computerized determination of the Allergology department is in
permanent use since March 1978. During 10 days the results of all measurements
were compared with the results obtained from the usual method. For each patient
the absolute and relative differences between these results have been calculated.
In tabel I the mean and the standard deviation (S.D.) of the absolute and the
relative difference of all these controle measurements are given. The difference
between the usual method and the computer method are unrelevant in the clinical
situation.

```
                    AUTOMATISCHE LONGFUNCTIEBEPALINGEN
      INTERNE KLINIEK , AFDELING ALLERGIE   LABORATORIUM VOOR MEDISCHE FYSICA
      ACADEMISCH ZIEKENHUIS GRONINGEN            RIJKSUNIVERSITEIT  GRONINGEN

      ALLERGIE V6H  13:42 21-FBR-78
      NAAM: ********
      AZG NR: *******
      STATUS NR: *****
      LENGTE: 186
      GEWICHT:
      GEB.DATUM: 600211
      GESLACHT: MAN
      ASSISTENTE: M

      HISTAMINEDREMPEL

      NR TIJD:    VC   VC/%VC    FEV  FV/%FV FEV/VC
      1      NORM 6,19  100,0%  4,99  100,0% 80,6%  (VC & FEV: 100%)

      2  11:19  4,45   71,8%  3,13   62,7% 70,3%
      3  11:21  5,26   84,9%  4,39   87,9% 83,4%  AD (VC & FEV: 100%)

      4  11:23  5,82  110,6%  4,88  111,1% 83,8%  1/2 MG/ML
      5  11:24  5,35  101,7%  4,56  103,8% 85,2%    2 MG/ML
      6  11:27  5,38  102,2%  4,48  102,0% 83,2%    8 MG/ML
      7  11:29  5,12   97,3%  4,00   91,1% 78,1%   16 MG/ML
      8  11:31  4,21   80,0%  3,34   76,0% 79,3%   32 MG/ML <== DREMPEL
      9  11:35  4,86   92,3%  4,22   96,1% 86,8%   NA  0:04
```

Fig. 3. Example of the final report of the Allergology program.

Table I. The mean and the standard deviation (S.D.) of the absolute and the
relative difference of the results obtained by the technicians and
the computer.

$$\Delta VC \quad = VC_{comp.} \quad - VC_{usual} \qquad \Delta VC \quad (\%) = 100 \times \Delta VC/VC_{comp.}$$
$$\Delta FEV_1 = FEV_{comp.} - FEV_{usual} \qquad \Delta FEV_1 \ (\%) = 100 \times \Delta FEV/FEV_{comp.}$$

		November 1975 173 patients		April 1976 139 patients		November 1977 1100 measurements	
		mean	S.D.	mean	S.D.	mean	S.D.
ΔVC	(l)	0.023	0.066	0.023	0.057	0.045	0.056
ΔFEV_1	(l)	0.006	0.039	0.025	0.038	0.032	0.073
ΔVC	$(\%)$	0.78	2.08	0.74	2.46	1.14	1.48
ΔFEV_1	$(\%)$	0.44	2.00	1.21	1.99	1.18	2.45

Conclusions and future plans

The experience at the Lungfunction department is quite satisfactory, so we want
to give each department an independent computer system, based on a microprocessor.

Remarks

An extensive description of the equipment and signal analysis has been internally
reported, 'On line computerized Spirometry' (1976). and 'Computerized Allergology'
(1978), which are available upon request.

References

Bouhuys, A., 1970. Bull.Physio-path.resp., 6, p. 561-578
Derret, C.J. and Brown, C., 1975. Thorax, 30, p. 674-677
Rosner, S.W., Abraham, S. and Caceres, C.A., 1969. Med.Rs.Eng. 8, p. 18-21
Shonfeld, E.M., Kerekes, J. Rademacher, C.A., Weihrer, A.L., Abraham, S.,
Silver, H. and Caceres, C.A., 1964. Diseases of the Chest, 46, p. 427-434

NATIONAL POLICY AND CO-ORDINATION OF HEALTH CARE EDP IN FINLAND

Ilkka Linnakko and Hilkka Seppälä
National Board of Health
Helsinki, Finland

Raija Tervo-Pellikka
The Finnish Hospital League
Helsinki, Finland

1. Health care system

One of the principles of Finnish society is the equitable distribution of social benefits and resources. Health care is a natural
right of the citizen and the society has an obligation to organize
the necessary health services. The health services system in Finland
emphasizes the principle of distributing services in such a way that
the needs of the entire population are satisfied as well as possible.

Local administrative units, the communes or the municipalities, have
primarily the responsibility to organize and finance the services
needed. At present, there are 462 local authorities (communes, municipalities), all with the same legal responsibility. These communes
have a relatively great autonomy and administrative power. Individual
communes or a few smaller neighbouring communes together have established 213 health centres, which guarentee the basic health services.
But the more specialized the service, the more the communes must
cooperate: hence, they have established associations to provide
the services needed.

The district hospitals (23 in number) provide special care services
for the population living in their spheres of influence. The central
hospitals (21) provide specific levels of special services. Five of
these are university hospitals which in addition to the services for
the population of the district also share country-wide responsi-
bilities. In addition, communes or associations of communes own and
manage mental hospitals (70) and tuberculosis sanatoria.

2. The planning system

In 1972, a new law for the organization of primary health services entered into force. It introduced the principle of medium-term or 5-year planning for the health sector.

A national plan is made every year for five calendar years. The National Board of Health does the preliminary work, but the final plan is issued by the government and has about the same significance as a statute. Before that, the plan is scrutinized and the resource limits adjusted by the Ministry of Social Affairs and the Ministry of Finance.

The local health boards produce their plans within the guidelines of the national plan and submit them for approval to the provincial government and the National Board of Health. If the local health centres follow the approved plans, the central authorities pay a share of the costs, but otherwise no such obligation applies. The state share is 40-70 per cent of the running costs, depending on the financial status of the commune.

Through this procedure the goverment can regulate developments along the desired lines, balance regional differences in health care services and supervise the engagement of new personnel, acquisition of new equipment, etc.

3. Development and co-ordination of computer activities

The report of the EDP Committee set up by the Ministry of Social
Affairs and Health was completed in 1973. In the same year, a chief
inspector's post was established in the National Board of Health for
co-ordination of the computer activities of hospitals. The committee
dealing with the computer activities of hospital laboratories completed its report in 1975. The proposals made by the committees were
concentrated into a country-wide 5-year plan to the extent that
definite, common development targets and areas of emphasis were
clear.

Each hospital, naturally, bears the main responsibility itself for
developing the automatic data processing and data processing methods
that it regards as necessary. However, the national plan defines
fairly accurately the kind of computer applications that can be adopted at hospitals of different levels and the staff and equipment resources that can be used to implement them. The plan emphasizes specifically the role of regional co-operation and the general applicability of the systems. Central areas of application are patient administration, clinical laboratory and financial EDP systems. Hospitals
may diverge from the targets propounded in the national plan, but at
the risk of forfeiting state subsidies. The development of computerization in hospitals has in fact followed fairly closely the principles presented in the national plan.

In accordance with the development goals presented in the plans,
special interest is being taken at present in regional computer activities and regional or country-wide uniform computing applications
such as
- information systems which serve regional planning and produce
  statistics and follow-up reports for planning;
- uniform applications serving health care activity and covering
  the whole region, such as pre-registrations and hospital admissions, automatic analysis of ECG, reporting of laboratory tests,
  etc.;
- intra-hospital systems which are similar within the region, such
  as appointments, payroll, stock control, accounting, etc.

University hospitals may within the scope of the plan select their development projects relatively freely and apply different technical solutions. They act in a way as development centres for hospital computing activities and there is continuous co-operation between them. For instance, there are regular joint meetings of the EDP heads of university hospitals which representatives of the National Board of Health and the Finnish Hospital League also attend. University hospitals are expected to give expert assistance and to sell computing services to health care institutions. In addition, they co-ordinate the computing activities of the hospitals in their region.

For small institutions, the systems developed do not require a special staff but can be operated by the existing staff with outside consulting assistance, e.g. from the central hospital. Hospitals may procure data processing equipment of their own, but the chances of engaging computer staff are fewer in small than in university hospitals.

4. Computer activities of hospitals

The electronic data processing activity of hospitals at the beginning of 1978 was managed by approx. 150 computer employees on the staff of the hospitals. About 40 per cent worked on EDP management, programming and training. There are also approx. 30 persons in service and maintenance centres engaged in EDP and computing services for the hospitals.

There are 11 general computers in six hospitals and a number of other computers linked to various measuring devices. In addition, many hospitals use the services of the computing centre and approx. 30 hospitals have an office computer. Applications in general use total about 20. The applications for patient administration total seven, for medical information four, for personnel administration two and for finance and material administration seven.

The computer applications developed by hospitals for finance and patient administration were prepared by different hospitals, the National Board of Health and the Finnish Hospital League in co-operation. The majority of them are owned by the hospitals and thus are at the disposal of all hospitals without separate charge. Most of the applications are programmed in the FAS programming language and this makes it possible to run them without major changes also on the hospitals' own computers. FAS is a high-level business-oriented programming language, independent of the computer type, evolved by the State Computer Centre.

5. The management group for hospital applications

The management group for hospital applications which is maintained
by the Finnish Hospital League supervises the use and development
of the applications owned by hospitals and developed by the State
Computer Centre. The management group for hospital applications is
the co-operation organ of the owner hospitals for matters concerning
the creation and development of EDP applications for general use and
makes suggestions and recommendations for the procurements of computer services and the conclusion of agreements relating to them.

Six application working groups have been established under the management group: the group for joint use of minicomputers and service
centres, and the working groups for patient administration, statistics, finance, material administration and payroll calculations.
The working groups collect proposals for the maintenance and development of the systems from users of the systems and prepare proposals
for the maintenance project. The working groups may also plan and
prepare training courses for the use of an application. They follow
the costs of using the systems.

The way in which the working groups operate is being developed as
experience is gained. EDP programmes are in principle products that
have been jointly developed by hospitals and the working groups enter
the scene when the programmes are to be taken further. This product
development is best done as a co-operation project in which the
opinions and development ideas of all the users of the product are
presented.

As the result of the activity of the management group general principles have been established for the development and maintenance of
systems of general applicability and for distribution of the costs
incurred.

6. Computer co-operation

The national guidelines mean in practice that EDP systems must be
planned jointly by different establishments in order to avoid duplicating work and costs. The systems should be such that different
computer solutions can be used to suit local conditions and that,
in addition to the planning work, co-operation is possible also in
the use of the computers and staff.

Good models have in fact already been created, but further development and experimental work is necessary. The EDP applications for
primary care also still require a great deal of study. Development
work usually begins at the institutional level from ideas and needs
arising out of pioneer projects. Local activity must therefore be
supported in order to find the best solution models which can then
be standardized and put into wider use.

The demands of co-operation and general applicability occasionally
cause local inconveniences when it is not possible to fit all the
needs and aims into the same system at once. However, there seems
at present to be a suitable balance and unanimity concerning the
content of the systems, and organisations have been created for
maintenance and development. The participants in this co-operation
have all realised the high costs of excessive individuality and
have adapted to development co-operation based on common, generally
accepted principles. In addition, the by-products of co-operation
are standardization of methods, exchange and learning of ideas and
better comparability of information.

SUMMARY

Centralised direction and control and fixing of goals rest with the
central government, while the responsibility for the operation of
computer activities lies with the communes and hospitals. State
subsidization is used as an instrument of control of EDP activities.
In this way, common goals accepted by all the parties concerned
have been established and hospitals have been able to combine their
development resources. An example is co-operation in programme development which has been made possible by the use of a programming
language (FAS) not dependent on the computer. The programmes and
the other software are owned by the hospitals and their use is thus
not business activity but co-operation which is of high motivational
significance.

THE IMPACT OF COMPUTER TECHNOLOGY

ON HEALTH CARE

J.A. Dinklo
Philips' Medical Systems
Medical Data Processing
Best, The Netherlands

1. Introduction

Health care can be considered as a system. In other words, health care is an
ordered structure of interrelated elements, aiming at the achievement of
optimal health for each individual.

Data processing is the way of structuring the elements within the health
care system concerning collection, entry, storage, transfer, processing and
retrieval of data. Although the computer has not yet penetrated into all
sectors of health care, the data processing structures are already partly
determined by the application of computers. Health care is patient-oriented.
The family doctor, the specialist, the laboratory, the hospital, the pharmacy
etc. can be considered as service bodies in the care of the patient.

Increasing specialization necessitates fast communication, making data available when it is required, in order to enable decisions to be taken. This
holds for several types of data; for example:

- data relevant to a particular patient, such as treatment results, or medication prescribed;

- data describing treatment duration;

- administrative or financial data.

The introduction of computers within the health care system goes on and will
continue to do so. The way in which this happens is mainly determined by the
possibilities provided by the computer. These, in turn, are determined by the
progress of computer technology. Therefore computer technology can be seen to
have considerable impact on the structure of data processing within the health
care system and, as a result, on health care itself. In virtually all countries the costs of health care are continually increasing, both in absolute
and relative terms, requiring an ever increasing part of the Gross National
Product. Meanwhile the prices of computers, in particular of the hardware,
decrease. Therefore an increasing application of computers in health care
seems an obvious decision.

However, the introduction of automated systems or subsystems in health care
may meet with objections. These objections may appear in several forms:

- automated systems present data in a format unfamiliar to the medical man;

- the confidentiality of medical data is not sufficiently guaranteed;

- mistakes made in early attempts to automation give rise to mistrust;
- automate systems threaten the economic and even professional security of
  medical people.

It may be stated, however, that modern computer technology and the expected
advances in that field in the near future, will enable - and even make desirable - its application in health care. It will become generally accepted as
an instrument in the improvement of health care.

In the following paragraphs the main characteristics of computer technology
and their impact on health care are discussed.

2. Health Care

Although the structures of health care may differ considerably from country
to country, functions may be distinguished which are more or less independent
of these structures. Whether or not automation will be introduced, and when
and how this will be done, is strongly dependent on the attitude of the local
authorities, who usually have to provide the funds.

If we restrict our subject to hospitals as an important element in health
care, three levels may be distinguished on which computers and automation may
be applied.

a. The computer is applied for a single medical task, often in such a way
   that both computer hardware and software are more or less hidden from the
   user. Some examples of these dedicated systems are:
   - The Treatment Planning System for radiation therapy. This type of system
     computes the radiation dose distribution and is an important link in the
     chain of activities in a radiation therapy department.
   - The Automated Catheterization System, which facilitates the catheteriza-
     tion process by means of an on-line data processing system.
   - The computerized ECG Analysis System, providing computer-controlled
     analysis of electrocardiograms.
   - Computerized Tomography or X-Ray Scanners. This type of system provides
     video display or image reconstructed from measured X-Ray absorption
     patterns. This image reconstruction system requires a fast computer.

b. System for departmental automation. Examples of this type of system are:
   - Data processing in medical laboratories, e.g. clinical-chemical labs,
     haematological labs, etc. Important functions provided are patient/
     sample administration, data collection and validation, reporting and
     management information.

- Automated Multiphasic Health Testing. The purpose of AMHT-centers is to report on a set of biological and physiological examinations, in a standardized and programmed, systematical form. These systems are not restricted to hospitals. They provide an important contribution in preventive medicine, as they are applied, for example, for periodical medical examinations.
- Automated Radiology Reporting System. This type of system provides fast generation of required reports, giving patient status and management information, and billing.

c. Hospital Information Systems. A hospital information system is a computerized system supporting the information flow and processing in a hospital environment. The main purpose is the improvement of the decision making process both qualitatively and quantitatively. Such an automated system has business aspects such as billing, payroll and stock control and medical administrative aspects such as patient identification and registration, appointment and resource planning. Medical information streams have also to be controlled. In this area we see data items such as medical essentials, index of diagnosis and treatments, laboratory results, diagnosis support data, etc.

Dedicated systems (a) and systems for departmental automation can also be incorporated in a HIS through on-line connections. In the on-line mode the end-user has direct access to the system via a terminal.

3. Computer technology

The evolution of computer technology is characterized by both decreasing hardware prices and an intensification of the use of software. The decrease of hardware prices is caused mainly by the advance of the integration of basic electronic components. In addition to LSI (integration level of over 100), VLSI (integration level of over 1000) is coming into the picture. At present, one of the results of this development is the microprocessor, of which the entire central processing unit is built into a single chip. The advance of the minicomputer and now also of the microcomputer, has made possible the application of computers for many purposes, including in particular within the health care industry, not least because of the small physical dimensions involved.

Before data can be processed by a computer, the data have to be collected after the observations have been made. The collected data must be input; this data input may take place either close to the computer or from a remote site (point of origin of the data).

The transfer of data can be done along telephone lines, which have a limited speed, or via special high speed data links. After processing the data by the computer the results have to be output to be made available to the user.

3.1. Networks

In the classical application of computers three main functions can be distinguished: input, processing and output. The introduction of terminals (keyboard and display) creates a function essentially new dialogue. This function is important to the extent that it entrances human influence on the computer system. Important parameters here are response times, speed of input, thinking time, etc. If remote terminals are connected to the transfer function mentioned above becomes relevant as well. From a terminal point of view there are many ways to connect terminals to a central system. The connection may be half duplex or full duplex; the connection may be semi-permanent (via switched lines) or permanent (via leased lines); it may be a point to point or a multipoint connection; use can be made of different types of line conventions; etc. When several computers - each serving a number of terminals - are linked together, the resulting system is called a computer network. A computernetwork can be defined as a system in which terminals, transport equipment and a number of computers at a distance from one another are interconnected. In such a network the user services and processing facilities are distributed over a number of computers. Via a transport network a number of terminals can communicate with the computers and the computers can communicate with each other. This type of network is of particular importance in health care. Using minicomputers, it is applied for keeping medical records in behalf of groups of hospitals. The network topology varies, although in health care a topology frequently occurring is the star structure. As regards the switching techniques, three types can be distinguished: circuit switching, message switching and packet switching.
Circuit switching and message switching are wellknown techniques, applied in the public telephone and telegraph networks respectively. Circuit switching implies the switching of a physical data path between transmitter and receiver before data exchange takes place. Message switching does not imply this data path: data exchange takes place by means of addressed messages. A message is a logical unit of information e.g. a letter, a program or a data file. Packet switching, which was introduced about ten years ago, aims at minimizing the delay and maximizing the throughput for conversational traffic with a high peak load and for bulk traffic. The unit of transport is called a packet, that is a block with a fixed length (e.g. 1000 bits) and a fixed format. Messages are split into two or more packets.

3.2. Compatibility

A computer system consists of hardware elements and software elements. Compatibility becomes important when elements of a computer system must be replaced by more or less equivalent elements or when elements of a computer system must be transferred to a different environment. The terms used in this context are "replacing" ("replaceability") for hardware and "transferring" ("transferability") for software.

Compatibility can be defined as follows:

if the interfaces of two computer elements towards the rest of the system are identical, both elements are mutually compatible (i.e. replaceable or transferable). Because for computer systems many interfaces can be discerned, many kinds of compatibility exist. Important kinds of compatibility are:

1. Program compatibility, which is important when programs have to be transferred, e.g. between hospitals.
2. Data compatibility. Data can be characterized by:
   - representation (format)
   - organisation of files
   - medium (carrier).

The type of compatibility is important for the information supply by means of exchanging of data between various bodies involved in health care. Differences in procedures, however, may still cause a situation in which the user must perform different actions to obtain the same data, when data compatibility exists.

3.3. Micro/mini

Technological developments such as the processor-on-a-chip, read-only memories and random access memories (ROM, RAM) based on large scale integration (LSI), microprogramming, small peripherals such as the floppy disc or the tape cassette, result in decreasing prices of hardware which, in turn, strongly influence the possibilities for application of the so-called mini and micro computer. Although both mini and micro computers are already being applied in many areas in health care, it is still difficult to establish the border line between mini and micro computer.

The mini computer descends from the general purpose computer; the term denotes a class of computer which has a number of limitations as compared with general purpose computers. These limitations, such as limited memory capacity, limited facilities for the connection of peripherals, limited software, resulted in a low-priced computer for a limited application area. Today, however, these limitations no longer exist, particularly for the big minicomputers.

The micro computer has grown out of the micro processor, which was originally a LSI development meant for electronic calculators. The combination of micro processor chips together with input/output chips and semi-conductor memory chips results in a micro computer. Addition of restricted software, such as a simple monitor, an assembler and, as the next step, a cross compiler for a high level language, such as BASIC, transforms the micro computer into a system which no longer shows essential differences with a small mini computer. The differences between micro and mini computers, therefore, are not of a fundamental or functional nature, but consist of differences in degree, in particular as regards costs, technology and software and, therefore, performance. So if the choice for a computer has to be made, the name - either micro or mini - may be considered irrelevant. The characteristics to be taken into account are mainly processor speed, memory capacity, peripheral support and software support.

4. The impact

Health care requires an adequate information supply on many levels (see chapter 2), for medical, medical-clerical, financial administrative and management purposes. Often the same data has to be collected, processed and transferred for different purposes. Two cases which may be distinguished here are:
1. the same programs used with different data, e.g. patient data from different hospitals, and
2. different programs used with the same data but for different purposes, for example, for the national registration of patient data.

4.1. Patient data

At all levels described in chapter 2 patient data is important; that means that patient administration systems, patient registration systems and patient identification systems are needed in different places. Computer Technology gives a lot of possibilities to develop such systems and to store and archive patient data. The advantages seem to be clear, but various developments in health care sometimes give incompatibilities between information systems. Exchange of programs and data will be very difficult and costly in such cases. In place of the planned and calculated decrease in costs, where such incompatibilities exist, an increase in costs may be the result. Discipline, standardization and management in health care are needed. A standard product from a well-known manufacturer guarantees maintenance, a very important aspect of software products.

This maintenance aspect is often forgotten by health care management.
A patient administration system is needed for
- identification; who is the patient?
- billing; who is paying?
- medical record keeping.

With the aid of a computersystem we can distinguish two modes of operation:
- batch mode; input-processing-output
- real time mode; conversational processing (dialogue).

A patient administration system operating in batch mode has the following
advantages:
- changes are easy
- validation is possible
- summary and statistics are also possible.
But disadvantages of batch mode are:
- registration has to be repeated
- matching patient with file is difficult
- data entry is needed.
In a patient administration system operating in real time mode registration
is needed only once and paper is not used anymore.

With the aid of minicomputers it is possible to build a network based on a
distributed concept for a number of hospitals. A central main frame gives
problems such as: back-up, too many lines and a large investment.
Distributed computing gives
- conversational applications in a hospital and
- data base control in the central system.

Besides the aspects mentioned, computer technology gives to patient administration systems:
- reliability, regarding input validation and copying of files
- security, regarding authorized and restricted access
- availability, to other hospitals, dedicated systems and departmental systems.

4.2. Open/Closed

Dedicated systems (chapter 2.a.) are often considered as so-called closed
systems i.e. systems with a computer dedicated to one application. Due to
technology and an increase on the user's part of know-how about computers and
programming, dedicated systems are made open.

This means that the computer of the dedicated systems will be used for programming applications other than the dedicated application for which it was intended. As example, we can mention the availability of a FORTRAN compiler on a dedicated system. It is difficult to predict the future of a closed/open system philosophy. The hidden computer power in a dedicated system asks for general use of the computer, but on the other hand the decreasing hardware prices and the implementation of microprocessors makes a closed concept very attractive as seen from the commercial point of view. On the other hand a medical terminal is easy to connect to an existing network of minicomputers.

5. Concluding remarks

The increasing costs in health care, together with the decreasing prices of computer hardware due among other things, to VLSI (very large scale integration) continues to have an increasing impact on attitudes to health care. The effects will not only be felt in the tools used for health care, but in organizational aspects as well.

A STUDY OF THE DEMANDS MADE ON CASUALTY SERVICES BY THE

POPULATION OF SOCIALLY DEPRIVED AREAS

J.A. FARRER, P.W. HARVEY, J. DYER,* J. ROBERTS

Royal Lancaster Infirmary
Lancaster U.K.

Attendance Profiles for a District General Hospital Casualty Department have been used with National Census information, local knowledge and statistics to identify areas and subsections of the community who could benefit from increased Health Care facilities.

INTRODUCTION

The Royal Lancaster Infirmary Casualty Survey has been in progress since 1968. The annual samples have been biased in different ways to cover various parts of Casualty activity. The current (1977) study has been carried out to compare the Attendance Profiles of patients from subsets of the hospital catchment area. The information collected from this survey of the Casualty attendances at our District General Hospital has been correlated with data from the National Census (10) for the same catchment area. A flexible computer package is used as the questions to be asked of the database are not known in advance (7).

INFORMATION SOURCES

The National Census information defines the types and standards of housing and details of occupancy within Enumeration Districts (ED) (areas of approximately 150 dwellings). Considerable information on the occupants and dwellings of each Enumeration District is available including such details as family structure and number of road vehicles per household and whether there are bathrooms, outside W.C.'s, and telephones, or hot and cold running water. Information extracted from the standard Casualty Department records has been detailed previously (1, 4, 6, 9). It covers time of attendance at Casualty and the delay between accident and arrival, a definition of the incident resulting in the visit and personal details about the patient – age, sex, General Practitioner, address and school.

DISCUSSION

These two surveys together with local knowledge, and statistics for (still) births, deaths and infectious diseases gives a general picture of areas where a high proportion of residents are 'at risk' and which are believed to show

*Health Offices, Lancaster District.

'accident-proneness'. These areas could benefit from increased Health Education and other social services. It is also expected that these investigations may suggest possible reasons for the varying uses made of Casualty by people from different areas of Lancaster.

An area which is lacking in basic facilities tends to give rise to a relatively high use of Casualty facilities (3, 5). By summating all those census factors that point towards relative deficiencies in life or living standards compared with the average for the City, areas of 'Social Deprivation' can be defined.

FIG.1: Examples of Census Factors

	Area X(1ED)	Area Y(3ED)	Area Z(2ED)
Occupied Households	148	618	344
No Hot Water	0	3	39
No Bath	0	4	94
No Internal W.C.	8	0	114
All Amenities	140	215	219
Under 3 rooms	1	2	8
3-5 Rooms	47	385	252
6 or more Rooms	98	172	82
Owner-Occupied	108	45	277
Council	1	560	3
Rented	37	8	63
One Car	64	173	99
Two Cars	57	14	13

A complete study of the Casualty attendances in the city of Lancaster has been carried out on a 5% random sample of the 20,000 cases received at the Royal Lancaster Infirmary Casualty Department in 1977. The trends observed confirm that the people living in the relatively more socially deprived areas of the catchment area make more frequent use of the Casualty facilities than the less socially deprived residents of other parts of the City. Two socially deprived areas showed a high attendance rate at the Casualty Department.

Area Y was of predominately Council-owned properties, built in the post-war period. Only three of the six hundred and eighteen houses had no hot water supply and four had no bath. Over sixty percent had four or more rooms. Twenty eight percent of households owned a car (two percent owned two vehicles).

The other was a late Victorian estate of small stone-built terraced houses with a high proportion owner-occupied (eighty percent). No less than a third had outside W.C.'s and a quarter had no bath;(Area Z)

Thus the Council housing estate had excellent housing conditions compared with the privately owned estate, yet nevertheless they had equally high accident rates. Whilst the type of housing on the Victorian estate may account for the domestic and road accidents, the only difference from the Council housing estate must be the characteristics of the residents.

The following calculation was used to give relative 'Accident Factor' indices for various areas under study:

$$\text{Accident Factor} = \frac{\text{No. of accidents presenting from this subgroup}}{\text{No. in this subgroup}} \times \frac{\text{No. in this group within City}}{100}$$

FIG. 2 The probability of presenting at Casualty - an example

	age 0-14	15-19	20-59	60 plus
Accidents in Cas. Survey (1 in 20 study)	275	161	498	156
Accidents presenting from addresses outside the city	121	71	246	116
Accidents from within city	154	90	142	40
Census numbers in groups within city	11083	3792	23014	11032
Accident factor (average) within city	1.54	0.90	1.42	0.40
Census numbers for Area X (high class residential)	110	64	208	78
Accident presentation	1	1	1	0
Accident Factor	1.01	0.59	1.1	0
Census numbers for Area Y (council estate)	670	327	792	292
Accident presentation	13	7	8	1
Accident Factor	2.15	0.81	2.32	0.38

The underlying causes of domestic incidents are legion. For instance lack of care with home medications, misuse of appliances and equipment (2) inadequate supervision of children, over indulgence, or lack of intelligent forethought. Over thirty percent of home accidents result in cuts, with a further ten percent producing dislocations or fractures. Stairs or steps, and floors are responsible for a large proportion of all home accidents which result in a visit to a hospital

It is thought that property in bad condition, badly lit or with steep stairs or
no garden can be a contributory factor in accidents. Homes which are overcrowded
or contain badly maintained electrical gadgets generate larger proportions of
accidents.

In areas where little attention is paid to the individual-large families,
in elderly groups or where people have psychological problems, a visit to Casualty
may be initiated by some trivial incident in order to attract attention and
receive sympathy and care. The larger proportion of elderly ladies presenting at
Casualty with minor ailments is probably due to their liking for a 'chat' and some
reassurance.

FIG 3. Age and Sex Distribution of Casualty Patients - an example

		0-14	15-19	20-59	60 plus
Census numbers in city	M	5797	2027	11096	4514
	F	5286	1765	11936	6518
Accident presentations in total survey	M	151	98	331	64
	F	122	63	166	92
Accident presentation from outside city	M	69	40	173	48
	F	58	31	77	69
Accident presentation from within city	M	82	58	158	16
	F	64	32	89	23
Accident Factor of City	M	0.82	0.58	1.58	0.16
	F	0.64	0.32	0.89	0.23
Accident cases from AREA Y (No. of cases in this subgroup)	M	8(325)	3(167)	7(382)	1(98)
	F	4(345)	4(160)	1(410)	1(194)
Accident Factors (AREA Y)	M	1.43	0.36	2.03	0.46
	F	0.61	0.44	0.29	0.33

Notes:　(i)　The figures for AREA X are low and statistically insignificant and
therefore not included.

(ii)　The low Accident Factor of women in the age range 20-59 adds credence
to the theory that 'housewives' and 'working mums' perhaps do not
present at Casualty because they cannot spare the time, as it
cannot be said that the females in the age range 20-59 are placed
in any less 'at-risk' situations than their male counterparts.

(iii)　Note the alteration in sex bias with the over-60's

Some trivial cases present at Casualty rather than their own G.P. because
the hospital treats the condition and is usually unaware of a history of hyper-
chondria or malingering. A G.P. may know too much about a patient for minor
ailments to receive a sympathetic hearing yet again! It is to be noted that a
Casualty Officer can "sign off" a patient for a specified period - that is give
him an official form to state that his absence from employment is for acceptable
reasons and thus the patient will not lose financially by taking the suggested

period to recover from his injuries.

Special note is taken of (suspected) non-accidental injuries to children and this information is passed onto the Social Services.

In retrospect the correlation of the Census and Casualty surveys has been used to assess the needs in certain areas of the town for additional health education and advisory services. Having a trained medical advisor, though not a Doctor, available for consultations on an informal basis is thought by local health care officers to limit the number of visits to Casualty for minor incidents.

The paydays of local factories can be deduced from the incidents involving alcohol and assault detailed in the Casualty survey. The less deprived show less 'out of the home' incidents, less electrical appliance problems and less domestic incidents, perhaps due to their habits of drinking at home not in public, not letting their children play in the street, and having domestic help or making more intelligent use of electrical or other appliances.

Socially lower graded people with injuries will either visit Casualty immediately without much forethought however trivial their injury may subsequently be found to be, or may leave progressive incidents - bad sprains, infections and the like until they become more serious, perhaps due to their reluctance to take time off work to recover and thereby suffer unacceptable loss of earnings. Panic through minor disease being unrecognised and allowed to develop has been seen more frequently in patients from 'deprived areas.'

Employers and schools send patients to Casualty frequently because of caution and lack of detailed medical assessment of an injury at the site of the incident.

A composite map of bad social conditions and the incidence of 'accidents' was produced. This identified 'at risk' areas which were found to be predominantly of certain identifiable subcultures - New Commonwealth persons, or single-parent families or elderly in unsuitable accommodation. The District Community Physician is coordinating the channelling of additonal resources to these areas when necessary.

Effects of distance between hospital and school and the evidence of truancy in areas of Lancaster have been investigated. 'Like breeds like' when scholars see others missing school because of minor or non-existant injuries.

The decision to visit Casualty rather than a patient's own G.P. surgery has little to do with the appointment systems now operated (8) but rather the distance between incident site, Casualty and the Surgery. Village dwellers tend on the whole to be more self-sufficient. Rural G.P.'s are accustomed to being more flexible than those with hospital facilities close at hand. Also, the effort required for rural patients to visit the hospital is greater and therefore not undertaken lightly. Such factors are important in the exploration of the possibility of establishing daytime Health Clinics staffed by 'paramedics' as first line medical care in outlying areas.

CONCLUSIONS

We have found that a definition of the study data must be complete in order to identify specific profiles of attendance at Casualty shown by differing groups of prospective patients in the hospital catchment area. The studies to be carried are not known in advance so a computer package is used to manipulate the data leaving time available for the actual interpretation of the results. A detailed knowledge of the catchment area is also needed in order to put the results of the analyses in their correct perspective.

Continued monitoring of the uses made of available Health Care resources will help to make the best use of the equipment and manpower so that a more efficient Health Service will be available to those most in need.

ACKNOWLEDGEMENTS

We acknowledge the kind interest of G. Balmer Esq. F.R.C.S. and his consultant colleagues as well as that of Dr. A. Davies, Senior Casualty Officer and her staff.
We are grateful to H. Carr Esq. B.E.M., F.C.I.S., F.H.A. and his staff for advice and encouragement and to Mrs Isabel Walker who has coded and collated the data as well as typing the text.
This study has been financed by a Research grant from the North Western Regional Health Authority.

REFERENCES

1. DALBY B.C.S., FARRER J.A., & HARVEY P.W.   Casualty Activity Analysis Coding
   & Computing. Computer Programs in Biomedicine 3 (1974)
2. The Home Accident Surveillance System. A Report of the First Six Months'
   Data Collection (1977) Dept. of Prices and Consumer Protection.
3. DYER J. FARRER J.A. HARVEY P.W. & ROBERTS J. The Demands made on Emergency
   Room Facilities by an Urban Population. Public Health (1978) In Press.
4. FARRER J.A. HARVEY P.W. & ROBERTS J.M. Problems Arising from the
   Classification in I.C.D. of Non-Fatal and Minor Conditions. MEDINFO '77
   North Holland Publishing Co. 289-292
5. HOLTERMANN S. (1975) Areas of Urban Deprivation in Great Britain – an
   analysis of 1971 Census data. Social Trends No. 6 Government Statistical
   Service.
6. HARVEY P.W. FARRER J.A. Investigation of the Work of the Casualty Department
   by Analysis of a sample of the Case Notes. MEDINFO '74 North Holland
   Publishing Co. (1974) 523-527
7. NIE N. BENT D. & HULL C.H. (1970) SPSS – Statistical Package for the Social
   Sciences (McGraw-Hill)

8. ROBERTS J.M. FARRER J.A. & HARVEY P.W. The use of a Computer System in the
    Study of the Attendance Profile in a District Hospital Casualty Department
    Computers in Biology and Medicine (1977) Vol. 7 No. 4
9. ROBERTS J.M. FARRER J.A. & HARVEY P.W. A Progressive Study of the Emergency
    Room Demand by the Community. Medical Inform. 2 (1977) No. 3 197-201.
10. Small Area Statistics (1971) Census, England and Wales 1971 (Office of
    Population Censuses and Surveys).

MONITORING OF ALIMENTARY AND RESPIRATORY INFECTIONS [+]

J. Radkovský

Institute of Social Medicine & Organization of Health Services,
Prague, Czechoslovakia

Infectious diseases are still one of important health problems
in the world. Although some of them were eradicated or supressed,
the others are still prevailing or endemic in all countries. These
are especially the infections of the respiratory and alimentary
tracts.

The first group is presented by influenza and other virus infections
of the respiratory tract, which are very difficult to control. Measures such as immunization and epidemiological control are not effective and further research is needed.

The second group , alimentary infections, are caused mainly by bacteria (salmonella, shigella and others) which could be identified in
a microbiological laboratory. The identification of the source of infection enables health services to introduce control measures, with
the aim of interrupting the strain of infection in the population.

But there are some problems with compulsory notification of these
diseases: some of them are without symptoms or not notified (more
than 90 %), the identification and final notification is late and
the exchange of informations between field physicians, laboratory
health and veterinary workers takes too much of the time needed for
control measures.

For these reasons, even the system of compulsory notification of
final diagnosis using telex and central data processing by computer,
introduced in our country in 1971 was not sufficient. Therefore the
daily monitoring of alimentary diseases was introduced in one district in 1973.

Problem analysis

The system of the control of alimentary infections depend in Czechoslovakia on the monitoring of the spread of infection in men & ani-
mals, preventive control measures done by health services, organized

[+]The project was designed by Drs K.Žáček & J.Radkovský in a working
paper from 1973; the programmes were prepared by Z.Roth, M.Šampalík,
V.Hynčica, Institute of Hygiene & Epidemiology, Prague; the implementation of the project in the field was organized by Drs. H.Mina-
říková, Epidemiologist, J.Ševčík, Hygienist, District Hygiene Station in Teplice and Vl.Verhun, Epidemiologist, Regional Hygiene Station
in Ústí n.L.

by epidemiological services and by veterinary control of meat and milk products.

We disregard cooking and eating habits, commune hygiene, water supply, level of hygiene knowledge of the population and other factors, which are also very important.

Process of the spread of alimentary infection

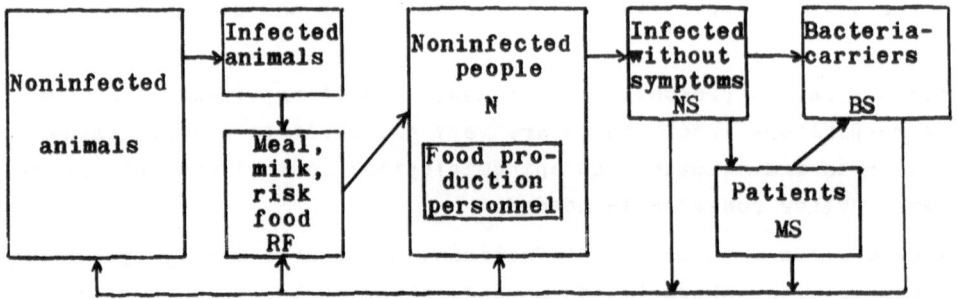

Population (N) is divided in three groups: not supplied and supplied by risk food, from these persons, who does eat it. From the above scheme it follows the possibilities of the interference in the process of the spread of infection:

Elements of the process	Health Services	Hygiene Services			Veterinary Services
		Epid.	Lab.	Food Hygiene	
Noninfected people		X			
Infected without symptoms		X	X		
Patients	X	X	X		
Carriers	X	X	X		
Food production personnel	X	X	X	X	
Infected animals					X
Meat & milk products			X	X	X
Risk food			X	X	

The Czechoslovak health services are organized in a system of polyclinics and physicians in a Public Health Centre serving a population of about 3000 and a Hygiene Station in district serving in average 100 000 population. This station has physicians and asistants specialized in epidemiology, microbiology and hygiene (commune hygiene, food hygiene, working hygiene etc.). The assistants can investigate the notified or suspected sources of infection, collect the material from patients and risk food.

The epidemiological measures organized by a Hygiene Station depend on timely introduced measures focused on the exposed group of population or contaminated food. Therefore the aim of monitoring is to supply the above workers with signals about the occurance of the focuses of infection.

The information system for control of alimentary infections

→ monitoring   ----> obligatory notification

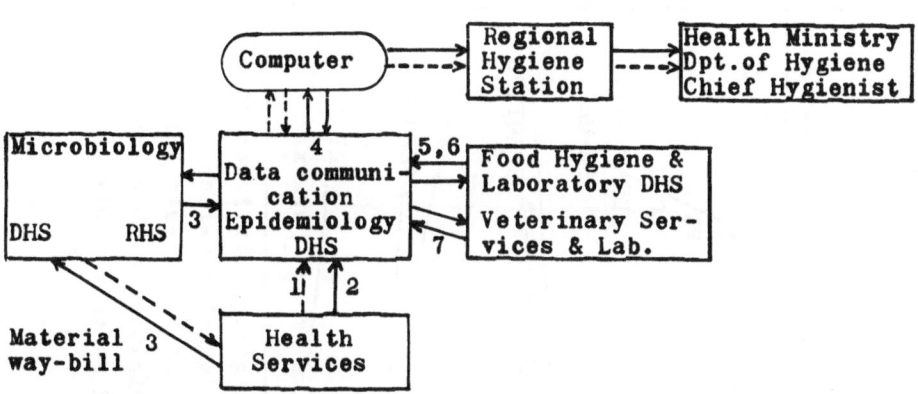

Input data:

1 Obligatory notification of infectious diseases.

2 Monitoring of acute alimentary diseases.

3 Data on the way-bill to material for microbiological examination and their findings.

4 Data from epidemiological examination of positive cases.

5 Data on food specimens for bacteriological examination and the findings of hygiene assistants.

6 Data on the bacteriological examination of food specimens.

7 Data on bacteria found in veterinary laboratory from meat and milk specimens.

Output from computer for District Hygiene Station (DHS):

- Signals on excess incidence of alimentary diseases in population served by Public Health Centres (PHC) in comparison with daily average in the district and average in previous week.
- Significantly higher incidence in groups of population supplied by some risk food.
- Weekly and/or daily incidence of alimentary diseases by PHC.
- Bacteriological findings in men and food.

Output from computer for Regional Hygiene Station (RHS):

- Daily brief report by districts.
- Weekly report of incidence of alimentary diseases.
- Weekly report on bacteriological findings.

Scheme of weekly cycle of monitoring of acute alimentary diseases

1) Bacteriological diagnostic and obligatory notification. 2) DHS - monitoring

	Monday	Tuesday	Wednesday	Thursday	Friday	Monday

Legend:

xxx Acute alimentary diseases treated in PHC

TTT Notification to DHS by phone

PT Control and dataprocessing on paper tape

DC Data communication by telex to computer centre

DP Data processing and communication to DHS and RHS by telex

ON Obligatory notification

EH Epidemiological and hyg.investigation following obligatory notification

MAT Collection of material for bact.examination

TYPE Typisation of bacteria (grouping type)

SEROTYPE Further typisation in the laboratory

Output for Health Ministry:

- Weekly report on incidence by regions and/or districts.
- In case of an epidemic daily concise information on the development of epidemiological situation.

From the above scheme of weekly cycle of monitoring of acute alimentary diseases follows the dependance of the clarification of the epidemiological situation on the early collection of material and bacteriological examinations. That requires to process the information every morning and to send the signals to the DHS workers before 24 hours after onset of diseases.(visit of PHC). Thus in their daily working schedule they may respect the recent epidemiological situation.

The previous system of epidemiological surveillance of alimentary infections was based on obligatory notification. The epidemiological assistants visited the patients or their family usually one week after onset of first symptoms and therefore the introduced measures had limited results. The compulsory notification sent by cable from DHS to Computer Centre sould save only one day in data processing.

The suspected focus of infection should be investigated bacteriologically and only the findings of bacteria of the same type in men and food samples could initiate the direct epidemiological measures. Thus the collection of all informations and their analysis allows the physician - epidemiologist and hygienist - interfere in the process of the spread of infection. If the feed-back of the information system leads to the shortening of the interval between the onset of infection and the introduction of epidemiological measures we could expect higher effectiveness of such measures.

The possibility that patients are visiting physicians in the working place or a physician who is not his normal PHC physician cause the incorrect values of incidence by PHC. Therefore the system was enlarged by the notification of names and adresses, eventually if the patient belongs to the children collective (crèche, kindergarten). This complicated, but more accurate notification enable the sorting by the PHC and other aspects.

The implementation of the simple system has shown that the assistants should visit every day about 5 PHC and follow there the data concerning the epidemiological situation in alimentary diseases. The later more accurate system increases the number of places which has to be visited, but the assistants have already the adresses and can select more exposed groups (families or collectives). On the other side the administrative work of nurses in PHC as well as in DHS is more complicated and time consuming.

The practical implementation of such notification has shown the decrease of the number of notified cases. In the present technical possibilities such system was found very expensive and difficult to execute and therefore not acceptable for the introduction in the large scale.

But the new situation could arise if the general information medical system could be based on the civic register of the population with birth number as identification number. In such a system the diagnosis only gives the possibility to start with the data processing and the monitoring by computer as personal data are known.

Problem quantification

N - population in the area
N_i - population served by PHC_i
S_k - bacteria: salmonellosis, shigellosis etc. (k)
NS_k - persons infected by bacteria S_k without symptoms
MS_k - infectious diseases caused by infections S_k
NS,MS- infected persons or infectious diseases without known type of bacteria S_k
M - number of patients visiting PHC (first visits)
MA - from these acute alimentary diseases
MAS - from these infectious alimentary diseases .

$NS+MS$ = total number of infected. Ratio NS_k/MS_k varies according S_k, thus information on MS from number of patients with acute alimentary disease (MA) is misrepresented by the number of patients not visiting PHC (MS-MAS) and by the number of patients with other acute alimentary diseases noninfectious (MA-MAS).

Information on infected persons (MS+NS) from number of patients (MS) depend on the manifestation rate $MS/(MS+NS)$. This question arise epecially in the case of conditional pathogens, e.g. citrobacteria.

Exposure to risk food

P_j - risk food by food-producers (j)

NP_j - population of the area supplied by P_j

MP_j - from these estimate of the population part which according epidemiological investigation consumed P_j (milk is consumed by many, some speciality only by few)

MP_j/NP_j - ratio of exposure to the P_j, if it is infected

Example: Infected meat was supplied to the area of 10 PHC from total 50 PHC in a district and consumed by 5 % of the population, thus 1 % was infected. With manifestation rate of 30 % the incidence would be .3 %. If only one half of patients visits PHC and notification rate would be 80 % than the notified incidence would be .003 x .5 x .8 = .0012 = .12 %.

Such low probability of notified cases means 2 or 3 isolated patients in few PHC, which dont give the idea about the spread of infection among larger area and population groups without the evaluation of the epidemiological situation including exposure to the risk food in supplied area.

The results of the monitoring

The data on the incidence of acute alimentary diseases were reported by phone from PHC to the District Hygiene Station between 11 and 14 hours every working day. Here were transferred to the paper tape and cabled to the Institute of Hygiene & Epidemiology each afternoon from Monday to Friday.

The next morning an evaluation by computer was sent as signal report by cable and the listing of results by post to DHS and RHS.

Beside this part of the problem the microbiological and epidemiological findings were reported from the laboratory and processed by computer.

The programme was written in FORTRAN IV and the data processing executed by the computer HP-2100.

The carrying out of this project from 1974 to 1977 has shown in few cases the usefulness of the monitoring of alimentary diseases for the more effective work of both epidemiologist as well as hygienist. On the other side the actualisation of data for monitoring is so difficult and expensive that new approach, e.g. multipurpose information health system using terminals in polyclinics could be only considered for larger use.

The monitoring of <u>respiratory diseases</u> is done by computer from 1965 by districts, age groups (before school-, school-age and adults) and complications.

The rates are tabulated and plotted in a chart automatically. The feed-back distribution of this material to all DHS and RHS enables them to follow the spread of influenza epidemics in the whole country.

THE TRANSFER OF OUTPATIENT CLINICS TO RURAL HOSPITALS:

A FEASIBILITY STUDY AND COST-BENEFIT ANALYSIS

I T Russell
University of North Carolina, Chapel Hill
(Present address — University of Newcastle upon Tyne)

Norma G Reid
London School of Economics

P R Philips
University of Newcastle upon Tyne

N J Glass
HM Treasury, London

R L Akehurst
University of Lancaster

Summary

This paper describes a research project designed to evaluate the transfer of outpatient clinics from general hospitals to rural communities. On the basis of three specially-designed surveys, we have estimated that, of 43,000 outpatient consultations which currently take place each year in Carlisle, England, it would be feasible to transfer 4,700 to one rural hospital. The transfer would generate additional attendances, perhaps as many as 2,000.

Cost benefit analysis suggests that, although the transfer is likely to increase NHS expenditure, this increase may be outweighed by benefits to patients and to the rest of society. However, this conclusion depends critically on the number of additional outpatient attendances; the fewer there are, the stronger the case for the transfer.

Introduction

In Great Britain, there are two information systems relating to hospital inpatients — Hospital Activity Analysis and the Hospital In-Patient Enquiry (Benjamin, 1965; Ashley, 1972). Despite criticisms (Acheson, 1968; Benjamin, 1977), these systems provide information relevant to the planning of inpatient services. In contrast, the only routine statistics relating to outpatient (OP) care — the SH3 returns — are voluntary (and hence unrepresentative), loosely-defined and restricted to the numbers of new and repeat attendances at each clinic. Hence if a decision affecting the organisation of outpatient services is to be well-informed, an ad hoc information system must be constructed.

In 1973, the outpatient facilities at the district general hospital (DGH) in Carlisle, were becoming increasingly congested. As the hospital serves a population of 175,000 of whom only 70,000 live in Carlisle, one solution proposed was to transfer clinics to nearby rural hospitals. This paper describes the information system set up to guide this decision and the resulting statistical and economic findings.

Method

Six specialties were considered as candidates for rural clinics — medicine, surgery, ear nose and throat surgery (ENT), gynaecology, orthopaedics and psychiatry. These specialties provided 44 weekly clinics — 40 in Carlisle and the remaining four (one in gynaecology and three in psychiatry) in Penrith, a town of 10,000 inhabitants 18 miles from Carlisle. We aimed to answer three questions:

(1) How many attendances *could* be transferred to rural clinics?

(2) What *would* be the effect of such a transfer?

(3) *Should* such a transfer take place?

Our information system consisted of three separate surveys. The *attendance survey* covered all 53,000 appointments in the six specialties during a period of 12 months. Data on the following variables were abstracted from clinic lists and from case-notes collected together for the clinic: date and location of clinic, consultant, whether the patient was 'new' or 'old', whether he attended, his hospital number, data of birth, sex, marital status, area of residence and general practitioner. These data were transferred to magnetic disc via punched cards, checked for internal consistency and linked to the other records for that patient.

The *patient survey* interviewed a two-stage stratified random sample of nearly 1000 outpatients, essentially using the attendance survey as a sampling frame. While waiting for their appointments, patients were asked about their number of companions, mode and cost of travel, time spent travelling, loss of earnings and preference between rural and central clinics. The *clinical survey* scrutinised the medical records of a retrospective random sample of 700 completed patient episodes, comprising more than 1600 attendances, for information on investigation and treatment.

Findings: Feasibility Study

Seven rural hosptials were origiñally considered as potential sites for outpatient clincs. In the interests of brevity this paper will restrict attention to the site which the study identified as most favourable — Penrith. Of the 53,000 appointments recorded in the attendance survey, some 2,500 took place rurally and a further 7,500 were not fulfilled. Three factors determine whether the remaining 43,000 consultations could have been transferred to Penrith:

(1) Geographical convenience. The patient survey asked each respondent which of the eight potential clinic sites (one central, seven rural) was the most convenient. Since the answers were consistent with the geography of the study area, they were used to define a notional Penrith catchment area, from which 7000 of the 43,000 attendances originated (Table 1, row (a)). Since very few of these were in psychiatry, the three existing clinics per week at Penrith are clearly adequate for that specialty. This paper will therefore consider only the remaining five specialties.

(2) Clinical considerations (Table 1, row (b)). Although the simpler medical procedures (Table 2, category I) can be provided at Penrith, the more complex procedures in category II can be provided only in Carlisle. There is a third category of procedures — those which need a separate journey to the district general hospital, either for practical reasons (e.g. when fasting is required) or because there is a waiting list; consultations which give rise to such procedures can also take place in Penrith.

(3) Patient preference (Table 1, row (c)). Of respondents for whom Penrith was both more convenient and clinically appropriate, 17% nevertheless preferred to attend in Carlisle.

TABLE 1 — Feasibility of Transferring Outpatient
Clinics From Carlisle to Penrith

Specialty	ENT	Gynae-cology	Medicine	Ortho-paedics	Surgery	Total
(a) Annual number of Carlisle attendances for which Penrith is geographically more convenient (1) (3)	1190	620	1230	2260	1750	7050
(b) Proportion in categories I or III i.e. for which clinical facilities at Penrith are likely to be adequate (2)	0.732	1	0.599	0.723	0.950	
(c) Proportion for which patient prefers to attend at Penrith (3)	0.846	0.797	0.809	0.855	0.870	
(d) Annual number of Carlisle attendances eligible for transfer to Penrith ((a)×(b)×(c))	740	490	600	1400	1450	4680
(e) Projected annual number of additional Penrith attendances likely to be 'generated' by the transfer of clinics	320	210	260	600	630	2020
(f) Projected annual number of additional Penrith attendances resulting from the transfer of clinics	1060	700	860	2000	2080	6700

Sources   (1) Attendance survey
         (2) Clinical survey
         (3) Patient survey

Taking account of all these factors, row (d) of Table 1 calculates that 4700 of the 43000 attendances per annum are eligible for transfer to Penrith. However, regular clinics at Penrith would bring specialist medical care some 14 miles closer to the average patient in the notional catchment area. It is difficult to predict how this would affect the demand for outpatient services. Although the referral rate within Carlisle is about twice that more than 15 miles away (Figure 1), this is partially attributable to concomitant differences in morbidity and consultation behaviour.

TABLE 2 — Availability of Medical Procedures at Outpatient
Clinics in East Cumberland

Category I   - Procedures available at rural hospitals

Specimens   - Urine, bacteriology, routine biochemistry, cytology, histology,
               haematology, serology.
Electrocardiography, proctoscopy, spirometry, simple hearing tests.
Surgery - Excisions, injection of varicose veins, etc.
Dressing, strapping, plaster, simple appliances.
Physiotherapy.
Removal of sutures.

Category II   - Procedures which are available only at the DGH and can take place
                 on the same day as the outpatient consultation.
Radiography - chest, other straight, extremities, skull.
Audiometry, sigmoidoscopy, special biochemistry.
Biopsy.
Special applicances.

Category III - Procedures which are available only at the DGH but cannot take
               place on the same day as the outpatient consultation. (The con-
               sultation itself may therefore take place at a rural hospital.)
Special radiography.
Audiology, electroencephalography, pathology.
Other surgery.

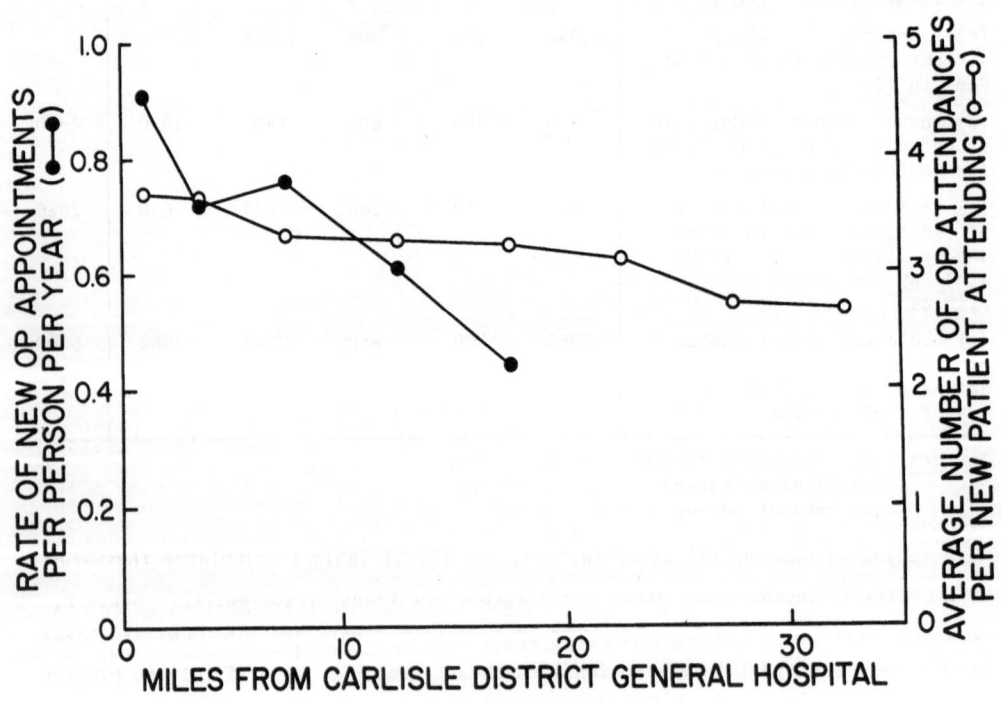

FIGURE 1 — Effect of Distance Upon Referral and Recall

We therefore predicted the number of additional attendances which would be 'generated' by regular clinics at Penrith by applying multiple regression analysis to data from both the attendance survey and the 1971 Census. Since the technical details will be reported elsewhere, we record only the prediction and two qualifications. In addition to potential statistical bias due to underspecification and multicollinearity (Johnston, 1972), referral and recall to rural clinics may turn out to be quite unlike that to central clinics.

Subject to these reservations, row (e) of Table 1 predicts that the 4700 transferred attendances would be joined by 2000 generated attendances. This would require that the existing weekly clinic in gynaecology be expanded and that five weekly clinics be transferred from Carlisle - two in surgery, one each in ENT and medicine, and one in orthopaedics in place of the existing monthly clinic at Penrith.

Findings: Cost-Benefit Analysis

The first column of Table 3 lists all the identifiable benefits and costs of transferring clinics to Penrith. (Note that this strategy was first proposed only as a means of achieving benefit B1.) Because this list includes essentially clinical benefits such as B3 and social costs such as C4, formal evaluation of the proposal requires the detailed application of cost-benefit analysis (Layard, 1972; Williams, 1974). Since the technical details will be reported elsewhere, we summarise the findings in Table 3 and comment selectively on the underlying economic considerations:

(B1) Reduced activity in the Carlisle outpatient department. Although the resources thus released could be used in many ways, we evaluate them on the assumption that staffing levels would be reduced.

(B2) Reduced travel for existing patients and their companions. This benefit comprises the (direct) saving in transport costs and the (indirect) value of the saving in travel time. In estimating the direct benefit, care is needed in identifying the beneficiaries.

If a patient driving his own car travels a shorter distance to a clinic, he and society as a whole gain to the extent of the petrol and wear saved. If he travels by ambulance, the NHS saves most but the expected saving is small unless he is the only patient carried. Finally, if the transferred appointment results in his getting off a bus at Penrith rather than Carlisle, the factors affecting the supply of rural bus services are such that there is no net (short-term) saving; although the patient has gained, the bus company has lost. These guidelines yield estimated direct benefits per patient transferred of £0.44 to the NHS, £0.76 to the patient and £1.13 to society with a balacing loss of seven pence to the bus companies. (All these sums represent 1973 prices, in common with all others quoted.)

In valuing travel time we distinguish between working time and leisure time. According to the theory of marginal productivity, the value of the 'goods' which would have been produced in working time is calculated not only from the employee's

TABLE 3 — Benefit and Costs of Transferring Outpatient Clinics From Carlisle to Penrith (Estimated at 1973 Prices)

Nature of benefit or cost	Estimated magnitude	Estimated average value per unit	Estimated annual value to		
			N.H.S.	Patient	Society
B1. Reduced activity in Carlisle OP department	240 less clinics	£4.58	£1100		£1100
B2. Reduced travel for existing patients and their companions	4700 transferred attendances	(a) £0.44 (NHS) (b) £0.95 (Patient) (c) £1.59 (Society)	£2050	£4450	£7450
B3. Increase in total number of OP attendances	2000 generated attendances	£0.21		£400	£400
C1. Increased activity at Penrith hospital	228 extra clinics	£10.31	-£2350		-£2350
C2. Increase in consultant time and travel	228 extra consultant sessions at Penrith	£14.55	-£3300		-£3300
C3. Patients mistakenly referred to Penrith rather than to Carlisle	170 mistaken attendances	(a) £0.42 (NHS) (b) £1.44 (Patient) (c) £3.00 (Society)	-£50	-£250	-£500
C4. Reduced number of opportunities for patients to visit Carlisle	4700 less opportunities	£0.41		-£1950	-£1950
C5. Increase in waiting time for appointments	3200 delays of about 1 week	£0.08		-£250	-£250
			-£2550	+£2400	+£600

wages but also from his employer's other costs (including the provision of facilities and the payment of pensions and national insurance). Thus the cost to society of working time lost in 1973 was on average 1.28 times the patient's wage-rate. However, the patient would have lost 0.65 times his earnings if paid by the hour and taxed at the standard rate but probably nothing if salaried.

In contrast, the Department of Transport currently recommends that cost-benefit studies of transport projects should value leisure time at 0.25 times the appropriate wage-rate. This figure has been derived from empirical studies of personal decisions on whether, where and how to travel, which route to take and how fast to drive (Harrison and Quarmby, 1972).

(C1) Increased activity at Penrith hospital. The cheapest method of housing the transferred clinics is in 'portable' accommodation at a capital cost of £4000, equivalent to an annual cost of £800 including depreciation. Staffing them would cost about £1550 per annum.

(C2) Increase in consultant time and travel. Given a 1973 mileage allowance of five pence, the direct cost of each consultant trip to Penrith is £1.80. Although the theory of marginal productivity is not entirely appropriate to consultants, there is no practical alternative method of valuing their time. In applying the resulting figure of £5.54 per hour, we recognise that the transfer of clinics requires consultants to spend additional time both in travelling and in treating generated attendances.

(C3) Patients mistakenly referred to Penrith rather than to Carlisle. Table 1 assumed that GPs can predict with complete accuracy the category (Table 2) into which every new consultation will fall. However, even if they were to err in as many as 20% of critical decisions, only 170 'unnecessary' attendances would result. This cost has been estimated in the same way as benefit B2.

(C4) Reduced number of opportunities for patients to visit Carlisle. Of respondents for whom Penrith was (geographically) most convenient, 17% nevertheless preferred to attend in Carlisle, for example to shop. By comparing individual preferences with the corresponding net benefit from transferring to Penrith, we estimate the average value of an opportunity to visit Carlisle as 41 pence. The increases by eight pence when the transfer causes a week's delay (cost C5), as it is likely to do for all specialties except surgery.

(B3) Increase in total number of outpatient attendances. By combining benefit B2 and costs C3, C4 and C5, we deduce from Table 3 that the average net cost to the *patient* of attending a clinic in Penrith is £0.42 (viz (£4450-£250-£1950-£250)/4700) less than in Carlisle. If we assume that GPs and consultants act (solely) in the interests of their patients, then the *a priori* expected net value of each generated attendance must lie between zero and £0.42. For if this value is negative, it is not in the patient's best interest to be referred or recalled even to Penrith; and if it exceeds £0.42, the patient should already have been referred or recalled to Carlisle. By further assuming that the expected net value of a generated attendance is uniformly distributed between zero and £0.42, we calculate that the average value is £0.21.

Discussion

We know of only two other studies which have set up an information system capable of guiding the location of outpatient services — Gruer (1971 and 1972) and Goldacre and Gatherer (1977a and 1977b). Goldacre carried out a survey very similar to our attendance survey, albeit for only one month. Gruer's information system was essentially a prospective version of our clinical survey and was used as the basis for a cost-effectiveness analysis of seven alternative configureations of outpatient services in the Scottish Borders. She restricted attention to travel costs (in particular to direct costs and loss of working time) and asserted that peripheral clincis invariably result in a reduction in patient travel costs greater than expenditure on consultant travel. Table 3 shows that we would have come to the same unequivocal conclusion had we been concerned only with benefit B2 and cost C2 (although our definition of these two effects is rather more comprehensive).

Because we wanted to consider all the identifiable benefits and costs of transferring clinics to rural hospitals, we designed a more extensive information system and adopted more sophisticated analysis than either Gruer or Goldacre. Even so, our system could have been improved in two ways. The attendance survey could have been based on a random sample of clinics; the clinical survey could have been based on the same random sample of patients as the patient survey, thus making it prospective rather than restrospective.

Table 3 suggests that the case for rural clinics is not as strong as suggested by Gruer and many others. An estimated net NHS expenditure of £2550 per annum generates benefits worth £2400 for patients and £750 for the *rest* of society, principally patients' employers. However, this conclusion is very dependent on our assumption that referral and recall to rural clinics (and, in particular, the effect of distance) can be predicted by observing central clinics, and on the resulting projection that the transfer of clinics would generate 2000 additional attendances. If there were to be only 1000 extra attendances, the net annual cost to the NHS would shrink to an expected £1450 but patients would gain an expected £2250.

Hence, the fewer attendances are generated by the transfer of outpatient clinics from district general hospital to rural hospitals, the stronger the case for that transfer becomes. Although this conclusion appears somewhat paradoxical, the explanation lies in the fact that, although the additional attendances cost the NHS more or less the same as the transferred attendances, the benefit they bring to patients is considerably less.

Acknowledgements

We are grateful to the DHSS for financial support and Mrs. Madge Moor, Mrs. Sheila Robinson and Mrs. Margaret Williams for assembling the data.

References

Acheson, E.D. (1968). *Journal of the Royal Statistical Society*, Series A, 131, 9-12.

Ashley, J.S.A. (1972). *British Journal of Preventive and Social Medicine*, 26, 135-147.

Benjamin, B. (1965). The Hospital, 61, 221-224.

Benjamin, B. (1977). *Journal of the Royal Statistical Society*, Series A, 140, 366-376.

Goldacre, M.J., Gatherer, A. (1977a). *The Hospital and Health Services Review*, 73, 14-16.

Goldacre, M.J., Gatherer, A. (1977b). *British Journal of Preventive and Social Medicine*, 31, 205-208.

Gruer, R. (1971). *Lancet*, i, 390-394.

Gruer, R. (1972). *Outpatient Services in the Scottish Border Counties*. Scottish Health Service Studies No. 23. Scottish Home and Health Department, Edinburgh.

Harrison, A.J., Quarmby, D.A. (1972). In *Cost-Benefit Analysis* ed. Layard, P.R.G. Penguin, London.

Johnston, J. (1972). *Econometric Methods* (2nd edition). McGraw-Hill, New York.

Layard, P.R.G. (1972). *Cost-Benefit Analysis*. Penguin, London.

Williams, A.H. (1974). *British Medical Bulletin*, 30, 252-256.

MODELS, INFORMATION SYSTEMS, AND THE MANAGEMENT OF
HEALTH CARE ORGANIZATIONS

G. A. Gorry, Ph.D.
Baylor College of Medicine
Houston, Texas, U.S.A.

Introduction

Concern that the health care system as currently constituted is incapable of adequately serving the needs of society has motivated a
reappraisal of existing organizational forms and functions and a
search for new, more effective configurations of services. Attention has been focused on innovations such as health teams, group
practice, prepayment, and taking health services out to the community. In some cases, the fruits of these efforts are already apparent
in neighborhood health centers, reorganized ambulatory care systems,
and health maintenance organizations. Experiments are underway to
evaluate the effectiveness of such organizations, and although such
experiments are fraught with many difficulties and definitive results
have yet to be obtained, it is apparent that variants of such organizations will play an important role within the health care system of
the near future. Although the general role of such organizations
is predictable, the precise shape they will take and the policies
which will govern them are less clear. Even if a clear picture were
available, there would remain the difficult task of altering organizational structures with a minimum of trauma to the system.

To cope effectively with this range of novel situations and demands,
decision makers within health care organizations need a better understanding of the systems they control and of the environments in which
these systems operate. Information scientists can help in the development of this improved understanding. For the best use of the
skills of information scientists, however, both they and the managers
of health care organizations need to reassess the role of information
science in supporting managerial decision making.

The major emphasis of information scientists in the health care

setting (and in many industrial settings as well) has been on providing managers with information of better quality, where quality is
measured along a number of dimensions such as accuracy or timeliness.
The presumption has been that improvements in the quality of information provided the managers will produce improvements in the quality
of decisions. In this paper it will be argued that, in the context
of health care organizations, this assumption is for the most part
invalid, and that this emphasis on extensive data collection is mis-
placed. In order to improve the quality of decision making at high
management levels, health care managers and information scientists
should focus more attention on model building than on data gathering.
The principle that will be developed in this paper is that model
building precedes data collecting and hence it precedes information
systems development. Any effort that is directed at data gathering
to support management decision making which does not have a firm
basis in a model for using that information is ill-conceived and
will undoubtedly have little positive effect on the organization.

In this paper managerial decision making will be viewed in a way
which relates modeling and information systems development. The
approach, which was used successfully in the analysis of industrial
uses of information systems (1), is decision-centered, relating the
role of information and models to different types of decisions within health services organizations. By concentrating on the decisions
to be made rather than on questions of organizational structure,
the approach underscores the variety of ways in which information
scientists can augment the abilities of health care managers to make
sound decisions. The framework which this approach yields may help
those managers allocate their resources more rationally and move
from an ex post facto justification of specific information science
projects to a coherent program more directly reflective of this
organizational goals.

A Framework for Decision Making in Health Care Organizations

A combination of two different perspectives on managerial decision
making (1) yields a useful view of the potential role of models in
the management of health care organizations. The first, proposed by
Anthony for understanding planning and control systems (2), emphasizes

the type of management activity involved. Anthony identifies strategic planning as being "... the process of deciding on objectives of an organization, on changes in these objectives, on the resources used to attain these objectives, and on the policies that are to govern acquisition, use, and disposition of these resources." Management control he defines as "... the process by which managers assure that resources are obtained and used effectively and efficiently in the accomplishment of an organization's objectives." As his third type óf management activity, Anthony defines operational control as "... the process of assuring that specific tasks are carried out effectively and efficiently". These are broad characterizations of fundamental management activities in health care organizations.

Whereas Anthony's view of planning and control activities emphasizes the nature of the management task, that of Simon (3) stresses the nature of the decision-making process involved, irrespective of the particular management task at hand. Simon identifies a continuum along which any management decision-making process can be placed. At one extreme are routine and repetitive decisions which are here termed structured; and at the other novel and consequential decisions which are here termed unstructured. As one moves from the structured end of the spectrum towards the unstructured end, one encounters in-creasing requirements for judgment and evaluation as well as more emphasis upon the development of proper problem definitions.

The combination of these two perspectives on managerial decision making yields the framework for the consideration of the role of models in the management of health care organizations. When the framework was developed to aid in the analysis of modeling efforts and information systems work in the private sector, it was observed that virtually all of the activity to date had occurred in the structured operational control area. This is true despite the fact that many of the most significant decisions within the organizations occur in the other areas of the matrix, and most high level managers devote virtually all their time to problems in the unstructured domain. In health care organizations, a similar concentration of model building and information systems effort on structured operational control problems can be seen, although, in

general, in the health care field these efforts have been less pro-
nounced and successful.

As in industrial organizations, the reasons for this relative imbalance
in the effort within health care organizations are several. First,
the term 'structured' implies that routine procedures have been developed for dealing with the problems in question, and these routine
procedures are often quite amenable to modeling. Second, the line
which divides structured from unstructured decisions shifts over time
so as to encompass in the structured domain those decisions which are
made more routine by the development of new analytical techniques.
Third, the more specific nature of the tasks involved in operational
control makes this area a more obvious target for model development
and adaptation. Often the problem of developing good models for a
structured operational decision is basically that of implementing an
existing model, drawn perhaps from the industrial setting, in a new
certain organizational context. In contrast, for the other areas of
managerial activity in health care organizations, far greater emphasis
must be placed upon the development of appropriate models through
which data can be organized and upon which decision making procedures
can be based. The lack of such models is one of the principal im-
pediments to the advancement of information systems in support of high
level management decision making in the health care sector.

Managerial Problem Solving

Not only does the current use of models vary across the managerial
functions of health care organizations, but so does the use of models
in problem solving within the context of a given managerial activity.

Many years ago, John Dewey identified three phases of problem solving
by associating each phase with a key question: "What is the problem?",
"What are the alternatives?", and "Which alternative is best?" Of
course, few important problems are dealt with through the strictly
sequential consideration of these questions. For example, difficulties
in defining reasonable alternatives may well invoke a whole new problem-solving cycle, and the definition of a particular problem itself

may require an extensive problem-solving activity. Nonetheless, these three questions do denote the major phases of problem solving and hence of managerial decision making.

Dewey's first question deserves special attention, because managerial decision making is characterized most often as problem solving with the emphasis being placed on the choice among given alternatives. It has been noted by various investigators of organizational behavior, however, that problem definition is an equally basic managerial task. The failure to identify important problems, the incorrect definition of problems, and the inappropriate assignment of priorities to problems all constitute potentially major deficiencies in the administrative function.

A static picture of the problem definition process is presented in Figure 1. The manager possesses a model of his environment which we shall term normative. The "environment" is some aspect of his organization exists, and the normative model is the manager's view of how that entity ought to function. This model generally is not a formal one; indeed it is most often a rather crude, implicit notion of "the way things should be." It may be based upon history, as in the case where the performance of some organizational function is measured against the past performance of that function. The model may reflect a belief that some aspect of his organization should perform comparably to a similar aspect of another organization. In some cases, the normative model may be based on little more than a "feeling" about the standards which should be achieved by certain individuals or groups.

By comparison, the manager's information system (computer-based or not) provides him with a descriptive model of the same segment of his environment. The descriptive model is an approximation to the way in which the particular entity in question currently is functioning. By comparing these normative and descriptive models, the manager can identify differences between the two, and some of these differences are problems for the organization to solve. The success of problem definition then depends on the validity of both the manager's normative model and the descriptive model provided to him. Deficiencies in either model or incomparabilities between the two can limit his ability to define problems properly. This, in turn, can cause him to squander resources (time, money, etc.) in a given situation.

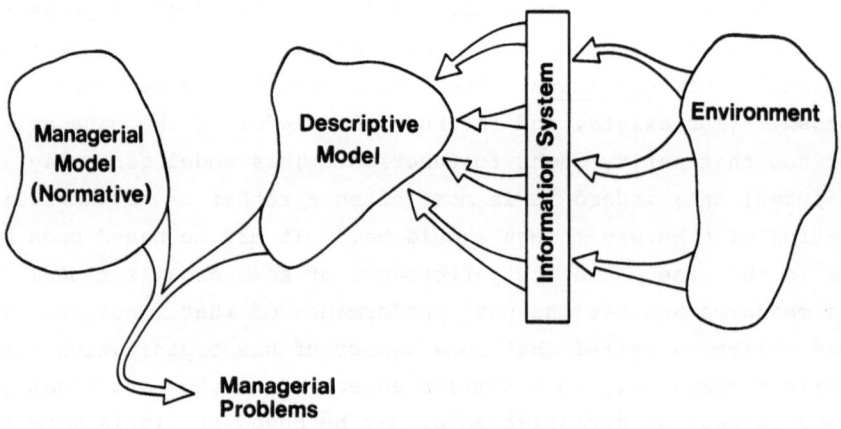

Figure 1.

Once a problem has been defined (and has been deemed worthy of
solution), the manager finds himself faced with Dewey's second question, namely finding alternative solutions. This can often be the
most difficult aspect of problem solving, particularly when there
exists a host of organizational constraints on any proposed solution.
Indeed in some instances, the fundamental problem may be to generate
any feasible alternative. Again, however, the models which the manager
possesses play an important role in determining the alternatives which
he investigates. Those "variables" which appear in these models are
the most likely choices for investigation. He will consider the
manipulation of these variables to achieve a reduction in the difference between the situation as it is and the situation as he wishes it
to be. In fact, the generation of alternatives may be synonymous
with assigning specific values to various model variables over which
he has control. It is difficult for him to consider alternatives
which require terms different from those appearing in his model.

The selection of the best alternative is of course the prospect of
problem solving which most often is identified with decision making.
From our brief discussion, however, it is clear, that this "moment
of decision" merely follows on several important previous steps. In
this phase inadequate models can have another detrimental effect on
the decision making process. His models may be too simple or they
may be simply incorrect so his subsequent predictions of the effects
of various alternatives may be in error. The model in question may
be inappropriately bounded; important variables aspects of the
manager's environment are not represented in the model. Hence, an
alternative which is deemed optimal in theory may well prove to be
a poor one in fact.

Model Building for Health Care Management

To improve the quality of decisions in health care organizations,
improvements in the quality of available information or changes the
decision process (or both) can be sought. Here the variety and importance of these uses of managerial models has been emphasized, and
the inadequacy of many of these models has been suggested. Although

an emphasis in data-gathering activities is appropriate for structured
operational control problems, it can retard the development of support
for unstructured problem solving; because it tends to attribute low
quality in decision making to low quality in information. More current,
more accurate, or more detailed information may be of little value to
the managers of health care organizations without improved models by
which they can apply that information to their problems. For this
reason, model development often should precede data gathering as
Forrester has repeatedly emphasized. Speaking of the analysis of
industrial operation, he noted (4):

> "...many persons discount the potential utility of models
> of industrial operations on the assumption that we lack
> adequate data on which to base a model. They believe a
> first step must be an extensive collecting of statistical
> data. Exactly the reverse is true...a model should come
> first. And one of the first uses of such a model should
> be to determine what formal data needs to be collected...
> before we measure, we should name the quantity, select
> a scale of measurement, and in the interest of efficiency
> we should have a reason for wanting to know."

This principle applies equally well to the public sector. The models
that we need to develop should be aimed as much at identifying information needs and providing a framework for the integration of
various judgments as they are at predicting the consequences of
various actions.

Information scientists, working in close collaboration with health
care managers, can develop the needed models. Although managers and
planners of health care organizations often lack the ability to
articulate a firm basis for their decisions in the complex environments within which they work, it should not be assumed that this
inability prevents them from contributing to the development of better
models. Our work and that of others has shown that in many cases,
health care managers constitute a rich source of descriptive information even when their decision-making performance is unimpressive
(5,6). Through the selective use of their judgments, a significant

data collection analysis effort may be avoided. After the sensitivity of a given model to the estimates of its parameters has been investigated, the value of refined estimates can be determined more rationally.

Along the same lines, it should be noted that the educative value of model building often is underemphasized. In their emphasis on improving planning and resource allocation decisions, many people, analysts and decision makers alike, tend to judge the value of a model in terms of specific decisions which must be made. Educative models however ultimately can improve decision-making effectiveness. First, the decision maker's ability to assess parameters may increase as he becomes more familiar with the model and the consequences it draws from his assessments (6). Additional benefits may accrue over relatively long periods of time in unanticipated ways. Although a concern for a definite immediate return from a modeling effort is understandable, it should not be allowed to divert attention from the need for a better understanding of the environment in general.

Conclusion

Models and information systems can play crucial roles in the development of health care organizations. The information scientist then, has a potentially important role to play in this development. By involving themselves more intimately in the analysis and refinement of managerial decision-making processes, information scientists can profitably enlarge the scope of their activities within health care organizations. One of the principal contentions of this paper is that such an involvement should emphasize model building as much as data gathering, because the quality of managerial decision making is presently limited more by the inadequacies in managerial models than in available data. Further, without an increased emphasis on the development of sound managerial models, little progress can be expected towards the effective use of information systems in the support of higher management functions.

Health care managers, too, should recognize the importance of model development. Without collaboration with managers, information scientists cannot be expected to produce models which are directly useful in defining and resolving higher level management problems.

In the final analysis, a new partnership between managers and information scientists is needed to help guide health care organizations through the difficult times ahead.

References

(1) Gorry, G.A., and Scott Morton, M.S.   "A Framework for Management Information Systems." Sloan Management Review. Fall 1971, 55-70.

(2) Anthony, R.N. Planning and Control Systems: A Framework for Analysis.   Boston, Harvard University Graduate School of Business Administration, 1965.

(3) Simon, H.A. The New Science of Management Decision. New York, Harper & Rose, 1960.

(4) Forrester, J.W.   Industrial Dynamics. Cambridge, Mass., MIT Press, 1961

(5) G. A. Gorry and Scott Morton "The Development of Managerial Models", Sloan Management Review, Winter 1971.

(6) Little, J.D., "Models and Managers: The Concept of a Decision Calculus," Management Science, Vol. 16, No. 6, (April 1970), pp. B46-B48.

The Patient-Service Scheduling System at the Dresden Medical Academy and its Further Development on the Basis of an ESER EDPS

W.-D. Grimm, M. DSc.

Medizinische Akademie "Carl Gustav Carus" Dresden

1. Introduction

The Dresden Medical Academy is a 2000-beds Medical School for medical and stomatological education. Since 1972, its hospital operates with a patient-oriented information processing system which represents an essential contribution to comprehensive computer application. The overall system is made up of the subsequently listed computer-aided procedures of patient-oriented information processing in the hospital:
- Basis processes of patient-oriented and administrative information processing
- Patient-oriented information and documentation
- Communication between user (ward, outpatient clinics) and service units (clinical laboratories, radiotherapeutic department etc.)
- Computer-aided decision finding.
At the time being, more than 15 of the largest medical units in the GDR are using EDP projects worked out at the Dresden Medical Academy. To further develop patient-oriented information processing in large hospitals it is now necessary to employ a more efficient EDPS of the ESER Series. The acronym "ESER" stands for "Unified System of Electronic Data Processing Technique" of the Socialist countries.
This generally applicable and complex information system has to be worked out with due consideration of the following requirements:
- Implementation of the data bank principle
- Modular structure of the overall system and of its components
- Adequate problem variablility of subsystems
- Use of telecommunication access and display techniques for work in conversational mode
- Development of a computer hierarchical system.

2. MADIS Information Processing System of the Dresden Medical Academy

The information processing system of the Dresden Medical Academy
(1) is based on a comprehensive functional centrlization; i.e.,
depending on the ESER Technique to be used, based on a centralized
computer configuration and on a central data bank. The thus obtained concentration in hardware and software is supplemented by small
computer or process control computer systems which handle subsets
of the necessary overall information; provided the specific characteristic of these sets does not indicate that processing on the
central computer seems to be more adequate. The I/O system must ensure that all relevant information is received and retained in a
central data bank, processed and finally made available to the decentralized subsystems or users. Employed as central is an ESER
1040 EDP System. In addition, some selected diagnostic and therapeutic units are fitted with suitable small computer system or process control computers that are prevalently used for automated medical data processing (Figure 1). The most significant components
of the Academy's information processing system are:
- MADAB Medical Data Bank System
- MADPIV Patient-oriented I/O System
- MADLAB Clinical Laboratory Information Processing System based
  on the use of the KRS 4200 Small Computer System
- MADRAS Inquiry and Evaluating System
- LIS Management Information System inclusive of hospital management
- MADRIS Dispensary and Register Information System.
The MAD Information Processing System is a modular assembly compri-
sing a variable number of subsystem which, in effect, are mutually
linked by the data bank. In part, however, these subsystems may al-
so take over independent functions in an isolated manner.

MADAB Medical Data Bank System

To obtain a scheduled structural presentation of all data residing
in the data bank, patient-oriented information is divided into four
categories, viz:-
(i)   Condensated fixed master data of the patients
(ii) Patient data collected during stationary treatment

(iii) Patient data collected in outpatient departments

(iv) Set of particular diagnostic and therapeutic data collected
      in the specialized departments of the hospital.

Object of stored data category (i) is the patient himself. Category
(ii) concerns stationary treatment of the patient within a given period (e.g., stay in hospital, specialized departments or wards). Data allocated to category (iii) are referred to a particular period
of time of outpatient treatment. Fixed, condensated patient data of
all categories reside in direct-access volumes to render them available in converational mode during admission of the patient to the
hospital. This data set is followed by further patient-oriented information gathered either during stationary (ii) or outpatient (iii)
treatment. It should be pointed out, however, that these data are directly accessible only for case of the current year. Data kept for
records are further managed within the framework of MADAB and may thus
be evaluated by batch processing. Evaluation in conversational mode
must also be prepared via batch processing. In compliance with the
structurized schedule the data bank is supplemented by a variable
amount of data files for special diagnostic and treatment records
(iv). Here the object referred to is the individual finding (e.g,
clinical and chemical laboratory findings, microbiological findings,
radiological consultation reports etc.) obtained in a patient who was
given treatment either stationary in the Dresden Medical Academy or
in one of the outpatient departments, and in a patient who is cared
for by another regional medical unit, respectively. Similar medical
findings are collected in filed allocated to the various specialized
diagnostic department. Findings pertaining to patients who were given
treatment either in the Dresden Medical Academy or in an outpatient
department will be added to patient data already stored in the categories (ii) and (iii), respectively. An extrem case is the data file
required for radiological therapy which - due to its complex nature -
has been set up as a partial autonomous data base. The basic principles of implementing the program technique are shown in Figure 2. User
and data base are linked on various levels with different technique
components, i.e.:

- MADPIV Patient-oriented I/O System
- MADRAS Inquiry and Evaluating System
- DBS/R Data Bank System
- OS/ES General EDPS Operating System.

MADPIV Patient-oriented I/O System

Continuous updating of the data bank is by a general I/O program
system which also includes the checking of patient-oriented data.
Up to a defined interface of the DBS/R Data Bank System, this program system operates almost independent. With the aid of such a User system, patient-oriented primary data (2) may thus be acquired
and input on either punched tape or punched card and marked documents, respectively. In the first completion stage, the following
information is acquired and output in the form of computer epicri-
ses, consultation reports, activity or inventory lists etc., viz:
- Patient master data
- Admission and dismissal reports
- Follow-up basic and specific medical reports totalling to 12
  applicatory cases
- Clinical and laboratory findings
- Reports on autopsy examinations
- Microbiological and cytolytic findings
- Special radiological findings inclusive of physical radiotherapy
  scheduling.

MADLAB Clinical Laboratory Information Processing System

This system operates with the KRS 4200 Small Computer System and,
at present, handles the following service activities:
- Informations processing in the fields of clinical chemistry and
  hematology
- Computer-aided quality control
- Data preparation for off-line pooling with the ES 1040 EDP System.
In the first phase, off-line data coupling is by magnetic tape. The
MADPIV I/O System transfer all patient master data to the laboratory
information processing system so as to create the necessary prerequisite to uniform patient identification in the subsystem. The small
computer system, on the other hand, passes on results, statistical
information and already processed data to the central data bank. In
the large-size computer these data may then be further processes
together with other patient-oriented information for generating a
cumulative report. In addition, specific laboratory files are made
available for special evaluation (i.e., quality control and scien-

tific work).

Planned in the second completion stage is the on-line connection of MADLAB to the ES 1040 EDP System as a first step towards the development of a computer hierarchical system. In this stage complete coupling is obtained between the subsystems MADLAB and MADPIV. Because the laboratory information processing system not only processes on-line data but - generated on various media either by manual input or laboratory equipment - also parameters of clinical chemistry and hematology, autonomy must be maintained by defined interfaces. This is the more so as such a system has to satisfy high demands with respect to time. The mentioned 32 K-byte process control computer and, in part, peripheral small computer systems (Model OLLI-3000) or microprocessors assist in splitting up the respective processing procedures.

MADRAS Inquiry and Evaluating System

One essential component of hospital information processing systems is a pack of almost immediately accessible search and evaluating programs. Although the data sets may be stored in any convenient manner, they must comply with a system of uniform data organisation. In the information processing system of the Dresden Medical Academy this is accomplished by a centralized medical data bank in connection with specialized data based and autonomous projects. To prepare such data, MADRAS provides a corresponding program system which - at a later date - will form part of an A. I. System for conversational processing without thesauri; using a medical language for the purpose. The nucleus of this inquiry and evaluting system comprises methods of descriptive and mathematical statistics based on preengineered program modules of VEB Kombinat Robotron (e.g., PP Statistics etc.). Facility for interactive work with this system will then be provided in a subsequent completion stage. Derived in agreement with this general task are the basic modules of MADRAS, viz:

- Descriptive module for data conversion to a uniform organizational structure
- Input and checking module for creating user-orientes evaluation matrices in a special evaluation file
- Retrieval module for selecting the data needed for evaluation in the sense of iterative working with the evaluating system

- Patch module for updating or correction of the special evaluation file
- Analysis module which comprises methods of descriptive and mathematical statistics
- Computing module for arithmetic, boolean and cumulative operations.

MADRIS Dispensary and Register Information System

It is a request of top priority to acquire and store patient-oriented information within the framework of a particular category of diseaese beyond the coverage of a medical unit on a regional or, if possible, national scale. Forms of medical care existing in the GDR - such as dispensary care, compulsory registration of certain diseases etc. - give a sound foundation for setting up such a specific register of grouped diseases (MADRIS) which allows the creation of administrative call and supervision systems as well as comprehensive medical evaluation (case histories, scientific interrogation etc.). In this way the physician will be able to gather current information on the individual patient and on the respective group of diseases within a very short time. Being developes as a computational base is the MADRIS Subsystem wich possesses a defined interface to the inquiry and evaluating system needed for special investigation which also offers facility for data transfer to the central data bank system.

Service to be rendered by MADRIS:
- Supported data input via any peripheral input unit
- Data checking according to User requirements by means of flexible checking module
- Data storage and management by a data base operating system independent of the central data bank and supported by facilities for file updating, data stock correction and data set extension.

3. Further Development of the Patient-oriented Information Processing System at the Dresden Medical Academy

The following aspects are characteristic of the advanced patient-oriented information processing system being under development at the Dresden Medical Academy:

- Extension of medical/problem-oriented solutions (biopsy findings, radiological consultation reports, functional diagnosticss etc.)
- Step-by-step substitution of batch processing by conversational mode processing of all components contained in the overall system; i.e., MADPIV, MADLAB, MADRAS and MADRIS
- Setup of a comprehensive computer hierarchical system in compliance with the three levels usually found in medicine, viz:
  (a) Microprocessor level
  (b) Small computer system or process control computer level (data concentration)
  (c) EDPS level
- Step-by-step incorporation of hospital information processing into a pooled regional computer system.

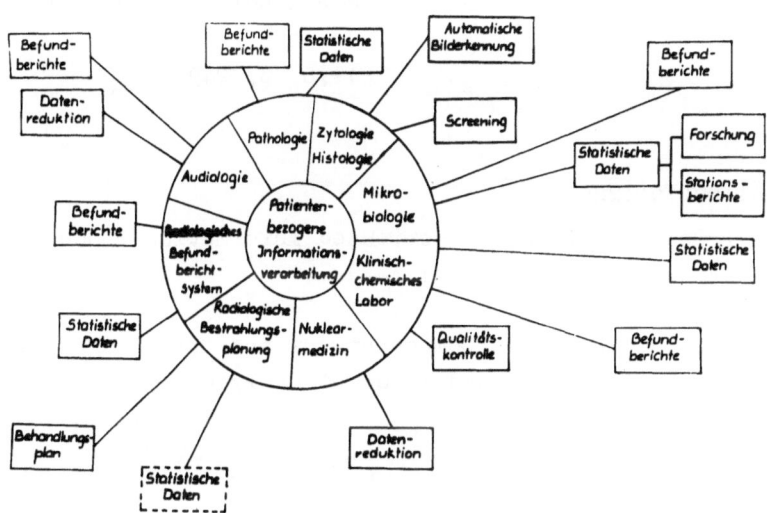

References

(1) Grimm, W.-D.   The Patient-oriented Infor-
                                    mation Processing System at
                                    the Dresden Medical Academy
                                    and its User Reactions
                                    7th International Congress
                                    on Medical Records, Toronto,
                                    September, 12 - 17, 1976

(2) Schmincke, W. et al.   Automatic Data Processing
                                    of Medical Records for the
                                    Increase of the Effectivity
                                    of Medical Care
                                    Information Systems for Patient
                                    Care (Ed. J. van Egmond)
                                    North Holland Publishing
                                    Company
                                    1976, p. 249 - 280

Legend to Illustrations

Figure 1:   Principle of Patient-oriented Information Processing
            at the Dresden Medical Academy

Figure 2:   Program Technique Components of the Data Bank System
            for Patient-oriented Information Processing

Address of author:

OA Dr. sc. med. W.-D. Grimm
GDR - 8045 Dresden
Rottwerndorfer Str. 3/1002

A COMPUTER PROGRAM FOR CALCULATING INTRAVENOUS FEEDING REGIMENS AND ITS

APPLICATION IN A TEACHING HOSPITAL AND A DISTRICT GENERAL HOSPITAL

by G.Shearing[1], P.D.Wright[2], R.M.James[3], J.M.Roberts[3],

R.I.Cooper[4], J.D.Bellis[5], P.W.Harvey[3] and A.J.Rich[2].

1. Introduction.

The provision of nutrients for hospitalised patients by routes other than oral can be expensive. The cost of infusion fluids for typical patients on intravenous feeding is about £30 per day and it has been estimated that one Regional Health Authority spends roughly £1 million a year on intravenous fluids alone, (1). The normal 'rule of thumb' management of short-term intravenous feeding relies on the innate clinical judgement of the experienced clinician and cost is not usually an important consideration in such cases. However, prolonged illness with its associated metabolic and nutritional problems is more difficult to manage since at least ten inter-related variables may need to be taken into account, often on an hour-to-hour basis. Without aid, calculation of intravenous feeding regimens for such patients in real time becomes almost impossible and costing is almost invariably disregarded.

The work on a computer program to calculate i.v. feeding regimens was started in 1974 in the Department of Surgery at the Royal Victoria Infirmary, (RVI), Newcastle-upon-Tyne, (PDW), in consultation with the University Computing Laboratory, (GS). The Northumbrian Universities' Multiple Access Computer, (NUMAC), in the form of an IBM 370/168 was available and much of the early development work was carried out on this machine using the Michigan Terminal System, (MTS),(2). This is a very powerful system and is ideal for developing large programs but is not so suitable for providing a full time hospital service. An interim report was published,(3) and consequently the group at the Royal Lancaster Infirmary, (RLI), became aware of the project. They then expressed interest in adapting the programs to their own particular needs.

Initially, no reports of similar work could be traced but while preparing this paper we have come across such a reference, (4). This work is based on a DEC PDP-8 mini computer and is aimed at providing a local hospital service.

---

1 Computing Laboratory, University of Newcastle-upon-Tyne, UK
2 Surgery Dept., Royal Victoria Infirmary, Newcastle-upon-Tyne, UK
3 Pathology Dept., Royal Lancaster Infirmary, UK
4 Pharmacy Dept., Royal Lancaster Infirmary, UK
5 Area Pharmacy Officer, Beaumont Hospital, Lancaster, UK

2. The General Intravenous Feeding Problem.

Most patients undergoing surgery are relatively well nourished and are able to compensate for excesses or deficiencies in their therapy without ill effects. For those patients who present longer term problems as a result of complications, proper calculation of precise fluid, electrolyte and nutritional requirements becomes more important. With more advanced knowledge of the complex requirements of patients it becomes increasingly difficult for adequate regimens to be prepared at the foot of the bed on a daily ward round. It is important not only to collect accurate data on the daily input and output of a patient, but also to be able to interpret the information and use it to the best possible advantage.

The calculations can be conveniently divided into two parts: 1) to calculate, for the following day, the patient's requirements of basic constituents, (water, calories, protein, etc.), and 2) given a list of available fluids and their composition, determine that combination which most effectively satisfies these requirements. These two problems are fairly independent and quite different. The former requires much medical knowledge and, by computer standards, not too much calculation. The latter involves a great deal of calculation but minimal medical content. So far, most progress has been made with the second problem.

Before describing the program for the second problem, it is appropriate to briefly review the methods used to solve the first. The general principles are well known and comprehensive accounts are given in several textbooks, for example (5)-(9). If a bedridden patient has no major physical problems then it is quite straightforward to calculate his requirements for water, calories, sodium etc. which will keep him 'in balance'. In practice problems arise due to:

1) the patient being 'metabolically depleted' initially,
2) the patient having a high temperature,
3) other fluid losses via vomit, diarrhoea, fistula drainage etc.,
4) chronic organic malfunction such as renal or hepatic failure,
5) severe burns.

Treatment consists of prescribing fluid therapy which will maintain continuing insensible losses, replace any extra losses and make up for previous deficits. Consideration must also be given to whether the patient can actually tolerate the proposed therapy, and whether there is a risk of contamination due to additives. Necessary information comes from biochemical tests on blood and urine in particular. A computer program, Dailyreq, has been written at Newcastle to solve this problem but it is currently rather rudimentary.

3. The Newcastle Infusions Program.

This section describes how the second problem has been solved by a computer program. The following simple example elaborates. Suppose that we know the requirements for water, sodium and calories of a patient on i.v. feeding. Suppose also that we have only three different types of bottle of infusion fluid. The contents of the available bottles and the patient's requirements are given in the following table:

Fluid	Abbreviation	Water,ml	Sodium,mmol	Calories
Normal saline	N/S	500	77	0
Dextrose 20%	D20	500	0	410
Dextrose saline	D/S	500	15	83
Requirements		1300	100	350

For nursing it is necessary to restrict the choice to whole-bottle combinations. Because of the water requiremnt, it is clear that only 2 or 3-bottle combinations need be considered. There are, in fact, 16 such combinations in this simple case. A good regimen is one bottle each of N/S and D20 which gives -23,-23 and +17 for the percentage errors of the 3 constituents respectively. If we add one bottle of D/S then these errors become +15,-8 and +41. Which combination is best? It all depends how you define 'best'. The second regimen is better with respect to sodium but worse for calories. Does it matter unduly if the patient has too many calories? Even if we decide that the second choice is better, it must cost more as there is an extra bottle. Therefore we should consider whether this extra cost is justified.

In a more realistic situation, the number of available types of bottle is 20 or 30, including small ampoules and we need to consider many more constituents. A computer program for solving this problem was first written a few years ago but many difficulties were encountered due to the 'combinatorial' nature of the problem. A satisfactory Fortran IV program now exists which runs interactively on an MTS terminal and is known as the Infusions Program.

Associated with the program are three computer files, (on magnetic disk storage), which give the program the specifications of the available fluids and other numerical information. A few records of the specifications file are:

```
KD/S     500    POTASSIUM CHLORIDE IN DEXTROSE SALINE
NA   30    K    30    CL    60    GLUC 40    H2O 1000  /
CCAL  164    TCAL  164
```

The first line defines the abbreviated name used by the program, the normal size of bottle and the full name. Subsequent lines define the amounts of the various constituents per litre. Here GLUC = glucose, TCAL = total calories, CCAL = carbohydrate calories and '/' is a continuation character. The order and precise format are flexible. Not all items specified need be used by the program for it contains its own list of those constituents which it needs. This master file is also used by other programs. Besides i.v. fluids it contains details of injections, additives, oral/tube feeds, blood products and bodily secretions.

The second file contains a list of names of i.v. fluids to be read from the main file, together with the sizes, costs and units used. Different users may have different versions of this second file but use the same main file. The third file gives the program other items of information such as numerical parameters for the fit function, (see below). The aim is to be as flexible as possible since this is important in hospital practice. It is easier to change files than programs.

The basic data for the program consists of the required values, RV, of 9 constituents, (some of which may be ignored). The program systematically examines combinations of the available bottles and calculates the fit function. This gives a measure of how good each trial combination is. Let CV be the calculated value of a constituent in a combination, then we define the relative error E by the formula

$$E = (CV-RV)/max(RV,tol)$$

and 'tol' is introduced so that an artificially small RV cannot produce a large E.

The fit function is given by

$$F = \Sigma\, w_i * E_i^2$$

and the weights w_i are chosen according to how important it is for that constituent to be fitted accurately. The value of the weight depends on the sign of E. The mixtures and constituents are arranged in an optimal order so that as many terms as possible of the fit function can be calculated at the earliest opportunity. (The external order of the constituents is as given in the example; the best internal order depends on the available mixtures and can be changed if necessary without altering the external appearance). As it proceeds the program stores details of the 40 best regimens found so far. As soon as a partial regimen is found to be worse than the worst of these 40 then the program abandons a whole group of potential regimens and 'backtracks'. The current program virtually guarantees to find the 'best' regimens, (according to its definition), very rapidly. It is now considered to be 'robust' enough to experiment with the fit function, introduce other constituents and so on. Previous versions were rather sensitive to such experimentation and also to different sets of mixtures.

The program is simple to use at a terminal. On the following page is an example terminal run as used for a real patient's data in conjunction with the current file of fluid specifications at the RVI. This should be fairly easily understood with the aid of the following notes:

1) Numerical input is in free format and is checked; if in error it can be re-input.

2) The program checks that all numbers are of reasonable size.

3) A minus sign on its own for a required value means that that constituent is to be omitted from the fit function.

```
RUN INFUSIONS                              *-------  User's input marked thus.
NUMAC-RVI INFUSIONS PROGRAM MARK 13  MAR '78
PATIENT NO.,DAY NO. & WEIGHT?
233347 5 43                                *-------
PLEASE TYPE IN THE REQUIRED VALUES OF:
   H2O  TCAL N    NA   K   PO4  CA   MG   CCAL
IN ML.       GM.  MMOL MMOL MMOL MMOL MMOL          Notation:
2420 2930 14.6 101 85 19 - 6 880           *-------
PATIENT'S WEIGHT = 43 KG.,INFUSION TIME = 24 HOURS  H2O    water
 2420.0 ML.  H2O                                    TCAL   total calories
 2930.0      TCAL                                   N      nitrogen
   14.6 GM.  N                                      NA     sodium
  101.0 MMOL NA                                     K      potassium
   85.0 MMOL K                                      PO4    phosphate
   19.0 MMOL PO4                                    CA     calcium
    6.0 MMOL MG                                     MG     magnesium
  880.0      CCAL                                   CCAL   carbohydrate calories
IS THE INPUT DATA CORRECT?                          GLUC   glucose
YES                                        *-------  I20    Intralipid 20%
WHICH MIXTURES ARE NOT AVAILABLE FOR THIS PATIENT?  BPO4&  buffered phosphate inj.
BA BB AX14 D5 D10                          *-------  AMFF   Aminofusin Forte
 40 POSSIBLE REGIMES                                MGCL&  magnesium chloride inj.
COST = 30.54 - 41.93 POUNDS                         AL10   Aminosol 10%
FIT =  0.0334 - 0.0944                              KCLG*  potassium chloride inj.
'FIT:COST RATIO'?                                   D5     dextrose 5%  etc.
0.5                                        *-------  BA     Baxter's solution A
MAX. % ERROR FOR PRINTING?                          BB     Baxter's solution B
7                                          *-------  AX14   Aminoplex 14
HOW MANY TO PRINT?
2                                          *-------
ALL REGIMES OF THE FOLLOWING GROUP,( 1 - 2),CONTAIN:
  2 *   500.0 ML.   I20
  2 *     8.3 MMOL  BPO4&
  1 *   500.0 ML.   AMFF
  2 *     2.0 MMOL  MGCL&
  1 *   500.0 ML.   AL10
  4 *     1.0 GM.   KCLG*
TOTALS & % ERRORS:
PO4   16.7 MMOL -12
CA     0.0 MMOL
MG     6.5 MMOL   8
FAT  200. GM. = 4.7 GM. /KG = 0.19 GM. /KG/HR
THE REMAINDER OF THE REGIMES ARE:
 1
 1 *   500.0 ML.   D50
TOTALS & % ERRORS:
CCAL 1118.1       27
GLUC  250. GM. = 5.8 GM. /KG = 0.24 GM. /KG/HR
COST = 31.40 POUNDS, FIT = 0.0334 COST-EFF. = 0.1763
 2
 2 *   500.0 ML.   D20
TOTALS & % ERRORS:
H2O 3044.0 ML.    26
GLUC  200. GM. = 4.7 GM. /KG = 0.19 GM. /KG/HR
COST = 30.98 POUNDS, FIT = 0.0503 COST-EFF. = 0.1958
HOW MANY MORE TO PRINT?
0                                          *-------
ANY MORE PATIENTS?
NO                                         *-------
```

Example run of Infusions program, (slightly abbreviated).

4) At various stages the user is asked questions for which a simple YES/NO answer is required. The program only needs to recognise whether the first letter is 'N' or not.

5) The 'fit:cost ratio', R gives a measure of the relative importance of fit versus cost. A small value means that the cost is more important, a large value that fit is. A value of 1 means that they are equally important and that the values of fit and cost are multiplied together to give the 'cost-effectiveness' value, CE. The general formula is

$$\log(CE) = A*\log(C) + B*\log(F+D)$$

where $A = 2/(R+1)$, $B = 2R/(R+1)$,
C = the cost,
F = the fit function value as defined above,
and D is a small constant.

The latter is introduced so that an artificially small value of F will not cause too much importance to be given to it, (we don't know exactly what the fit function should be because of uncertainties in the original required values).

6) If several regimens are printed they usually share a 'common sub-group'. The program therefore attempts to economize by printing this sub-group once only.

7) Further economy of output is achieved by allowing the user to specify a threshold value for the percentage error of any constituent below which the totals and errors are omitted. Both these output-saving devices make the program more complicated but are worthwhile on a slow teletype.

8) Note the range of costs and fits. In practice we have often found a considerable variation in both.

4. Adaptation and Use at the Royal Lancaster Infirmary.

It was possible to use the existing Infusions program by dialling up NUMAC on a remote teletype. This experiment was highly successful and provided valuable experience for both parties. The RLI group were sent the Fortran source of the Infusions program with a view to trying it out on the NWRHA ICL 1900 computer at Prestwich which was available to them. Thirdly, and most important, the RLI group agreed to try out the system in another hospital and make any necessary adaptations to make it more suitable for use in a District General Hospital.

The Newcastle Dailyreq program was not considered suitable for use at the RLI so the Lancaster group wrote a similar program in BASIC based upon standard textbooks, (5)-(9). Initially this was also run on the NWRHA machine but was later rewritten for a Hewlett-Packard 9810A Desk Top Calculator available in the department. It was obviously desirable to have all the calculations done on the same computer so the original NUMAC Infusions program was considerably simplified for running on the very limited desk top machine.

The 'COMPUTAFEED service' was established after many discussions between biochemists, computer programmers, pharmacists, clinicians and nurses. A standard request form is sent from the ward to the Biochemistry Laboratory early in the day with a blood sample and a collection of all the available fluids lost during the previous 24 hours, (urine, aspirates, drainage fluids etc). Eventually a recommended regimen for the next 24 hours is returned to the clinician. The clinician is, of course, ultimately responsible for the regimen actually used. It is just one of the routine services provided to assist the treatment of patients. The complete procedure is fully described elsewhere, (10),(11).

5. Experimental Results.

An investigation was carried out at Lancaster to ascertain whether the regimens recommended by Computafeed were actually being prescribed on the wards. The results showed that after some initial hesitancy the advice of the Pathology Laboratory was usually accepted, though modifications were made as a result of clinical circumstances. An important factor was a flexible interactive program which enabled clinicians' preferences to be incorporated without difficulty. Previously, long term therapy had been managed in the RLI by standard 'menus'. Use of specially calculated regimens tailored to the needs of the individual patient was not only acceptable to the clinicians but also produced tangible financial benefits, (10).

Some simple calculations have been done at Newcastle on data from surgical patients. Detailed data on 54 such patients are stored on the NUMAC machine. From this data a small group of 6 was chosen which had fairly complete intake, output and blood analysis records for two consecutive days. Complications such as blood transfusions and dialysis were deliberately avoided. The actual intake and losses of water, sodium etc. were calculated and the first days' results used as input to the Dailyreq program. This allowed comparisons to be made between, 1) the second day's input as recommended by Dailyreq, and 2) the therapy actually given to the patient. Any suspect results due to known limitations of Dailyreq were discounted. The average percentage absolute differences are given in the following table:

Constituent	Water	Calories	Nitrogen	Potassium
No. of cases	6	5	5	5
Average abs. difference %	45	31	20	58

It was not considered worthwile doing anything more elaborate than this. These figures tentatively confirm what had been suspected, namely that clinicians seem to be better at, or concentrate more on, getting the nitrogen and calories right.

Using clinical data retrospectively, it is not possible to compare the Infusions Program's performance with clinicians because we cannot tell what they were attempting to prescribe in terms of basic constituents - or indeed, whether such calculations had actually been made.

A second set of calculations was done with this same data. Using the intravenous therapy actually given to these patients on the second day, the Infusions program was run with this as input data. The costs of it's recommended cheapest regimens were compared with the actual costs. For each patient, the 'fit' of the computer's regimen was quite good - the worst discrepancy being 23% for sodium in one case. The result of this test was that the program did, on average, 12% better than the clinicians for cost; the range was between 2 and 25%. This test is heavily biased against the program because the actual regimen given and not the (unknown) requirements was compared with the program's regimen. Even so, by accepting a slight discrepancy of fit, significant potential cost reductions can be shown.

After examining this program's output for many other cases we have noted that it is comparatively rare to find a constituent with a disrepancy worse than 30% in the 40 best regimens calculated. One way in which this program has an advantage is that it always takes account of electrolytes in amino acid solutions. The wider the choice of solutions and factors considered, the greater is the computer's advantage.

6. Discussion.

Although development of this project is still continuing, several important lessons have been learned. A clinician using a computer to assist with the management of patients on intravenous feeding has a great potential advantage over unassisted medical staff. It is possible to achieve accurate replacement of all the requirements of an individual patient without the 'see-saw' effects of over-hydration and excess electrolyte replacement that may be seen when nutritional requirements are adequately fulfilled. Current costings, often not available to the clinician, are taken into account and may result in a saving of up to £10 for a single day's feeding.

The association of computer techniques with clinicians and nurses has brought to light limitations on the methods of collection of medical data and on the application of rigid formulae to material subject to biological variation. For example it became apparent that accurate timing was essential in the collection of urine samples since a 15-minute error in voiding time gives rise to a 1% error over a 24-hour period. Intake data were often found to be quite seriously in error if the clinician had done the conversion calculations from the nursing records himself, (12). This can be rectified by using the original nursing records as computer data. However, it is a non-trivial exercise to set up the necessary specification data in standard form on a computer, particularly for blood products and oral/tube feeds.

A limiting factor in the use of any computer program is the quality of data supplied. When the computer is first used to prepare regimens for a patient, the initial requirements must be calculated with care to eliminate the risk of a vicious circle developing if the patient had recently been suffering from fluid overload. In these circumstances, the simplistic computer program would tend to replace the apparently excessive water loss, so perpetuating the state of over-hydration.

An important factor which influences the cost of the regimen chosen is the proportion of fat to carbohydrate as a calorie source. 20% Intralipid has a similar calorific content to 50% Dextrose but is about seven times as expensive. The exact proportions may be modified depending on clinical considerations, but most clinicians tend to use fat to supply between 25 and 50% of calorie requirements.

A significant feature of the Infusions Program is that it presents the preferred regimens in terms of whole bottles and ampoules. While this must produce a less accurate regimen in terms of the fit function, this disadvantage is far outweighed by the ease of use by the nursing staff and the minimum of interference required with the solutions before infusion.

A particularly valuable feature of this study was the opportunity to apply the program to two different hospital environments, a teaching hospital and a district general hospital, with their different facilities and requirements. The Lancaster group were able to modify the Newcastle programs, incorporating original ideas of their own, for use on a mini-computer. The service which they provided was found to be highly acceptable to clinicians, nurses, biochemists and pharmacists.

This project is a good example of how working with a computer forces fundamental rethinking of problems and raises some debatable questions. For instance whether it is better to use a cheaper calorie source like 50% Dextrose, which should be infused via an expensive central vein catheter, or a more costly Intralipid which is suitable for a peripheral vein. Similarly, is a larger selection of fluids, which allows the program to satisfy the requirements more accurately, preferable to a smaller selection, which allows the pharmacist to control his stock better?

In order to provide a computerised intravenous feeding system, a multi-disciplinary team is necessary. Clinicians, nurses, dieticians, pharmacists, biochemists and computer scientists must all be involved.

As the 'micro-processor revolution' continues to advance and computer hardware costs fall, it is inevitable that more mini-computers will find their way into hospitals. As knowledge of intravenous feeding improves and better fluids become available, the expert and motivated clinicians in the field will take many more factors into account when devising therapy. For this advanced knowledge to be made available to the majority of busy clinicians, it seems to us that the use of computers in this field will become more desirable.

7. Acknowledgements.

We wish to acknowledge the help and advice of the following: Professor

I.D.A.Johnston and Mr.A.W.Goode of the Department of Surgery, RVI, Mr.R.Elder and Mrs.A.Saunders of the RVI Pharmacy, Mr.H.Carr, District Administrator, Lancaster, and our colleagues on the wards at both hospitals. Financial assistance has been provided by research grants from the NWRHA and the Newcastle AHA,(Teaching). Finally, we would like to thank members of the Documentation Group in the Computing Laboratory at Newcastle for technical assistance with the preparation of this paper which has been done entirely on the computer.

8. References.

1) J.D.Bellis, 1976, Personal Communication.

2) D.W.Boettner and M.T.Alexander, 1975, 'The Michigan Terminal System', Proc. I.E.E.E., vol. 63, no. 6, p. 912.

3) G.Shearing, 1976, 'The NUMAC-RVI Infusions Program', Computing Laboratory, University of Newcastle-upon-Tyne.

4) V.Blackmore and D.Morrison, 1977, 'Computer Aided Fluid Therapy', in 'Biomedical Computing', W.J.Perkins, (ed), p. 325, Pitman Medical Publishing Co. Ltd., Tunbridge Wells, UK.

5) F.D.Moore, 1959, 'The Metabolic Care of the Surgical Patient', Saunders Co., Philadelphia.

6) H.A.Lee, (ed.), 1974, 'Parenteral Nutrition in Acute Metabolic Illness', Academic Press, London.

7) W.F.Walker and I.D.A.Johnston, 1971, 'The Metabolic Basis of Surgical Care', Heinemann, London.

8) J.E.Fischer, (ed), 1976, 'Total Parenteral Nutrition', Little Brown and Co., Boston.

9) W.A.Wilkinson, 1973, 'Body Fluids in Surgery', Churchill Livingston, London.

10) J.D.Bellis, R.I.Cooper, P.W.Harvey, R.M.James and J.M.Roberts,   1978, 'Computerised Intravenous Feeding Regimes', Pharm. J., (in press).

11) R.M.James, J.M.Roberts, P.W.Harvey, J.D.Bellis and R.I.Cooper, 1978, 'A Computerised Scheme for the Preparation of Parenteral Nutrition Regimes', Medical Informatics, (in press).

12) A.W.Goode, 1976, Personal Communication.

COMPLIANCE ASPECTS OF A COMPUTER-ASSISTED
ANTICOAGULATION CONTROL SYSTEM

Albert M. Vossepoel; Leiden University Medical Centre,
Department of Biomedical Information Processing,
Lab.voor Fysiologie, Wassenaarseweg 62, 2333 AL Leiden, The Netherlands.

1. INTRODUCTION

In order to prevent thrombo-embolic phenomena, treatment with oral anticoagulants is widely used. The pharmacological aspects are reasonably well
understood in general. But the patient's response to oral anticoagulants
is highly individual. The average dosage required for the maintenance of a
therapeutic effect differs enormously from patient to patient. This precludes
the use of a generally applicable fixed dose of these drugs.
Moreover, the individual response may change over time. This makes it
necessary to check the patient's blood coagulation time intermittently /1/.
The coagulation time should be within the limits of a therapeutic range set
for the patient in accordance with existing (contra-)indications. If the
coagulation time is outside the therapeutic range, the physician may adjust
the dosage or the appointment period, or both. He should do so very
carefully, because a small dosage adjustment has a relatively large and
slow effect. Intercurrent factors - such as changes in the use of other
medications, or in eating or drinking habits - also may cause rather
dramatic changes in individual response.
Because of these factors, anticoagulation treatment requires much attention
and experience. That's why most physicians in The Netherlands delegate an
important part of this treatment to regional specialized thrombosis centres.
At Leiden Thrombosis Centre (LTC) the physicians employ a Computer-
assisted Anticoagulation Control System (CACS) in every-day therapeutical
routine since spring 1975 /2,3/. CACS computes suggestions for dosage
of phenprocoumon tablets and the next appointment period for over 5000
out-patients of the centre.
CACS is part of the fully conversational real-time Information System for
Thrombosis Centres (ISTC), which is in operational use since spring
1974 /4/. ISTC shares the facilities of the integrated Hospital Information
System (HIS) of Leiden University Hospital: a double PDP11/45 computer
configuration, and a special-purpose operating system and database
management system /5,6/.

The communication between ISTC and its users is strictly conversational, in contrast with current practice elsewhere /7,8,9/. Video Display Units (VDU) are used to exchange information with physicians and nurses of LTC. The dialogue is balanced between clearness and brevity, ease and speed of use. Besides, the absence of intermediary personnel decreases the risk of errors and information loss /10/.

The suggestions computed by CACS are presented to the physicians as a part of the patient's printed medical history. Approval is effectuated implicitly, avoiding a terminal conversation for every single prescription. If a suggestion has to be changed, the physician only keys in a 3-digit serial number on the VDU. This displays in reply a short version of the printed medical history from the database. The suggested average daily dosage of phenprocoumon, the appointment period and/or the remarks may now be changed at choice. The input data is checked on consistency and validity, it is processed and a dosage rhythm, appointment period and remarks, adjusted or not, are displayed for approval. If desired, these data may be changed again conversationally. The actual appointment date is adjusted by a specialized subsystem that accounts for holidays, vacations and the workload of LTC.

After approval, a dosage list is printed for every individual patient, showing the number of prescribed tablets for each day of the next appointment period. These lists - 300 to 400 daily at present - are mailed to the patients on the same day they visited LTC.

The required accuracy of the dosage prescription is achieved by modeling it to a rhythmic dosage schedule consisting of 0, $\frac{1}{2}$, 1, 2, or 3 daily tablets. CACS replays this schedule, which results in a prediction of the coagulation time for the next appointment date. The difference between the measured and the predicted value of the coagulation time is then used to adjust the patient's response parameters. This adjustment is balanced between effective noise suppression and fast response to gradual or step-wise changes, by means of both statistical and syntactical filtering. If a step-wise change in the patient's response is detected, or if remarks are entered by a nurse, the dosage needs special attention of the physician. In this case, CACS suppresses the display of the dosage suggestion, thereby forcing the physician to use the same procedure as when changing a suggestion.

CACS will not try to counteract a suddenly weaker response by a higher dosage suggestion, as the patient presumably did not adhere to his dosage schedule. Instead, CACS then suggests continuation of the previous dosage schedule with an appropriate remark ('sermon') to the patient.

2. COMPLIANCE ASPECTS

The process of computer-assisted anticoagulation control has three basic relations between the participants involved: patients, physicians and CACS.

Each of these relations shows compliance aspects:

- patient compliance, i.e. the degree in which the patients adhere to the physician's prescriptions;
- user compliance, i.e. the degree in which the physicians adhere to CACS' dosage suggestions;
- system compliance, i.e. the degree in which CACS reacts to the patients' measured coagulation time and related data.

2.1. Patient compliance

As already mentioned in section 1, CACS provides - as a by-product - predictions of the patient's blood coagulation time resulting from the actual dosage prescription. Patient compliance may be analyzed by studying the frequency distributions of the deviations from the predictions, as a function of changes in average dosage. This results in a two-dimensional histogram, with classes of relative change in average dosage along the horizontal axis and classes of relative deviation from the predicted blood coagulation time along the vertical axis.

For most classes of relative dosage change, a bell-shaped distribution of deviations is found with a mode at or near to the horizontal axis, i.e. with zero deviation. This distribution represents the combined effects of measuring errors, intercurrent factors and lack of adherence to the dosage prescriptions.

Given this distribution, it is interesting to test the hypothesis that many patients do not comply with changes in their dosage prescriptions, i.e. they simply stick to their previous prescriptions. To this end, the histogram of all deviations from the predicted blood coagulation times is taken as the "expected distribution".

The histogram of deviations for a single class of dosage change may now be compared to the expected distribution, in order to find significant systematic differences. To this end, the expected distribution is scaled with respect to the central elements of the single class histogram of deviations, the scaled elements are subtracted from those of the histogram and divided by the square root of the sum of the elements involved in the subtraction, yielding a quantity q. The division is performed in order to give an indication of the significance of the difference, assuming Poisson statistics for the number of counts in one class of the histogram. In order to find coherent regions in the resulting array of quantities q, it is processed by iterating a median-smoothing procedure /11/ until a steady state is reached.

Applying this procedure to approx. 57000 dosage records, two regions were found where the quantity q was greater than 1. The position of these regions confirmed the hypothesis for dosage changes greater than approx. 10%. For these classes of dosage changes, the differences with the expected distribution within the regions amounted to approx. 15% of the total number within each class of dosage change, corresponding to a compliance of approx. 85%. In the further development of CACS, it may well be wise to consider this figure significant for all dosage changes.

2.2. User compliance

Of the approx. 57000 dosage suggestions mentioned in section 2.1, 69% were displayed to the physicians. The remaining 31% were suppressed by CACS because of one of the reasons mentioned at the end of section 1. Of the displayed suggestions, 86% were accepted without change, i.e. 59% of the prescriptions involved were produced without physician intervention.

It is interesting to evaluate the individual variations in user compliance of the four physicians involved, and to see if these variations have any influence on the result of the prescriptions. To this end, a prescription is defined as successful if the resulting blood coagulation time, measured on the next consultation, is within the limits of the therapeutic range set for the patient concerned.

The results of the evaluation are summarized as follows:

TABLE 1.

Physician nr.:	1	2	3	4	total
Prescriptions involved:	11606	9161	7087	11070	38924
Accepted suggestions:	99%	89%	78%	74%	86%
Successful prescriptions:	84%	85%	85%	85%	85%

It is clear from this table that the large variations in user compliance - from 74% to 99% - have virtually no influence on the success of the actually prescribed dosages. From this may be inferred that a vast majority of the changes applied to the dosage suggestions is at least unnecessary. If one bears in mind that changing a dosage suggestion takes from 10 to 20 seconds, whereas approving one takes only 2 seconds on an average, low user compliance represents a considerable waste of time and effort.

2.3. System compliance

In principle, system compliance is fully predictable, because CACS has a deterministic structure. However, a detailed analysis goes beyond the scope of this paper. Therefore, system compliance is defined here more restrictedly as the fraction of dosage suggestions counteracting a deviation from the target coagulation time, i.e. different from the previous dosage prescription.

This fraction turned out to be 29% of the displayed suggestions, and 26% of all computed suggestions. It is interesting to compare these figures with the fraction of previous prescriptions actually changed by the physicians: 32%. Bearing in mind that patient compliance is far from ideal (cf. section 2.1.), changes in dosage prescription should be kept to a minimum. In the further development of CACS, this means that suggestions should be kept equal to the previous dosage as long as there is only a small risk that the blood coagulation time will go beyond the limits of the therapeutic range set for the patient concerned.

Another important comliance aspect of CACS is in its reaction towards remarks entered by nurses. Until now, CACS only reacts to such remarks by suppressing the display of the dosage suggestion. A more sensible reaction would be the presentation of a dosage suggestion that accounts for the contents of the remark. In order to achieve. this, a retrospective study has to be undertaken towards the systematic deviations from the predicted coagulation times related to various remarks.

3. FURTHER DEVELOPMENTS

After discussing the findings of section 2 with the medical staff of LTC, it was concluded that more profit could be gained from CACS by printing dosage suggestions with all medical histories.

The suggestions that are displayed up to now have proven to be acceptable to a high degree. They will be printed in a separate output stream and may then be handled by one of the physicians with high compliance.

The display of the remaining -"experimental"-suggestions has the immediate advantage of saving time and effort for every suggestion that needs not be changed. This is because prescribing a dosage otherwise - without the suggestion - would have taken approximately as much time as changing a suggestion (cf. section 2.2.).

In the long run, the advantages are greater, especially when the remarks relevant to dosage prescriptions are coded distinctly, i.e. not as the free text used for this purpose at present. The feed-back of critical comments provoked by the display of "experimental" suggestions will provide an important means of improving CACS.

Eventually, certain classes of "experimental" suggestions may be transferable to the output stream of "acceptable" ones. By this, the physicians will have an increasing opportunity to devote their attention to the really difficult and extraordinary prescriptions. The shift in allocation of tasks between physicians and CACS will most probably result in a more efficient treatment of all patients of LTC.

REFERENCES:

/ 1/ Weiner, M. (1962) Pharmacological considerations of antithrombotic therapy, Advanc. Pharmac. 1, 277-293.

/ 2/ Wiegman, H. and A.M. Vossepoel (1977) A computer program for long-term anticoagulation control, Comp. Progr. Biomed. 7, 71-84.

/ 3/ Vossepoel, A.M., and H. Wiegman (1977) Computer assisted medical practice in anticoagulation control: theory, practice and evaluation, in: Medical Computing, eds. M. Laudet et al. (Taylor & Francis, London) pp. 375-389; also in: Med. Inform. 2, 125-140.

/ 4/ Wiegman, H. (1976) A real-time information system for thrombosis centres, experiences and conclusions, in: Information Systems for Patient Care, eds. J. van Egmond et al. (North-Holland, Amsterdam) pp. 327-348.

/ 5/ Snitker, P.P. (1975) Description of a real-time operating system for information processing, Proc. DEC Users Soc., The Hague, pp. 117-122.

/ 6/ Bakker, A.R. (1977) Implementation approach and evaluation of the use of Leiden university hospital information system, in: Medinfo 77 eds. D.B. Shires and H. Wolf (North-Holland, Amsterdam) pp.943-947.

/ 7/ Sheiner, L.B. (1969) Computer-aided long-term anticoagulation therapy, Comput. Biomed. Res. 2, 507-518.

/ 8/ Hoffer, E.P., K.D. Marble, P.M. Yurchak, G.O. Barnett (1975) A computer-based information system for managing patients on long-term oral anticoagulants, Comput. Biomed. Res. 8, 573-579.

/ 9/ Visser, J. (1976) Manual for automation of out-patient anticoagulation treatment, (in dutch: Handleiding voor automatisering van poliklinische antistolbehandeling), (Ziekenhuis de Weezenlanden, Zwolle).

/10/ Collen, M.F. (1970) General requirements for a medical information system, Comput. Biomed. Res. 3, 393-406.

/11/ Abele, L.W., and F.M. Wahl (1977) A digital procedure for boundary detection and elimination of background in cytologic images, in: Medinfo 77, eds. D.B. Shires and H. Wolf (North-Holland, Amsterdam) pp. 1035-1038.

IS A LARGE COMPUTER SYSTEM OF VALUE IN THE

INTENSIVE CARE UNIT?

A E S Goh and B Richards

Department of Computation,

U.M.I.S.T.

The fact that a patient is in an Intensive Care Unit usually indicates that his condition is such that it requires close surveillance and this is reflected by the high staff-to-patient ratio and the amount of monitoring performed in the unit. One of the most important functions of the unit is the monitoring of respiratory functions and other related variables, for example, biochemical and haemotological measurements. The quantity of available information pertaining to each patient is far in excess of what would be measured if he were in a general ward. In order to process this information and consequently to aid the clinicians, a computer system designed specifically for intensive care data processing was developed.

Before going on to discuss the role of a large computer system in such an environment, there is a need to define more precisely what we mean by the term 'large computer system'. We refer to not just the size of the central processing unit but to the size of the total configuration, including fast backing stores, terminals, and other peripherals. The requirements are that of any real-time system where interactive computing and fast response are needed. A schematic diagram of the features of a typical system is given below. The paper will elaborate on the usage of each feature.

Various types of computers have been employed in the Intensive Care situation, including those of a small dedicated nature which attempt to assess specialised data. Though useful, such machines are limited by the size and capability to future program extensions. An example of this is the use of desk-top computers for evaluating blood-gas measurements (1,2). There are also computers with large backing storage which are used mainly for handling and storing patients' particulars but are limited in the amount of actual processing and usage of the data (3,4). There are also highly specialised systems involving hybrid machines that enable analogue to digital conversions of pressure, fluid output, and other measured values as well as computer controlled transfusions and infusions (5). The high outlay costs and the quantity of extra equipment involved in such systems may be factors which have deterred their wider use.

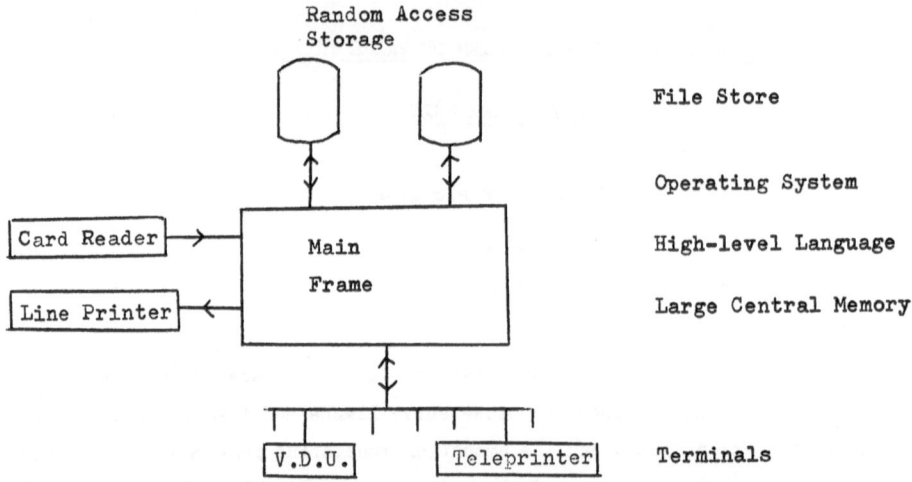

Fig. 1 <u>Features of an Intensive Computer System</u>

From our experience of computing in the Intensive Care Unit, the following advantages of features in a large computing system have been found.

1.   A large central processing unit which permitted the input program not only to accept raw data but performed error checks and correction and further calculations from the available information. Tasks like the checking of the normality or otherwise of a measured value are more complex than may initially be thought. Normal values are dependent on age, sex and other factors (6,7,8) and as each of these considerations are taken into account for every measured value, the size and complexity of the program grows to beyond what a small desk-top machine would be able to cope with. We have been using the CYBER 72 mainframe which has 64K words of central memory.

2.   Random access file stores are used to keep the data-base and various text files. In order to use the biochemical and other data in the diagnostic process, a list of aetiologies and their corresponding biochemical patterns are stored in a matrix (9). There are more than 4000 elements in the matrix but increase must be allowed for as more aetiologies may be added to the list and further tests performed. The program has to be able to access this data-base quickly and efficiently.

```
        HB(GM%)     PCV(%)      BODY TEMP(C)     FIO2(%)
?        9.2        26.9           39               60
ARTERIAL VALUES
      LAB TEMP(C)      PH      PCO2(MM HG)      PO2(MM HG)
?        37          7.46       37.8               58
VENOUS VALUES
       PH      PCO2(MM HG)      PO2(MM HG)
?     7.43      41.7              36
. . . . . . . . . . . . . . . . . . . . . . . . . . . .
ARTERIAL BLOOD VALUES CORRECTED TO A BODY TEMP OF 39 C
PH= 7.431     PO2= 66.53 MM HG    PCO2= 41.09 MM HG     SAT= 91.53%
. . . . . . . . . . . . . . . . . . . . . . . . . . . .
RESULTS IN 60% OXYGEN
INSPIRED PO2       = 424.4 MM HG
ALVEOLAR PO2       =381.6 MM HG    O2 CONT= 13.47 VOL%   SAT= 99.85 %
ARTERIAL PO2       = 58   MM HG    O2 CONT= 11.48 VOL%   SAT= 91.65 %
MIXED VENOUS PO2 = 36 MM HG        O2 CONT= 8.666 VOL%   SAT= 69.41 %
ARTERIAL PCO2      = 37.8 MM HG    CO2 CONT= 56.07 VOL%
MIXED VENOUS PCO2= 41.7 MM HG      CO2 CONT= 58.17 VOL%
CALC A-V PO2 DIFF= 22 MM HG        A-V O2 CONT= 2.809 VOL%
CALC V-A PCO2 DIFF=3.9 MM HG       V-A CO2 CONT= 2.109 VOL%
ALV-ART PO2 DIFF = 323.6 MM HG
ARTERIAL HCO3     = 26 MMOL/L
CALCULATED R.Q.   = .7507
CALCULATED SHUNT = 41.54 %
. . . . . . . . . . . . . . . . . . . . . . . . . . . .
PULMONARY CONSTANTS IN 100% OXYGEN
     R.Q.    A-V O2 DIFF(VOL%)  V-A CO2 DIFF(VOL%)    SHUNT(%)
?    .78           3.1                2.4                36
     PO2 (MM HG)
? 145
TO ACHIEVE A PO2 OF 100 MM HG, A FIO2 OF 94% IS SUGGESTED.
```

Fig. 2 Part of the Pulmonary Function Program

Text files containing diagnostic statements are also stored in this media. An acid-base map based on the serum pH and PCO_2 parameters was developed (10). The map was divided into 28 sectors and corresponding to each sector is a diagnostic statement which describes the blood-gas status of the patient. Since the diagnosis could vary if the patient is being mechanically ventilated, there exists a further set of 28 statements. These are but two of the collection of text files which include aetiology lists, biochemical test names, etc.

3.   A high level language enabled the program to be written so that it is both readable and easily utilised by non-computing personnel. A language which allows for string manipulation, for example text insertions and concatenations, is needed. As the data is processed, warning statements and further questions may be asked and this is made more flexible by the availability of these text manipulation functions (11,12). Furthermore, in the calculation of more

THE FOLLOWING VALUES ARE ABOVE THEIR UPPER NORMAL LIMITS:-

	UPPER NORMAL	LOWER NORMAL	MEASURED	
SERUM OSMOLALITY	295	285	320	*
SERUM PHOSPHATE CONC.	1.3	.6	2.24	*
SERUM ALKALINE PHOSPHATASE	85.5	15	241	*
ALT	46	5	67	*
SERUM TOTAL BILIRUBIN CONC.	20.5	1.7	82	*
SERUM UREA CONC.	6.9	2.4	28.6	*
SERUM CREATININE CONC.	.114	.051	.56	*

THE FOLLOWING VALUES ARE BELOW THEIR LOWER NORMAL LIMITS:-

	UPPER NORMAL	LOWER NORMAL	MEASURED	
SERUM CHLORIDE CONC.	106	98	94	*
SERUM GLUCOSE CONC.	10	5	3.5	*
SERUM ALBUMIN	48	32.65	26	*
24 HR. UREA EXCRETION	600	250	147.4	*
24 HR. CREATININE EXCRETION	15.48	9.29	6.16	*
URINE CREATININE CONC.	15	6.66	5.6	*
SERUM HAEMOGLOBIN	17.29	13.4	11.3	*

   * THE VALUE IS BEYOND + OR - 3 STD. DEV. OF THE MEAN

ON THE EVIDENCE SUBMITTED, THE MOST LIKELY DIAGNOSES ARE:-

	SCORE
LIVER DAMAGE	65
IMPAIRED RENAL FUNCTION	54
PULMONARY DISEASE PRODUCING HYPOXAEMIA	50
HEPATIC COMA	50

THERE ARE ABNORMAL VALUES RECORDED WHICH SUGGEST THAT
THE FOLLOWING CONDITIONS MAY BE PRESENT:-

	SCORE
MANNITOL THERAPY	44.75
SEVERE RENAL INSUFFICIENCY	41
INFECTION	32
ACUTE PANCREATITIS	29
EXCESS BICARBONATE ADMINISTRATION	28

Fig. 3 Differential Diagnoses based on Biochemical Data

values, numerical techniques may have to be used in the solving of non-linear
functions. An example of this is the calculating of the required inspired
oxygen concentration in order to achieve a certain arterial oxygen tension,
given that the shunt and other pulmonary constants are known. Another
example of the need for numerical analysis is in the calculation of "standard
bicarbonate". This is illustrated below.

$$M = -1.0285 + 0.0051Hb - \left(\frac{3.542 + 0.6105Hb + 0.009Hb^2}{SB} \right)$$

$$Q = (\log (40/PCO_2)/M)$$

$$SB = 40 \times 10^{(0.4328pH_a + 0.0406pH_a^2 - 5.64 + 0.4328Q + 0.0812pH_a \cdot Q + 0.0406Q^2)}$$

Fig. 4 An example of the Need for Numerical Techniques in the Solving for Standard
       Bicarbonate Value

The program must be able to cater for the multiple function calls in order to iterate to the required answer. The language that has been used in the system is BASIC. Such high level languages offer greater portability in that it is easier to transfer the program to another machine than if the programs were written in machine-dependent code.

4. An operating system with facilities for file maintenance and program handling is required. Amendments to the text files mentioned above are made possible by the existence of an editing package. Macros which 'call down' and attach program and text files aid in making the program initiation very simple for the user. In this system, which has a range of available utility programs, for example, for diagnosis, or therapy, the ability of a particular program to hand control from one program to another without user intervention is most useful. There is therefore no need to explicitly issue commands to fetch, compile and run the next required program. The NOS operating system of the CYBER 72 provides all these facilities.

5. Terminals which are portable proved to be convenient in that they are able to be transported from one room to another within the unit. Access to the computer may be via telephone lines on terminals with speed of 10 to 30 characters per second. Hard copies of the interactive sessions are obtained for immediate consultation and for future reference. One terminal currently used is the Telex 300 which, with a heat sensitive writing head, produces the output silently, unlike a conventional teleprinter.

6. Potential extensions to the system are numerous and so there must be an ability to deal with increased needs without having to purchase further hardware and consequently involving problems of transferring existing software. Research possibilities exist in the areas of pulmonary function tests, real-time monitoring of operations, treatment of diabetics, etc.

7. More terminals can be connected to the system for teaching purposes in the training of medical students and nurses. This can be said to be a 'by-product' of the ICU system. It serves as an interesting test for the user to ascertain as to why certain decisions and conclusions were made by the program on the basis of the information which formed the input data (13).

Conclusion

In this short paper, we have not been able to give details of all the programs referred to. However, in the presentation, the results of repeated runs on the various programs will be given.

It is felt that much of the potential of large computer systems to Intensive Care applications has remained untapped. It is not feasible from the economic and space point of view for individual Intensive Care Units to own such systems, hence, it is suggested that use be made of current resources by linking up with existing large computers which may be presently in use elsewhere or in use in the hospital for administrative purposes, provided that the functions do not interfere with one another. This is not to say that, in many cases, there is not a place for the micro-computer after the research and development work has been carried out on a larger machine and the final software specifications are known.

References

1. Grogono, A W. Assessment of Acid-base disturbances employing a desk-top computer. Br Med J, 1:381 (1973).

2. Rowberg, A, and Lee, S. Use of a desk-top calculator to interpret acid-base data. Am J Clin Path, 59(2):180 (1973).

3. Franklin, C B. Living with someone else's computer. "Real-time computing in patient management" (Payne, J P, and Hill, D W, eds), Peter Peregrims Ltd 1976.

4. Ashcroft, J M, and Berry, J L. The introduction of a real-time patient data display system into the Cardio-thoracic Dept at Wythenshawe Hospital. Medinfo 74, North Holland Pub Co 1974.

5. Robicsek, F, Masters, T N, Reichertz, R L, Daughty, H K, and Cook, J W. Three years' experience with computer-based intensive care of patients following open heart and major vascular surgery. Surgery 81(1):12 (1977).

6. Bold, A M, and Wilding, P. Clinical Chemistry: Conversion scales for SI units with adult normal reference values. Blackwell Scientific Pub 1975.

7. Scientific Tables. (Diem, K, and Lentner, C, eds) Giegy Pharmaceuticals, 7th ed. 1970.

8. Kelman, G R. Calculation of certain indices of cardio-pulmonary function using a digital computer. Resp Physiol 1:336 (1966).

9. Hobbie, R K, and Reece, R L. Computer interpretation of laboratory test results. Fed Proc 34(12):2152 (1975).

10. Richards, R, and Goh, A E S. Computer assistance in the treatment of patients with acid-base and electrolyte disturbances. Medinfo 77. (Shires, D B, and Wolf, H, eds) North Holland Pub Co 1977.

11. Bleich, H L. Computer based consultation. Am J Med 53:285 (1972).

12. Richards, B, Doran, B R H, and Goh, A E S. Computer assistance in an Intensive Care Unit. Intensive Care Med 3(3):395 (1977).

13. Dickinson, C J. A computer model of human respiration. M.T.P. 1977.

THE STRATEGIC ANALYSES AND INITIAL IMPLEMENTATION
OF THE SHARED HOSPITAL INFORMATION SYSTEM

A. Gunji

The office of Medical System Development

The Medical Affair's Bureau

The Ministry of Health and Welfare, Japan

1. Preamble

This article is the report on the shared hospital information (SHIS) which is promoted by the government as one of its R&D projects on medical informatics in Japan since 1974.

There had been much ·expectation for the computer application in hospital activities in its early days and a vast amount of research and development has already been done in many countries, but now we have to accept the fact that the successful cases are quite modestly small in number compared with the expectation for it.

The criteria for the judgement between success and unsuccess is always full of confutation but it should be acceptable to say that if the project is aiming at a product for practical usage and it is not widely used, then the project is not yet successful. If we accept this, it entails that the economic fator is crucially improtant for the project to succeed. This economic factor barred the hospital information system from being judged as complete success in spite of its technological refinement. Nevertheless, it seems that HIS is begining to settle down, centred round administrative and managerial jobs in hospitals in many countries. Unfortunately, the economic and organisational system of health care is quite different from country to country, and this fact makes it difficult to exchange the precious experiences among different countries. It denotes, however, the necessity for more communication rather than the devaluation of each experience.

2. The Status of HIS and Problems

1) The survey on computer usage in medical facilities

In 1974, at the outset of the project, the survey was carried out on the computer usage in medical facilities in Japan by the author himself. In this survey, the computers which were used for research work were excluded.The numbers in talble 1 show the sets of computers of each size, which were implemented in each year. The classifications of the computer, such as large, medium, small and

	large	midium	small	mini	others	total
1963		1				1
64						
65						
66						
67		1	1			2
68	2	1		4	2	9
69		2	3	3	1	9
70	1	3	2	14	1	21
71	1	3	4	26	5	39
72	3	2	10	24	3	42
73	3	3	22	67	9	104
unknown			2	5	1	7
total	10	16	44	153	22	233

Table 1, The number of computers implemented in medical facilities in Japan.

management	134
billing of insurance	87
statistics	16
medical record	11
payroll	10
inventory control	6
appointment	4
clinical laboratory	47
physiological examination	60
EKG	29
EEG	10
PCG	5
RI	5
dose calculation	5
others	6
ICU	3
CCU	1
AMHTS	24
miscellanea	20

Table 2, The field of application in 1973.

mini, were quite conventional but it was enough to know the facts as follows.

a) The introduction of computers in medical facilities was exponentially increasing in number, but

b) this increase was mostly caused by small size computers.

Looking at the field of application in table 2, it was outstanding that the majority of them were devoted to managerial usage and especially to the clerical work imposed by the health insurance scheme of the government. The next prevalent usage was in the clinical laboratory and it was one of the characteristics in Japan that the application for medical record keeping was quite rudimental. It was also noteworthy that the number of computers had no correlation with the scale of the hospital. This proliferation of small computers coincide with the fact that several companies began to deliver small dedicated machines with or without the back-up of the large system for the single purpose of clerical work of health insurance in hospitals and clinics.

Since then, a similar survey was carried out after two years, but the tendencies were unchanged, by and large.

2) The survey of opinions

The survey of opinions were carried out next, among specialists of medical informatics. This asked their opinions on various applications and showed up the differences between the stages at which they ought to have been and those at which they actually were at that time. In short, it said that the administrative and managerial applications of HIS were delayed but on the other hand, those of AMHTS and ICU had gone too far, compared with the advancement of related knowledge and technologies.

3) Need for HIS

Many countries, especially those in which insurance is the dominant financial system of health care, are suffering from the growing scale and complexity of its clerical work. Japan is a paradigm of deterioration of this sort. Roughly speaking, medical expenditure has been increased six fold from 1965 to 1975, when it was 4.33% of GNP and about 80% of this was covered by insurance. Every hospital and clinic has to send bills of services which they have delivered in a month to the "Health Insurance Payment Organisation" at the end of the month, where they do clerical checks and peer review, and then they remit the cash to each medical facility on behalf of different insurance organisations. It is said that the number of bills issued every month in Japan is now around 35 million. In order to try to visualize the amount, suppose that they were piled up, they would become higher than the highest mountain in Japan, Mt. Fuji, the summit of which is 3776 meters(about 12,400 feet) high. About 97% of bills are written manually and the other 3% is of computer output.

The insurance payment system of Japan is based on "fee-for-service", and it requires the bill to have the list of diagnostic and therapeutic services done to the patient, to have these priced and sum up according the statutory price list which is in the form of a book and government regulations. The logic for calculation is fairly difficult to be programmed becouse of its complexity and is getting more and more so to meet with claims from every quarter.

Nowadays, it is already so complex that even a minor change in the logic could have a strong impact on the clerical work in facilities, especially to cashiers who have to calcuate the fee of the patient instantly, and practitioners who have no clerical employee in their office.

I am afraid I have digressed from the main topic, but I think it is now clear that there is a definite need for information processing on the financial aspect of the health care system in Japan

In order to rationalise the whole system, it is essential to input data at each hospital and clinic, where the source of information flow is.

4) Constraints

The major constraints in implementation of EDPS in hospitals are economic. Reasons may be epitomized as follows.

 a) The ownership of each hospital in an area is usually different and there is no single authority which can command or influence them to implement information processing devices.

 b) Each hospital has to be self-supporting. Therefore, the implementation has to be cost beneficial to the hospital. This condition is more stringent than if it has to be globally cost beneficial.

 c) If the system has a module to calculate the bills of patients at each point of payment, it has to have large online files such as the patient registration file, the price list, the logic of calculation and so forth. This entails that the system has to be fairly large and is consequently expensive.

5) Problems of status quo

From the other point of view, it can be said that the revenue side of the hospital is controlled to some extent by the statutory pricing, but the expenditure side is decided by the free market pricing machinery. Therefore, the financial situation of the hospital is chronically difficult. It is the major concern of the financial management of the hospital, but most hospitals tend to be in the red. Therefore, there is a strong need to improve managerial efficiency by any means such as computers, but on the other hand, they tend to use the machines specifically for the purpose of printing the bills of insurance at the end of the month. This is the reason why the small computer is proliferating in Japan.

It could, however, be anticipated that this phenomenon might cause some problems as follows.

a) Since prices and the logic of insurance are to be revised annually in principle, the maintenance of the system is inevitable. It is usually difficult to maintain a single purpose system.

b) If the proliferation of these systems goes too far, the revision of the rules may in turn lead to repercussions and thus, increase the rigidity of the whole system of insurance.

c) It may be impossible to solve interface problems, when integration of these systems is intended.

d) The general purpose computer costs too much money, manpower and time for each hospital to plan, implement and maintain it.

This is the situation which we have to break through deploying the funds of the government. It is clear that other functions and modules may be added to this basis.

3. The Objective of SHIS Project

The objective of SHIS project can be stated as to develop HIS, making it cost/effective by the sharing of facilities and personnel among as many hospitals as possible throughout the country.

Technologically, the project presupposes computer network. The basic idea is to try to maximize cost/performance by distributing the standard functions to the large central machine and local processing to the small devices which would be in the hospital and interface with the environment of the hospital. This system is to bring about the following merits.

a) High cost/performance

b) Hospitals are released from the burdens of planning, implementation and maintenance.

c) Planning stage is shortened.

d) Hospitals can use a system of high reliability.

e) Sharing of data will be facilitated.

4. Analyses of Alternatives

We had to do various works of assessment and evaluation, and to develop the methodology itself. They can be classified into three actvities; 1) technological analyses of the terminals, 2) optimization of the system design, 3) economic analyses. They are interrelated very strongly.

1) Technological analyses of terminals

    The functioning of the terminal is all important for users of
this type of system. Hitherto, the selection of hard ware tends to
be biassed by subjective judgement of decision makers and specification is decided more or less on trial-and-error basis. This is
partly because there is no reliable methodology to evaluate the
functioning of the terminal objectively. The team of Professor T.
Ishii applied a motion analysis for this purpose and found   the
method is extremely effective. Using devices of their own development, they examined three systems of different terminals, which had
been implemented successfully. I do not go to detail because I think
it will be fully reported elsewhere but the contribution of this
research was that it showed up clearly the following facts.

    a) CRT terminal is superior to POS terminal(bar code reader) and
key matrix terminal interms of efficiency, learning effect and veri-
fiability.

    b) The efficiency of CRT terminal is crucially dependent on the
kind of job and software specification, and it is quite common that
unnecessary operations have to be performed before the essential
one is reached. These results have given far reaching contributions
to the process of system design. This method will also be effective
in evaluating the function of SHIS terminals after their implementation.

2) Optimization of system design

    The basic problems which had to be solved in the course of
system design were to make decisions on;
    a) the candidate hospitals which are supposed to implement SHIS,
    b) the specifications of terminal's functions,
    c) the number, the position and the scale of central facilities,
    d) whether 'Kanji'(Japanese ideographic character) processing
system should be applied from the outset or not, and how to input
the diagnoses, and
    e) how to distribute the processes and files among the machines of
centres and indivual hospitals.

    Regarding the problem a), the Ministry of Health and Welfare
decided to implement SHIS in its 94 acute hospitals first and 147
long term care hospital afterwards. Since these hospitals are about
8% of the whole in terms of the number of beds, we may expect more
candidates. Experts of each job involved in the system met together
to define the specifications getting the feed back from the research

groups. Models were built to solve the problem c), and two centres
produced a minimum cost. The problem d) had some philosophical
aspects and technological difficulties, but the steering committee
decided to tackle these positively.

The most complex problem to be solved was e). As I think the
whole result will be published elsewhere, I do not go into details
here, but it proved the fact that an appropriately distributed
design would result in reducing costs to between 65% and 71% of the
cost of the centralized system which has only the terminal control-
ler in the individual hospital, and it also gives a quicker response time.

3) Economic assessment

The following criteria were set.
 a) Total cost for the system does not exceed 1% of each hospital
revenue.
 b) Higher cost/benefit compared with manual system.
 c) The price is comparable to commercial system.

A research team was set up and detailed to investigate these
points. They showed that SHIS would satisfy these criteria, but a
difficulty might arise in the future from the fact that SHIS is
still more expensive than we expected and seems to be relatively
more expensive for the smaller hospital.

It was decided to implement SHIS and since the first of July
in 1977, it began to operate to a limited extent in the National
Centre Hospital for Cardio-vascular Diseases. It is to be implemented in at least 4 hospitals in the 1978 fiscal year. This project
is now managed by the non-profit organisation, the Medical Information Development Centre(MEDIS-DC) which was organized by the
government for the whole R&D projects of medical informatics in Japan.

5. Summary

 1) There is strong need for HIS in managerial use, especially the
job imposed by the national insurance scheme in Japan.
 2) Small single purpose computers seems to be answering to this
demand but their proliferation seems to be problematic.
 3) The results of strategic analyses, showed that SHIS with distributed functions between central facilities and individual hospital
devices gives higher cost/performance than any other alternatives.
 4) Technological evaluation using motion analysis proved to be

effective in evaluating the functions of the terminal.

5) The system was implemented in one hospital in 1977FY and is going to be implemented in four other hospitals at least in 1978FY.

6) In future, other relevant programmes can be added to the system.

Acknowledgement
    This project is now being carried out in collaboration with many organisations and experts. I am in an administrative position for the project and I was given the honour and privilege of reporting on it while I am in this country. Therefore, I would like to express acknowledgement of the organisations and people who have been contributed to this project: Dr. M. Oshima, the Chairman of MEDIS-DC; Prof. K. Atsumi, Prof. T. Ishii, Prof. K. Kiikuni, Prof. T. Furukawa, these professors are the leaders of the research groups; the colleagues of MEDIS-DC, the Nippon Telephone and Telegraph Corporation and the Ministry of International Trade and Industry.

ON-LINE SUPPORT FOR BASIC MEDICAL INFORMATION IN A LARGE
UNIVERSITY HOSPITAL

R. Klar, J. Haase, C. Th. Ehlers
Lehrstuhl für Medizinische Dokumentation u.Daten-
verarbeitung
Universität Göttingen
Robert- Kochstr. 40
D- 3400 Göttingen

Abstract
At the Göttinger University Hospital, an interactive basic medical
information system has been developed. The main part of this system
consists of the automatic coding of diagnoses using the German KDS-
classification, which is compatible with the ICD. The aims of the
system are improving the treatment of the current case, storing
data for exact morbidity statistics and supporting supervision of
students and less experienced physicians.

Introduction
The Göttinger University Hospital consists of twelve different
hospital disciplines with more than 30 departments, about 1500 beds
and nearly 1000 outpatients per day. In the last 5 years, a computerized hospital information system has been developed using
IBM 370/158 MP3, 3270 and 3750 terminals, IMS database and data
communication system. This hospital information system contains
typical application, e.g. online registration and identification
in the admission office for in- and outpatients, automatic printing
of labels and covers of patient charts, patient scheduling, on-line
support for patient medication and laboratory reports (1),(2).
Beside these frequently described computer applications in medicine,
we have also introduced a special on-line method for entering and
displaying basic medical information, such as diagnoses, risk
factors and bloodgroup.

The Aims of the Basic Medical Information System
There are three main reasons for the development of this an new
system:
            1. to support the flow of information of all these

medically significant items about the same patient, gathered at different times and locations in order to improve the treatment of the current case and assure high quality care.

2. to store data for exact morbidity statistics, which is not obligatory in West Germany, and for support of medical research.

3. to support the supervision of students and less experienced physicians with respect to diagnosis.

To meet these aims in an appropriate manner, it is necessary to avoid large amounts of paper handling and terminal activity by physicians and to take advantage of the larger hospital information system.

Free Text and Coding Systems

The diagnosis is one of the most important pieces of information about a patient and there are two methods for EDP- support of diagnosis documentation:

1. free text analysis
2. coding

The free text method has been well developed especially in North America with complex nomenclatures like SNOP and SNOMED (3),(4). But in Germany free text systems are less common and following problems of this method are still unsolved: the thesaurus development is rather difficult and time consuming, the comprehensive text analysis by computer leads to high response times in on- line dialogs and entering of data often requires the use of highly qualified personal. Especially for a multi- disciplinary hospital like the University Hospital Göttingen coding methods are more suitable (5).

The disadvantages of coding, for example, difficult and time-
consuming manual encoding with high rates of mistakes, can be
avoided by on- line methods (6,7).
The coding classification KDS (Klinischer Diagnosenschlüssel from
IMMICH (8)) has been chosen for our basic medical information
system. KDS and ICD are the most frequently used coding classifications in West Germany, thus allowing us to compare our diagnoses
with data from other hospitals. The KDS with its 5 character
notation is compatible with the ICD (International Classification
of Diagnoses) and has been extended to include a suffix of 4
characters for new diagnoses and a synonym notation of 2 further
characters.

Flow of Information
During the process of inpatient admission at the Göttinger
University Hospital, the physician receives a computer printout
of a condensed medical history of any patient who has formerly
visited the hospital. The physician describes the current case
by entering in free text form further diagnoses and risk factors.
While most of the medical units require the complete KDS catalog,
some, like the Neurology ,use only an extended subset, which includes the most frequently used diagnoses.
While such catalogs are not always necessary, they are a useful
tool in assisting new physicians and students to learn the unit's
diagnostic approach. In a recursive process these catalogs are updated and lead to a first level of medical standardization.

Once more it is to be emphasized that it is not necessary for any
one in the hospital to encode diagnosis using a large reference
containing all possibilities. Hence, a ward clerk receives the
completed printout from the physician and is able to enter the
diagnosis text, bloodgroup and risk factors at a display terminal
for any patient currently resident on that ward.
The encoding dialog with the help of the computer is divided into
three steps:
    - the entering of diagnosis
    - the lightpen selection of a diagnosis from a list
      presented on the display
    - the control of the encoding.

The diagnoses can be qualified by means of abbreviations which indicate whether it is confirmed or suspected. In addition, the physician may also protect the diagnoses against patient-specific retrieval; in this case they may only be read anonymously for statistical purposes.

Every ward physician, or any other person who meets the comprehensive interactive password and privacy checks, can obtain an immediate overview of the basic medical information about requested patients in display or hardcopy form.

Each discipline has an experienced physician, the so-called revisor, who receives computer printouts. These printouts are oriented either to wards, patients, physicians or diagnosis and include not only basic medical information but also medication notes and lab results. These lists make it clear for which patients diagnoses either not been formulated or are insufficient. The revisor is than able to contact the diagnosing physician in order to improve the diagnosis and treatment of the current case. Among the benefits derived from such lists are good overviews of the morbidity rate of the whole discipline or hospital, immediate retrieval of risk factors of single patients, especially in emergency cases, etc. This on-line support of computerized medical records ensures that the system may be used as an integral part of the patient's care, and not as a scheme to retrospectively document the patient's visit once (s)he is discharged.

The Method of Automatic Diagnosis Encoding
When the ward clerk has finished entering the diagnosis text, the encoding process begins with the removal of non-essential words from the entered text. The first five letters (key) of each remaining word are used in a search of an IMS data base. Every data base record consists of the key itself and a data field. The data field contains the numerical notations of all entries in the KDS, in which at least one word contains the referring key (see Fig. 1).

DIABE

84405000002	00401000001	00401000002	00401000003	00403000001
04401000001	04401000002	04401000003	04402000001	04403000001
04407000001	04408000001	04409000001	04409000002	05403000001
14401000002	14401000003	18421000001	24401000001	24401000002
25403000003	68401000001	68405000001	71401000001	71401000002
80401000001	84405000001	84405000003	...	

DIAL

01267000006

DIAMO

13675000001

.
.
.

MELKE

04110000002   21381000001   93291000002

MELLI

68401000001   68405000001   84405000003

MEMBR

| 36101000006 | 36639000001 | 36639000002 | 37618000001 | 42622000001 |
| 64623000001 | 65631000001 | 83726000001 | 83764000001 | ... |

.
.

Fig. 1: Part of the key data base
The keys DIABE and MELLI of the diagnosis " diabetis mellitus "
to be encoded, are underlined as well as the 11-character-
numerical notations of the extended KDS of those diagnoses containing at least one of these both keys.

If there were n keys in a text, n key records are accessed and
n quantities of KDS- notation occurrences are formed. The intersection of these n quantities of KDS occurrences are formed and the
referring diagnosis text is retrieved out of a KDS data base and
presented on the display in descending order of frequency of the
found keys. The clerk finds the correct KDS- formulation of the
diagnosis with a high probability in the first lines of the display and selects it using light-pen. The corresponding KDS notation
is then stored in the patient data base in order to present a
condensed medical history for subsequent visits of the patient, to
support statistics etc.
Normally such intersections are made by sequentielly comparing
every element of a quantity with all elements of the other quantities.
This method would be too slow for an on-line dialog program.
Hence, the KDS numerical notations are used as keys in a direct

access method and the degree of intersection is stored. This random access methods is further accelerated by using only the main-storage.

Additional Supports and Extensions

If a diagnosis text cannot be found in the presented list, it is assigned a preleminary code number. The revisor controls these preleminary codes. (S)he can either use the KDS notation of a known diagnosis or create a new KDS entry for this new diagnosis. If (s)he chooses to use an existing KDS notation the revisor contacts the diagnosing physician in order to explain the structure and medical basis of the KDS or the discipline-specific catalog. If, however, (s)he decides to include this diagnosis as a new one in the KDS, the four character suffic of the KDS notation provides an automatic extension to the key.

A special update mode permits the user to correct typing errors, complete   diagnosis or change a suspected diagnosis to a confirmed one, etc. Frequently used synonymous diagnoses are registered to ensure that only one of the synonyms is presented independent of which synonym has been entered.
There are some people who quickly learn the KDS code numbers corresponding to frequently occuring diagnoses. They may use these numbers instead of the full text and for a control purposes the text belonging to KDS numbers will then be presented.
The topological and nosological parts of the KDS offer the possibility of searching only with one of these parts. Interesting results have already been achieved in this way.

Conclusions

With all these possibilities, this kind of on-line processing of basic medical informations combines the advantages of free text analysis and coding methods and ensures high data quality. Currently, internal medicine (the largest disciplin of the Göttinger University Hospital) and neurology are connected to this on-line support. The other disciplines will follow stepwise. A year successfull application of this system justifies the extention to other disciplines and further medical dokumentation fields such as surgical operation notation.

References

(1)   EHLERS, C.TH.:
         Einpassung eines EDV-Systems und seiner Planung
         in das Funktionskonzept eines Großklinikums.
         21. GMDS-Jahrestagung, Hannover 26. - 28.9.76

(2)   KLAR, R.:
         Hierarchische strukturierte Datenbanken in
         der Medizin. 21. GMDS-Jahrestagung, Hannover
         26.- 28.9.76

(3)   WHITE, W., BARKMAN, B., BERNIER-BONNEVILLE, L.
         COUSINEAU, L.:
         A method for automatic Coding of Medical Information
         in Patient Records.
         Meth. Inf. Med. 16 (1977) 1 - 10

(4)   WINGERT, F.:
         Das Textverarbeitungssystem von PRATT.
         in: Reichertz, P.L., Holthoff, G. (Hrsg.):
         Methoden der Informatik in der Medizin.
         Springer-Verlag, Berlin - Heidelberg - New York,
         (1975) 216 - 223

(5)   HOLTHOFF, G.:
         Aufbau einer multidisziplinären, zentralisierten
         Medizinischen Basisdokumentation.
         Diss., Hannover, (1976)

(6)   ENGELBRECHT, R., SCHERTLEIN, G., REICHERTZ, P.L.:
         AKOS - Allgemeines Kodierungssystem.
         in Fuchs, G., Wagner, G. (Hrsg.): Krankenhaus-
         Informationssysteme.
         Schattauer Verlag, Stuttgart (1972) 95 - 100

(7)   HÖLZEL, D., KARRER, R.:
         VERDI - Ein Programmsystem zur Unterstützung der
         Verschlüsselung von Diagnosen.
         Hrsg.: Institut für Medizinische Informationsver-
         arbeitung, Statistik und Biomathematik (ISB),
         Technischer Bericht Nr. 4, München, (1976)

(8)   IMMICH, H.:
         Klinischer Diagnosenschlüssel.
         Stuttgart: Schattauer (1966)

AN APPROACH TO EFFICIENT ON-LINE MASS STORAGE OF PHYSIOLOGICAL
PARAMETERS IN AN INTENSIVE CARE ENVIRONMENT

H. Schillings, B. Scharnberg, R. M. Sabean, C. Th. Ehlers
Lehrstuhl für Medizinische Dokumentation
und Datenverarbeitung
Universität Göttingen
Robert-Koch-Str. 40
D 3400 Göttingen

Abstract

From the data processing point of view, monitoring critically ill
patients by computer is primarily a problem of reduction of mass
data.

This paper describes a way of reducing data for storage purposes
which results in a minimum loss of accuracy. The reduction factor
is 1:5 on an average for fast varying parameters and up to 1:100
for slowly varying parameters.

Our approach is to store trend information rather than averaged
data. The algorithm transforms a continuous input of data in
equidistant time intervals to an output in trend format. High compression on quasi-static data input and a fast reaction in case of
relevant changes are the main characteristics.

This algorithm is part of a data path in a decentralized mini-
computer system for intensive care, the Göttingen Information System
for Intensive Care "GISI".

Introduction

A computer system running in an intensive care environment has to
handle different kinds of patient related data:

    (i)   physiological values such as ECG, temperature and
               blood pressures

    (ii)   care related data such as medication plans, lab
               results and nurses' notes

    (iii)   administrative data

Looking at data input rates, the category of the physiological
values represents the most important one. In our case, as many
as 10 physiological parameters could be analyzed per patient.
This results in a maximum data input of about 15,000 data items
per patient per day.

Nevertheless, from the clinician's point of view, all three
classes of data are important to provide an overview of the
patient's status. Moreover, all data must be easily and quickly
accessible (1) and should not be compressed in such a way that
significant changes are lost.

The Göttingen Information System for Intensive Care "GISI" meets
these requirements by breaking up the input data into two logically different categories:

(i)   Real time data input.
        This category includes nearly all
        data handling of physiological values.
(ii)   Additional input.
        This category deals mainly with the not-time criti-
        cal input classes of care-related data and ad-
        ministrative data.

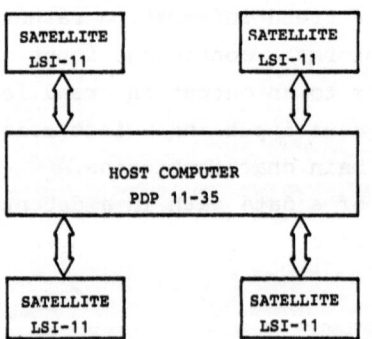

Figure 1:
GISI system components

Corresponding to these two input categories, the hardware used by
the "GISI" system is a distributed mini-computer network in two
levels as shown in figure 1. "GISI" supports

(i)   four remote LSI-11 micro-computer satellites for
patient monitoring. Each satellite is a stand-alone
system and performs automatic data acquisition,
analysis and representation of a patient's vital
signs.

(ii)   a PDP 11-35 mini-computer host system with the data
base management system MUMPS-11. All satellites are
hierarchically connected to the host system (2,3).

Data processing of the physiological values is done in a data path
which runs through both parts of the GISI-System.

The Satellite's Data Path

All branches of the data path originate in the satellites. Each of
the four satellites currently in use processes 10 physiological signals with a parameter specific sampling rate, varying from 10 Hertz
to 100 Hertz. Executing up to five cycles per second, the satellite's
internal real-time analysis programs refer to the samples' buffers
when evaluating the derived physiological signals from the input
samples.

The data is buffered in the derived parameter buffers. The consolidator, called once per second, does a first compression of the
resulting input data by a simple averaging over one second. The output data of the consolidator is used within the satellites for further
processing and display.

The data output buffers of the consolidator are input to the·
satellite's data logging system. The data logger is called once
per minute and keeps track of the satellite's data base structure.
Before updating the satellite's data base with a new set of values,
the data logger compresses the data to one value per derived parameter per minute.

At this stage of data reduction, the data path is split into two
different ways relevant to the subsequent handling of the data:

    -     further data path in the satellite itself
    -     data path in the host system.

As all data processing in a satellite is tailored to the needs of patient monitoring, the results will provide a quick patient status and an overview of the last few hours. To meet these requirements, it is not necessary for the satellite's internal data path to keep this data without further compression. Internally, the satellite compresses data according to its age three more times using an averaging procedure. All data is stored in a ring-buffered data structure; data older than 72 hours is overwritten.

Only the host system can provide long time storage of the results as well as a time window effect for any time slice and any parameter.

Data handling in the host system deals with pre-processed data items only. Thus, the input to the satellite's data base is identical to the input to the host's data path (see figure 2).

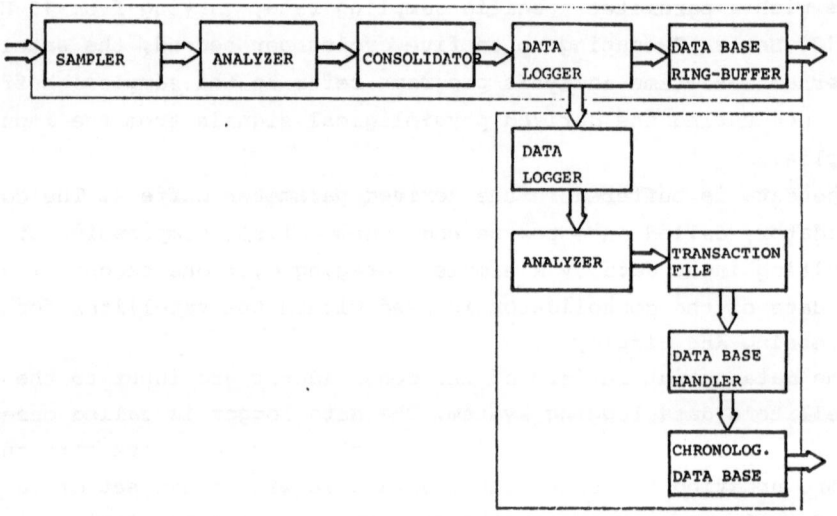

Figure 2:
Data path in satellite and host system. Data reduction increases in horizontal direction.

The Host's Data Path

The first module of the host's data handling routines is the clock handler. It initiates the host's data input mechanism in fixed time intervals by starting the logger programs. The logger switches from satellite to satellite to receive each patients actual physiological signs. According to a data definition file, a rough prefiltering of this data is done in order to avoid processing of badly transmitted data.

For each satellite, e. g. for each patient being monitored, the logger now calls an analysis program. The analyzer has to decide whether the incoming data should be stored or not. The algorithm used for compression is identical for each kind of input data. Only relevant changes within a physiological signal will be stored.

When data storage is required, the result will be written into a transaction file. The transaction file serves as a data entry file to the patient data base as well as a 24-hour backup to all data entries for the patient data base.

The data base handler which is invoked by the clock handler in periodic time intervals has exclusive control of all data input to the chronological patient data base. In addition to other data, the final results of the patient's physiological values are stored in this chronological patient file in time ascendant order.

The Data Reduction Algorithm

The main problem of the whole data path in the satellites as well as in the host itself is the handling and storage of mass data. It is unrealistic to assume that in a system in which several patients were being monitored, each pre-processed physiological value could be stored, even if the host system had access to large mass storage devices. An algorithm must be used to reduce the data while maintaining the highest possible accuracy in order to provide a time-window effect when retrieving data.

Our storage approach in the host's data path is to store trend information rather than averaged data. The basic idea is that any continuously measured physiological signal is somehow a continuous waveform with more or less smooth changes in small time intervals. Storing trend information means that the algorithm defines a line with an optimized slope which replaces a series of physiological values within a certain time slice as shown in figure 3. This process is continued as long as the difference between the calculated graph and all values within this series does not exceed a previously defined deviation ε_{max}.

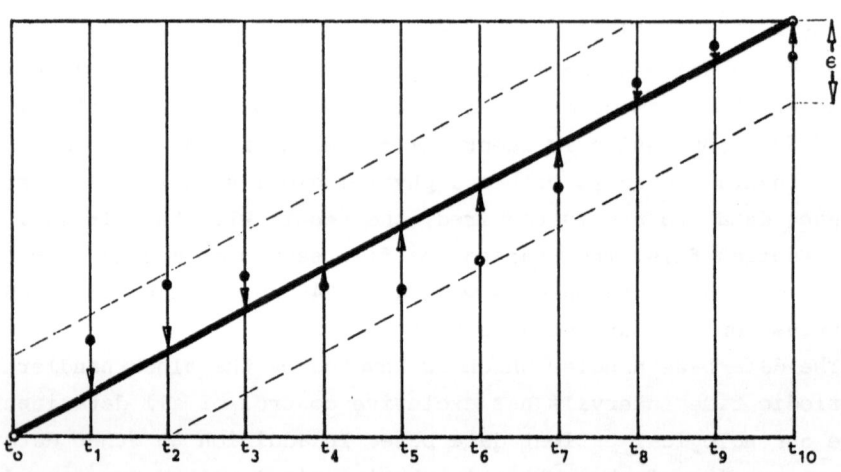

Figure 3:
Optimized graph $f_i(t)$ replacing a series of physiological values. The interval length t_j-t_{j-1} is fixed by the logging frequency.

In the interval (t_o, t_k), the curve is defined as

$$(1) \quad f_i(t) = a_1 \cdot t + a_o$$
$$t_o \leq t \leq t_k$$

The problem is now to find an optimized slope a_1 in order to minimize the absolute deviation.

$$\sum_{j=1}^{k} \varepsilon_j^2 \rightarrow \text{Min}$$

where ε_j is the difference between the graph and the actual value y_j for $t=t_j$.

This leads to an optimized slope $a_1(k)$, which meets equations (1) and (2).

$$a_1(k) = \frac{\sum_{j=1}^{k} j(y_j - a_o)}{\sum_{j=1}^{k} j^2}$$

To ensure that a relevant change in the trend will be recognized, a suitable ε_{max} is defined to

$$\varepsilon_{max} = \varepsilon(a_o) = \delta \cdot a_o \qquad , \quad 0 < \delta < 1$$

The choice of ε should be done carefully, since it has a direct impact on the correlation between storage space and accuracy. The tolerable error for any point of the graph will then be

$$\varepsilon_j = y_j - f(t_j) \qquad , \text{ where } \quad j = 1...k$$

A graph will not be continued if an ε_j is evaluated which does not match the initial error definition

$$|\varepsilon_j| < \varepsilon_{max} \qquad , \text{ where } j=1...k$$

In this case the current optimizing process is stopped. The last value y_{k+1} is not taken into consideration when the final optimized slope a_1 is calculated. The whole series of k+1 values is now reduced to one tupel of information $(f_i(t_k), t_k)$, called switch data.

The next optimizing process will be initialized recursively using
the last point of $f_i(t)$ as a common point to both graphs by rede-
fining it to a_o of the new graph $f_{i+1}(t)$.

$$f_i(t_k) = f_{i+1}(t_k)$$

This condition must be met, because two consecutive graphs must always have one common point (see figure 4).

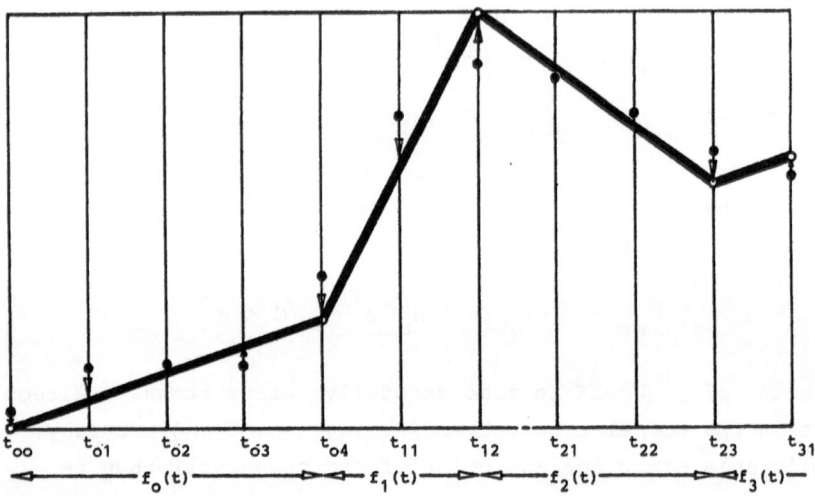

Figure 4:
Series of consecutive graphs.
The continuity conditions are met for $t_{o4}=t_{10}$, $t_{12}=t_{20}$, $t_{23}=t_{30}$.

As a line is completely determined by two tupels of coordinates,
n optimized lines will be represented by n+1 tupels of switch data.
Any intermediary point of a graph can always be reconstructed with
a deviation less than ε.

Discontinuous Graphs

The only limitation to the algorithm being discussed is continuity.
The logger is supposed to deliver values for a parameter each time
it is invoked. This, of course, is not always true. There are many
constellations for which the logger cannot give any concrete result.
In order for the algorithm not to malfunction on non-continuous
signals, it must be expanded to work on both types of waveforms.
This means that each switch point is not only a tupel $(f_o,t_o)_i$, but
a three dimensional vector $(f_o,t_o,c_o)_i$ with c_o defined as a flag for
continuity.

Per definition, all two dimensional graph vectors are regarded as
continuous graphs and all three dimensional ones as discontinuous
graphs. The result is, that the following switch conditions must be
defined:

$(f_o,t_o)_i - (f_o,t_o)_{i+1}$	defines a continuous curve between t_{oi} and t_{oi+1}
$(f_o,t_o)_i - (f_o,t_o,c_o)_{i+1}$	defines a continuous curve between t_{oi} and t_{oi+1}. It is discontinued after t_{oi+1}
$(f_o,t_o,c_o)_i - (f_o,t_o)_{i+1}$	the graph is undefined in the range between t_{oi} and t_{oi+1}

The results of the trend-storer are switch points. If a parameter
is always continuous, the curve can easily be reconstructed by simply
connecting the switch data.

If a data entry is flagged with a discontinuity flag, it indicates
that from this time until the next value can be found, a connection
between two following data is illegal since no data could be meanwhile evaluated.

The Resulting Reduction Factor

The reduction factor resulting from this algorithm cannot be determined theoretically, since the algorithm performes a dynamic data
compression. The most important factors on which the reduction factor depends are

    (i)   the waveform of a physiological signal

    (ii)   the choice of the maximum deviation ε_{max}.

The waveform of a physiological signal is not predictable. Nevertheless, a suitable choice of the tolerable deviation will lead to a high data compression on quasi-static data input of any physiological parameter. Slowly varying parameters, such as temperature, tend to be quasi-static over a longer time period. Theoretically there is no lower limit of the minimum storage frequency.

In case of rapidly changing waveforms within any physiological signal, the trend-storer algorithm is capable of a quick adaption of its storing frequency to the needs of the signal input. The upper storage frequency is the logging frequency, e. g. the frequency with which the algorithm gets its data input.

A paramter with a direct impact on the resulting reduction factor is the choice of the tolerable deviation. There are two ways of defining ε.

- ε is a parameter-specific constant
- ε is not a function of the physiological parameter but dependent on the initial value a_o of a graph.

Both types of definitions contain some disadvantages, leading to non-optimal storage. When defining ε to a parameter specific constant, the algorithm may malfunction on some non-standard data input, either too low or too high in it's absolute values. The resulting storage frequency will not be dynamic in all ranges of a physiological signal.

On the other hand, an ε not being dependent on the physiological signal itself will lead to an unnecessarily high storage frequency in some cases. When thinking of temperature, for example, a difference of $1^{\circ}C$ is an extreme increase. Nevertheless, this change is only about 2% of an average initial value, whereas a relative change of 2% is too small a range for other parameters such as heart rate.

During our tests it became clear that a mixed solution is best. Generally, ε is set to 5% of the initial value of a graph. This gives a fair compromise between storage space and accuracy. Exceptions to this rule are made for temperature and multiple parameters derived from the same original signal such as arterial systolic, -mean and -diastolic pressure.

A typical reduction factor for a fast varying signal such as an ECG of a postoperative coronary care patient, is about 1:5 (see figure 5). Over a one hour period the maximum reduction practically evaluated using the same signal, was 1:16 and the minimum reduction was 1:3.

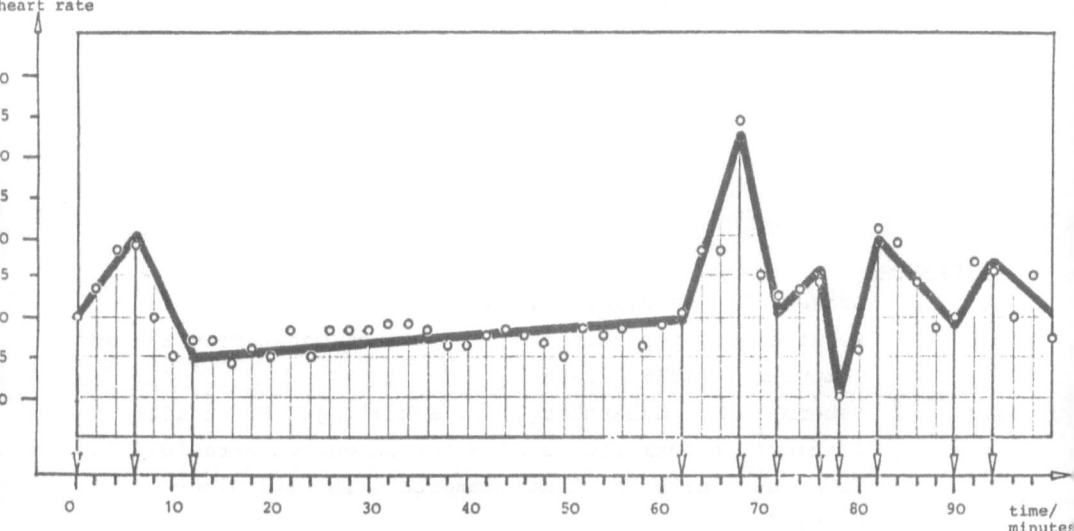

Figure 5: Analyzer output and real patient data.
All stored switch data is marked.

Discussion

The main disadvantages of the storage algorithm being described are:

- it works effectively only for continuously measured parameters, e. g. saving storage space
- the storage algorithm always needs a temporary help file for data buffering during the evaluation of a graph
- output data is stored not in equidistant time intervals. Therefore, retrieval of this trend data is rather complicated.

On the other hand there are some important advantages of this algorithm, that cannot be denied:

- high compression on quasi-static data
- a fast reaction in case of relevant changes within a signal
- no important peak within a waveform is smoothed by averaging
- dynamic storage
- good total reduction for all parameters.

References

(1)   Drazen, E., Wechsler, A., Wiig, K.:
Requirements for computerized patient monitoring systems.
Computer 1 (1975) 22-26

(2)   Sabean, R.M., Scharnberg, B., Schillings, H. et al.:
Göttingen information system for intensive care "GISI".
To appear in: Proc. Conf. Computers in Cardiology
Rotterdam 1977.
New York: IEEE Computer Society.

(3)   Scharnberg, B., Sabean, R.M., Schillings, H. et al.:
A data base for intensive care units.
In.: Shires, D.B., Wolf, H. (Eds): MEDINFO 77, Vol. 2
p. 1063
Amsterdam: North Holland Publ. Co., 1977

A NEW APPROACH TO EVALUATION IN THE NHS

EXPERIMENTAL COMPUTER PROGRAMME

B. W. H. Molteno, Regional Management Services Officer

Trent Regional Health Authority

1. The Problem

In the 1960's the NHS was able to employ computers for purposes which had previously been tried and tested in industry - e.g. payroll and accounting. At the same time it was recognised that computers might also assist procedures required to run hospitals and health centres, and that these procedures had no parallels in industry or commerce. Experimental computer projects were therefore started in fourteen hospitals and in a health centre and, subsequently, a careful attempt to evaluate these experiments was started. By the end of 1976 enough work had been done to suggest that evaluation was no simple task, and an Evaluation Working Group was set up to consider the problems outlined in the report "Interim Report on the Evaluation of the National Health Service Experimental Computer Programme (DHSS 1977)". The Working Group formulated a hypothesis and commissioned a study to test it. A full explanation was published in the Working Group's report in the summer of 1977.

It had been assumed that, because a successful computer project ought to improve the working of the hospital or health centre, measurements taken before and after the introduction of the computer should yield a predictive statement about the improvements which could be achieved elsewhere by the installation of a similar computer. The attempt to use this approach met with the following problems:

a)   During the considerable time required to develop computer systems, many other causes of change operate. It is impossible to isolate changes caused solely by the computer, except in matters which are only a means to an end, such as the timely and accurate presentation of information.

b)   Even if the effect of a computer in one hospital could be precisely identified, there are good reasons to doubt any simple prediction of the same results elsewhere. No two hospitals are alike. Improvements achieved in the first hospital with the help of a computer may have been achieved already in the second, before a computer has been considered.

A further difficulty encountered in the first phase of evaluation was that the "improvement objectives" against which evaluators set out to take measurements were lists of possible improvements drawn up logically and chronologically after the prior decision to install an experimental computer. They were lists of desirable improvements, rather long and detailed lists which were unlikely to match any statement of the top priorities for change which might have been derived from a prior analysis of any major problems facing the hospital or health centre before a computer project was proposed.

2. Objective

Computers ought to be installed in hospitals and health centres in order to deal with problems already perceived or improvements already desired by those responsible for hospitals or health centres. If we can identify the criteria by which these responsible people decide what problems or opportunities for improvement exist, evaluators can make relevant measurements, thus avoiding the problem described at the end of the paragraph above. However, "before and after" measurements cannot be predictive because of the complexity (a) and variability (b) of hospitals and health centres. As an alternative, it is suggested that criteria could be used to measure the effectiveness of those activities within hospitals and health centres which can be supported by computers. Such measurements would enable comparisons to be made between effectiveness in hospitals or health centres with computers and in those without. The comparison would not in itself define the contribution of the computer to effectiveness: those responsible would have to make judgements about that in the light of all circumstances at the existing and potential computer sites. The project here reported was set up to test the hypothesis that useful performance criteria for this purpose can be identified such that their validity will be generally recognised at all levels in the service. "All levels" were interpreted to mean people in hospitals and health centres, DMTs, ATOs, RTOs and DHSS.

3. Scope

Although the remit referred to "areas of NHS activity" (an almost limitless field) we decided to start with nine areas of activity which have been supported by experimental computer systems, namely:

    inpatient administration
    outpatient administration
    waiting list management
    medical records
    nursing records
    pathology services
    pharmacy services
    x-ray services
    health centre records

It was easy to identify the people we should consult as "decision-makers" in DMTs, ATOs and RTOs, i.e. a sample of all members of such officer teams. Within DHSS we were to be guided by advice from the Computers and Research Division. The aspect requiring judgement was consultation with the "users" of computer systems. It may be argued that the entire staff of a hospital or health centre will be affected in some way by a computer system, and that any of them may have relevant opinions to which a sensible decision-maker should listen.

However, it was impossible to consult everybody, and a few types or disciplines of user could be identified who ought to be consulted separately. Various sub-divisions were attempted, but in the end the list derived was:

Hospital clinicians - physicians and surgeons
Consultant medical staff providing diagnostic services
General Practitioners
Nurses
Administrators, including Medical Records Officers
Professional and Technical staff

It was assumed throughout the study that each of these disciplines might legitimately hold different values, and that any attempt to analyse a total hospital or health centre view would have to include any issue of importance to any one discipline regardless of whether other disciplines agreed or valued that issue or not.

4. Method

Project team members already had considerable collective experience of all nine topics and could have offered lists of potential criteria for consideration by the people consulted (referred to as "respondents" in the rest of this paper). Alternatively, respondents could have been asked to give a list of criteria. The former approach was rejected because it would lead respondents into pre-determined modes of thought and the latter because it would not stimulate wide or deep thought. To meet both these considerations an interview structure was designed to deal with all topics in a broad exploration of objectives and problems. Interviews using this structure were found acceptable to respondents and useful to interviewers. Lists of potential performance criteria were drawn up on the basis of these interviews.

Having created lists of possible criteria, we then critically examined them. One important consideration deliberately excluded from this analysis was the question of measurement. Health Service activities could be judged against some criteria (e.g. cost) which could be measured fairly easily. Others might be expensive to measure (e.g. patient satisfaction) or virtually impossible to measure (e.g. health outcomes). An alternative study could have stated the cost and feasibility of measurements and then asked respondents to say which criteria they would "buy" first, given a quantum of money. We rejected this approach and sought simply those criteria which respondents would think important regardless of the cost and feasibility of measurement. This allowed unbiased judgements in principle, but leaves the measurement question to be examined outside the scope of this study.

We had also to exclude considerations which are very important in particular situations but impossible to generalise as demanded by the aims of the study.

Despite these exclusions we were faced with some long lists, and two important considerations seemed to justify shortening them. First, it is possible to set up a number of criteria which are really only various ways of measuring performance under a single conceptual heading. It was essential to use this consideration cautiously: any radical attempt to delve into the underlying concept could lead to the sterile conclusion that there is only one fundamental criterion, i.e. cost-effectiveness. We tried to exercise judgement about this first consideration in a balanced way across all topics.

The second consideration was more precisely definable. Any performance criterion which was insulated from the effects or potential effects of computer systems would be of no relevance to the study. Those receiving evaluation information will require a profile of the whole situation evaluated, but fixed profile data are not criteria. Thus outpatient arrangements may vary in their effectiveness according to their accessibility to the population, or according to the level of provision of diagnostic services. We tried to refine our lists of potential performance criteria so that they only contained criteria which were "system sensitive", i.e. criteria against which improvements could reasonably be expected from changes in supporting systems, whether manual or computer-assisted. This search for the potential causal link suggested that all ultimate criteria such as health outcomes should be excluded. Only in this sense was our decision to avoid the question of feasibility of measurement modified.

We were going to consult DHSS and members of RTOs, ATOs and DMTs who could be required to consider the interests of the citizen in order to fulfil their own roles. The preamble to the main consultation therefore asked respondents to reply as holders of posts, not as citizens.

Ideally each respondent should be asked both to rank all potential performance criteria in order of importance and to place each one on a scale such that the extent of differentiation as perceived by that respondent could be compared with the perceptions of all other respondents. Methods are available to achieve this, but more time and manpower would be required than were available.

To meet these difficulties we developed a method based on experience in market research, but modified to suit the purposes of the study. In its initial form this consisted of a preference sheet for each topic with 7 positions ranging from "most important" at one end to "least important" at the other. Potential performance criteria were written onto cards, one card for each criterion, and respondents were asked to allocate them on the preference sheet in order of importance. So far, this procedure is analogous to a questionnaire with seven tick-boxes, but there is already an important difference. With cards, it is much easier for the respondent to modify early decisions in the light of later ones, thus all judgements are more likely to be made in a balanced way over a whole topic.

Respondents' markings on questionnaires tend to follow different patterns. Some are weighted to the centre, others to either or both of the extremes. Average marks from a group of respondents are therefore not very useful. By controlling the number of cards respondents are allowed to place in each preference box, the results can be directed into a common framework which can, with justice, be aggregated into a group average or median score for each card.

The pattern of cards in preference boxes had to be uniform for all respondents. We preferred the simplicity and naturalness of a uniform distribution. Respondents were therefore asked to place one seventh of the cards in each box on the preference sheet, with one extra card in as many boxes (starting from the least important end) as were required to distribute the number remaining after the total number of cards had been divided by seven.

Although this constraint had the advantage that it allowed group results to be aggregated, it caused some acute dissatisfaction among those respondents on whom we tried it. They felt that it implied fixed relationships that did not correspond with their judgements. Thus it might imply that cards in the sixth box were twice as important as cards in the third. Also some felt that a significant proportion of the cards were entirely unimportant. We therefore provided respondents with tokens with which to weight the results after they had sorted the cards as prescribed. This enabled them to show equality, if they so wished, between cards in adjacent boxes, and to allocate no weights to boxes containing cards which they thought unimportant. By restricting the number of weights to a fixed total, the results were kept within a consistent range which would still allow group results to be obtained.

As described, the whole game of sorting and weighting sounds elaborate. In practice we found that respondents understood it readily and seemed to find it a satisfactory way of expressing their views quickly.

We now had a predetermined method of consultation, a fixed timetable and a defined project team. The total number of people we could afford to consult would be less than a thousand. The varieties of viewpoint in the NHS are so numerous that statistically reliable samples of all of them would total to more than a thousand people. We could not afford to search for statistical validity: the sample could only be defined on the basis of general intuitive judgement. The main aim was to ensure that we did not fail to consult any significant sector of opinion.

The sample included health centres, large hospitals, small ones, teaching hospitals, hospitals with and without computers, consultant physicians and surgeons and providers of diagnostic services, general practitioners, nurses both in administration and in wards and departments, on day and night duty, Area and hospital pharmacists, unit administrators, medical records and patient services officers. All these and other more detailed discriminations are recorded in

working documents. The main analysis, however, is based simply on the main disciplines, with a minimum achieved sample size on any one topic of six people.

Top management, i.e. members of DMTs, ATOs, RTOs or DHSS faced with a computer proposal supported by evaluation evidence, would require other information
as well. Evaluation evidence would simply give the benefit side of the case.
Also required would be costs, feasibility, availability of finance and nature of
conflicting claims for it, climates of opinion etc. These matters were thought
to be outside the scope of the study, and the consultation concerned only the
potential performance criteria as prepared for the consultations in hospitals
and health centres.

The method of consultation described above was too detailed at this level,
and a few officer team members were asked whether we ought to consult their
colleagues by presenting short-lists of criteria selected by respondents in
hospitals and health centres. The advice given was clearly against this. Decision-makers would have quite different views about the relative importance of
criteria. They would have to be shown the whole lists.

It seemed fair to assume that decision-makers would expect their colleagues
in hospitals and health centres to examine evaluation evidence in detail, and
confine themselves to broadly based judgements. Therefore, instead of a seven-
place preference sheet and 28 weights, decision-makers were asked to review all
the cards for a topic and simply select any which appeared either specially relevant or specially irrelevant. This method of consultation enabled us to consult
each decision-maker on up to 3 topics.

5.   Results

Using Kendall's Coefficient of Concordance we verified our prior judgement
that there would be more consensus within than between disciplines. Thus a method
of combining group rankings was required. Neither a mean of the group median
weighted scores nor a mean of the group rankings seemed appropriate, because both
methods would mask strong feelings of individual disciplines. The rankings have
therefore been used to create bands in such a way that the band number for any
criterion is given by the highest rank number from any discipline. The banding
method implies that all disciplines are equal and that every discipline has the
right to push its own priorities up the combined list but no right to push the
priorities of other disciplines down.

It is very difficult to give a proper account of the results without reproducing all the tables in the project report (about 40). A single example is here
used to illustrate the material from which we drew the following conclusions.
(see Annex).

a)   Sufficient consensus within disciplines exists to support the claim
          that the report reflects a true and useful picture of NHS judgements about

the topics considered.

b)   No simple short-lists can be provided. All potential criteria presented for consideration in the study are, in fact, valid criteria.

c)   There are valid reasons for the relatively light contribution to this study from top management (members of DMTs, ATOs, RTOs and DHSS). This does not detract from the value to them of the result.

d)   The banded lists of criteria provide a useful starting point for any plan to measure the value of the NHS Experimental Computer Applications. Priority should in general be given to criteria in higher bands.

e)   The analysis provides only one consideration among many. The plan to measure must be modified by careful consideration of all the facts, many of which are available in the working papers of this study.

f)   The study provides a starting point for considering a better research basis for the planning and monitoring of health services.

6.   Next Steps

As many measurements as resources allow need to be made in hospitals and health centres with and without computers, and the results offered for consideration by the same types of people who were consulted in drawing up the criteria. This large task has been started.

TOPIC INPATIENTS   ANNEX

Band (1)	Performance Criteria (2)	Order of Choice by Respondent Group						
		SP (3)	PR (4)	GP (5)	N (6)	A (7)	PT (8)	TM (9)
1	BED USAGE: Bed usage measured by one or more of the following a) turnover interval (average time bed remaining empty) b) occupancy c) patient throughput (discharges and deaths per available bed) d) average lengths of stay (27)	6		11	4	6		1
	TIMELINESS OF DISCHARGE LETTERS: Average delay between discharge and discharge letter being dispatched to GP. (02)	2		1	25	1		6
	PATIENT SATISFACTION: Patients' and relatives views concerning inpatient procedures (21)	15		7	1	3		15
	'MISSING' CASE NOTES AND X-RAYS: Proportion of case notes and x-rays not available at time of admission (06)							
2	TIMELINESS OF DISCHARGE SUMMARIES: Average delay between discharge and discharge summary being dispatched to GP. (03)	3		3	18	2		8
	CO-OPERATION BETWEEN DISCIPLINES: Views of admission/discharge/ ward clerks and doctors/nurses/other staff towards degree of co-operation between them (20)	13		10	2	7		16
	THEATRE USAGE: % of available theatre time used (excluding closures due to infection, staff shortages, industrial action or renovations). (28)	8		15	21	10		2
	COMPLETENESS OF DISCHARGE SUMMARIES: Frequency with which important information is omitted from discharge summaries (04)	7		2	27	15		17

No								
3	LEAD TIME OF INVESTIGATIONS: Average time between admission of patient and initiation of preliminary investigations (23)	4		9	3	16		10
	TOTAL COSTS: The cost incurred, including revenue expenditure, indirect costs and resources used for which financial cost statements would be inappropriate (31)	21		16	32	19		3
4	CO-OPERATION BETWEEN HOSPITAL & GP: GPs and hospital staffs views on degree of co-operation (19)	5		4	14	4		12
	MEAN LENGTH OF STAY: Mean length of stay analysed by specialty and/or standardised for specialty mix (24)	20		18	22	29		4
5	LENGTH OF INPATIENT WAITING LIST: Length of inpatient waiting list analysed by specialty, sex and urgency (25)	11		6	20	20		5
	ACCURACY OF DOCUMENTATION: Rate of procedural errors (e.g. failure to register a transfer) and/or rate of transcription errors over specified period of time (01)	14		13	19	5		14
	LENGTH OF OUTPATIENT WAITING LIST: Average number of weeks necessary to wait for non-urgent clinic appointments analysed by specialty (26)	16		5	31	11		7
	TIME SPENT BY NURSES ON ADMIN & CLERICAL DUTIES: Time spent by nurses on the ward on administrative and clerical duties which are not nursing functions (e.g. excluding nursing records, pharmacy ordering etc.) (17)	10		23	5	32		18
6								

7	VOLUME OF WORK/STAFF RATIO: Staffing levels required to administer inpatient procedures for a given workload in terms of discharges/deaths and/or throughput per bed. (11)	25		17	7	18		11
8	USEFULNESS OF DISCHARGE SUMMARIES: GPs views concerning usefulness of discharge summaries received (07)	9		8	30	24		21
	STAFF SATISFACTION - TURNOVER/ ABSENTEEISM: Staff satisfaction as measured by turnover rates and absenteeism among admissions, discharge and ward clerks (13)	19		20	8	21		26
	LEGIBILITY OF DOCUMENTATION: Subjective assessments by admission, discharge and ward clerks of legibility of admission, transfer and discharge documentation (05)	27		24	16	8		23
9	CALIBRE OF STAFF EMPLOYED: Calibre of admissions, discharge and ward clerks as measured by qualifications and experience (12)	12		12	9	13		29
	TIME TAKEN TO ADMIT PATIENT: Average time between planned admissions entering hospital and arriving on the ward (22)	17		19	24	9		22
10	COMPLAINTS: Number of officially recorded complaints from staff and patients regarding inpatient procedures over a specified period of time (30)	29		14	10	12		13

NEW TOOLS FOR EVALUATION : THEIR APPLICATION TO COMPUTERS

Rachel Rosser
Department of Psychiatry
Charing Cross Hospital Medical School
Fulham Palace Road
London, W.6.

Tim Benson
Computer Evaluation Unit
Charing Cross Hospital
Fulham Palace Road
London, W.6.

Expenditure on experimental computer application in NHS hospitals so far exceeds £26 million (see Committee of Public Accounts 1976) and expenditure on evaluation alone exceeds £750,000. The measures which have been used for evaluation of computer systems include reductions in the time spent by patients in clinics, the turn-round time of laboratory reports, the quality of information provided (its accuracy, completeness and ease of use) and the time spent by hospital staff on tasks which are affected by computer systems (DHSS 1977). It has been assumed that improvements in these intermediate outputs would lead to improvements in the accuracy and timeliness of clinical decision-making and hence improve the quality of care given with benefits for the health of the patients treated.

The relationships between these intermediate outputs and the end output of effects on a patient's health is illustrated in figure 1. The priorities assigned to improvements in different intermediate outputs should depend on their contribution towards improving the patient's health. However the tools available for measuring changes

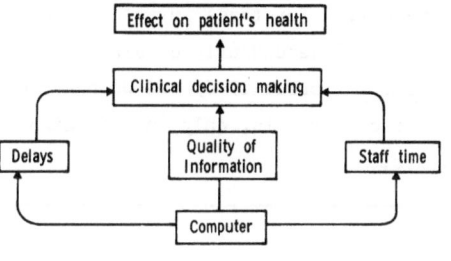

Figure 1.

in a patient's health which could be related to the intermediate outputs have been inadequate. This paper describes some progress that has been made in developing tools for measuring changes in the health of patients during episodes of hospital care. They have been developed as part of the preparatory work for a comprehensive evaluation of a computer system.

The need to relate improvements in intermediate outputs to the end result, improvements in health care, has become more pressing because of the recent development of integrated computer systems which bring information more directly to the clinician. This may be leading to a situation in which accurate information is being presented to the clinician but his decision-making and action-taking may be no faster nor precise than before the introduction of a computer.

Measures of the quality of medical care have already been developed to examine the benefits derived from other NHS activities. The stimulus for their development has been the increase in the demand for medical care and the rapid rise in its cost since the Health Service was set up in 1948. Conventional indicators such as mortality statistics have not demonstrated a conspicuous improvement in the state of the health of the population despite this expenditure. Therefore, questions have been asked about what return we are getting on a substantial investment. Similar questions have been raised about the output of other aspects of public expenditure such as road-building schemes, education and housing. Such questions lead to the idea of social indicators (Abrams 1976) one of which might be an index of the state of health of the community (Fanshel and Bush 1970, Berg 1973, Culyer, Lavers & Williams 1971).

Operational researchers became interested in the problems of the Health Service in the late fifties. To develop planning models with the purpose of allocating health service resources they needed a measure of what the health service was aiming to optimise i.e. a measure of what it was producing (Torrance 1970). Economists also entered the health field but were unable to calculate cost-benefit ratios without a measure of benefit (Prest & Turvey 1965). Hence the need for a measurement of output became apparent. For these purposes a method was required for quantifying the health of a population independently of diagnosis. Such methods have come to be known as global measures (Rosser 1976) and we hope to use one to compare the outputs for two similar sets of patients, only one of which has been treated with the assistance of a computer system.

DISABILITY

1 No disability.
2 Slight social disability.
3 Severe social disability and/or slight impairment of performance at work. Able to do all housework except very heavy tasks.
4 Choice of work or performance at work very limited. Housewives and old people able to do light housework only, but able to go out shopping.
5 Unable to undertake any paid employment. Unable to continue any education. Old people confined to home except for escorted outings and short walks and unable to do shopping. Housewives only able to perform a few simple tasks.
6 Confined to chair or wheelchair or able to move around in the house only with support from an assistant.
7 Confined to bed.
8 Unconscious.

DISTRESS

1 No distress.
2 Mild.
3 Moderate.
4 Severe.

Figure 2. Classes of Disability and Distress.

The tools we have developed have been based on one of these global measures: that of
Rosser and Watts (1972).   Their paper describes the application of a <u>scaled classification of states of illness</u> to the measurement of the output of a London hospital.
The classification is shown in figure 2.   It defines two major dimensions of illness:
<u>disability</u> i.e. what the patient is unable to do, and <u>distress</u> i.e. the patients'
subjective suffering.   There are eight categories of disability and four of distress
and, on the assumption that the unconscious patient does not suffer, there are 29 combinations of disability and distress.   The classification has been shown to be
reliable in use by doctors and nurses who have been trained in the use of the method
and know the patients.   A simple explanation of the method is not sufficient, practical training exercises using real patients as examples are required and the
results are discussed until a consensus is reached.   We shall also use a reliable
classification of <u>prognosis</u> (figure 3).

The scale places valuations on the states of illness defined by the classification,
indicating the severity of each state relative to every other state, as perceived
by selected judges.   It has been derived by a psychometric method which has
demonstrated a consensus about the relative severity of the 29 states as perceived
by judges with different personal characteristics (Rosser and Kind 1978).   The
<u>scale</u> is shown in figure 4.   There is evidence for the validity of this scale and
when it is applied to classification of patients in a hospital it gives very similar
results to an earlier published scale which was derived by the analysis of legal
awards   (Rosser & Watts   1975).

PROGNOSIS

To be completed as soon as a diagnosis
is made; with the <u>present</u> treatment in
one year's time the patient is most
likely to be:

1   Recovered
2   Better
3   Same
4   Worse
5   Dead

		DISTRESS			
		1	2	3	4
DISABILITY	1	0	1	2	6
	2	2	3	5	14
	3	4	6	9	18
	4	7	9	12	30
	5	11	13	20	60
	6	25	31	64	200
	7	65	87	200	520
	8	406			

Figure 3. Classification of Prognosis.   Figure 4. Scale values.

The classification and scale are used to measure output in the following way. Each
patient is classified at the beginning and end of an episode of medical care and the
scale valuation is then applied to the initial and final states. The difference
between the two is calculated and these differences are summed for all the patients
who are treated during the period of the evaluation. This measure provides a
comparison between different hospitals or units with similar case mixes and/or a

hospital or unit over time. However the measure does not take into account the natural history of a disease or how difficult it may be to treat and this places a limit on the value of the measure for comparing hospitals or units with very different case mixes.

This method of measuring hospital output is extended to examine not only the extent to which patients are cured but differences in the care they receive from day to day, by daily classification of disability and distress. Thus two patients who may be cured to the same extent may none the less suffer to very different degrees whilst in hospital; one may be relieved of distress early in his stay, while the other continues to experience pain until just before discharge. This difference may seem even more important where cure is not achieved; for instance, in a case of terminal care, one patient may experience a "good death" whereas another has suffered to a much greater extent. It is not too far fetched to suggest that computers may sometimes affect the speed at which suffering can be relieved; rapid transmission of results of laboratory investigations, drug interaction information and so on may speed up the whole decision making process so that a specific intervention may be made earlier during treatment. Even in the case of terminal care results of an investigation such as tissue biopsy at bronchoscopy might arrive a little earlier from the laboratory and, once the diagnosis is known to be one of malignant disease, the doctor may be more willing to prescribe effective but potentially addictive analgesics.

	Purpose	Source	Frequency	Data
1.	OUTPUT	Nurses	Daily	Disability, distress
		Clinicians	Admission	Disability, distress, prognosis
			Discharge	
			Follow-up	
2.	CHECKS FOR	Other	Once per	Patient details:
	COMPARABILITY	Sources	episode	age, sex, occupation etc.
	OF PATIENT			Episode details: length of
	MIX			stay, diagnoses, operations etc.

Figure 5. Information for each episode care profile.

The basic information to be collected for each episode is shown in figure 5 together with its source, frequency of collection and purpose. It might be thought that the reliability of the classification would be difficult to demonstrate because no two nurses or doctors can ever have the same knowledge of all their patients, observation is not continuous and the condition of patients can change rapidly. There are also difficulties in assessing a patient's distress, since some patients are stoical and others react more openly to suffering. However, we have encountered remarkably few such problems. The classification has now been tested on over 4,000 ratings of patients by some 90 doctors and nurses and reliability has been excellent. With a little practice it takes less time to classify a patient than to write down his name.

The method, which is simple and quick to use, has stimulated considerable interest amongst doctors, nurses and administrators. The daily classification of disability and distress by nurses provides a summary in the nursing record of each patient's progress during the episode to date which may be used to help nurses unfamiliar with the patient and others such as doctors, physiotherapists etc. to assess and communicate the patient's condition and progress. This potential benefit has helped to secure its acceptance. Its application could be extended to research and teaching.

SAMPLE RESULTS

We present the results in three ways:

(1)   The day by day progress of individual patients is followed through an episode of illness. We refer to this as the episode profile.

(2)   The state of a group of patients (a ward, an institution or a community) is summarised on a particular day. We refer to this as a state spectrum.

(3)   The day by day progress of groups of patients are followed for defined periods of evaluation. We refer to these as Ward or Hospital profiles.

1.   Episode Profiles

In figures 6, 7 and 8 episode profiles are shown for three patients, a surgical patient A admitted from the waiting list, an acute medical case, B and an acute orthopaedic case, C. The vertical axis represents severity of illness using the psychometrically derived scale (figure 4). These care profiles have been discussed with the doctors who treated the patients and were found to reflect accurately clinical decisions and other events during the episode of illness.

When information is available for many similar cases, typical profiles should be obtainable. Comparisons could then be made between typical profiles for the same condition treated in different wards, units or hospitals and between these "typical profiles" and "standard profiles" based perhaps on the observed average, the observed optimum or a theoretical ideal.

Patient A (figure 6):

This 30 year old female civil servant was
admitted for a cholecystectomy after 4
months on the waiting lit. She was admitted two days before the operation for
cross matching of blood and for chest
physiotherapy.   The operation took
about two hours and the next day a chest
infection was diagnosed and responded to
treatment immediately.   The slight
reduction in severity on the 8th day
after admission was a reduction in the

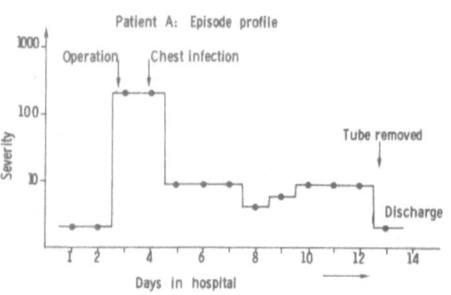

Figure 6.

patient's distress.   On the 13th day her drainage tube was removed and she was then
discharged.   When seen in outpatient follow-up clinic she appeared to have recovered
completely.

Patient B (figure 7):

This 69 year old woman living alone was
brought to hospital by ambulance suffering from an acute exacerbation of chronic
bronchitis and asthma. She was treated
with antibiotics, physiotherapy, oxygen
and prednisone (steroids) and her condition improved. On the 10th day the
dose of prednisone was doubled to 40mg
which led to further improvement.   The
prednisone was then gradually reduced
to 10mg and she was discharged on the

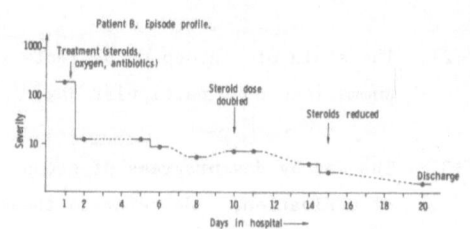

Figure 7.

20th day.   Four months later, when she was seen in out-patients, her condition was
satisfactory and the prednisone dose was further reduced to 5mg. Her residual
disability was the result of permanent lung damage due to chronic bronchitis.

Patient C (figure 8):

This 97-year old woman, who was living with
her daughter, fell and fractured the base
of the neck of her right femur and was
brought to hospital by ambulance. Later
that day the fracture was internally
fixed, the operation lasting one and half-
hours.   The patient needed a blood trans-

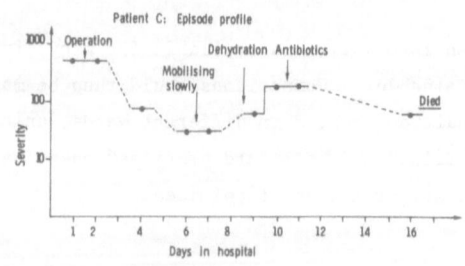

Figure 8.

fusion immediately after the operation.   Mobilisation was slow, she became dehydrated and developed infections of the urinary tract, eye and chest.   These were treated with antibiotics but she died from bronchopneumonia sixteen days after admission.

SURGICAL WARD

27 Patients   DISTRESS

		1	2	3	4	
DISABILITY	1	7	11			18
	2					-
	3		22	4		26
	4		22			22
	5		11			11
	6		11	4		15
	7			7		7
	8					
		7	77	15		

Scaled severity   :   698

Patient mean   :   25.9

MEDICAL WARD

22 Patients   DISTRESS

		1	2	3	4	
DISABILITY	1	5				5
	2	5	9			14
	3	5	9	9		23
	4		13	5		18
	5		9		5	14
	6		13	5		18
	7			5		5
	8	5				5
		20	53	24	5	

Scaled severity   :   928

Patient mean   :   42.2

Figure 9.   State Spectra.   Percentage of patients in each state.

2.   State Spectra

Figure 9 shows the states of patients on a medical ward and on a surgical ward for the same day. The mean severity on the medical ward (42.2) is higher than on the surgical ward (25.9).   On the surgical ward only 33% of patients are in disability state 5 (only able to perform a few simple tasks) and above, while on the medical ward the equivalent figure is 42% including one patient in a coma (state 8, 1). Similarly there are nearly twice as many patients in moderate or severe distress (states 3 and 4) on the medical ward (29%) as on the surgical ward (15%).

3.   Ward Profiles

A three-week ward profile for a 26-bed surgical ward is shown in figure 10. The state of the ward fluctuates considerably but this can be explained by the severity of the operations carried out and the recovery rates of patients. The profile shows a pattern which appears to be cyclical

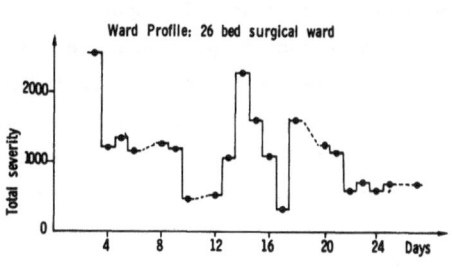

Figure 10

but the variations are not obviously predictable. With such daily changes it is
clearly difficult to allocate the appropriate number of nurses to meet the precise
needs of the ward. This particular problem does not have an obvious solution but
such profiles (with brief reports, summarising their implications) could be returned
to the wards from time to time to inform nursing officers and ward sisters. They
could be value for example in drawing attention to shifts in the nature of the nursing
care appropriate at times when distress is very prevalent in contrast with other
occasions when disability may dominate.

DISCUSSION

Evaluation of computer system requires measurements to be carried out both where the
computer is being used and where it is not. This can be arranged in three ways.
Firstly, some patients being treated in one unit can be allocated randomly to computer-assisted treatment while others are treated using traditional methods. This
approach is suitable for the evaluation of specialised applications such as computer-
assisted diagnostic aids. Secondly, a "before and after" approach may be used.
Measurements can be taken before implementing a computer system and repeated after
the system is fully operational and has settled down. This approach is suitable for
evaluation of the effect of transferring a fully developed computer system to a
previously uncomputerised institution, but in the principal experimental sites, such
as Charing Cross Hospital, the development and implementation periods have been so
protracted that this is no longer meaningful. The third approach is to compare two
similar units, one of which uses a computer system and the other of which is dependent solely on the best available manual information system. Such a comparative approach is open to the objection that the inevitable differences in case mix, organization and even personalities may obscure the differences due to the presence of a
computer in one of them.

The tools described above could be used in all three of these situations. The evaluation study in which we are currently involved falls into the third category. Because
of the problems of attributing the differences to individual causes we shall be collec-
ing data about a number of intermediate outputs and likely contributory factors. This
implies detailed knowledge of a proportion of episodes of care.

In considering the impact of computers on medical care we have devised tools for evaluation which themselves provide doctors and nurses with new information about each
patient's progress and outcome. This information may itself help to improve quality
of care and the impact of this could be greater than the effect of the computer which
we set out to detect. However if the process of evaluation were not seen to be useful
in itself then it is unlikely that we would have received cooperation and encouragement
from doctors, nurses and administrators. This additional effect may not matter if it
is the same for both sites.

Computer professionals, whose work we are evaluating, have not shown as much interest in these new tools as doctors, nurses and administrators. This may be because their attention is confined to the extent to which the computer performs its specified tasks and does not go beyond this to ask whether these tasks are the most appropriate ones to computerise nor whether the information provided is being used effectively. For example, information about patients may be reaching the doctor earlier than it would by conventional methods but he may not be making his decisions earlier because he is not thinking sufficiently quickly or perhaps because he is not on the spot to receive the information. If there were such problems at the computer-user interface, then they would have implications for planning doctors' working schedules and far-reaching consequences for medical education and practice. They could perhaps also be remedied to some extent by more elaborate software. For example, the doctor might receive, not only the results of laboratory investigations, but suggestions as to the differential diagnosis and other investigations which might be ordered. In some situations, the tests could be ordered and scheduled automatically unless the doctor specifically cancelled them.

In summary, the computer evaluator has not completed his task until he has measured, not only what information the computer can deliver accurately, quickly and relevantly, but also whether this is being put to use to the patient's benefit. The tools we have described in this paper will contribute to this process.

ACKNOWLEDGEMENT

This work is supported by a grant from the DHSS.

REFERENCES

Abrams, M (1976) "A Review of work on Subjective Social Indicators 1971-1975" SSRC Survey Unit, Occasional Papers in Survey Research No.8. London.

Berg, R.L. (editor) (1973) Health Status Indexes Hospital Research and Education Trust, Chicago.

Culyer, A.J, Lavers, R.J. and Williams Alan (1971) "Social Indicators: Health", Social Trends 2, 31-45.

Committee of Public Accounts (1976) "Sixth Report (1975/6 Session)", HMSO, London.

DHSS (1977) "Interim Report on the Evaluation of the National Health Service Experimental Computer Programme" Department of Health and Social Security, London.

Fanshel, S and Bush, J.W.(1970) "A Health Status Index and its Application to Health Services Outcome", Operations Research 18 1021-66.

Rosser, Rachel (1976) "Recent Studies Using a Global Approach to Measuring Illness" Medical Care Supplement, 14 5, 138-147.

Rosser, Rachel and Kind, Paul (1978) "A Scale of Valuations of States of Illness: Evidence for a Social Consensus" in Press.

Rosser, Rachel and Watts, V.C (1972) "The Measurement of Hospital Output", International Journal of Epidemiology, 1, 361-368.

Rosser, Rachel and Watts, V.C. (1975) "Disability: a Clinical Classification" New Law Journal, 125, 323-328.

Prest, A.R and Turvey, R (1965) "Cost Benefit Analysis - A Survey." Economic Journal 75, 683.

Torrance, G.W (1970) "A Generalised Cost-Effectiveness Model for the Evaluation of Health Programmes" Research Series: No.101, Faculty of Business McMaster University.

EVALUATION OF THE DIAPHANE DIALYSIS REGISTRY

DEGOULET, P., GOUPY, F., BLAMOUTIER, A., HIREL, J.C.
Inserm U 88, Méthodologie Informatique et Statistique
en Médecine, and
Centre Interuniversitaire de Traitement de l'Information (CITI2), 91, bd de l'hôpital, 75634 Paris

AIME, F., REACH, I., JACOBS, C., LEGRAIN, M.
Service de Néphrologie, Groupe Hospitalier
Pitié-Salpétrière, 83, bd de l'hôpital
75634 Paris

I. INTRODUCTION

Since June 1st, 1972, the medical records of several hundreds patients
treated by chronic haemodialysis have been processed by the "Diaphane Dialyse Informatique" system .on the computer of the CITI 2 (Centre Interuniversitaire de Traitement de l'Information 2) (9). In 1978, Diaphane is used by 34 dialysis centers, and
2000 patients have a record in the Data bank. After 6 years of experience, this
paper is intended to describe the present status of the system and to emphasize the
major problems encountered during those years.

II. AIMS

Diaphane has been implemented with two aims :
- first , to help in the medical management of patients thanks to   periodic reports
  on the patients' status and the functioning of each dialysis center.
- second, to build up a national data bank for epidemiological research studies.
  These studies are either defined on a nationwide basis or specific to each dialysis
  center which has the ability to access the data bank.

III. DESCRIPTION OF DIAPHANE

3.1. Data acquisition

The standard record is made up of four main questionnaires :
- an identification questionnaire (80 items) contains administrative data and the
  patient's medical history ;
- a dialysis session questionnaire (100 items) is directly filled in by the nurses
  during each dialysis session. It contains technical, clinical and biological data,
  questions about the hazards which may occur and treatments given during the session. A space is kept for medical comments that do not need to be taken into account by the computer (Fig. 1). In volume, the items contained in the session

questionnaire represent more than 90 % of the data which are stored in the data
bank.
- a quartely health status questionnaire (100 items) is completed by the physician.
It is a checklist of major problems which may have occured to the patient ;
- a termination of dialysis questionnaire is completed in   case of a transfer
to another center, kidney transplantation or death.

Specialized questionnaires corresponding to each body system (cardiovascular, pulmonar, neurological, endocrinological, ...) are available to the users
who wish to detail some particular topics (in a research environment for example).

Each questionnaire has a duplicate sheet (Fig. 1) : a copy is sent to the
computing center, the other being kept in the patient's record in the dialysis center.

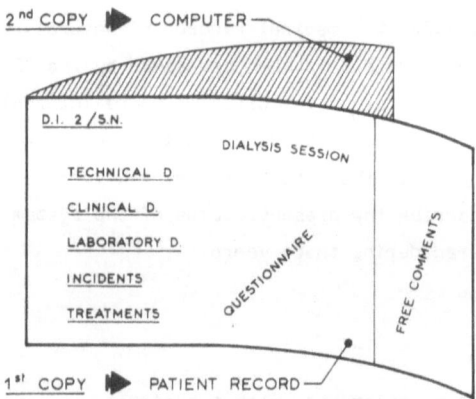

Fig. 1 : Dialysis session questionnaire

3.2. Data processing

Data are handled by "CHRONOS" system which is a set of parametrized programs
devoted to the management of evolutive medical records (9, 10). The retrieval procedure is generally carried out in three steps :
1. choice of the population
2. choice of a set of items
3. for each evolutive item, definition of the period of study and of the
function to be calculated (e.g. mean, standard deviation, maximum, ...).
Results may be edited in a fixed format in order to be processed by
statistical packages.

CHRONOS programs are written in Fortran IV or Assembler Macro X and run on
the DEC PDP 10 computer of CITI 2.

3.3. Periodic computer reports

3.3.1. Patient-record

For each patient, the dialysis center receives monthly :

- an identification (for each new patient)
- clinical and biological summaries of the dialysis sessions
- reports with the evolution month after month of the means of main clinical and biological data (weight, blood pressure, blood urea, ...)
- eventually the quartely health status report which is a cumulative report of the absence or presence of major problems in a tabular form.

3.3.2. Dialysis center record and quality control

The dialysis center record includes : monthly tables of biological averages, quartely summaries of blood transfusions and of various problems which may occur during dialysis sessions. In each case, the center receives its own means and the national mean and is able to compare its results with those achieved in other centers.

IV. EPIDEMIOLOGICAL RESEARCH STUDIES

4.1. National statistics are published each year in a monograph (6, 7). The aims of these statistics are :

- to give an epidemiological profile of chronic renal failure treated by maintenance haemodialysis,
- to provide medical authorities with statistical data concerning chronic renal disease and its treatment with the hope of defining a better health policy.

4.2. Specific research programs

In addition to the national research program, each dialysis center has access to the data bank. This access is free for its own patients : to get information involving another dialysis center necessitates a written agreement with the corresponding center. Forms help the user to define his statistical work. Results may be printed or transferred on a magnetic tape in order to be processed on a local computer.

V. DISCUSSION

5.1. Present interest of the system for patient follow-up and treatment

Several systems which have been described are oriented towards immediate help (2, 5, 14). Diaphane mainly provides intermediate and long term assistance for medical care. Intermediate assistance is provided by the different periodic summary reports. For example, the interest of the monthly center reports is twofold :

1. to enable each center to compare its results to those achieved in the other centers and to highlight the factors which may account for diffe-

rences in the treatment of patients ;

2. to point out the specific problems (e.g. a too high incident rate, a too low mean hematocrit, a bad control of acidobasis disturbances, ...).

The long term assistance is provided by the statistical analysis of the data bank. In 1978, 2000 patients have a computer record and more than 400 000 dialysis sessions performed in 34 different dialysis centers may be considered for analysis. With a six years follow-up, the data bank has to be considered by the physician as a valuable tool for epidemiological studies.

5.2. Users acceptability

Computers systems are inducing modifications in the traditional medical activity. The main risk is that costly and unused computerized systems might be added to an imperfect but functional traditional system.

5.2.1. Nurses acceptability

In most dialysis centers the computer sheets and computer printouts have totally replaced the traditional dialysis booklet which has been withdrawn. In those centers the session questionnaires, which represent the most important part of the input documents, are directly completed by nurses during the dialysis session. Therefore, nurses have a primary role in the generation of the data bank.

In order to evaluate the nurses' acceptability (4), a questionnaire was sent in mid 1976 to 71 nurses of a sample of 11 dialysis centers. Some results of this survey are shown in table III. 83 % of the nurses find questionnaires completion easy, but 39 % have difficulties with coded questions and 37 % consider questionnaires filling as a certain waste of time. Most of the nurses (66 %) consider the computer system as progress for patients' treatment. Few nurses (17 %) consider the continuation of the present system as troublesome.

5.2.2. Physicians acceptability

A similar evaluation questionnaire was filled in by 50 physicians of 29 dialysis centers at the end of 1977 (table I). Physicians have few problems with questionnaires filling. However, it must be stated that they are only concerned by the identification questionnaire and the quartely health status questionnaire which represent in volume less than 10 % of the computer record. More than 80 % regularly examine the patients reports. A majority of them find an actual influence of the computer system on patient follow-up, but not directly on patient care. About 30 % of physicians interrogate the data bank for their own research studies. This failure is not explained by a lack of information since 94 % of the concerned physicians are aware of the computer interrogation facilities.

5.3. Data reliability

Data reliability is one of the most important features of a research oriented data bank for two main reasons :

1. it conditions the precision of the data bank interrogation

2. It conditions to a great extent the users' acceptability.

In Diaphane system, the data bank content is obtained from questionnaires which are filled in by nurses and physicians. Reliability of the users' answers depends on the precision of the questions. However, whatever the precautions taken in defining the questionnaires, some questions fail to be understood and are sources of error. In January 1975 and June 1977, completely new sets of questionnaires were implemented. The reasons of this change were :

- improvement of quality of the input procedure

- evolution in the medical activity

Such modifications were facilitated by the parametrized features of "Chronos" programs (8).

Reliability depends further on the accuracy of answers. Mistakes are likely to appear at each level of data input procedure :

- errors on the patient identification

- errors or omissions in questionnaire filling (e.g. errors in biological units)

- key punched errors

Table II shows the errors and omissions in a sample of 800 session questionnaires checked in the Nephrology Department of the Pitié-Salpétrière school of Medicine. Except for questions with complicated codes, such as dialyzer codes (more than 50 different commercialized and available dialyzers), the error is largely under 1 %. Omission rate is generally under 5 %.

A particular problem may occur with the interpretation of laboratory investigations. Most of investigations, even simple or important for the patients' follow up (eye fundies, bone radiography, ...) are not systematically performed, but only when the clinical context suggests an abnormality. In this case the frequency of pathologic results is overestimated. Table IV explicits this problem by showing the cumulative actuarial rate (1) of the data base filling for simple laboratory investigations. After four weeks of follow up more than 90 % of the patients have at least one hematocrit value in the data base, but less than 50 % a cholesterol value or a measurement of nervous conduction velocity.

5.4. Computer records limits

Utilization of standardized records renders the development of multicenter studies possible. However standardization limits the interrogation depth of a data bank. In multicenter registries (3, 12, 13) such as the European and Dialysis Transplant Association (E.D.T.A.) registry or the American National Dialysis Registry, questionnaires are limited to a few number of first level data (age, sex, etiology of the nephropathy, causes of death, ...). Diaphane system tries to integrate second level data and so to participate more closely to the patient follow up and patient

care management. However the statistical analysis of results needs an extreme care-
fulness and the user has an important role in interpreting   the results. For example
if significant differences may appear between the results of a dialysis center and
those of others centers, the final explanations may only be found by the concerned
centers : variations may be due to small differences in measurement techniques,
questionnaire filling, or in the dialysis session management.

5.5. Financial evaluation

     In 1977, exploitation costs are of 13 $ /month/patient. Those costs include
key punch, data input procedure, the processing of patients' centers' reports,
national statistics, but not the specific research programs of each dialysis center.
Since 1974, exploitation costs are charged to the dialysis centers. The approximative cost/dialysis session of 1 $ represents approximately 0.5 % of the total cost
of a dialysis session.

CONCLUSION

     Diaphane is a computerized system   developped on a national basis for
patients treated by maintenance haemodialysis with a double aim : to make possible
epidemiological research, but also to directly help the physicians in the medical
management of their patients.Six years after the system implementation, the initial
aims may be considered as reached to a large extent. The data bank is used as well
as by physicians as researchers.Present objectives are :
- the decentralization of the data bank access and of the processing for research
  studies
- the extension of the present system to the overall follow up of advanced renal
  failure.

REFERENCES

1. ANDERSON, R.P., BONCHEK, L.I., GRUNKEMEIER, G.L., LAMBERT, L., STARR, A. : the
   analysis and presentation of surgical results by actuarial methods. J. Surg.
   Res. 1974, 16 : 224-230

2. ALBERTAZZI,A: Informatica ed emodialisi periodica. Min. Nefr. 20 : 334-341, 1973

3. BARNES, B.A., BERGAN, J.J., BRAUN, W.E., FRAUMENT, J.F., KOUNTZ, S.L.,
   MICKER, M.R., RUBIN, A.L., SIMMONS, R.L., STEVENS, L.E., WILSON, R.E. : the
   12th Report of the Human Renal Transplant Registry. J. Amer. Med. Ass. 1975, 33 :
   787-796

4. BOURGEOIS, P., PELEGE, J., BOUILLAGUET, D., DARONAT, M.C., ROBIN, A.M., OFFRET, C.
   Computer methods and maintenance hemodialysis : the critical role of nurses.
   Presented at 5th Annual Conference of the European Dialysis and Transplant Nurses
   Ass. 1976, june 22-25, Hamburg

5. DEGOULET, P., MARICHAL, J.F., COURNOYER, G., MELOCHE, H., LAPIERRE, L., PIETTE, Y.
   Applications de l'informatique à la surveillance des malades traités par

hémodialyse périodique. Un. Med. Canada 1976, 105 : 1217-1222

6. DEGOULET, P., PROULX, J., AIME, F., BERGER, C., BLOCH, P., GOUPY, F., LEGRAIN, M.
   Programme Dialyse-Informatique. III - Données épidémiologiques. Stratégies de
   dialyse et résultats biologiques. J. Urol. Néphrol. 1976, 82 : 1001-1042

7. DEGOULET, P., REACH, I., AIME, F., BERGER, C., GOUPY, F., JACOBS, C., ROJAS, P.,
   LEGRAIN, M. : Programme Dialyse-Informatique IV. Rapport cumulatif. Epidémiolo-
   gie des complications. J. Urol. Néphrol. 1977, 83 : 925-983

8. GOUPY, F., HIREL, J.C., BLOCH, P., BERGER, C., : CHRONOS : a data bank for physicians and researchers. Comp. Prog. Biomed. 1976, 6 : 149-165

9. GOUPY, F., HIREL, J.C., DEGOULET, P., LEGRAIN, M. : Diaphane, une banque de
   donnéees sur l'hémodialyse itérative. Bilan de deux ans d'une étude coopérative
   réalisée à l'échelon national. Journées d'Informatique Médicale. Toulouse 1975.
   Institut de Recherche d'Informatique et d'Automatique. Le Chesnay 1975, tome 1,
   pp. 291-298

10. GOUPY, F., DEGOULET, P., BERGER, C., HIREL, J.C., PLOUIN, P.F., MENARD, J. :
    Artemis : follow up of hypertensive patients. In MEDINFO 77, ed. by D.B. Shires
    and H. Wolf, North Holland Pub. C°, Amsterdam, 1 vol., 529-532, 1977

11. GREMY, F., DEGOULET, P. : Some aspects of information handling in medicine. In
    Physical Techniques in Medicine. J.T. Mc Mullan Ed., John Wiley and Sons, New
    York,vol 1, 1977, pp. 1-50

12. JACOBS, C., BRUNNER, F.P., CHANTLER, C., DONCKERWOLCKE, R.A., GURLAND, H.J.,
    HATHWAY, R.A., SELWOOD, N.H., WING, A.J., : Combined report on regular dialysis
    and transplantation in Europe VII, 1976. Proc. Europ. Dial. Transpl. Ass.
    Pitman Medical, Bath, 1977, 14 : 3-70

13. KRUEGER, K.K. : Report on the National Dialysis Registry. Proc. 7th Annual
    Contractors' Conference, 1974 : 197-206

14. SABATIER, J., RORIVE, G. : Evaluation of an interactive computer medical and
    management system for hemodialysis. In MEDINFO 77, D.B. Shires and H. Wolf eds.
    North Holland Pub. C° , Amsterdam, 1977, pp. 963-966

SUMMARY

        The Diaphane system is a data bank devoted to patients treated by mainte-
nance haemodialysis. The system is operational since June 1972 and computer records
are now currently used by 34 dialysis centers throughout France.

        Diaphane was designed to facilitate the medical management of chronic dia-
lysis patients thanks to periodic reports about the patients' clinical status and
the management of dialysis centers. It also enables epidemiological research
studies on a nationwide basis. The main problems raised by the implementation of
Diaphane are emphasized and an evaluation of the system acceptability and the data
reliability is given.

Table I

Physician acceptability
(1977, 50 physicians, 29 dialysis centers)

	YES	$\frac{+}{-}$	NO	Response rate
Questionnaire filling is easy ?	81 %	19 %	0 %	86 %
Do you have difficulties with coded questions ?	28 %	17 %	55 %	92 %
Does the computer represent an extra work load ?	36 %	4 %	60 %	90 %
Do you follow computer feed back editions ?				
. patients' reports	81 %	13 %	6 %	96 %
. dialysis center reports	69 %	17 %	15 %	96 %
Are you interested in national statistics ?	80 %	12 %	8 %	98 %
Have you already questioned the data bank for your own research studies ?	33 %		67 %	96 %
Do you know that the data bank is available for your own research studies ?	94 %		6 %	100 %
Present influence of the computer system for patients' follow up ?	43 %	24 %	33 %	98 %
Present influence of the computer system for the patients' treatment ?	35 %	24 %	41 %	98 %
Is the computer system a progress for patient follow-up and treatment ?	76 %	20 %	4 %	100 %
Any suggestion to improve the system ?	58 %		42 %	80 %

	Number of checked questions	Errors rate/question	Omissions rate/question
Questions with complicated codes (dialyzer, blood vessel access)	5	2.60 %	0.43 %
Clinical and biological data	20	0.18 %	1.63 %
Incidents	1	0.13 %	5.38 %
Treatment	3	0.13 %	4.00 %

Table II

Filling errors and omissions (rate/question in 800 session-questionnaires)
(Nephrology Department, Pitié-Salpétrière Hospital)

Table III

Nurses acceptability
(1976 - 71 nurses, 11 dialysis centers)

	YES	NO	I do not know	Response rate
Is the questionnaire filling easy ?	83 %	17 %	-	97 %
Do you have difficulties with coded questions ?	39 %	61 %	-	97 %
Does the computer system represent an extra work load ?	37 %	46 %	17 %	100 %
Do you examine computer reports ?	67 %	33 %	-	68 %
Is the computer system a progress for patients' treatment ?	66 %	17 %	17 %	97 %
Present influence of computer work for patients' follow-up and improvement of treatment ?	51 %	33 %	16 %	97 %
Is continuation of the present system troublesome ?	17 %	75 %	8 %	99 %
Any suggestion to improve the system ?	52 %	48 %	-	84 %

	4 weeks	3 months	6 months	1 year
Hematocrit	96.6 ± 1.1	99.3 ± 0.6	-	-
Blood urea	92.7 ± 1.5	97.2 ± 1.1	-	-
Uric acid	53.5 ± 2.9	78.4 ± 2.8	85.9 ± 2.5	-
Hb_s antigen	51.7 ± 2.9	80.8 ± 2.5	85.8 ± 2.2	-
Cholesterol	44.5 ± 2.8	61.4 ± 2.9	69.2 ± 2.9	74.6 ± 2.9
Nerve conduction velocity	32.4 ± 2.6	49.6 ± 3.0	65.2 ± 3.2	76.8 ± 3.5
Bone radiography	40.5 ± 2.8	52.2 ± 3.0	62.1 ± 3.1	80.8 ± 3.5

Table IV

Data base filling
(Cumulative actuarial response rate, 1975-1976, 330 patients)
Actuarial rate ± standard error, Greenwood's method (1)

THE RELATIONSHIP BETWEEN

NURSING AND MEDICAL INFORMATICS

by

Kathryn J. Hannah, R.N., M.S.N.
Assistant Professor
The University of Calgary
Calgary, Alberta, CANADA

1. INTRODUCTION

Before attempting to identify the existance of a relationship between these two
disciplines, it is necessary to first establish operational definitions regarding
the nature of nursing and of medical informatics. While the art of nursing in
the sense of "attempting to cure by care and treatment"[1] is as old as man, the
profession of nursing is an emerging, professional, practice discipline. Nursing,
as perceived by its practitioners, has as its goals:

(1) the promotion of man's adaptation in health and illness[2]

(2) the facilitation of man's achievement of his highest
     possible individual state of health.[3]

Among the roles which the practitioner of nursing assumes are that of interface
between the client and the health care system and that of client advocate. The
functions of present-day nursing can be divided into three major categories:

(1) Managerial, which includes establishing nursing care plans,
     keeping charts, transcribing orders and requisitions and
     time scheduling.

(2) Medically orientated tasks, which include physical treatments
     and administration of medications under the direction of a
     physician.

(3) Hands-on therapy, which includes the use of interpersonal
     communications skills, application of the psychological
     principles of client care and the provision of physical care
     to clients based on the initiative and judgement of the
     professional nurse.

The term Medical Informatics first became acceptable and legitimate in 1975 when
it was used to describe "those collected informational technologies which concern
themselves with the patient-care, medical, decision-making process."[4] Another
definition was proposed in the first issue of the Journal of Medical Informatics
which stated that the term represents "the complex processing of data by a
computer to produce new kinds of information."[5] The first definition seems to
be preferable in that it is more precise, however, the question arises, does the
word *medical* refer only to physicians or does it refer to all of the health care
professions? The premise in this paper is that the word medical in the definition
refers to all health care professions and that a parallel definition of Medical
Informatics might be *those collected informational technologies which concern*

*themselves with the patient-care, decision-making process performed by health
care practitioners.* Thus, since nurses are health care practitioners and are
involved in the patient-care, decision-making process which by our definition
utilizes information technologies, there is a relationship between nursing and
medical informatics. The purpose of this paper is to demonstrate this relationship.

2. <u>CONTRIBUTIONS OF MEDICAL INFORMATICS TO NURSING PRACTICE</u>

The literature clearly demonstrates the contributions of Medical Informatics to
the practice of Nursing and to client care. In this aspect of the relationship
nurses are the *consumers* of developments in Medical Informatics.

2.1 <u>Automated Charting of Nurse's Notes</u>

Good nurse's notes are usually lengthy, narrative, handwritten, unbiased observations. At worst, they are inaccurate, inconsistent, incomplete or consist of such
trivia as, "Had a good day." Automated methods for recording of nursing observations have been developed by information specialists and are now commercially
available from computer vendors. The researchers who developed these approaches
to the automated method of recording nursing observations claim numerous advantages
for client care.[6, 7, 8, 9, 10] Better observations, that is, increased number,
accuracy and reliability of observations, facilitates better assessment, planning
and evaluating of nursing care. Less time spent writing the notes provides more
time for assessment, planning, implementing and evaluating care, that is, for the
nursing process. Increased use and accuracy of interpretation of the notes
facilitates consistency and continuity of the plan for nursing care. Statistical
analysis facilitates research which would ultimately lead to refinements in the
nursing process and to improvement in patient care.

2.2 <u>Automating Nursing Care Plans</u>

In most health care settings the Kardex or some similar tool has been the repository
of nursing care plans. These have had drawbacks similar to those encountered with
nursing notes and other drawbacks that are unique to the Kardex alone. The nursing
care plans, if indeed they ever get entered in the Kardex at all, are usually
outdated, illegible, inconsistent, and incomplete. Notations are made by all
levels of nursing personnel from aides to head nurses. Written patient care
assignments are usually accompanied by verbal explanations which are often
forgotten during a tour of duty.

The advantages of automated approaches for development of nursing care plans[11, 12, 13]
can be related to nursing practice. Time saved in the preparation and communication
of care plans means more time available for assessment, planning, implementing and
evaluating care; that is, more time for the nursing process. Increased account-

ability for care improves nursing practice because documentation is available to evaluate quality of care and thus quality of practice. The benefits to patient-care of decreased errors and omissions and increased consistency of care include more rapid diagnosis, more valid assessment, and more rapid recovery, all of which reduce the cost of health care for the patient and open the system to more patients. Placing the responsibility for nursing judgements clearly on the shoulders of the professional nurse assists in defining nursing practice and helps the profession in its search for a clearly delineated identity.

2.3 Automated Patient Monitoring

The major area of development of automated patient monitoring has been coronary care. In coronary care units and pacemaker clinics, computers are used to monitor electrocardiograms, analyze the information and reduce the volumes of data formerly produced to manageable proportions (generally some type of graph). The computers have also been programmed to recognize deviations from accepted norms and to alert attending personnel to the deviation by some indication, for example, an alarm or light.[14, 15, 16] Also, commercially available are automated systems which perform functions involved in monitoring the irradiation of patients with malignancies. These automated approaches to monitoring free the nurse from the technician role of watching machinery and permit her to focus her attention on the patient (including both his physiological and psychosocial needs) and on the nursing process.

2.4 Interdepartmental Scheduling and Communication (Hospital Information Systems - H.I.S.)

Health care institutions today generate massive volumes of information which must be collected, transmitted, recorded, retrieved and analyzed. The problem of managing all of these activities for clinical information has become monumental. As a result, medical informatics has contributed by the development designing and vendors are now marketing computer-based hospital information systems (H.I.S.).[17, 18, 19, 20] The purpose of H.I.S. is to provide a computer-based framework to facilitate the communication of information within a health care setting. Essentially, a H.I.S. is a communications network linking terminals and output devices in key patient care or service areas to a central processing unit which coordinates all essential patient care activities. Thus, H.I.S. provides a communications system between departments (for example, dietary, nursing units, pharmacy, laboratory, etc.); a central information system for receipt, sorting, transmission, storage and retrieval of information; and, a high speed data processing system for fast and economic processing of data to provide information in its most useful form.[21]

The advantages[18, 19, 20] of an H.I.S. in relation to nursing practice are much the same as the previously identified advantages of automation. Time saved from manual information processing tasks provides more time for the nursing process. More complete patient records and greater accuracy and speed of information transfer facilitate the nursing assessment. More effective use of personnel and continuity of care result in better quality of patient care.

2.5 Automated Personnel Time Assignment

Each day, innumerable head nurses and supervisors spend countless hours "doing the time." Manual scheduling of personnel work rotations cannot eliminate the possibility of bias in assigning days off or shift rotation, the difficulty in establishing minimum staffing to avoid wasting manpower, or the dependence on the memory of individuals within the nursing administrative structure.[22] In an effort to alleviate these problems researchers in medical informatics have automated the scheduling of personnel work assignment.[22, 23, 24] In order to accomplish this automation, patient care needs are first quantified to assess staffing needs, personnel policies are clearly delineated and a computer program is designed for scheduling of staff within the foregoing constraints. When the program is run the result is a printed staff time schedule. The documented advantages of automated scheduling of personnel include:

(1) Easier recruitment and increased job satisfaction of the staff because schedules are known well in advance.

(2) Less time spent on manual scheduling thus providing more time for the nursing process.

(3) Advance notice of staff shortages requiring temporary replacements.

(4) Unbiased assignment of days off and shift rotation.

(5) Work station printouts available for staff inspection and for ward assignment worklists.

(6) More effective utilization and distribution of personnel.

(7) Documentation of the effect of staff size on care quality arms the nurse with data to justify requests for staff increases.[21, 22, 23]

2.6 Gathering of Epidemiological and Administrative Statistics

Batch-oriented retrieval modules have been designed and are being refined to retrieve statistical information for administrative and epidemiological purposes. Such outputs as number of patients treated, classification of diseases that patients are presenting with, or number and type of nosocomial infections developed by patients can be retrieved almost immediately. The emphasis in these reports is on graphic displays (histograms, time-series charts, map plots, etc.).[25, 26, 27]

The advantages for nurses of this contribution by medical informatics lie mainly in the speed with which such data can be retrieved, compiled, summarized, and presented in a meaningful and comprehensible form. The relationship of these advantages to the practice of nursing is found primarily in the availability of data for research purposes -- research being the means by and through which the profession of nursing will continue to develop, expand and define its practice.

3. CONTRIBUTIONS OF NURSING TO MEDICAL INFORMATICS

What is it that the discipline of nursing has to contribute to the development of those collected informational technologies which, by its definition, are the essence of the discipline known as Medical Informatics? Nurses can and should contribute in the areas of research, education, and practice. In the area of research nurses with doctoral preparation have participated in developmental projects, for example, as consultants to companies developing computer systems for use in health care agencies and as project directors of government funded investigations studying the effects of the implementation of such systems on health care delivery and nursing practice.[28] In the area of health care delivery, nurses have traditionally provided the interface between the client and the health care system. Thus, in the discipline of Medical Informatics, nurses with Masters or Baccalaureate preparation can and should participate in deisgn selection of the systems to be implemented. For example, they serve as the interface between the client and the automated health care system; they should also articulate for the computer program designers and systems engineers the needs of health care professionals and of clients relative to automated systems. In the area of education, nurses with appropriate preparation should be teaching and interpreting the jargon and basic tenets of modern nursing for the information specialists. They should also be preparing (through both basic and on-going education programs) their professional colleagues for the inevitable widespread implementation of automated information systems. Nursing contributions to medical informatics are imperative in two specific areas; systems design and moral-ethical issues.

3.1 Systems Design, Architecture and Programming

It must be remembered that computers are merely machines whose capabilities are limited by the knowledge and imagination of their creators and of the authors of their programs. Thus, in order for information systems to best assist in the process of patient-care, decision-making by nurses, medical informatics must receive and respond to input from nursing regarding the development of information systems which produce the types of information needed by nurses in their practice. Information specialists and nurses must establish a dialogue which results in each understanding the needs and constraints under which the other functions.

The more complex the system, the higher the cost of change, and therefore the more rigid and inflexible the system.[29] Thus, caution in the designing and the implementation of any information system is essential; future nursing needs must be anticipated and provision made for flexibility in the design of programs and in the information system selected for use. Again, a general understanding is needed between nurses and information specialists as to the functions and limitations of computers and the dynamic nature of nursing in order to select flexible hardware and design satisfactory computer programs to meet the changing needs of nursing and of client care.

3.2 Moral-Ethical Issues

Among professionals and lay people alike, there is a growing concern about possible moral abuses such as breach of confidentiality, individual right to privacy, and professional ethics related to the introduction of computerized processing of information about individuals. The concern stems from the belief that personal information should be more accessible to the public at large, but that this might also make information available to those who would make improper use of it and that individuals would suffer where information was used to their detriment. These apprehensions are not without substance and nurses, as patient advocates, should clearly articulate these concerns to information specialists:

> "we, as health professionals, should support all laudable
> attempts at legislation that prevent the storage and
> misuse of incorrect personal data and provide legitimate
> access to files. However, we should ensure that such
> legislation does not carry with it the potential danger
> of overburdening the practitioners of health care, of
> diminishing the value of clinical service, of exposing
> us to new legal risks and on the bottom line, of
> increasing the suffering of our patients."[30]

4. SUMMARY

Research has demonstrated clearly that medical informatics provides numerous advantages for nursing practice and many improvements in nursing process. The use of computers frees the nurse from tedious clerical chores and provides more time for the nursing process, that is, for the assessment, planning, implementing and evaluation of patient care. Computers facilitate nursing research. Computers assist in reducing errors and omissions and promote consistency and continuity of patient care. The use of computers in nursing places responsibility for nursing judgements with the professional nurse. This assists in defining nursing practice and helps the profession in its search for a clearly delineated identity. Thus, the research has clearly demonstrated the advantages of medical informatics for nurses.

Nursing's contributions can and will influence the evolution of medical informatics. The contributions of nurses hinge on the anticipation of the expansion and develop- ment of medical informatics, and the provision of leadership and direction to ensure that medial informatics evolves to benefit the client, that is, to improve the quality of health care provided.

Thus, the relationship between nursing and medical informatics has its conception in the common goal of better health care for the client. But the relationship will only grow if nursing provides input to developments in medical informatics as well as receiving output by being consumers of the developments of medical informatics.

REFERENCES

1. Webster's Seventh New Collegiate Dictionary, edited by G. and C. Merriam Company, Springfield, Mass., Thomas Allen and Son Ltd., Toronto, Ontario, 1969.
2. Roy, Sister Callista. Introduction to Nursing: An Adaptation Model. Prentice-Hall, Inc., Englewood Cliffs, New Jersey, 1976.
3. Rogers, Martha E. An Introduction to the Theoretical Base of Nursing Practice. F. A. Davis, Philadelphia, 1970.
4. Greenburg, A. G. "Medical Informatics: Science or Science Fiction," unpublished manuscript, November 1976.
5. _____. "Editorial," Journal of Medical Informatics, Volume 1, No. 1, April 1976.
6. Rosenberg, Mervin and Carriker, Delores. "Automating Nurses' Notes," American Journal of Nursing, Volume 66, May 1966.
7. Stein, R. F. "An Exploratory Study in the Development and Use of Automated Nursing Reports," Nursing Research, Volume 18, January-February 1969.
8. Olsson, D. E. "Automating Nurses' Notes - First Step in a Computerized Record System," Hospitals, Volume 41, June 16, 1967.
9. Rosenberg, Mervin and others. "Comparison of Automated Nursing Notes as Recorded by Psychiatrists and Nursing Service Personnel," Nursing Research, Volume 18, July-August 1969.
10. Knight, J. E. and Streeter, Jacqueline. "The Computer as an Aid to Nursing Records," Nursing Times, Volume 66, February 19, 1970.
11. Speed, E. L. and Young, N. A. "SCAN-data Processed Printouts of a Patient's Basic Care Needs," American Journal of Nursing, Volume 69, January 1969.
12. Somers, J. B. "A Computerized Nursing Care System," Hospitals, Volume 45, April 1971.
13. Cornell, S. A. and Garrick, A. G. "Computerized Schedules and Care Plans," Nursing Outlook, Volume 21, December 1973.
14. Wolff, G. A. "Computer Watches Heartbeat While Nurse Watches Patient," Modern Hospital, Volume 117, August 1971.
15. Shilling, Esther. "Pacemaker Evaluation Clinic," American Journal of Nursing, Volume 73, October 1973.
16. Tolbert, S. H. and Pertuz, A. E. "Study Shows How Computerization Affects Nursing Activities in ICU," Hospitals, Volume 51, September 1977.
17. Kelsay, R. C. "Computerized H.I.S.: A Control Mechanism," Hospital Progress, Volume 51, April 1970.
18. Cook, Margo and McDowell, Wanda. "Changing to an Automated Information System," American Journal of Nursing, Volume 75, January 1975.
19. Bartel, G. J. and Fahey, J. J. "Nursing Station is Home Base for Phone-printer System," Modern Hospital, Volume 113, November 1969.
20. O'Kane, K. C. and Kelly, V. M. "A Review of Medical Information Processing Systems," Journal of Clinical Computing, Volume 4, May 1975.
21. Kelsay, op. cit.
22. Murray, D. J. "Computer Makes the Schedules for Nurses," Modern Hospital, Volume 117, December 1971.
23. Morrish, A. R. and O'Connor, A. R. "Cyclic Scheduling," Journal of Nursing Administration, Volume 1, September-October 1971.

24. Jelinek, R. C. and others. "Tell the Computer How Sick the Patients Are and it Will Tell How Many Nurses They Need," Modern Hospital, Volume 121, December 1973.
25. Gentles, W. "Sunnybrook's New Acute Stroke Unit (a Biomedical Engineering Viewpoint)," Hospital Administration Canada, Volume 17, May 1975.
26. Hosking, D. J. "The Computer Assisted School Health Program (CASH): A Field Unit's Viewpoint," Canadian Journal of Public Health, Volume 64, November-December 1973.
27. Tolbert and Pertuz, op. cit.
28. Farlee, Coralie. "The Computer as a Focus of Organizational Change in the Hospital," Journal of Nursing Administration, February 1978.
29. Singer, J. P. "Hospital Computer Systems: Myths and Realities," Hospital Topics, Volume 49, January 1971.
30. Shires, D. B. and Dunean, G. "Freedom of Information Legislation and Medical Records," Canadian Medical Association Journal, Volume 118, February 1978.
31. Given, C. W. and Given, B. "Automation and Technology: A Key to Professionalized Care," Nursing Forum, Volume 8, No. 1, 1969.

NURSING INTERVENTION SCORING SYSTEM:
A CONCEPT FOR MANAGEMENT, RESEARCH, AND COMMUNICATION

A. G. Greenburg, M.D., Ph.D.; Douglas K. McClure, B.A., M.S.; Cheryl A. Janus, R.N.; and Judith A. Stubbs, R.N. Depts. of Surgery, Veterans Administration Hospital and the University of California, San Diego, CA (92161)

Surgical intensive care units are particularly complex systems whose functional objective is the provision of high level care for seriously ill patients. Beneficial system effects and functional improvement can be achieved through effective resource distribution, especially nursing allocation. For the past few years we have been particularly interested in the Surgical Intensive Care Unit (SICU) as a system (1, 2, 3, 4, 5, 6) and have pursued a variety of techniques to evaluate and improve its function.

In the design stage of a major digital simulator of the SICU (7, 8) the "system function index" created to acquire data regarding type and distribution of nursing interactions by patient state of health appeared to have more generally applicable characteristics, particularly for management and communication. We have recently expanded that concept and transformed it to a working adjunct within the unit. This paper describes the concept, its application, and the preliminary results obtained from the initial implementation with reference to its use as a management, research, and communication adjunct within an active SICU.

The Concept:

Our Nursing Intervention Scoring System (NISS) is an extension and rational expansion of the TISS concept previously presented by Cullen and co-workers (9, 10). We believe NISS provides a more accurate and complete description of nursing tasks well beyond those related to therapeutics. Close examination of the various TISS factors reveals that not all items are nursing intervention or even SICU tasks! Some items are patently patient related (e.g., cardiac arrest) and usually generate a great deal more intervention than is reflected in a set number of points. Although critical of the structure functional organization and components of TISS, we applaud its concept and impact. Significant basic information relating cost and morbidity as well as unit function has been gleaned and made useful at a practical level.

In the detailed analysis necessary for construction of complex digital simulation models we realized the system function index was the basis for a more accurate metric of nurse utilization. As an index it was more descriptive of how the nurse's time was distributed or utilized than TISS.

Generation of the Nursing Intervention Scoring System (NISS) followed the multidisciplinary analysis of SICU function. Identified individual tasks, 108, were rearranged into 12 categories based on functional or physiologic system requirements. To these we added two categories of tasks for which SICU nursing personnel were not directly involved with patient care related functions and a single category of description in terms of perceived fatigue.

With the nursing personnel of the unit serving as "experts", rearrangment of the task lists into workable and functional categories was readily accomplished using the principles of the Delphi Method (11). This resulted in 90% of the tasks being consistently grouped by all personnel. The remaining 10% of tasks were distributed after further "executive" consultation. Thus we arrived at 15 categories of tasks which were greater than 95% effective at describing nursing utilization within the SICU. Some items of previous lists were deleted because they were not directly patient related or could be handled by paraprofessional personnel such as the ward clerk who is present 12-16 hours per day and to whom all telephone communication is directed. The final categories are shown in Table 1.

Table 1. NISS Task Categories and Number of Tasks Per Category

Monitoring	13	
IV Lines	5	
Medication	14	
Fluid Intake	6	
Blood Therapy	4	
Fluid Output	11	
Metabolic Management	10	
Respiratory Management	13	
GI Tract Management	4	
Wound, Skin Care	3	
Miscellaneous Therapy	10	
Miscellaneous Task	15	108
Patient Events	4*	
Non-ICU Services	3*	
Nursing Factors	2*	9
		117 Total

*Not "scorable" items--no points assigned

The component items for each category are shown in Tables 2 through 13, along with the number of "points" per task. In Table 14 we have the three non-point categories candidated.

"Points" are assigned to tasks based on amount of nurse time required for task completion. Obviously tasks are not "pure"; most are multi-component having at least an associated clerical task or requiring two or more steps to complete. Based on the data acquired in the preliminary studies used for definition of the simulation model, each "point" represents between five and eight and one-half minutes of nursing personnel time. Statistically the mean is 6.75 ± .5 minutes.

Table 2. Monitoring Tasks

Task	Number of Points	Task	Number of Points
ECG, Rate	1	Neuro Vital Signs	3
Vital Signs, Q1H	1	Measurement of Cardiac Output	4*
Vital Signs, Q30M	3	Left Atrial Pressure	3
Vital Signs, Q15M	4	Intra-Cranial Pressure	4
Peripheral Arterial Line, B.P.	1	Peripheral Pulses - Doppler	3
C.V.P.	2	ECG, Rhythm	2
Pulmonary Arterial Line, Pressures	3		

*Dye dilution; 2 if thermal

Table 3. Intra-Vascular Lines

Task	Number of Points	Task	Number of Points
3 or more	2	Continuous Arterial Infusion	4
2	2	IV: Keep Open	1
1	1		

Table 4. Medication Related Tasks

Task	Number of Points	Task	Number of Points
Intermittent: 3+ Antibiotics	2	Cardiac Rhythm/Tone Infusion	4
Intermittent: 1,2 Antibiotics	1	Non-Cardiac Infusion	2
Intermittent: Narcotics	1	Bolus IV Meds (2+ per 24 hrs.)	3
Intermittent: Cardiotonic	2	IV Meds (1,2 per 24 hrs.)	1
One-time IV Meds: 3+ per 24 hrs.	2	Intra-Muscular Meds	1
Anti-Metabolite Rx	1	P.O. Meds	1
Acute Digitalization	3	Epidural Catheter	3

Using hospital parenteral preparation facilities and "unit dosing".

Table 5. Fluid Intake

Task	Number of Points	Task	Number of Points
Hyperal/Renal Failure Fluid	3	Tube Feeding: Gastro, Jejunostomy	2
Replacement (6+ Liters per day)	2	Potassium Repl/Suppl (IV, hourly)	3
Tube Feeding: N/G or Ped-Feed	2	Diabetic Mgmt (Fract. + Insulin)	4

Table 6. Blood Therapy

Task	Number of Points	Task	Number of Points
Platelet Transfusions	3	Acute Anti-Coagulation	3
Freq. Infusion of Blood Products	3	Chronic Anti-Coagulation	1

Table 7. Fluid Output

Task	Number of Points	Task	Number of Points
N/G Tube	1	Drainage (1,2 Chaffin-Pratt)	1
Urinary Catheter	1	Hemovac (1 or 2)	1
Pleurovac (2+) + Blood Balance	4	Colostomy - Fresh (5-days)	3
Pleurovac (1) + Blood Balance	3	Colostomy - Old	2
Chest Tubes (72- Hrs, Draining)	3	Abdominal Irrigation (Drip/Suck)	3
Drainage (3+ Chaffin-Pratt)	2		

Table 8. Metabolic Management

Task	Number of Points	Task	Number of Points
Standard I&O (Q4 hrs)	1	Standard Chems (2 per 24 hrs.)	2
Complex Metabolic Balance, I&O	3	ABGS (1,2 per day) No Art. Lines	2
Active Diuresis	3	Serial Potassium Chems (3+/Day)	1
Mult. ABGS (4+ per 24 hrs.)	3	Frequent Stat Chems	3
Mult. Stat Labs (4+ per 24 hrs.)	3	Rx: Metabolic Acidosis/Alkalosis	1

Table 9. Respiratory Management

Task	Number of Points	Task	Number of Points
Controlled Ventilation with Peep	4	Icentive Spirometry/Blow Bottles	1
Controlled Ventilation, No Peep	3	Trans-Tracheal Catheter	2
Muscle Relaxants	4	E-T Suctioning (Nonintubated Pt)	4
Assisted Respiration with IMU	4	Tracheostomy Care (48+ Hrs)	2
Assisted Respiration, No IMU	3	Tracheostomy Care (48- Hrs)	3
Respirator Weaning	4	Tracheostomy Weaning	4
O_2 Supplement (Nasal/Mask)	1		

Table 10. G.I. Tract Management

Task	Number of Points	Task	Number of Points
P.O. Antacids	1	Lavage of Acute G.I. Bleeding	3
Maintenance of Intra-Gastric pH	3	Enemas (Neomycin, K-Exalate)	3

Table 11. Wound, Skin Care

Task	Number of Points
Dressing Changes (3+ per day)	3
Dressing Changes (2+ per day)	2
Decubitus Rx	1

Table 12. Miscellaneous Therapy

Task	Number of Points
Induced Hypothermia (Blanket)	2
Atrial or Ventricular Pacing	4
Circle Bed/Stryker Frame	2
Complicated Orthopedic Traction	1
Peritoneal Dialysis	4
G-Suit	4
Thora-, Para-, Pericardio-Centesis	3
Balloon Tamponade of Varices	4
Phlebotomy	3
Intra-Aortic Assist Balloon	4

Table 13. Miscellaneous Tasks

Task	Number of Points	Task	Number of Points
Transport Patient to Ward	2	Set-Up 2+ Transducers	3
Transport Patient to Radiology	3	Set-Up 1 Transducer	2
Accompany Patient to O.R.	2	Change Bedding	1
Give/Receive Reports	3	Feed Patient	1
Nursing Discharge Note	4	Zero Bed Scale	1
Nursing Notes (2+ per shift)	3	Ambulate Patient	4
Nursing Notes (1 per shift)	2	Sit Patient Up in Chair	3
Set-Up Swan-Ganz	4		

Table 14. Non-Scorable Tasks/Factors

Patient Events:
  Cardiac Arrest or Counter Shock
  Emergency Operation (Last 24 hrs.)
  Delirium Tremens
  Encephalopathy
Non-ICU Services:
  Hemodialysis
  Chest PT, IPPB, Inhalation Rx
  Endoscopy
Nursing Factors:
  Perceived RN Emotional Factor
  Perceived RN Fatigue Factor

Implementation

An interactive data acquisition subsystem enabling us to collect a description of the tasks performed by personnel to patients was implemented on our existing computerized patient monitoring system. Each category is displayed as a "frame", and using numeric keyboard coded entry, applicable items are entered and stored for later use. Reports are generated at the completion of data entry either as descriptive outline format notes or as an NISS report summarizing the number of points for each task for the patient in question. Each form of output has a different application, the former for communication, the latter for management.

In practice, the NISS communication format has been implemented on a once-a-day basis in the morning for use at the regular 16:00 and 24:00 shift changes. The unit director and charge nurse daily review each patient's order set and enter the data interactively via the video display and keyboard. The report is then generated for hard copy and data collection and is scheduled for routine 'output' on the printer at 15:30 and 23:30 for use by on-coming personnel.

Every patient admitted to our SICU between 1 May 1977 and 1 February 1978 (nine months) has had at least one NISS compilation per day while resident in the SICU. In this period we admitted 317 patients with an average stay of 3.6 days and 17%, 60 patients stayed 5 days or longer. In addition to the NISS evaluation we also employ a "state of health" assessment index derived from a multisystem complex of physiologic and pathologic descriptions. Each patient admitted to the SICU has this assessment upon admission and just prior to discharge. Daily and dynamic assessment awaits refinement of our monitoring system to incorporate trend detection algorithms.

Results

A sample of 100 NISS scores for 38 patients, all resident in the SICU for less than four days, was evaluated. Scaled to represent an integer on a 1 to 10 scale, state of health index was significantly and positively correlated to initial admission state of health ($r=0.81$). The correlation was not as good between discharge NISS score and discharge state of health index ($r=0.61$). Patients discharged with scores above 30 returned with greater frequency; that is, they required readmission to the SICU with greater frequency than patients with scores below 30 (12:1). Thus it would appear that the NISS score is useable in planning discharges and could be utilized directly in that effort.

The NISS score decreases between 5 and 10 points per day for routine major postoperative patients. A "fresh" postoperative cardiac surgical case usually has a NISS score around 52-55 points on admission. Without complications this is 43-48 by day 1 and 35-39 by day 2. Discharge by day 4 is reasonable. A major vascular case, aorto-femoral bypass or aneurysmectomy, usually has an entrance score of 42-48 NISS points and similarly decreases daily. Complex emergency situations (e.g., pancreatectomy for hemorrhagic pancreatitis) may score as high as 65-68 NISS points and the daily decrease is only 4-5 points per day. Thus NISS appears a mechanism for potentially predicting load and discharge which could be utilized to fine-tune SICU function and regulate its input vis-a-vis control of elective surgical procedures.

Different patient groups seem to require attention in various categories. Emergency admissions and septic problems demonstrate high utilization of Intake/ Output and metabolic management segments while cardiac and vascular surgical patients generally utilize monitoring and respiratory segments with greater frequency. Indeed, for the first twenty-four hours of the latter patient population fully 30-35% of care required is in only three categories.

It is critical to note that patients with NISS scores near 60 represent a significant personnel drain on the SICU staff, especially if the census is full and the general PT:RN ratio of 2:1 is preserved. Simple calculation of minutes involved in the care of a patient with 60 NISS points indicates that at least 400 of the 480 available minutes are accounted for which leaves little room for unexpected events. Operating at 83% utilization, not counting time for lunch or break, leaves a small margin of safety and if maintained for long periods of time, results in fatigue (physical and psychological) and job dissatisfaction.

Use of the NISS report for inter-shift communication has been a significant advantage. The on-coming or "receiving" nurse receives a complete statement of each of her patient's care requirements. The systematic format is used to note specifics (e.g., which drugs, what infusion rate). The NISS report serves as a prompter to promote a more complete, accurate, and efficient transfer of necessary information. More importantly, because it is perceived as useful and useable, it is being used with regularity.

Discussion

The NISS concept appears to be a useful adjunct for management, research, and communication. By definition of "nurse utilization" in a standardized reference framework, shift-to-shift or day-to-day changes in nurse allocation can be achieved. This dynamic allocation ability would be of particular importance in units that have significant day-to-day census and type of patient variation. Intensive care units rely heavily upon the nursing staff for their functional capabilities and it is essential to have available methods that can allow appropriate and efficient allocation of this critical resource.

When correlated to state of health the NISS metric in some ways reflects "system utilization" and thus serves as a measure of cost-benefit. NISS clearly reflects nurse utilization but also intrinsically indicates which "support services" are utilized and to what extent. A search of the data base of collected NISS entries sorted by state of health, primary operation, major disease process, or whatever other/or combination of retrieval criteria is desired, will yield to the manager/planner necessary data about support service utilization so that alternatives can be generated and evaluated in preparation for problems should they develop.

From such a collected data base it is possible to develop predictors of unit utilization and thus provide management hard data for future planning. Such a dynamic prediction is, of course, only a future prospect but now closer to reality because this type of data can be acquired and subjected to close scrutiny and analysis.

As a communication tool the NISS report is serving a very needed function. In

our digital simulation models we avoided modeling the "shift-change" for we did not
then nor do we now know the complete interactions and dynamics of that situation.
What we have noted, quite simply, is that NISS appears to be a time-saver. The NISS
report is a rather complete <u>outline</u> or process guide of a patient's care requirements,
only the specifics need be provided (e.g., type of antibiotic). Nurse time is saved
by not repeating the obvious and perhaps better and more complete significant information is transferred between staff because of this. Independent of the rationaliza-
tion, this adjunct has been one of only a few we have implemented within our monitoring capability that reflects utilization and about whose absence the nursing staff
complains when the system is down!

The concept and implementation is obviously useful in our hands and appears to
contribute to over-all SICU improved function. It should be a transferable and useful adjunct to others in the same modes it helps us. One can argue the categoriza-
tion of tasks and even rearrange them into different groups, application site dependent. But these are minor components of the concept. We suspect one could enlarge
the task lists and in general we would agree. However, since the first version we
have added only 3 tasks in 6 months and thus do not anticipate others experiencing
difficulties were they to implement the program. We do recognize this is SICU oriented and might require extensive revision for application in other critical care
areas (e.g., neo-natal, coronary, medical).

If adopted by other SICU's, even if locally modified, a set of data can be generated which will allow objective comparison of these units by provision of a standardized inter-unit metric. This concept is most appropriate in large care delivery
systems, such as the Veterans Administration Hospitals, where upper level management
is always seeking referenced comparative methods. This concept obviously represents
a desirous extension of the application not yet implemented.

The systems engineer-designer can also utilize NISS when asked to evaluate a
particular unit, for the data is helpful in generating alternatives when one is asked
to improve an existing SICU or create a new one. The data obtained assists in problem identification because it elicits detail which is often overlooked because of
rare occurrence, infrequent use, or non-availability. The task lists thus serve as
prompting devices to make explicit what may be implicit or even obvious to personnel
but which they fail to communicate when asked.

Conclusion

We consider NISS a major adjunct for our SICU and have found it useful for unit
function, unit management, and research on unit function. We consider it to be a
transferable and useable concept for others as well. Its appeal as a standardized
metric of nurse utilization with the capability of correlating this measurement to
"state of health" or "systems support demands" cannot go unnoticed by designers,

planners, and managers of the complex SICU environment. We believe appropriate analysis of the data gathered by this device can only result in functional improvement in SICU's everywhere with the implied, but as yet unproven, proviso of improved patient care. For now, NISS is more than a data acquisition device in our SICU. It is a functional, useful, used, communication adjunct between personnel and between management and personnel. The staff perceives it as a significant aid to performance of their functions. What more could one ask of an adjunct?

References

1. Greenburg, A.G., McClure, D.K., Fink, R.M. and Goldberg, M.: Evaluation of a computerized intensive care monitoring system: An application of information utilization monitoring. Proc. of the Annual San Diego Bio-Med. Symp. 14:297,1975.

2. McClure, D.K., Fink, R.M. and Greenburg, A.G.: Computerized patient monitoring--A critical evaluation. Proc. of the Annual San Diego Bio-Med. Symp. 14:289, 1975.

3. Greenburg, A.G., McClure, D.K., Fink, R., Stubbs, J.A. and Peskin, G.W.: Computerization of the surgical intensive care unit: Improvement of patient care via education. Surg. 77:799, 1975.

4. Greenburg, A.G. and Peskin, G.W.: Monitoring in the recovery room and surgical intensive care unit. In: Monitoring in Anesthesia, Saidman and Smith, Eds., Chap. 10, pp 221-246, J. Wiley and Sons, 1978.

5. Greenburg, A.G., McClure, D.K., Goldberg, M. and Peskin, G.W.: Systems science, computers and the surgical intensive care unit. In: Systems Science in Health Care, Coblentz and Walter, Eds., pp 277-282, Taylor & Francis, Ltd., 1977.

6. Greenburg, A.G.: Computerization of the surgical intensive care unit: A new view for design. Proc. Medinfo '77, Shires and Wolf, Eds., North Holland Publishers, pp. 901-905, 1977.

7. Greenburg, A.G., Goldberg, M., McClure, D.K., Janus, C.A. and Stubbs, J.A.: Systems science, simulation and the surgical intensive care unit. Proc. of the 10th Simulation Conf., Tampa, Florida, pp 129-137, March, 1977.

8. Greenburg, A.G. and Goldberg, M.: Alternative surgical intensive care unit configurations: Evaluation by simulation. Proc. Medinfo '77, Shires and Wolf, Eds., North Holland Publishers, pp 437-441, 1977.

9. Cullen, D.J., Civetta, J.M., Briggs, B.A. and Ferrara, L.C.: Therapeutic intervention scoring system: a method for quantitative comparison of patient care. Critical Care Medicine 2:57, 1974.

10. Cullen, D.J., Ferrara, L.C., Briggs, B.A., et al.: Survival, hospitalization charges and follow-up results in critically ill patients. New Engl. J. Med. 294:982, 1976.

11. Linstone, H.A. and Turoff, M., Eds. The Delphi Method: Techniques and Applications. Addison-Wesley Publishing Company, Inc., Reading, Mass., 1975.

IMPLEMENTATION OF A PATIENT MONITORING SYSTEM

AT HERLEV HOSPITAL

Bo Svarre Nielsen

&

Per Andersen

The Data Processing Department
Copenhagen County Hospitals, Denmark.

1. INTRODUCTION.

In April 1977 a Patient Monitoring System was started up at Herlev Hospital. The system covers the intensive care unit, the
delivery unit, and the operating theatre.

The Department of Data Processing and the software company CHR.
ROVSING A/S have developed the system in close collaboration
with the Department of Anesthesia and the Department of Gyneco-
logy and Obstetrics.

2. PURPOSE OF THE SYSTEM.

The aim of introducing computers in patient care is to improve
the quality of care. The major reasons for such an improvement
to take place are:

a. Decisions regarding therapy can rely on more complex computa-
    tion.

b. A quicker detection of variations in physiological parameters
    recorded on-line can be carried out.

c. Automation of basal monitoring and calculation routines
    leaves additional time for patient care, for the nurses as
    well as for the physicians.

d. With the introduction of computer automated procedures daily
    working routines in general become more systematical.

e. Eventually, sufficient information of variations in physiolo-
    gical parameters, measured and calculated, can be accumulated
    in order to arrive at a higher degree of predictability as to
    the clinical course.

3. SYSTEM.

Based on Hewlett Packard's 5600 A computerized Patient Data Management System, the system runs on a HP 21 MX minicomputer.

In fact, the system supplied by Hewlett Packard was not exactly applicable at Herlev Hospital. This was due partly to the non-standard I/O equipment chosen and partly to the fact that all communication between the nurses and the system was in English. A major translation task was necessary, and the programs were changed concurrently to support the special I/O equipment.

Functions very much desired by the department involved were not included in the basic programs, so in order to meet these requirements the system was extended considerably.

4. CONFIGURATION.

The system was composed of equipment from several manufacturers. The computer configuration consists of two Hewlett-Packard 21 MX minicomputers each equipped with 32 K words of main memory and 5 Mbyte disc storage. One computer handles the routine applications, the other one is used for program development, special applications and as a back-up for the first computer.

The peripheral equipment includes 10 terminals, 2 plotters, 2 slow printers and various equipment for reading analog data.

The intensive care unit is served by 6 terminals, a plotter, and a printer. A terminal is placed at the bedside in four rooms for that particular patient's data. These terminals are used by the clinical personnel for entering data manually and for data reviewing. One terminal, the printer and the plotter have been placed at the central station. Here the secretary admits and discharges patients, enters laboratory data, besides requesting reports and plots.

Automatically measured data from the bedside equipment are transmitted to patient display generators, which continually display the parameters on TV monitors. From these generators the patient's data are transmitted in serial, digital form (V 24) to the computer.

The delivery unit has been equipped with two terminals, a plotter and a printer. One terminal is placed at the central station together with the plotter and the printer. Two terminals are placed in delivery rooms. All data from deliveries are at the moment entered manually by the midwives, who also request displays and reports.

The operating theatre is served by a terminal, a videogenerator connected to a TV display and facilities for reading analog data.

5. BASIC SOFTWARE.

The HP 5600 A was delivered with a certain amount of basic software, which forms a framework of application programs.

The software package is executing under the RTE II operating system. The most important features of the 5600 A are:

> terminal handling
> specialized file structures
> output spooling
> basic patient handling.

Terminal handling includes methods to construct and control series of menus, which guide the user to the application program he wants. Special function keys can be defined to enter a predetermined keystroke sequence, giving rapid access to the application.

Two special file structures are supported by the system, one for data entering at regular intervals, e.g. automatically measured data, and one for data coming at random intervals, e.g. manually entered data. A set of subroutines allows the user to store and retrieve data at a specified time and date or to search for data within specified intervals.

A report system implements output spooling to slow printers and thus allows several terminals to share the same printer.

The basic patient handling programs provide for admission, discharging and transfer of patients.

6. APPLICATION PROGRAMS SUPPLIED BY HEWLETT-PACKARD.

The HP 5600 A system includes a number of programs covering a range of application. The programs selected by the involved departments were divided into three groups:

> a. Requisition and presentation of manually
>   and automatically measured data.
>
> b. Administration of laboratory tests.
>
> c. Input and retrieval of free form notes.

At present the following five parameters can be measured automatitically: Heart rate, temperature, systolic, diastolic, and venous pressure. The monitoring rate is specified by the nurse from a choice of 0,5, 2,5, 5, 10, or 15 minutes. Manually measured parameters can be entered to extend and supplement the automatically measured data. The data presentation can be either in digital values or in trend plots.

Laboratory data are entered by the secretary at the central station. The results can be displayed at the bedside or used in other application programs. Comments to the trend plot or to the patient's state in general are entered in free form by the nurses and printed in connection with various reports.

7. PROGRAMS DEVELOPED LOCALLY.

When purchasing the 5600 A system it was considered essential that the system from the very start had the application programs necessary to be of use in a day's work.

Various working groups were formed to define projects for extension of the system, and from the large list the following projects were chosen to be implemented initially:

        a. A fluid balance system.
        b. A surveillance record for the ICU.
        c. A program to handle delivery data.
        d. A data transmission system to the
            central computer.

7.1 FLUID BALANCE SYSTEM.

Management of fluid is one of the more important aspects of intensive care therapy, so it was natural to extend the 5600 A system with programs for fluid balance. This subsystem presents:

A. A current summary of volume, sodium (Na), and potassium (K) inputs and outputs including instantaneous balances on a visual display.

B. Accumulated vol-Na-K and nitrogen balances including laboratory results to keep with the patients file.

C. A graphic summary showing body weight, accumulated vol-Na-K and nitrogen balances, intake of calories, urine output and creatine clearance.

The fluid balance system is updated by means of a display which presents a list of possible intakes and outputs from which the nurse can choose. The intake record includes 13 commonly used

standard solutions. The contents of Na, K, N, and calories are
known by the computer. In the output record only fluid volumes
(lost as urine, blood etc.) are entered. The contents of Na, K
and N in these fluids are calculated automatically on the basis
of laboratory results entered by the secretary. Thus, an updated
summary of fluid and electrolyte totals and balances always is
available.

7.2 SURVEILLANCE RECORD FOR THE ICU.

One of the reports generated by the system is the surveillance
record. The aim of the report is to give a graphic presentation
of the most important patient data within a certain period.

All automatically measured parameters are plotted as curves,
and manually measured parameters are marked as crosses or squares.
The following parameters appear on the record: Heart rate, respiratory rate, systolic, calculated mean and diastolic pressure, central and peripheral temperature, venous blood pressure and diuresis.
The latter is printed as a numerical value but not plotted.

At the buttom of the record events are marked relating to the
notes written by the nurses. Each event is labeled with a letter
referring to a corresponding note in the right column of the report.
The report is generated every morning at the central station.

A special version of the report is used when the patient is discharged. All parameters are here plotted as curves and no discrimination is made between manually and automatically measured values.
All remarks are printed on separate sheets.

7.3 PARGRAM.

In the baby delivery unit a birth summary is produced after each
delivery by the assisting midwife. As this procedure is completely
uniform and always includes the same calculation procedures, it has
been found suitable for automation.

The pattern of cervical dilation, especially early during the
birth and the pattern of fetal descent are useful parameters for
early identification of complications. It has therefore been
found convenient to have a graphic presentation of these parameters
as a function of time.

The program falls into three main sections:

1. Input of data   2. Presentation of surveys   3. Reports.

Input of data. The data for survey and records are entered manually on the display terminal through an interactive process in which the user is guided by the system.

Presentation of survey. The surveys which the system can present are:

1. A survey of the size of orificium and the position of the presenting part of the fetus shown in chronological order.

2. A survey of interventions and treatments, medications and analgesia/anesthesia.

3. A Partogram, which is a graphic presentation of the cervical dilation and the position of the presenting part of the fetus as a function of time. Time markings consists of actual time, time from the start of birth and reference to the cardiotocograph as well as to events occurring during labor.

Reports. The reports generated by the system are:

1. A partogram plot.

2. A typewritten birth summary.

7.4 DATA TRANSMISSION SYSTEM.

The original 5600 A system keeps the data for a certain maximum time or until the patient is discharged. When discharging the patient all data are purged. In order to make data available for statistical analysis a data transmission system was designed. This system transmits all patient data to the central IBM 370 computer, when the patient is discharged. Here data are archived on magnetic tape in a form suitable for the statistical standard system running on this computer.

8. CONCLUSION.

The system has now been in full operation for more than a year. Being fully integrated in a day's work it is now used extensively by both departments. It relieves the wards of tedious routine jobs and it is gratifying to see how the departments depend on it and look forward to every enlargement. Future plans include an interactive fluid balance system and various programs for physiological measurements, e.g. respiration, cardiac output and compression of cardiotocograph signals.

-- ooOoo --

A Review of The National Standard Child Health
Computer System and its Potential Benefits

J. S. Parkinson

Welsh Health Technical Services Organisation
Cardiff, United Kingdom

Summary

This paper describes briefly the development and
current state of the National Standard Child Health
Computer System. An outline of the system function
and probable future developments is given. Some
potentially valuable uses of the data collected
and likely problems associated with such uses are
mentioned. The possible longer term developments
are outlined. A brief technical synopsis is provided.

The need for a system to record and monitor information about the
health and developmental progress of newly born and young children is
a common health management problem. It is often associated with the
need to administer vaccination and immunisation programs and to
provide screening facilities. Provision of such a system has been
approached in a variety of ways using different degrees of technology
and with varying degrees of success by many individual health authorities in the United Kingdom. Following the reorganisation of the
Health Services in England and Wales in 1974 it was found that most of
the fifteen resulting "regions" (fourteen English Regional Health
Authorities plus Wales) were developing or had already developed at
least one and sometimes several different systems of their own. These
encompassed both manual and computer supported systems. The transfer
of responsibility for many aspects of child health from local authorities to the new health areas also meant that many existing computerised systems being run on local authority machines would need new
support facilities and transfer to the Regional Health Authority
computer centres which were being set up. It was apparent that
considerable duplication of effort in design, development and support
existed and there was little evidence of a common approach being
adopted. (This was a problem common to other major computerised
systems).

It was therefore decided, wherever possible, to adopt a system of centralised development whereby a single region would design, develop and test a standard system which would then be distributed to other regions. Support and maintenance would continue to be provided centrally. It was thus hoped that a greater degree of expertise would be developed at the responsible site and that a better return on resources invested would arise. In accordance with this approach the National Standard Child Health Computer System for England and Wales has been produced by the Welsh Health Technical Services Organisation (WHTSO) as Centre of Responsibility (COR) under the auspices of the Computers and Research Division on the Department of Health and Social Security (DHSS). Based on an initial design produced under contract by the National Computing Centre (NCC) the system was intended to be run on any Regional Health Authority standard computer installation. User involvement in the design and development of the system was by means of a steering committee and two technical sub-committees that allowed both medical and computing issues to be debated before their inclusion in the system. A modular design approach was adopted, with four units (Birth Registration, Vaccination and Immunisation, Pre-school Health and School Health) of which the first two are now in live use and the third is undergoing pre-design discussion with implem-entation planned for 1979. After a fairly lengthy trial period in Wales, during which the initial systems design was extensively modified by WHTSO to rectify operational shortcomings the system was released to English users and is currently in use by 11 out of 14 (January 1978) of the RHA's encompassing about half of the Area Health Authorities (AHA's) in England. (It has also been "exported" to Scotland). WHTSO, as a centre of responsibility, has continued to modify and "tune" the system to cater for individual requirements and the development of new techniques, such as computer output to microfiche (COM). Within Wales the system has been adopted by five out of the eight Health Authorities and it is hoped to take on the remaining three by the end of 1978. A comprehensive training package is now available for both new and exis-ting users. For those who are interested, some brief technical details are given as an addendum to this paper.

The heart of the system is a pair of master files. Records for each child born are created from the statutory birth notification form, completed by the doctor or midwife attending the birth and submitted, via the health authority within 36 hours. This creates a 100% birth register containing all known identification details and a certain

amount of social and medical data about mother and baby. This information is used to create a Child Register (CR) record and a Birth Details
(BD) record on respective masterfiles. At a later stage the BD record
is extended to hold Vaccination and Immunisation (VI) information.
Data is added to the records as it is collected by Health Visitors or
community physicians at child health clinics. The system automatically
requests follow-up data on premature births and monitors inputs outstanding beyond pre-specified periods.

As part of the normal post-natal care program the Health Visitor obtains
the parents' consent for some or all of the standard Vaccination and
Immunisation program offered to all children. The mother also chooses
whether to have her child immunised by her own General Practitioner or
at an authority run child health clinic. Details of all possible
sites are held within the system and when the child is old enough to
participate in the VI program (usually at six months), the system will,
optionally, schedule appointments (using a choice of scheduling methods)
for them to attend the clinic or GP of their choice to receive the
appropriate course. Participation by GP's is voluntary and no appointments are scheduled for those not participating. The system produces
postcard notifications to parents for whose children appointments have
been made and clinic lists for GP's and clinics. All results of courses
given, whether by participating GP's or not are collected by the health
authority and input to the system to update the VI records. A check
is kept on outstanding results and reminders issued as necessary. The
system provides comprehensive management facilities including the means
to generate registrars' lists of new births and GP payment lists; cancel
or suspend clinics; change GP, health visitor or clinic references in
records and alter or add to the file holding details of GP's and clinics.
Age/sex registers can be constructed by area or practice and states of
protection data produced. Comprehensive statistics are produced for
both births and the immunisation program at quarterly and yearly intervals. A facility to produce a print of each child's recorded details
on either paper or microfiche is also available, for single records
(on paper only) or the whole file. A shortened version of the record
can be printed as an option.

A recent extensive evaluation and review study of the system has shown
that the approach adopted, while not being entirely satisfactory at
the outset has developed well and has produced major financial savings
in development and support costs. The currently available version of

the system offers a cost effective alternative to manual methods and provides significantly greater facilities than would be possible without computerisation. While the overheads of providing a range of options within a standardised framework are greater than those associated with the provision of purely local facilities, the cost of running the national system still compares very favourably with locally developed systems, and this comparison will shortly be further improved by a partial rewriting and internal redesign of the computer programs to improve efficiency and ease of maintenance. This will also facilitate the introduction of the pre-school health module in 1979. Detailed design of this new module is currently underway and although details of the Pre-School Health Module have not yet been finalised the system will be similar in outline to the VI module, based on an extended Birth Details record and holding results of scheduled examinations and screening tests carried out up to the age of 5 years. It is anticipated that a fourth module will then be added (in 1980 or 1981) to allow scheduling of and recording of results from school health examinations up to the age of 18 years. It will, of course, be around 1993 before this situation of complete pre-adult coverage can arise, unless considerable effort is expended on the computerisation of existing manual records, but the need to allow for the use of the system over such an extended timescale has necessitated the consideration of probable changes in hardware and hence forward compatible software. It has also been important to allow for the growth in the volume of records involved (over half a million in Wales by 1990 requiring some 5400 megabytes of storage) and the consequent increase in computing power required to run the system. However, with a new generation of hardware about to be introduced and the associated improvements in storage devices these problems will hopefully not become too pressing before their technological solution is available.

We may therefore look forward to a time, hopefully around 1980, when the fifteen regional computer centres in England and Wales have, between them, a complete and ongoing register of births and are beginning to accumulate significant amounts of medical and demographic data about children under five. The value and potential for use of this information is much greater than appears to be appreciated by many of those involved in the introduction of the system and I would like to mention just a few of the possible benefits to be gained. I am sure that you can think of others. The most obvious areas of use are in epidemiology and health planning, both on a regional and a national level. A real problem in both areas in the past has been lack of accurate and comprehensive information of which to base studies or formulate strategies for resource allocation. With a complete computerised birth register available much of the cost associated with even the limited data collection exercises needed to obtain information will be removed and it will become feasible to undertake regular studies on fertility, population mobility and infant morbidity (as opposed merely to mortality) for use in planning the siting and extent of both maternity and paediatric facilities. It might also be possible, for the first time, to measure reliably the effectiveness of different care regimes and their associated resources, all hopefully, improving the way in which we provide health care for mothers and their children.

The potential uses, however, are not confined to health care. Since the rational planning of educational facilities depends on knowledge of the numbers and distribution of children in particular age groups, as far as possible in advance of the time when they need education (to allow for new building and the recruitment and training of teachers, both of which take several years), use of the complete birth register to provide this information could help to avoid the cycles of glut and scarcity that have been a feature of the last two decades. Finally, information about family size could be used to help plan housing programs and the provision of recreational facilities which often seem to be rather haphazard at present.

All of these uses, of course, depend not only on the information being available, but also on its being used. This in turn requires that those who are in a position to use it are made aware, both of its existance and of the ways in which it could be used. In doing so, however, a number of new problems arise, especially for those concerned with aspects of security and confidentiality of the data and the appropriateness of the uses to which it is to be put. In this context two points need to be made. The first is that nearly all the data collected and held by the computer system already exists on manually maintained record keeping systems and a good deal of it (details of birth certificates etc) is fairly readily accessible to the general public. All that the use of a computerised system has done has been to make logical access to large amounts of the information easier to achieve. In general, it has made phyical access more difficult since it is easier to control the use of computer held information than that held in a variety of insecure locations on more familiar media. The second point

in that, for the majority of the uses described here, information
about individuals is not required. Only demographic details would be
supplied and while it is possible, in rare cases, to identify individuals from such data, the numbers involved make this a very unlikely
occurrence. Where the nature of the usage demands that personal identification information is necessary, in for instance, an at risk register
access would normally be restricted to those health care providers who
need to use the data in order to provide for the child, such as GP's
and school health doctors, and the associated administrators. The
problem really devolves upon the question of who controls the access
to the data and who decides what types of access are to be allowed.
In this area, both as a profession and as a society we are only just
beginning to feel our way, and while a potential danger for misuse
does exist, I feel that it is rather overstated at the present time
and that considerations of security should not be given so great a
weight as to destroy all the very great potential benefits of the
child health computer system.

To finish with, I would like to say a few words about other collections
of health information and how they may interact with the child health
system. Generally speaking the other main sources are the general
practitioners records (and the associated family practitioner committee
lists) and hospital records, possibly at a number of different sites.
Work on the computerisation of both hospital and GP systems has been
going on in England and Wales for some ten years, but as yet few cost
effective (rather than technically enterprising) solutions have been
achieved. Only one attempt to link the two types of record has been
undertaken and although this has succeeded in showing the value of an
integrated record, it has also shown that only the advent of cheaper
storage and computing technology can achieve a widespread affordable
system. It therefore seems likely that the national standard child
health computer system will be the first comprehensive health register
and record system to be widely available, and consideration should,
perhaps, be given now to the possibility of using it as the basis of a
lifetime medical record, available, in whole or in part, to the various
health care providers with whom an individual may have contact. It
should be said that this is probably not yet technologically feasible
(the data storage volume required would probably be two orders of
magnitude greater than that envisaged for child health alone!) and
may not be socially acceptable for the reasons mentioned above. However
as the costs of storage and of access, especially real time access

continue to fall, it may not be too long before such a system is feasible and the child health computer system could well be a sensible starting point for it.

This has been a very brief review of the existing state and possible future usage of the first and currently most widely adopted of the national standard computer systems within the National Health Service. It would be misleading to claim that the introduction of computer methods into record keeping has been without its problems, but as users become educated to the benefits of automated information processing and as WHTSO continues to extend and improve the system most problems have been overcome. We now have to look ahead to the twin challenges of a new range of hardware and the design and introduction of pre-school and child health modules. It is to be hoped that, in parallel with this, users will come to realise the value of the information being collected and will make further use of it, so realising at least some of the very great potential benefits and helping to make better use of our limited resources.

Technical Notes

The National Standard Child Health Computer System consists of four
interdependant modules, the first two of which have now been released.
These modules form a suite of 32 programs linked together to form a
total of 17 runs involving over 50 processes (including sorts, dumps,
etc). All system programs are written in ICL 1900 Cobol utilising
forward compatibility standards. They are designed to run on ICL 1900
series processes in the range 1903T, 1904A, 1904S under executive,
George 2 or George 3 operating systems. They are supplied to users
as object programs plus necessary job descriptions on a magnetic tape.
The programs currently require a maximum of 32K words of core store,
3 or 4 EDS 60 disc drives and two magnetic tape decks, a line printer
and a slow input peripheral. Key-to-disc or key-to-tape input is
expected for the majority of the data. The master files use index
sequential access methods and there are two other permanent files associated with the system - an appointments master file, that may be held
on disc or tape and the file of GP and child health clinic details,
which is held on disc. A number of work files are used by the system
and under George 3 these are temporary filestore files. (In the event
of very high volumes of throughput exofiles may need to be used).

The training package consists of a tape/slide program plus wall charts,
introductory leaflets and sets of procedure cards. User, operations
and system manuals are also provided.

Outlines of the clerical procedures involved in the Birth Registration
and V.&.I. modules are given below.

CHILD REGISTER CLERICAL PROCEDURES

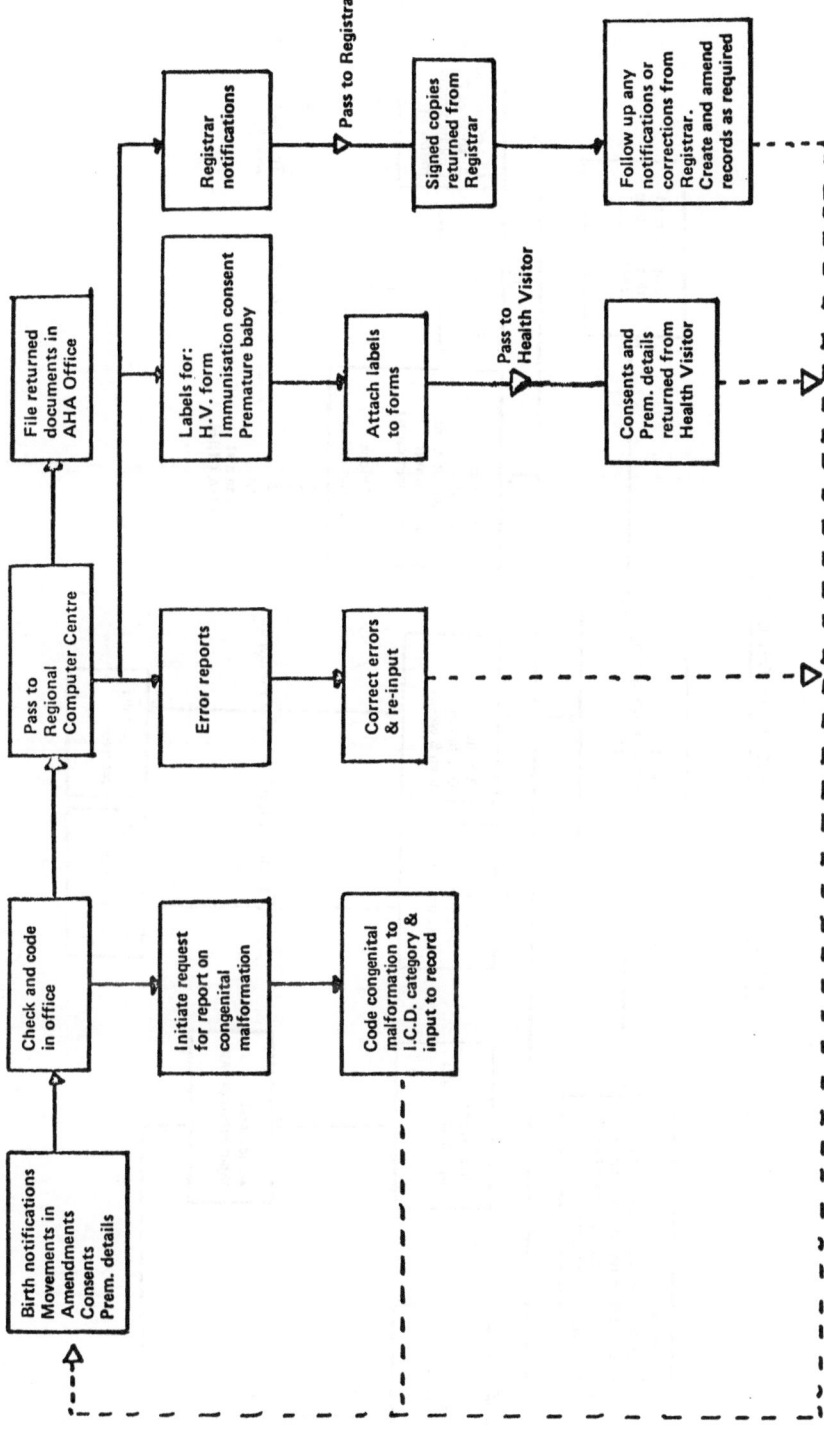

IMMUNISATION – CLERICAL PROCEDURES

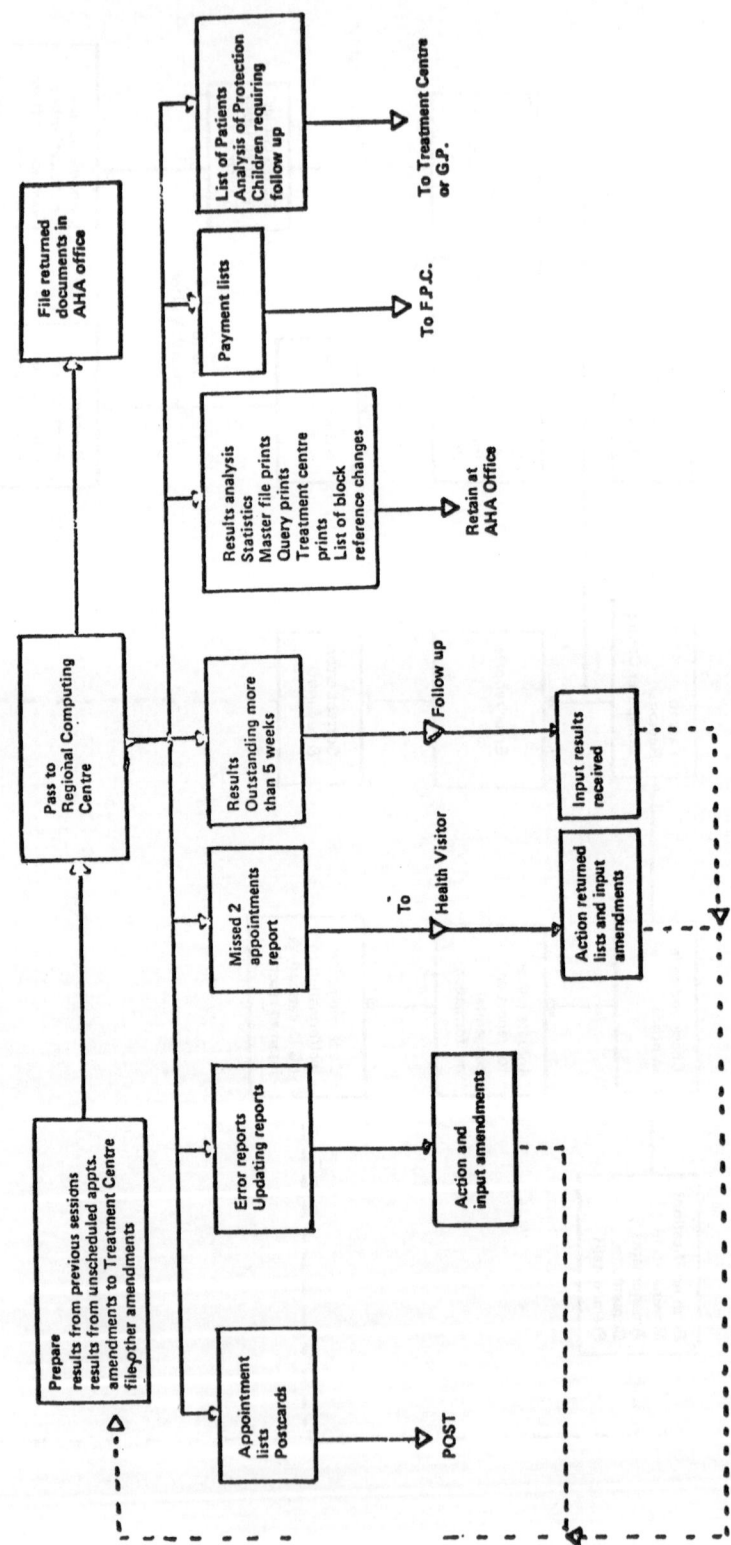

REFERENCES

1. Standard Child Health System User Manual.

2. Report of the Royal Commission on Child Health.

3. Report of the Committee on Privacy. CMND 5012 HMSO JULY 1972.

4. Computers and Privacy. CMND 6353 HMSO DECEMBER 1975.

5. Computers: Safeguards for Privacy. CMND 6354 HMSO DECEMBER 1975.

6. Research Methods in Health Care. J. Mckinley (ED). Milbank Memorial Fund 1973.

7. General Practice Record Keeping Using a Real Time Computer. Bradshaw-Smith. ECHSCP. MEDCOMP 77.

8. Real Time Record Management in General Practice. Grummitt. Int. J. Bio-Medical Computing 1977.

9. Standard Child Health System: Evaluation Report. WHTSO 1978.

A REVIEW OF THE USE OF COMPUTERS IN HOSPITAL AND

COMMUNITY INDEXES IN THE UNITED KINGDOM

J. R. Bryant and S. M. Fenlon
Computer Unit
Addenbrooke's Hospital
Cambridge England

1. HOSPITALS - THE BASIC CONCEPTS

1.1 The Medical Records Department

The modern Medical Records Department covers a very wide range of activities (1).
It is important to remember, however, that the prime responsibility of such a department is to undertake the custody, classification and confidential preservation of
the patient's case history, and it is in fulfilling this responsibility that the
importance of indexes is highlighted.

Most hospitals use the unit system of records in connection with patients' case
notes. On first attendance at hospital a patient is allocated a number. The number
is not subsequently discarded and thus acts as a means of permanent indexing, tracing
and filing, and as a reference throughout the hospital.

There are three basic methods of filing: alphabetical, chronological, and numerical.
For the patient's medical record, alphabetical filing can be used successfully only
in very small hospitals or health centres etc. where the quantity of material is
small and the turnover low. Its lack of elasticity and the difficulty of maintaining
good alphabetical order makes it unsatisfactory in large systems. In addition problems are created in complying with the aforementioned unit principle where the
prevention of duplication is essential and demands constant checking. Numerical
filing overcomes the problems of lack of elasticity by allowing for continuous expansion with planned and orderly growth of the files. It is also compatible with the
unit system of record keeping. Chronological filing is not satisfactory when dealing
with case notes as it would preclude use of the unit principle and make any access
difficult. It is more commonly used when related to waiting list and follow-up
systems. It is a fundamental feature of numerical and chronological filing that,
unlike alphabetical filing, they are not capable of standing alone, and require an
index to allow access to the material contained in the system (with the exception
of up-to-date filing used when the patient is present).

2. MANUAL INDEXES

2.1 Introduction

Since most hospitals use a unit system of numerical filing for case notes, an alphabetical index is also required as a means of entry to the contents of the overall system. The recorded information for this type of master index is usually minimised, consisting of the basic patient identification details, surname, forenames, address, date of birth, and sex. Master indexes can also contain further information such as religion, date of initial registration, G.P. name etc., hence encompassing the ability to perform other functions according to demands.

An index may take a variety of forms. It may be of card, with or without punched edges, or strip, or loose leaf type. It may have a variety of devices attached or inserted in it to aid quick retrieval. It may employ visible or non-visible signals to denote some special factor or action date. The standard hospital master index, because of its size and need for accuracy, usually consists of vertical cards well interspersed with alphabetical guides. Although it is possible to use phonetic sequence, grouping like-sounding names together irrespective of actual spelling, for example, Eliot and Elliott, Barrie and Barry, it is customary to maintain strict alphabetical sequence by the insertion of new cards in their correct position. It is also normal to adhere to the British Telephone Directory convention for names beginning with Mc, Mac, St. etc., and also for hyphenated names.

The available methods for physically storing a master index tend to be limited by two factors - the size of the index and the cost of the filing equipment. Whilst strip indexes and cardwheels are not suitable for large indexes, some elevator and carousel type files are expensive. In general, most indexes are held on cards and use either elevator files (for the larger hospital indexes) or some form of drawer filing. It is worth noting that large indexes are often divided according to sex. This is done for two reasons, firstly it improves physical access and halves the search time, and secondly, if achieved, for example, by card colour it reduces the amount of information to be recorded.

3. USING COMPUTERS

3.1 Introduction

The introduction of the use of computers in the area of medical records has had
wide-ranging effects. In this paper, however, we shall restrict our attention specifically to the effects of using computers to assist in medical records indexing.
The general benefits to be expected here can be classified under two main headings:
(a) improvement in the quality of the index and associated reduction in clerical
work, and (b) improvement in patient care. The first category of benefits arises
from the detection of existing duplicate records (at the conversion stage), the
considerable reduction in the possibility of future duplication, the elimination
of misfiling, and the improved presentation of the index data. In the second category the improved index substantially reduces the chances of a patient being treated
without knowledge of his previous medical history.

There are three main types of computer system: (a) on-line, (b) batch processing,
and (c) hybrid. On-line systems are systems in which all input/output operations
are performed, usually in real time, by equipment directly under the computer's
control, for example a visual display unit (VDU) linked directly to the computer.

Batch processing is a method of processing data in which transactions are collected
and prepared for input to the computer, for example on punched cards or paper tape,
for processing as a single unit. There may be an appreciable delay between the
occurrence of the original events and the eventual computer processing of the transactions. Hybrid systems, which are becoming increasingly common, usually consist
of an intelligent terminal which captures, partially validates and stores input
data locally and then goes 'on-line' for one or more brief periods during which the
data is transferred to a central computer. Output is usually from the central computer and is either in printed form or on microfiche.

3.2 On-line Systems

A typical on-line system consists of one or more terminals linked directly to the
computer which holds the master index on a random access storage device. Enquiries
or searches are made by the user entering the known details of the patient, usually
some combination of the patient's surname, forename, sex and age or date of birth.
The computer compares this information with the data held in its master index, and
where a match is found, displays at the terminal the details from the computer file.
A search can be made when the user does not know all of the patient's details. Most
systems have some minimum search criteria consisting usually of the patient's surname
and either sex or first initial. The computer then searches for all patients whose
details satisfy the given search parameters regardless of any other possible parameters. There are systems in operation for indexes that require only the first letter of the patient's surname plus the first initial in order to carry out a search.

If the computer system's file handling software is sufficiently sophisticated, or
if database techniques are being used (2), the file structure can be organised in
such a way as to provide the additional capability of phonetically orientated searching. This enables the computer to search its master index and display details of
any patient whose details match or are similar to those input including spelling
variants of the surname. Probably the most widely used procedure for achieving
this is the Russell-Soundex code (4). The principle of this system depends upon
the fact that most errors in the spelling of names involves vowels or certain alternative consonants such as C and K, or D and T. The first letter of the surname is
retained intact and subsequent consonants except H, W, and Y are assigned a digit
between 1 and 6 which places them in phonetic groups. The second of any pair of
repeated digits (i.e. those occurring without any intervening vowels), and all vowels
are then eliminated. The result of this is that many common variations in the spelling of a surname have the same code, for example Barratt, Barrett and Baratt.

An alternative approach to surname coding is to restrict the initial search parameters to say the first three characters of the surname plus the first initial.
This would obviously enable the search to detect certain types of mis-spellings.
Other parameters including sex, date of birth, full surname and first part of address
can then be used to refine the search responses to a suitable level.

A typical on-line master index will also be 'inverted'. This means that the user
can retrieve a patient's details from the computer by inputting that patient's hospital (or unit) number. In general, on-line indexes are kept up to date by inputting
amendments and additions directly to the computer via the terminals, thus making the
new information immediately available to all users. There is no reason, however,
why batch processing cannot be used to maintain the master index, although the index
is always lacking the information in any batch awaiting processing.

One area in which on-line systems require special consideration is that of providing
some alternative, or backup, for times when the computer system is unavailable,
either deliberately or as a result of some malfunction. This backup is usually
provided in the form of a straightforward alphabetical index - either printed or
held on microfiche. For large indexes the production of such a backup facility may
need to be cyclic.

3.3 Batch Processing Systems

Batch processing systems lack some of the advantages of on-line systems described
above, such as the detection of duplicates at the time of entry. Nevertheless,
such duplicates can be reported when the file is updated, and batch systems have the
considerable advantage of being economical to run, since a medium to large index
held on-line will generally require a dedicated disc drive. They may also be advantageous for small special purpose indexes, that is at ward or specialty rather than
hospital level, where accuracy and presentation are of greater importance than the

maintenance of a completely up-to-date index. Alternatively, a master index system sometimes uses pure batch processing as a prelude to an on-line or hybrid system during the conversion phase.

3.4 Hybrid Systems

Major advances in cost effectiveness in the areas of computer output on microfilm (COM) and intelligent terminals have led to the rapid development of hybrid systems. These types of system are characterised by the fact that they carry out some functions in an on-line mode and others by batch processing. In general they may be sub-divided according to the following criteria:

(a) whether or not on-line searching of the master index is provided,

(b) whether or not COM techniques are used,

(c) whether or not intelligent terminals are used to maintain the master index.

Although certain specific combinations of the above criteria are more commonly used, all combinations are theoretically possible. Before considering the commonly accepted systems, however, it is useful to describe COM and intelligent terminals in more detail.

COM is a procedure for transferring information stored on computer magnetic tape directly onto microfilm ranging in format from 16mm to 105mm. The 105mm format is used for producing microfiche - microfilm cards that each store up to 208 pages of computer printout. Information is read from the microfiche by use of a special viewer. Using this technique a typical large hospital master index of half-a-million patients can be stored on approximately 50 fiche, with each fiche containing details of up to 11,000 patients.

A number of systems people now believe that the "intelligence" of the system should be distributed farther and farther away from the large central processor. A major step in this direction arising from technological advances in the fields of mini-computers has been the incorporation of a processing unit, programmable memory and local file storage in the terminal itself - hence the 'intelligent terminal'. Terminals with these facilities can perform such functions as:

- formatting of input and output,

- syntax checking,

- complex buffering and polling,

- editing,

- pre-processing of input, and

- local data storage, for example on cassette tape or floppy disc.

There are various ways in which hybrid systems can be implemented. The master index

is usually held on a medium-to-large central computer with updating carried out
remotely using intelligent terminals. The main master index fiche are reproduced
as frequently as is required. If the fiche production is carried out on a cyclic
basis, an 'updates' fiche is produced, say weekly, and the most recent amendments
either printed daily or held 'on-line' in the terminal. The intelligent terminal
is connected on-line to the central computer for one or more brief periods each
day during which the data in local storage is transferred to the central computer
file.

4. COMMUNITY INDEXES AND RECORD LINKAGE

Outside the hospitals, the use of master indexes is somewhat different in emphasis.
Most GP practices and health centres employ alphabetical filing to organise their
smaller numbers of records and therefore do not require a master index as such.
The move towards the use of computers in this area has had far less momentum and
consequently very few computer index systems exist. The systems that have been
developed have tended to originate from two different starting points. On the one
hand there is the type of system primarily designed to enable the GP to maintain
his patients' medical records, usually in real-time via on-line terminals (3), and
to provide him, using COM and portable microfiche readers, with an accurate and
highly flexible medical records system. In this area, record linkage has tended
to lag behind other developments in the areas of recall systems and repeat drug
prescription systems.

Progress has also been made from a second starting point, that of medical record
linkage (5,6). Here the objective has been to provide a computer method of linking
together the various data concerning patients' health care, both in the community
and in the hospitals. In this case the function of the master index is to control
and cross-reference many different filing systems unlike the hospital's master index
which generally aims at controlling a single filing system.

A third starting point is currently being considered in a number of health districts.
This is the concept of a District patient index, that is, a master index cross-
referencing the medical records departments of all the hospitals in that district.

5. CONVERSION TO A COMPUTER INDEX

One of the major problems associated with computerised indexes is that of converting
the existing manual index to machine-readable form. The problems are, in general,
those of organisation due to three factors:

(a) the size of manual index (in the case of large hospital indexes),

(b) the confidential nature of the information, and

(c) the fact that the information is in constant use.

There are three general methods by which this conversion can be achieved.

The first method is to use standard data preparation techniques and batch processing
to convert the index. This usually entails the removal of small parts of the index,
one part at a time, to a data preparation bureau with special arrangements for retrieval of data from the missing part. The conversion must be organised in such a
way as to ensure that subsequent additions and amendments to that part of the index
already converted are not omitted. The problem of removal of part of the index can
be overcome by micro-photographic production of data preparation documents instead
of using the index itself.

The second method is to use on-site intelligent terminals. In this way the data
need not be physically removed from the index site. This usually implies both the
use of more terminals than would be needed for the operational system and the hiring
of temporary keyboard operators to undertake the work.

The third method is to use on-line VDU's. This is obviously worth consideration
when the operational system is intended to be on-line. This method, however, also
poses the problem of physically removing data from the manual index if the intended
operational siting of the VDU's does not coincide with the site of the manual index.
Under these circumstances some temporary reconfiguration of the connections between
the computer and the VDU's may be necessary.

6. CONCLUSIONS

The use of computing techniques for patient master indexes has been shown to provide benefits (7) in both the quality of the indexes themselves and their ease of use. Most implementations of computer master indexes report benefits (8,9) including the elimination of index mis-filing, reduction in time actually searching the index, reduction in the time needed to maintain the index, improved legibility of data, and reduction in the number of multiple registrations (that is patients who have been inadvertently allocated more than one hospital number). The quantification of these benefits has been difficult but reports indicate improvements in search time of 38% for computer printed indexes, 58% for on-line searching and 62% for microfiche, all as compared with card indexes held in elevator files. Additional benefits of using computing techniques arise from the ability to produce computer printed identification labels and other routine documentation, and from the ease with which automatic weeding and size reduction techniques can be applied based, for example, on date of initial registration, date of last attendance, or death. It is also worth noting that VDU's and microfiche readers occupy considerably less space than the elevator files that they replace (although space must of course be found somewhere for the computer).

The use of on-line techniques has shown additional benefits in terms of multiple registrations, for example an 80% improvement, due to the use of sophisticated file searching and phonetic coding techniques. It is important, however, to realise that file searching based on phonetic spellings can be expensive in terms of disc accesses unless the file organisation is specifically designed for this purpose.

Quantitative evaluation of the Russell-Soundex coding technique has shown significant benefits. In one study (10) the procedure dealt with two-thirds of all discrepant spellings of surnames, reducing the total number of records not selected for consideration from 4.4% to 1.6%. More recent work (9) has shown that of the total number of successful searches of a typical computerised on-line hospital master index, 5.6% were found through Soundex coding. It is interesting to note that in this second case, the majority of successful Soundex searches showed that one omitted or inserted letter was responsible for most of the normal search failures.

It should also be pointed out that the use of on-line techniques for such master indexes almost certainly cannot be justified in terms of cost-effectiveness unless, as usually happens, the index forms a building block for some integrated system containing many other applications.

The increasing use of microfiche in the area of patient indexes is based largely on cost and filing convenience. It is generally accepted that microfiche is cheaper than printed output if three or more copies of the same information are required, and that the cost-effectiveness grows rapidly with larger numbers of copies. A microfiche reader can be purchased for as little as £100. Also a microfiche index occupies far less storage space than its printed equivalent. The major disadvantage of using COM for a master index arises from the need to keep the index completely up to date. It is more economical to cycle the process producing new fiche containing the latest amendments and thus to have an 'amendments' fiche and a daily cumulative amendments record. Thus three separate locations may have to be searched if the index is being properly used. This can be both time consuming and a source of errors.

A similar problem arises from considerations of whether or not to convert the existing manual index. It can be a long expensive task to totally convert a large card index. Alternatively if not done an extra location is added to all index searches for many years.

It is also true that work in the area of medical record linkage and community indexes has made considerable progress with the aid of computing techniques. Indeed, it is difficult to see any other way in which such progress could have been made. The major problem in this area is one of pure size and organisation. The question of just which aspects of geography, demography and health care should be included is difficult to answer due to the number of possibilities. How much information from, for example, hospital records, waiting lists, general practice records, various screening and follow-up systems, birth and death registration, drug records etc. should be included? Ideally all of it, but the size of the task is enormous!

This paper attempts to summarise the methods of computerising Master Indexes which are currently in use in the United Kingdom. It would be difficult to provide a comparative evaluation of the techniques used, both because the varying requirements of hospitals dictate different solutions to the problem, and because of the difficulty of putting a cost on the non-quantifiable benefits involved. It is hoped, however, that this review is of use at least in presenting in one place information which could be used as a starting point for those interested in Master Indexes in health care.

7. ACKNOWLEDGEMENTS

The authors gratefully acknowledge the helpful comments of Miss B. Marshall, District Patient Services Planning Administrator, and the assistance of Mrs. H. Scarle during the preparation of this paper.

8. REFERENCES

1. Benjamin, B., (1977), Medical Records, Heinemann.
2. Bryant, J.R. and Fenlon, S.M., (1976), The design and implementation of an on-line name index, Proceedings of the Database Technology Conference, London.
3. Bradshaw-Smith, J.H., (1977), General practice record keeping using a real time computer, Proceedings of the MEDCOMP 77 Conference, Berlin.
4. Knuth, D.E., (1969), The art of computer programming, Vol. 3, Sorting and searching, p.p. 391-392, Addison-Wesley.
5. Acheson, E.D., (1967), Medical Record Linkage, Oxford University Press.
6. Martin, K.B., Scott, J.H., Angus, J. and Hopkins, R.T., (1976), The Tayside master patient index, The Tayside Health Board.
7. Department of Health and Social Security, (1977), Interim report on the evaluation of the National Health Service experimental computer programme.
8. Computer Evaluation Unit, Charing Cross Hospital, (1975), The microfiche master index.
9. Addenbrooke's Hospital Computer Evaluation Team, (1977), Master index second level (soundex) searches, A56.
10. Newcombe, H.B., and Kennedy, J.M., (1962), Record linkage making maximum use of the discriminating power of identifying information, Comm. of the ACM, 5, 563.

COMPUTERIZED SUPPORT OF ACTIVITIES AND IDENTIFICATION OF RELATED DATA IN KIEL KIS

G. Griesser and M. Jainz

Department of Medical Statistics and Documentation of the
Hospital of Christian-Albrecht-University Kiel, Germany
(Head: Prof. Dr. G. Griesser)

1. Hospital Activities

In a hospital environment each activity to be performed in care units, functional units, e.g. laboratory, X-ray department etc., or management is dedicated to distinct objects. In this context objects may be
- persons as individuals,
- persons as currently treated inpatients (cases),
- specimens taken from inpatients, radiographs etc.,
- physicians,nurses, paramedical personnel and managerial staff,
- payers (as a third party).

The problem to be solved is the unique assignment of activity to object and vice versa. Since more than one activity may be performed for one object at the same time, the many-to-one correspondence of activities to objects requires the unique identification of all activity and object related data. However, this problem of assignment has been discussed for many years,first in connection with medical record linkage (1,2). Yet due to the increasing application of computer-aided information systems in hospitals and the complexity of the information to be processed, the problem was becoming more and more urgent and serious. First of all the increased number of various records of data precludes the usual way of rather simply identifying items and their connection. This fact has led to highly complicated data structures like tree or plex structures. Using direct computer representations of these complex data structures necessitates the usage of sophisticated database management software. Those "Database systems run the danger of becoming cumbersome, inflexible, and problematic" (6).

Viewing the currently treated patient as a system,the patient oriented activities may be classified as system observing actions or system influencing ones, e.g. diagnostic or therapeutical measures respectively. The hospital stay of an inpatient may be viewed as a time series of patient-physician-encounters, named events,during which the patient's status is evaluated and possibly changed and which in turn may result in the initialization of further activities.

All other activities are of organisational, logistic or fiscal nature and comprise the efforts to enable the hospital to render the above mentioned services to the patient and to keep running the hospital as a system itself.

Activities occur in logically defined working areas and are delivered by the members of the
- care units
- medical staff
- functional units (laboratories, X-ray unit, operation theatre, physiotherapy etc.)
- management and administration.

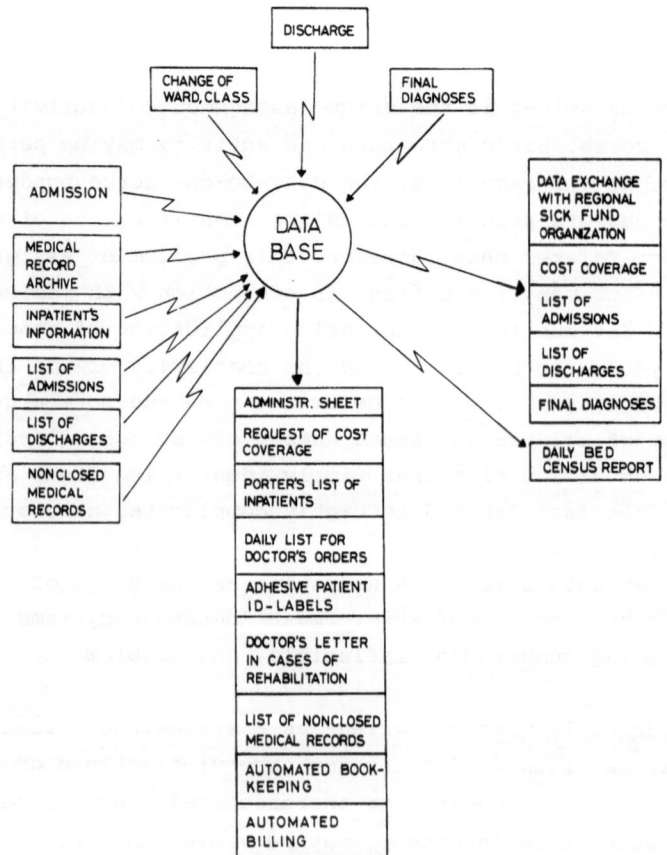

Figure 1: Supporting functions provided by KIEL KIS (5)

Although these theoretical considerations formed the starting point for the design of the information system of the Kiel University, we have to face the fact that only a rather limited number of the activities mentioned above can be directly performed by the operational hospital information system (HIS) itself. The majority of activities in a hospital are delivered by the personnel of the logically defined working areas. These activities can be only supported by the functions of a hospital information system in providing the acting persons with those information in edited format, that are needed for fulfilling their professional tasks.

Figure 1 gives a survey of the supporting functions provided by KIEL KIS in its current developmental phase to the departments of the University Hospital (4,5).

However this figure does not provide any insight into the interdependencies between working areas, activities, objects, which the activities are dedicated to, and data related to and needed for the performance of the functions.

2. Data Structure Model

The attempt to structure the patient oriented data led to the design of a logical structure model of medical data which was published by SAUTER et. al. and is shown by figure 2.

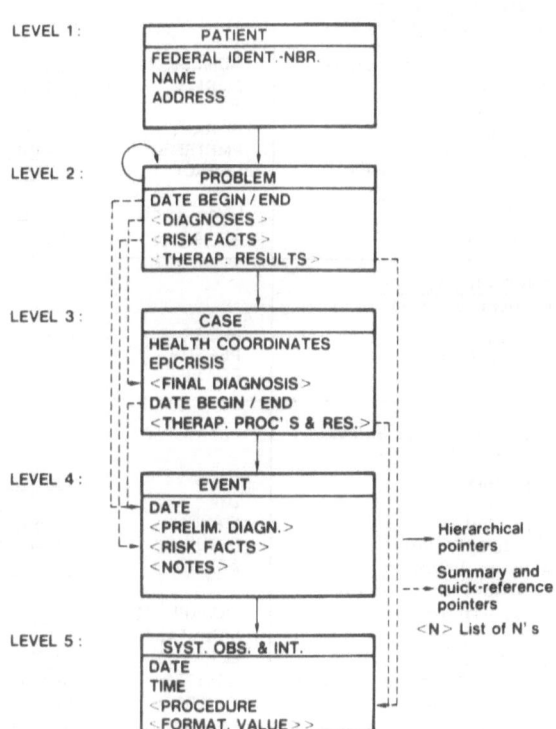

Figure 2:
Logical structure model of medical data (8).

In order to achieve insight into interdependencies mentioned in chapter 1, a cross-examination of the subjects mentioned above is necessary. A more detailed description of the data is given in table 1, where the database is depicted logically in the form of a relational data structure model. The degree of complexity of the relationships in our environment would lead to a description that would be similar to a highly entangled cobweb if the notions of tree or plex structures were applied. The main reasons for adopting the notions of relational databases are simplicity and clarity(3,6).For the same reason some relations have been simplified in their contents,especially the detailed information carrying items have been summarized as "Data". Additionally some types of relations like patient master record transactions and laboratory activities, which originally contain differently structured data items like testvalues, medical findings, notes, dates, have been put together under a common name. Compare figure 2 especially. The reason for this was to get a clear picture of the general overall structure of the database which otherwise would have been confused by too many details.

KIEL-KIS DATA BASE	RELATION	CONTENTS (keys underlined)
1.TEMPORARY PART (case-oriented)		
Admission-Serial-Number	ADMSER	DEPT, SER#
Patient-Master-Record, Fixed Portion	PMRFIX	ADMNO, PK, Name, Ward, Division, Data
PMR-Activity-Indicators	PMRACT	ADMNO, Activity Indicators
PMR-Transactions	PMRTRNS	ADMNO, TRTYPE, TRNS # Data
Laboratory-Activity-File	LABACT	ACT # LAB# WORKPL # ADMNO, Data
Laboratory-Activity-Serial-Number	LABACTSER	LAB#, SER #
Billing File	BILLS	BILL# Data
2.HISTORICAL PART (patient-oriented)		
PK-Serial-Number	PKSER	BIRTH, SER#
Patient-Register	PERSON	PK, Birth-Name, Risk-Factors
Former Case(s)	FCASE	ADMNO, PK, Data
3.ORGANIZATIONAL PART (resource-oriented)		
Department	DEPT	DEPT # Data
Division	DIV	DIV#, DEPT# Data
Care Unit	WARD	WARD #, DEPT #, Data
Functional Unit	FCTUNIT	FUNIT #, DEPT # Data
Activity Dictionary	ACTLEX	ACTTYPE, Data
Working-Place Activity-Cross-Reference	WORKPLACT	ACTTYPE, WORKPL #
Medical Staff	MEDSTAFF	EMPLOYEE #, DIV#, Data
Bed Census	BCENSUS	DEPT # WARD #, Data
Table of Costs per Activity	COSTTAB	ACTTYPE, PRICE, Data
Table of Payers	PAYERTAB	PAYERID, Data

Table 1: Database, its Relations and Contents

The model consists of three main parts, of which

- the temporary part (according to SCHNEIDER and BENGTSSON (7)) is oriented towards the current inpatients (case), and
- the historical part (7) towards individuals comprising all former cases per patient, whereas
- the third part describes the organization and the resources of the hospital for patient care.

WORKING AREA	1. ACTIVITY	2. OBJECT	3. SUPPORTING FUNCTION	4. RELATED DATA	5. KEYS
CARE UNIT	—	—	—	WARD	WARD ✦
	Preparation of Physician's Visit and Booking of Doctor's Orders	Case	Daily Visit List	PMRFIX PMRTRNS DEPT, WARD	ADMNO ADMNO, TRTYPE DEPT✦, WARD✦
	Labelling Specimens, Prescriptions etc.	Specimen Case	Adhesive Labels	PMRFIX	ADMNO
	Preparation of Lab-Specimens and Taking Specimens	Specimen	Preparative Reference-List for Lab-Tests	PMRFIX LABACT	ADMNO ACT✦
	Ordering Lab-Test	Case	Mark-Sensing Sheets	PMRFIX LABACT	ADMNO LAB✦, ACT✦
MEDICAL STAFF	—	—	—	MEDSTAFF	EMPLOYEE ✦
	Taking Medical History	Patient	Short Medical History	PERSON FCASE	PK PK, ADMNO
	Regarding Endangering Facts	Patient	Indication of Risk-Factors	PERSON	PK
	Message of Admission and Requirement of Cost-Coverage	Payer ADOSH	for ADOSH-Inpatients Automated Procedure	PMRFIX PMRACT	ADMNO ADMNO
	Doctor's Ward Round and Doctor's Orders	Case	Daily Visit List	PMRFIX PMRTRNS DEPT, WARD	ADMNO ADMNO, TRTYPE DEPT✦, WARD✦
	Decision on Lab-Results	Case	Cumulated Lab-Report	PMRFIX PMRTRNS	ADMNO ADMNO, TRTYPE
	Doctor's Letter for Rehabilitation	Company physician	Rehabilitation-Letter	PMRFIX PMRTRNS	ADMNO ADMNO, TRTYPE
	Documentation of Final Diagnoses and Endangering Facts	Case Patient	Discharge Diagnoses Entry Dialogue	PMRTRNS FCASE PERSON	ADMNO, TRTYPE ADMNO PK
	Message of Discharge and of Final Diagnoses	Payer ADOSH	for ADOSH-Inpatients Automated Procedure	PMRFIX PMRTRNS PMRACT	ADMNO ADMNO, TRTYPE ADMNO
	Closure of Medical Record in Due Time	Head-Physician	Auditing of Nonclosed Medical Records	PMRFIX PMRACT	ADMNO ADMNO

Table 2a: Interdependencies between Activity, Object, Supporting Function, Related Data and Keys for the Working Areas: Care Unit and Medical Staff.

WORKING AREA	1. ACTIVITY	2. OBJECT	3. SUPPORTING FUNCTION	4. RELATED DATA	5. KEYS
FUNCTIONAL UNIT (Laboratory)	—	—	—	FCTUNIT WORKPL	FUNIT✦ WORKPL✦
	Preparation of the Current Tasks	Specimen Case	Working-Place-Oriented Lists of Ordered Tests	LABACTSER LABACT PMRTRNS	LAB✦ SER✦ LAB✦, ACT✦ ADMNO, TRTYPE
	Separation and Labelling of Specimens	Specimen	Adhesive Labels	LABACTSER LABACT PMRFIX	LAB✦ SER✦ LAB✦, ACT✦ ADMNO
	Communication of Lab-Results	Medical Staff Specimen Case	Result-Entry Dialogue	LABACT ACTLEX PMRTRNS	ACT✦ ACTTYPE ADMNO, TRTYPE
	Writing Lab-Reports	Specimen Case	Cumulated Lab-Reports	LABACT PMRFIX PMRTRNS	ADMNO ADMNO ADMNO, TRTYPE
MANAGEMENT	Admission	Case Payer Patient	Admission Dialogue	PMRFIX PMRACT ADMSER PKSER	ADMNO ADMNO DEPT✦ BIRTH
	Requesting Cost-Coverage	Case Payer	Cost-Coverage	PMRFIX PMRACT	ADMNO ADMNO
	Change of {Payer Ward Class}	Case	Update Dialogue	PMRFIX PMRTRNS	ADMNO ADMNO, TRTYPE
	Examination of Bed-Occupancy	Case	Bed Census Report	BCENSUS	DEPT✦, WARD✦
	Discharge	Case Payer Patient	Discharge Dialogue	PMRFIX PMRTRNS FCASE	ADMNO ADMNO ADMNO
	Billing/Accounting	Payer	Automated Billing	PMRFIX PMRTRNS BILLS COSTTAB PAYERTAB	ADMNO ADMNO, TRTYPE BILL✦ ACTTYPE PAYERID

Table 2b: Interdependencies between Activity, Object, Supporting Function, Related Data and Keys for the Working Area: Functional Unit (Laboratory) and Management.

3. Relationships between Data and Activities

Tables 2a and 2b display the attempt of a systematic analysis of the
interdependencies mentioned above. For each working area, selected
activities are presented in connection with their dedicated objects
(columns 1 and 2). This is followed by the corresponding supporting
function provided by the information system (column 3). The final
columns 4 and 5 name the data,needed for the performance of the functions and their identifying keys.

Returning to the basic problem of the unique assignment of activities
to objects, tables 2a and 2b represent the means to identify
- objects,
- activities dedicated to those objects, and
- resources used to perform these activities in the
- various working areas.

The identification mechanism thus provided takes care of all types
of relationships, like one-to-many, many-to-one, many-to-many. As a
consequence the redundancy in data storage is limited to the provision of secondary keys for cross-referencing. Nevertheless the description given in this paper is only a logical model and does not
prejudice applicable techniques of physical storage. The peripheral
user should only identify the data he needs according to his knowledge, which means the externally known identifying keys. The aim of
the logical description in the user's view is clarity of the data ,
which should not be confused by describing access paths, i.e. how the
specific data items are retrieved in the database.

B i b l i o g r a p h y

1. ACHESON, E.D. (ed.) (1968) Record Linkage in Medicine.
              Livingstone, Edingburgh

2. ACHESON, E.D. (1968) Linkage of Medical Records.
              Brit.Med.Bull. 24, 206-209

3. CODD, E.F. (1970) A Relational Model of Data for Large
              Shared Data Banks.
              Comm. ACM. 13, 377-387

4. GRIESSER, G., (1976) Presentation and Use of Medical Basic
              Information in KIEL KIS
              In: van Egmond, J., P.F. de Vries-Robbé
              and H.A. Levy: Information Systems for Pa-
              tient Care.North-Holland, Amsterdam,

5. GRIESSER, G. M. JAINZ, H.-P. STRAACH and J.D. VOSS (1977)
             Kiel University Hospital Information System
             Proceed. MEDINFO 1977, North Holland,
             Amsterdam, pg. 1047

6. MARTIN, J. (1976)Principles of Data Base Management.
             Prentice-Hall, Englewood Cliffs, pg. 95 ff

7. SCHNEIDER, W. and S. BENGTSSON (eds.) (1975). The Application of
             Computer Techniques in Health Care, with
             Special Regard to Hositals.
             Comp. Progr. Biomed. 5, 171-249

8. SAUTER, K. (ed.), G. GRIESSER, M. JAINZ and W. SCHNEIDER (1976)
             A Data Structure Model for a Health
             Information System.
             Comp. Progr. Biomed. 6, 171-177.

COMPUTER SYSTEM FOR BLOOD DONORS MANAGEMENT

J. Vaqué
Sección de Informática
Ciudad Sanitaria de la Seguridad Social
Barcelona, Spain

INTRODUCTION

The object of this paper is to present the blood donor filing system, which is now functionning in two medical centers of the Social Security in Barcelona.

Each center has a blood bank which carries out the extractions from the voluntary blood donors. Each bank also has one or several mobile units which perform blood extractions in different firms, commercial centers and in towns or villages in the area.

As a whole, it is an informatic system supported by a central computer to which are connected the terminals situated in the respective blood banks. The computer operates on a time-sharing basis, a fundamental part of which is conversational, and can be used during the blood bank's working hours. At the present date the system has 24.000 active donors, and 32.000 donations are registered yearly. A large proportion of the said donations are carried out by sporadic donors who do not figure in the files of the active donors. Compared to other important informatic donor-control systems (1), this is a system of medium volume, but its consultation and updating conversational possibilities endow it with certain advantages in respect to the clasical batch systems (2).

ACTUAL PROBLEMS AND THE SOLUTIONS ADOPTED

Before establishing this system, the situation was the following:

- Each blood bank had a manual file with the demographic and medical information of its regular donors as well as that of the sporadic ones. But as a donor could (and can) present himself indistinctly at either one bank or the other, according to his personal preference, the two files very often contained repeated names.

- If a donor was rejected by one bank (because of a pathological case-history, sickness or arterial hypertension, etc.) the other bank might still keep him on as an active donor, as the information in one bank was not transmitted to the other. Likewise, the information of the donors from a firm or a town or village which has been obtained by one of the bank's mobile units, was not accesible to the other bank.

- At a given moment it may have been very important to rapidly obtain the list of a group of people with a given blood type and Rh factor, in conditions to perform a donation and ready to be called. Because of the faulty updating of the manual files, and due to the fact that the donors who had been called had just given blood at the other bank, the method used did not function at all well.

- There was a great overload of work in respect to making out the donor's identification papers and filing-cards, which were listed according to blood type, place of residence, printed matter and reports on the weekly, monthly and yearly donations, apart from different statistics, labels and remarks on merit.

- It was possible to foresee the immediate opening up of new blood banks with the same philosophy of performance.

And the following problem still exists:

- Due to the fact that a system for summoning donors does not exist, advantage is not taken of the extensive possibilities of obtaining blood, because the donors only present themselves spontaneously, and it is very likely that a year goes by without them having carried out a donation.

The aforementioned problems was solved in the following manner:

First stage:

- One and only central file of the donors was made, supported by the computer in one of the hospitals.

- Updating and consultation of the said file by means of terminals situated in the blood banks.

- Central information retrieval of the donors on the list, of reports, labels, statistics, etc.

- A one and only established rule of performance for the present and future blood banks. This stage has been funtionning since June,1977.

Second stage:

- A special file with three or four addresses and telephone numbers of donors likely to be called at any time of the day or night. This point requires a careful selection of the donors and of their information, and this is being carried out at present.

- Setting to work of the appointment scheduling system for donors. In Spain there is no blood bank that summons its members beforehand, which is why the establishing of a system of this kind requires careful planning and trial stages in order to test people's response. (This issue is under development).

- The question of a control of the stocks and an exchange of blood flasks from one bank to another presents no problem to either bank,

777

which is why no informatic intervention on its improvement or modification has been required.

METHOD USED

The computer which supports the application is a Univac 1106 that operates on a time-sharing basis. In each blood bank there is a terminal screen of cathodic rays, and a slow printer which in practice only allows for the emptying of the data on the screen.

The flow of information is the following:

If a person presents himself with the intention of giving blood at any one of the extraction centers, it is recorded whether it is the first time he is going to give blood, or whether on the contrary he has already done so before, the reason for this being that the information that must be obtained is different in each case. In the first case, the personal data of the individual will be taken down(christian and surnames, address, date of birth, etc.) according to a form designed for this purpose; on another sheit the date referring to the donation will be taken down (previous illnesses, weight, arterial tension, etc.). If the person is a regular donor, the second form only is made out, except in the case of modifications in the personal data (change of address, etc) which were recorded on the first form. Once the donations have been completed with the results of the blood test, the information is fed to the computer through the screen. This process generates the corresponding list of errors, as well as a report of the daily activity.

The blood donors are given a card that guarantee thet they are such, and they are asked to hand it in at the moment of the donation in order to obtain the donor's number (sequential number according to order of seniority) and to check the blood group and the Rh factor.Once in possession of the donor's number, a screen consultation is carried out, in which it is noted whether that particular donor is in conditions to perform a donation, or whether he is temporally or definitively disqualified. If the donor has not got his identification card with him at that moment a search by surnames is made in the Master File of Donors.

The mobile units whose fundamental job it is to perform extractions in partner firms they visit periodically, have at their disposal an up to date list of the donors belonging to the firms that they are going to visit on a given day; this list contains the medical information of the latest donation, together with other information of general interest.

In all cases, therefore, once the donor has been identified and the possibility of him giving blood confirmed, the extraction is then carried out, and the forms that have already been mentioned are filled in.

The blood donor's card is made out after the second donation, a pro-
provisional card being made out at the moment of the first donation
(sporadic donors). For legal reasons and also in the case of impossibility of consulting the computer (breakdown in the electric supply,
for example) each center has a file of all the donors with their personal data and donations they have performed (donors' book). Once a
month, the computer prints the identification cards of the donors who
have performed a second donation, or new ones for those who have mis-
laid theirs; it also prints the information of the new donors (donors control sheet), or those of regular donors whose personal data
is modified. These cards are produced in duplicate and a copy is sent
to each center. In this way both centers possess the same information
on any donor, and what is more, this information is up to date.

The computer produces, as well as the list of firms that was mentioned before, statistics, monthly and yearly donation summaries, and
the list of donors who have performed a given number of donations in
order to include them in the expressions of gratitude on behalf of
the Donors Organization. Also in the case of campaigns which are carried out in the towns and villages of the province, the computer do
prints letters addressed to those who gave blood in the previous cam-
paign, informing them of the date when the mobile unit will be in their town.

The system has two important files: the Master File of Donors that
has been mentioned, and the Donation File.

The Donors' File is a direct access file and the key of access is the
donor's number. Its initial creation presented certain difficulties.
It contains demographic and medical information of each donor. This
information was obtained from the manual files in the respective blood banks. Originally a manual selection was made, chosing the files
of donors who were really active, eliminating all donors who had not
given blood for two years, and those who had given blood inside that
period, but only once. The proportion of filed cards that were accepted in respect to all the existing cards was 40% approximately. However, a large number of these records corresponded to the same person, who had a given number in one bank and another number in the o-
ther bank.

The selected records were perforated and their data was fed into the
computer. Previously a filtering programme made it possible to highlight any error due to perforation. Another programme detected the
different donors with the same donor's number which corresponded to
the same medical center, and in the same manner the donation numbers
that were repeated (number given in sequential order from the first
of January of each year).

Once the previous stage had been carried out satisfactorily, on pro-
ceeded to detect the donors who had different numbers while being the
same person. The CIP (Internal Code for Access to the Population)was
created as a result corresponding to each donor, based on surnames,
sex, date and place of birth; with the CIP it was possible to group

together all donors with similar identifying data, for example, those with both surnames the same, and those whose dates of birth showed 80% identical digits, etc. The programme responsible for the operation produced a list in which figured the groups of donors likely to be the same person. According to this listing, it was decided manually which donors were one and the same person; in order to do this a document intended for perforation was made out, stating the Center and number of the donors that were to be united. Finally, we proceed, by means of another programme, to classify, according to the date of the first donation, all donors who had passed through the previous stages, and then to give a new number, stating with number 1, to each donor; the result of this whole process formed the Master File of Donors.

The Donations File contains information of all the donations carried out during the year, recording for each one the number of the corresponding donor and the date of the donation. The object of this file is to produce the periodic reports and the donation statistics, because if they were to be retrieved by reading through the whole donors' file, too much computer-time whould be consumed. Is a sequential-index file, classified by a code, result of applying a storage algorithm on the center code and the donation number. The inverse algorithm allow information retrieval of the same.

The Master File has a capacity allowing data storage of the five latest donations. The system have also other   files, among them: the CIP's File who make possible the quick retrieval of donors by surnames, sex and birth date, the Historic File of Donations, and the Free Numbers-Donors File who allow to assign the relative number to each new active donors.

The application is based on five Cobol Programme dhains:

Chain I: Intended for the initial creation of the donors' files.

Ch.   D: Performs the process of updating the donors' files and files related to the same.

Ch.   C: Contains the consulting programmes from terminal.

Ch.   L: Includes the programmes that performs listings of different kinds.

Ch.   U: It is a utility chain.

Apart from information retrieval, in interactive form, by the donors' number, by surnames and by the donation number, it is also possible to obtain screen information on a limited number (30-50) of donors in condition to give blood (of given blood type and Rh).

DISCUSSION

The system has proved to be effective, above all because it provides

autonomy to each blood bank. The banks know at any given moment the
exact situation of each donor and are conscious of the good or bad
quality of information registered in the master file; they are totally responsible for the same, as anybody unrelated to the blood
bank intervenes while information is being fed in the computer. It
has also signified an important alleviation by enabling voluminous
manual files to be got rid of.

Consultation, in this system, through the screens, is very simple
and is used as much by doctors as by nurses and hospital assistants;
in spite of which it is necessary to be very careful when introducing
data in order to update the files, and in each blood bank there is a
trained person to perform this operation.

The central production, in the computer center, of listings, which
are subsequently distributed, is a delicate part of the system because the listings cannot always be produced when needed (excess load
of central printer) and exterior delays never totally disapear.

The system as it has operated up to now is mainly orientated towards
a better management of the blood bank, allowing for information retrievals similar to the systems described by LUDWIG (3) and MOORE (4),
the costs and profits being the same as those refered to by these au-
tors. In each blood bank it has been possible to eliminate the labour
of one person.

In synthesis the objectives that have been reached are:

- Fusion of the donors of the blood bank, eliminating redundancy (repetition of data), by grouping all information on one donor, eliminating non-active donors, and by creating only one Master File of Donors.

- On line updating of the Master File and the related files.

- Fast access to a donor's information through conversational terminals.

- Retrieval of multifold reports and listings, which facilitates e
normously the work of the administrative staff of the blood bank.

- Automatic making up of the identification cards and the "donors'
control sheets".

- New blood banks are easy to connect to the system.

The next implementation of the appointment scheduling system of donors, and the creation of donors, and the creation of an emergency
donors' file, will allow for important progress to be made inside the
framework of what has been achieved so far.

REFERENCES

(1) CASSEMAR B. RAMGREN O. Ten years of an edp System for blood transfusion, Medinfo 1974, pp. 965-967.

(2) HALL P. Current status of the Karolinska Hospital Computer System, Hospital Computer Systems. Ed. Morris F. Collen, John Wiley & Sons, New York, 1974, p. 591.

(3) LUDWIG H.R. An interactive computer-based donor management system. Computers in Biology and Medicine, Vol. 5, Pergamon Press, 1975, pp. 69-76.

(4) MOORE R. A computer-assisted method to retrieve information about blood donors. Computers in Biology and Medicine. Vol.3, Pergamon Press 1973, pp. 63-70.

FEED-BACK IN AN OBSTETRIC DATA BASE

O.J.S. van Hemel[1], F. Schutte[2], J.H. van Bemmel[2] and A.M.M. Chang[3]

[1] St Hippolytus Hospital, Delft, The Netherlands
[2] Free University, Dept. Medical Informatics, Amsterdam, The Netherlands
[3] Siemens Nederland N.V., The Hague, The Netherlands

1 INTRODUCTION

As of 1972, in the Departments of Obstetrics of 11 clinics spread all
over The Netherlands, a co-operative project under the name GVR
(Gemeenschappelijke Verloskundige Registratie, i.e. Co-operative
Obstetric Registration) is being used which involves the coding and
processing of about 100 obstetric data for all deliveries preceded
by amenorrhea lasting 17 weeks or longer, a total of over 10,000
deliveries per year.
The degree of reliability of the recorded data determines for what
purposes the data can be used. Some examples of use are:
- *for scientific purposes*: an investigation into the effects of
  induced abortion on a subsequent pregnancy
- *to help set general European policy* : a study of the treatment and
  results of breech deliveries in The Netherlands
- *from the point of view of social obstetrics*: a comparison of the
  perinatal morbidity and mortality in different population groups in
  The Netherlands.
In this contribution attention will be paid to two feed-back mechanisms
having a positive effect on the reliability of the acquired data:
(i) a plausibility program and (ii) a computer-printed discharge
letter. Some examples of the contents of the data base are shown,
and implications of the GVR project are discussed.

2 ROUTINE DATA HANDLING

The daily routine in the 11 clinics and the data handling in the Dept.
of Information Processing of the hospital 'Onze Lieve Vrouwe Gasthuis'
(OLVG) in Amsterdam is shown in fig. 1.

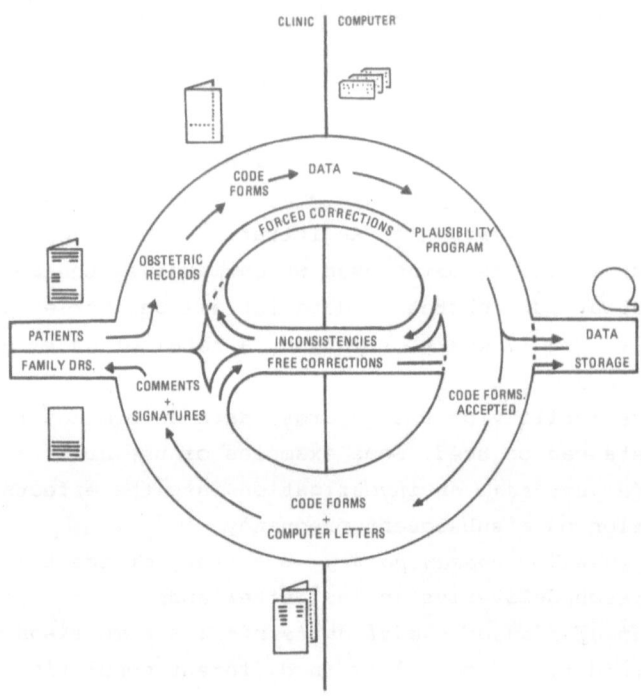

Fig. 1 Collection of obstetric data with feed-back mechanisms

During pregnancy, data are entered in a patient record. These data,
together with data on preceding pregnancies and the delivery, are
coded by the obstetrician on the special code form during delivery.
An example of part of this code form is given in fig. 2. Pages 1 and 2
are commonly used by all participating clinics. The lower part of
page 2, and page 3 are different for each clinic and contain data of
specific interest to the clinic involved.
After 7 x 24 hrs, taking into account perinatal mortality, the code
form is completed and sent to the OLVG, where the data are input in a
Siemens 4004-26 computer via punch cards at least two times per week.
The input data are verified by a plausibility program and when found
to be free of internal contradictions stored in the data base. The
code form, together with a computer-printed discharge letter for the

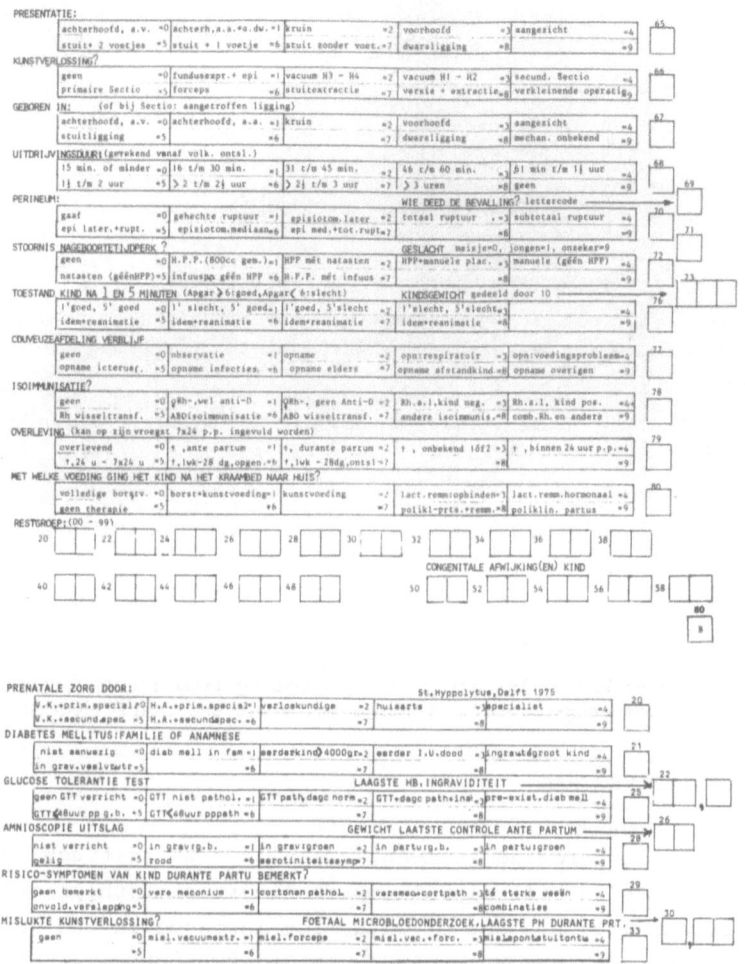

Fig. 2 Code form of the GVR system, page 2

general practitioner of the patient are returned to the clinic by
return mail. Data items, in which the plausibility program detects
improbabilities or even impossibilities are indicated and have to be
corrected by the obstetrician (fig. 1: *forced* corrections). Furthermore, comparison of the discharge letter with the medical record may
result in *free* corrections. These corrections are sent to the OLVG
and will be input as added data to the data base. The discharge letter
is appended with a conclusion and an advise, signed by the obstetrician,
and sent to the general practitioner. In this way, 5 days after discharge of the patient, this letter can arrive at the general practitioner. In fig. 3 a time-table of this obstetric data processing is
given. Compared to other systems, this time is relatively short:
Tuck et al. (1976) use 7–15 days, South and Rhodes (1972) about 24 days,
and Cope (1974) about 42 days.

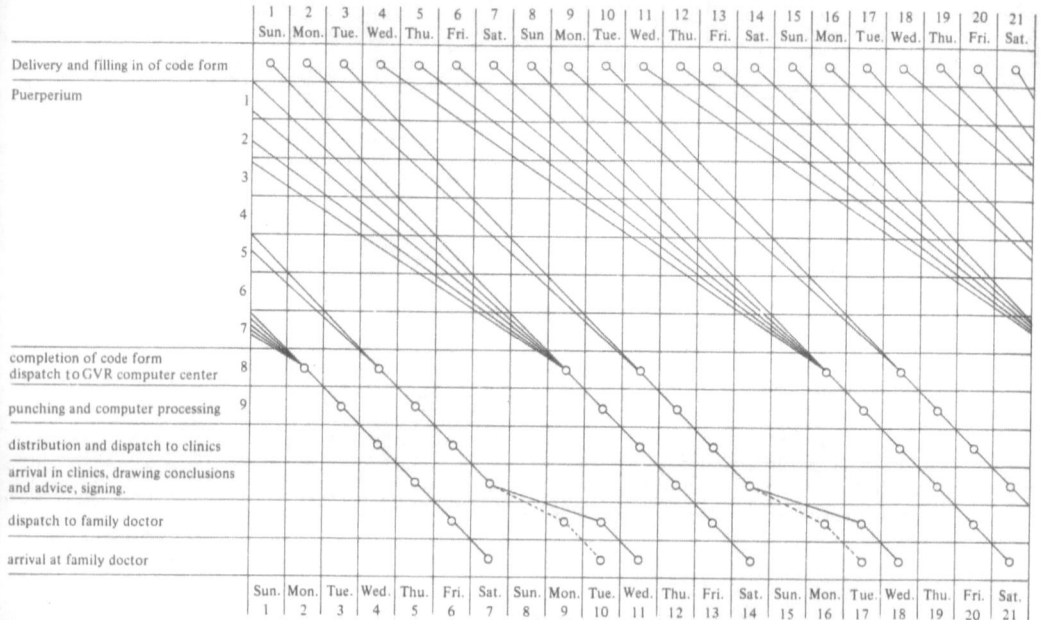

Fig. 3   GVR time-table of obstetric data processing from delivery up to arrival
of the computer-printed discharge letter at the family doctor

3 PLAUSIBILITY PROGRAM

By a plausibility program is meant a set of test instructions for the
computer so that it will signal improbable relationships or internal
contradictions within a set of data, for instance in the data of a
single patient. In the GVR project, about 60 checks are being carried
out. In fig. 4 the frequency distribution of reports from this
plausibility program applied to each of the approx. 15,500 patients
in 1974 and 1975 is given. The checks can be subdivided into 5
categories on the basis of the type of error being looked for:

1 *check on the correct interpretation of conventions and definitions*
   For example, if underdevelopment during pregnancy is noted, this
   may, according to the definition used, only be coded as 'negative
   discongruence' if there has also been fetal monitoring in the form
   of estrogen determinations in the 24-hr urine or cardiotocography.
   Checks of this type promote the standardization of concepts used.

2 *check on errors of observation and recording*
   A check on the coding of items as unknown on the code form when these
   items could have been known and probably also were known, such as
   the degree of dilatation at the time of active rupture of the

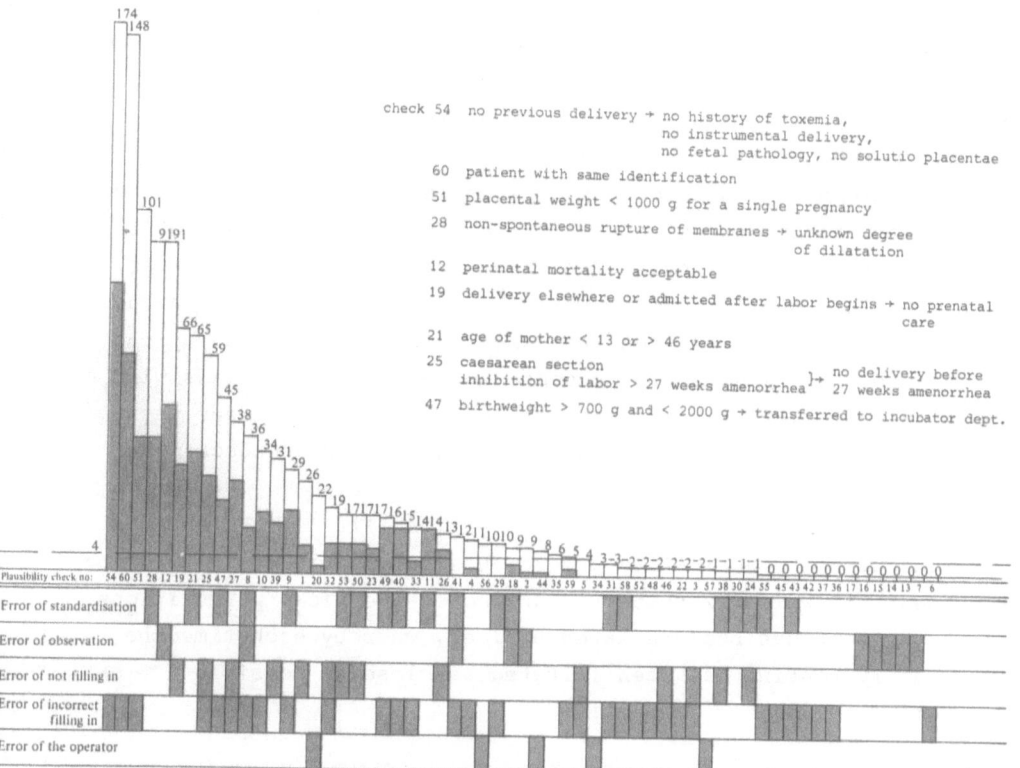

Fig. 4 The frequency distribution of reports resulting from 60 plausibility checks applied to approx. 16,000 patients in 1974 (grey) and 1975 (blank)

membranes. Pointing out the unjustifiable use of 'unknown' on the code form has a favorable effect on the observation and recording of such items.

3 *check on incomplete coding*

For example, failure to answer the question on survival of the child, or failure to enter the condition of the newborn infant as shown by the Apgar score. Each question should be answered with 1 out of max. 10 possibilities, 'no' and 'not applicable' included.

4 *check on incorrect filling out*

For example, data on the current pregnancy may be coded in the space on the code form allocated to the obstetric history (preceding pregnancies), and the coding of a caesarean section at a preceding pregnancy combined with the coding of a nullipara implies that either the coding of the section was done at the wrong location of the code form (should be this pregnancy) or that nullipara should be multipara.

5 *check on operating errors*

For example, the input of punch cards has been out of sequence.

In fig. 4 the checks are plotted in the order (left to right) of
decreasing frequency of error messages of the plausibility program.
The columns represent the absolute numbers of messages as a result of
the processing of data of 15,542 deliveries in 1974 (grey) and 1975
(blank). Forced corrections have been carried out in 1312 records, i.e.
in 8.4%. Checks with a frequency of 4 or less on these 15,500 records
may be replaced by more effective checks, unless the result of the
reported error is very severe for the integrety of the data base.
It is striking that per check the number of reported inconsistencies
during 1974 and 1975 has been the same. This can be caused by the fact
that a number of clinics are academic hospitals or hospitals with an
educational task: there is a flow of participating resident physicians.
In this way the plausibility program has a continuous educational
effect.
A similar percentage of improvement of reliability of the data as
generated by the plausibility program has been obtained in a coding
experiment, in which 72 obstetricians coded identical parturitions.
This experiment has been repeated 5 times, whereby each time the
normal daily routine has been imitated as close as possible
(Van Hemel, 1977).

4 COMPUTER-PRINTED DISCHARGE LETTER

In section 2 (fig. 3) it has been pointed out already that within 72
hrs after sending the code form to the computer center the obstetrician
receives a computer-printed discharge letter, based on the data input
from the code form. An example of such a discharge letter is given in
fig. 5.
It turns out that this feed-back mechanism has as much influence on
the reliability of the final data in the data base as the above
described plausibility program has. Alderson (1973) postulated this
mechanism as follows: forcing the coder to examine the stored data
makes him an interested party, which motivates him to accuracy. Subsequently, the accuracy of the stored data again determines how they
will be used, in the short run as part of a discharge letter and in
the long run for the drawing of statistical conclusions. Prerequisites
are (i) immediate processing of the code forms, having the output
available at the moment that a more conventional type of letter
should be typed anayway, and (ii) sufficient acceptation of the
computer-printed discharge letter for the recipient with respect to
readability and information contents.

CO-OPERATIVE OBSTETRIC REGISTRATION

ST.HIPPOLYTUS HOSPITAL DELFT

DEM

NOO

DATE OF DELIVERY:29-02-76

DELIVERY NO: 0154

DATE OF BIRTH: 23-07-46

MULTIPLE PREGNANCY, CHILD 2

```
*****        G E N E R A L        *****   *****        D E L I V E R Y        *****
BLOOD GROUP MOTHER B POSITIVE             AT AMENORRHEA OF 35 WEEKS + 1 DAY
AGE 29 YEARS                              CARDIOTOCOGRAPHY PERFORMED
BOOKED CASE (MEDICAL INDIC. ANTE PARTUM)  SURGICAL RUPTURE OF MEMBRANES
                                          CLEAR AMNIOTIC FLUID,RUPTURED 6-8 CM
*****      P A R T I C U L A R S     *****  MEMBR. RUPTURED LESS THAN 7 HRS (CERVIX)
VARICOSE VEINS                            PRESENTATION BREECH + 1 FOOT
DIABETES MELLITUS IN FAMILY               SPONTANEOUS DELIVERY
                                          BREECH DELIVERY
*****    GYN-OBST  H I S T O R Y    *****  2ND STAGE 15 MIN OR LESS(FULL DILAT=DEL)
GRAVIDA 2
PARA 2 (ALL DELVRS >16WKS AMEN,THIS INCL  *****     T H I R D  S T A G E     *****
1 PREMATURE DELIVERY (28-38 WKS AMEN)     SPONT PLAC DELIVERY,NO PPH OR I.V. DRIP
DATE PREVIOUS DELIVERY 15-11-73           PERINEUM INTACT
1 DYSMATURE CHILD, ALIVE, IN HISTORY      PLACENTA WEIGHT 1190 GR (EXCL MEMBR+CORD

*****       P R E N A T A L        *****   *****     P U E R P E R I U M      *****
REGULAR MENSTR, 28 DAYS, LMMP CERTAIN     LOWEST HEMOGLOBIN 13.7 GMX IN PUERPERIUM
LNMP 28-06-75                             HORMONAL LACTATION INHIBITION
HOSPITAL PRENATAL CARE FROM 18 WKS AMEN
TOTAL OF 17 WKS HOSPITAL PRENATAL CARE    *****       N E W B O R N         *****
PRENATAL CARE MIDWIFE,LATER OBSTETRICIAN  BOY
NORMAL GLUCOSE TOL.TEST IN PREGNANCY      APGAR 1' POOR, 5' GOOD;NO RESUSCITATION
LOWEST HEMOGLOBIN IN PREGNANCY 12.0 GMX   TRANSFER TO INCUBATOR DEPT,SEE OTHERDATA
BODY WEIGHT 68 KG AROUND 20 WKS AMEN      BIRTH WEIGHT 2300 GRAMS
HEIGHT 187 CM                             BLOOD GROUP NEWBORN B POSITIVE
DIASTOLIC PRESSURE:MAXIMUM 75 MM OR LESS  BIRTH WEIGHT 25-75%-TILE KLOOSTERMAN
MAX WEIGHT GAIN IN 1 WK 700-799 GRAMS     -PEDIATRIC CONSULTATION
LABOR INHIBITION AFTER 27 WEEKS AMEN      LIVE CHILD, 7x24 HRS POSTPARTUM INCL
ADMISSION TO HOSPITAL DURING PREGNANCY
ESTROGEN  ESTIMATION PERFORMED
```

C O N C L U S I O N   A N D   A D V I C E

Dear colleague,

One dysmature child in history, no diabetes of pregnancy found.
Twinpregnancy, admission for premature labor.
35 weeks: 1. girl, 2460 gram, vertex presentation, apgar score good,
           2. boy, 2300 gram, breech presentation, apgar score good.
Mother discharged 7th day, blood pressure 120/80.
Pediatrician's discharge letter follows.

Yours sincerely,

O.J.S. van Hemel,
obstetrician & gynecologist

Fig. 5   Example of a computer-printed discharge letter

The GVR concept fullfills the first requirement (cf. fig. 3). The
second one has been investigated by sending a questionnaire to 578
general practitioners, who on a regular basis receive computer-printed
discharge letters. A total of 324 reactions (i.e. 56%) have been
received; 62% of those GP's (N=201) completely read both discharge
letter and conclusion and advise. From these 201 GP's 43% prefers this
method of reporting, whereas 26% has an indifferent opinion whether to
prefer this method of reporting or a conventionally typed discharge
letter. This can be seen as a degree of acceptation of 69%.
Of the 38% (N=123) receivers who only read the appended conclusions
and advise, 18% prefers this concise report, and 28% has an indifferent
opinion, resulting in a degree of acceptation of only 45%.
Tables 1 and 2 give the reasons why the computer-printed discharge
letter was considered to be poorer or better than the conventional
discharge letter.

	Total N=109 %	Readers of contents+summary N=54 %	Readers of summary only N=55 %
POORER, because			
READABILITY			
difficult to read	28	26	27
unclear presentation	26	28	24
impersonal	15	20	9
unreadable	8	4	13
readable at the cost of much energy/time	5	7	4
poor typography and structure	4	4	5
less clear	3	4	2
boring	2	2	2
INFORMATION			
irrelevant information	5	5	5
too much information	4	–	9

Table 1   Reasons why the computer-printed discharge letter was considered to be poorer than the conventional discharge letter

	Total N=87 %	Readers of contents+summary N=71 %	Readers of summary only N=16 %
BETTER, because			
READABILITY			
better organized presentation	18	18	12
clearer	6	7	–
less time needed	3	3	6
easy to read	1	3	6
INFORMATION			
more information	37	40	32
more complete information	13	8	32
uniform information	10	10	12
relevant information	7	8	–
more complete and with better contents	5	6	–

Table 2   Reasons why the computer-printed discharge letter was considered to be better than the conventional discharge letter

5 OBSTETRIC DATA BASE

In this section, the frequency distributions of two items of the GVR data base, being essentially independent of the individual policies of the clinics involved and none of which affected by more than one variable, are presented graphically. In these graphs, the results of three years are superimposed, each with its own line of symbols. In connection with the low frequency in the extremes of these distributions, these could only be visualized by adjusting the scale. The results are shown in terms of the percentage of the total number of deliveries per clinic.

For clinics no. 1-11, inclusive, the total number of deliveries can be grouped into four classes:

deliveries per year:	ca. 250	ca. 500	ca. 750	ca. 1000
clinic no.:	1 + 2	3	4[1]	5 - 11[2]

[1] data available only for 1973 and 1974
[2] for clinic no. 8 data are available only for 1975

5.1 *Age*

The age of the mother at the time of delivery is not filled out by the coder but is calculated by the computer from the patient's date of birth and the date of delivery. Fig. 6 shows, for each of the 11 clinics, the frequency distribution of this item for the years 1973 - 1975.

It can be seen that those clinics with approx. 1000 deliveries per year all show a good resemblance in the age distribution. The differences can be explained in part by the regional composition of the population and by the location of the clinic in relation to an academic hospital.

For the age groups below 17 and above 39 years, the vertical scale has been magnified 10-fold. In addition, the figure shows the absolute number of patients per clinic over the three-years period.

It turns out that the number of patients below 17 years of age in clinics with approx. 1000 deliveries per year show definite differences from clinic to clinic: a total of 42 patients in 3 years in clinic no. 5 compared to 3 patients in clinic no. 8. These marked differences are not due to the reliability of the data, but are plausible since they can be explained in part by the ethnic composition of the population around the clinic. The data of the GVR reveal appreciable differences in ethnic composition of the patient population between some of these clinics.

As far as the number of patients older than 39 years in the larger clinics is concerned, it turns out that these are all fairly comparable: from 30 patients in 3 years in clinic no. 8 to 38 patients in clinic no. 9. The two exceptions (clinic no. 7 and 11) can be explained by a different composition of the patient population resulting from the presence of a university hospital in the district.

Apparantly, the referring midwives and family doctors consider a delivery at an age of 40 years or over to be something pathological, while an age below 17 years is looked upon as physiological. The plausibility program checks on patient's ages of less than 14 years or more than 45 years at the time of delivery. These threshold values are also shown in the figure (the dashed vertical lines). Referring to fig. 4(21) we can conclude that the data of approx. 100 deliveries in 3 years were sent back to the originating clinic to be reviewed. From fig. 6 we see that only 9 of these patients remained after review and were entered

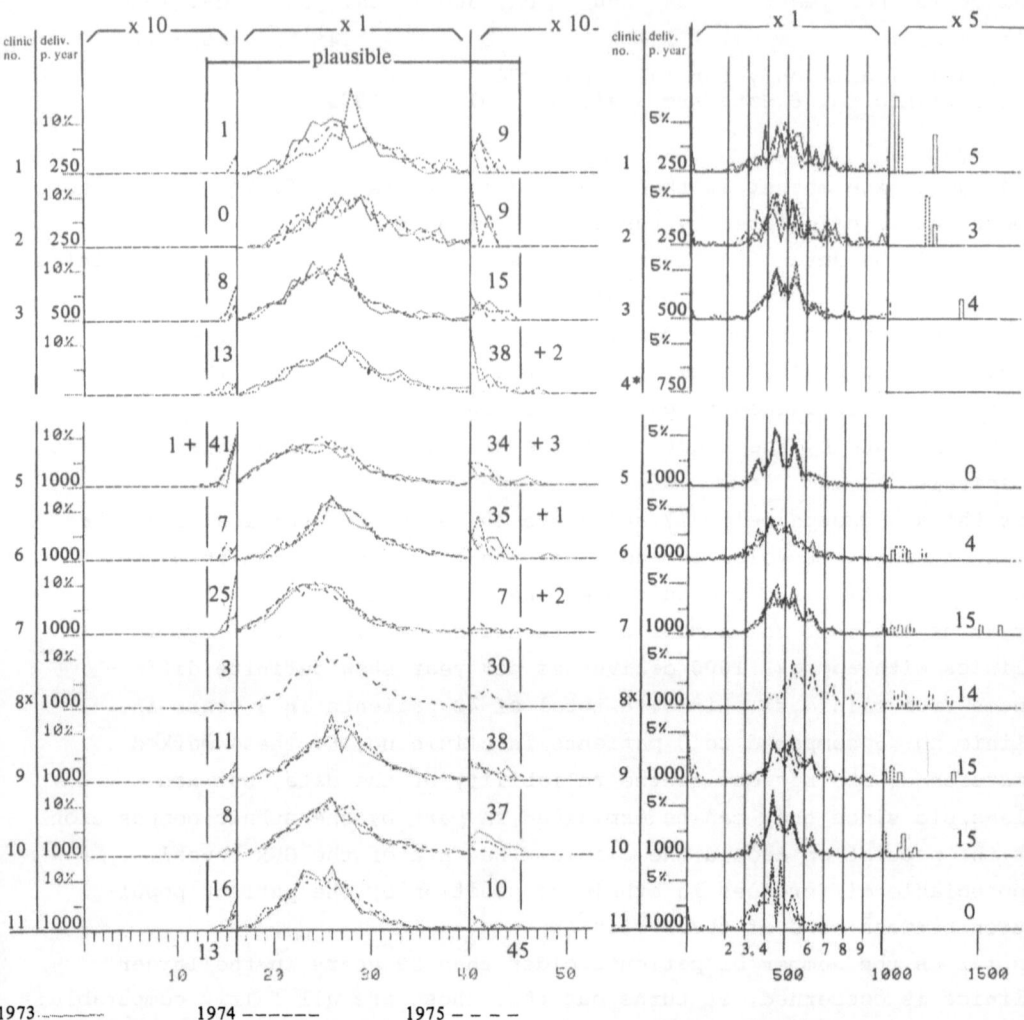

Fig. 6 Frequency distribution of the patient's age

Fig. 7 Frequency distribution of the net placental weight

recorded over 3 years from 11 clinics with a total of approx. 23,000 patients

into the data base with the originally indicated age, thus yielding a ratio of 1:10.

5.2 *Placental weight*

The placental weight, i.e. the net weight, without umbilical cord and membranes, can be coded immediately post-partum. Fig. 7 shows a graphic representation of the distribution of the net placental weight in each of the 11 clinics over the years 1973 - 1975. In view of the low frequency of weights above 1000 grams, the scale has been magnified 5-fold in this range. To the right of the plausibility threshold,

above 1000 grams, there are 81 placental weights, 21 of which are from
a single pregnancy. These weights could only be entered into the data
base on the second attempt, after review.

The figure also shows the absolute number of placentas weighing more
than 1000 g in each clinic. It is striking that this number is about
15 in 4 of the 6 larger clinics. All the clinics show a consistent
pattern from year to year. Certain clinics show a distinct maximum at
certain placental weights during each of the three years: for weights
of 450, 550 and 650 g in clinics no. 3, 5, 7, 8, 9 and 10. This
phenomenon is most obvious for clinic no. 5. This presumably is to be
explained by inaccurate weighing of the placenta.

6 IMPLICATIONS OF THE GVR SYSTEM

An operational GVR system has various implications which can be ordered
along a time scale. A summary of the implications of such use over a
period of days, approx. one year, several years and many years is given
in table 3. The advantages of using the GVR system in this way will
be discussed in this final section.

Time	Use	Implications
days	1. Plausibility reports	o forced corrections o education
	2. Computer-printed discharge letter	o free corrections o extramural communication o standardization
approx. one year	3. Annual statistics per clinic	o information about the preceding year o local management on the basis of annual trends
several years	4. Follow-up of children	o epidemiology of congenital mal- formations o evaluation of perinatal morbidity o obstetric policies
	5. Periodic coding	o revision of the code form o revision of the plausibility program
	6. Peer review	o analysis of comparable samples
many years	7. Research	o advice as to obstetric policies o indications for directed scientific research

Table 3   Implications in time of an operational GVR system

re 1 and 2: *Error messages and computer-printed discharge letter*
The feed-back mechanisms of error messages from the plausibility program and the computer-printed discharge letters lead to corrections in
the data on approx. 15% of all recorded deliveries. In addition to
their correcting effect, the forced corrections resulting from the
error messages also have a continuing educational influence.

As can be concluded from sections 3 and 4, the computer-printed discharge letters play a role in extramural communication. Since the text
of these letters also contain definitions, this form of communication
also has a standardizing effect.

The reliability can also be improved by still further increasing the
rapidity of communication. By sending in the initial data immediately
after delivery, followed by additional information on the puerperium
and neonatal period on the 8th day post-partum, the currency of the
information is improved and the number of days between discharge and
availability of the discharge letter is reduced. This can be achieved
by using an interactive terminal for the input of the data.

re 3: *Annual statistics per clinic*

A comparison, from year to year, of the frequency of occurence of
certain pathological findings or of the use of certain methods of
treatment within a clinic, of the data on perinatal and maternal
mortality and morbidity, can result in a more detailed analysis or even
in timely modifications in the procedures. The possibility of direct
access to the stored data at any desired moment results in more
frequent use of these data. The routine surveys which are presented
regularly result in a need for answers to specific questions on the
basis of the stored data. The creation of a direct possibility for
posing such questions favors the analysis of the policies in the
clinic concerned. This type of use is therefore also an argument in
favor of the use of an interactive terminal.

re 4: *Follow-up of children*

Rapid feed-back in connection with an increased incidence of congenital
malformations can lead to the timely detection of teratogenic
influences. Significant results can probably only be expected with
active participation of pediatricians for the retrospective entry of
data on subsequently discovered congenital defects. By making it
possible to study the results of follow-up of a large number of
children in relation to standardized data on the corresponding deliveries, well-founded modifications can be made in obstetric policies.

re 5: *Design of the GVR system*

In the future, a periodic coding test will be necessary to make
possible a continual evaluation of the reliability of the data of the
GVR system. Meanwhile, attention can be given to the following:
- improvement of the design of the code form,
- introduction of new plausibility checks, and
- revision of the lay-out of the computer-printed discharge letter.

re 6: *Peer review*

In section 5, attention was directed at the striking consistency, within each clinic, in the frequency distribution of some quantifiable and measurable items in each of the three years investigated, while there was significantly less agreement between the various clinics. Peer review can therefore not be carried out on the basis of a comparison of the over-all results from different clinics. It should become possible, however, after a period of several years, to select certain groups of patients per clinic on the basis of a large number of criteria which have been fed into the computer and thus attempt to form comparable groups. Terminologically speaking, the expression *peer review* is preferred to *medical audit* since the latter refers to a type of evaluation which can seem threatening to the doctors concerned. Whenever the providers of the information begin to feel threatened, then a decrease in accuracy of the data submitted must be expected due to bending of the truth.

re 7: *Research*

Those data of the GVR system which are to be used for scientific research must meet the highest standards of accuracy in the way in which they reflect the clinical reality. A number of types of data can meet such standards. For example, the percentile distribution of the birth weights corresponding to a predetermined duration of pregnancy, divided by Kloosterman (1970) into data for boys and girls from primiparae and multiparae, respectively, could well be revised periodically on the basis of GVR data. When using such quantitative data, however, one must constantly keep in mind that they are derived from hospital deliveries. On the basis of the curves showing the composition of the obstetric patients (cf. fig. 6), an evaluation can be made as to in which clinics the patients are more or less representative of obstetrics in The Netherlands as a whole. On the basis of the results of such a study, all of the items which have not been investigated must be examined carefully to determine whether they can be used directly for scientific conclusions or whether they are only suitable for deriving indications for prospective investigations.

CONCLUSION

In conclusion, the implications of the operational GVR obstetric data base system on the reliability of coding, extramural communication and standardization, local medical policies, the epidemiology of congential abnormalities and the evaluation of obstetric policies in relation to perinatal and maternal morbidity and mortality have been discussed as a function of time.

On the basis of this discussion, it is clear that feed-back mechanisms are very important, as there are the plausibility checks and the computer-printed discharge letter, both for individual patient care and, on a long-term basis, for the formation of obstetric policies. With regard to the GVR system, it is clear that any registration system must be continuously adjusted within a constantly changing system of health care as a function of an ever clearer insight.

REFERENCES

Alderson, M.R. (1973): Medical information systems and computer. Roma, Seminar Computer Applications in the Field of Medicine

Cope, I. (1975): Five year's experience with regional computer-based obstetric records in Sydney and Melbourne; Journ. Clin. Comp. 3,6,441-467

Kloosterman, G.J. (1970): On intra-uterine growth; Int. Journ. Gyn. and Obst. 8,895-912

South, J. (1971): Computer services for obstetric records; Brit. Med. Journ. 4,32-35

Tuck, C.S. (1976): The use of a computer in an obstetric department; Brit. Journ. Obst. and Gyn. 83,2,97-104

Van Hemel, O.J.S. (1977): An Obstetric Data Base - human factors, design and reliability; thesis Free University Amsterdam

REPLICABLE, MULTI-PURPOSE PATIENT INDEX SYSTEMS -

AN ANALYSIS OF SOME NECESSARY FEATURES

A.R.Wills
Chief Systems Designer
The London Hospital
(Whitechapel)

1. Introduction

Numerous situations arise in the health-care field when information about
a patient is stored, and subsequently retrieved or added to. It is then
imperative to devise a reliable mechanism for discovering any existing
record for a patient, every time new information is to be stored for
future reference. With files containing details for several thousand or
more patients, a local record number is usually allocated to each patient,
to assist in the practical problems of distinguishing between people with
a similar or identical name, and to provide a compact and reliable
cross-reference to the record for most day-to-day purposes. However, one
cannot entirely avoid the need to discover the local record number, based
only upon imprecise information about the identity of the patient; a
"patient index" is the usual basis for this task.

When a specialist hospital department wishes to build up a register of
patients with information relevant to that discipline, it is convenient
to base their register upon patient identity as defined in a more widely
applicable index, most frequently the index to hospital case-notes
maintained by the hospital's Medical Records department (Assoc.Clin.
Path; Caville; Wills). In the United Kingdom, such specialist
departments increasingly provide services on an Area or Regional basis,
whereas hospital case-notes are managed on a single-site or District
basis.

There is therefore a need to develop index systems that are more
appropriate to the needs of the developing health services. Such systems
should be designed to be appropriate in differing situations and
locations, should provide for real-time interrogation and updating, and
should be capable of supporting a wide variety of possible record systems.
Indeed they should not even be specific to patients, as there are
similar problems in personnel management.

Above all, such systems must be adaptable, so that they can be
effectively modified to meet new requirements and types of usage. The
file design and programs should also be straightforward to implement
effeciently on differing types of computer hardware and file management
software.

2.   Problems with existing Patient Indexes

The London Hospital(Whitechapel) has been using a Patient Index system on
a Computer since 1972, and is now introducing a more extensive index,
capable of supporting a District-wide case notes system. Experience has
highlighted many problems including those listed below.

2.1.   The reliability of information

i)   Few, if any, of a patient's details can be regarded as
absolutely permanent, accurate and reliable.

ii)   The record number allocated to case notes for a patient
attending a hospital is more reliable than personal
details, but not entirely foolproof.

iii) Record numbers are rarely quoted in more than 70% of
service requests for patients in hospital.

iv)   A patient sometimes receives more than one record
number. Occasionally the same number may be re-used
for a different patient!

v)   Temporary registrations may be issued(e.g in
Casualty) which may need merging with a pre-existing
registration.

vi)   Any identification details may be mis-quoted or
missing, including registration number and even
surname.

2.2   Technical complications

i)   Simple alphabetic searches based on surname may be
adequate if the index has up to 50,000 entries. Most
complete operational indexes have between 500,000 and
1,500,000 entries, requiring a much more sophisticated
approach to the selection of entries which closely
match the details available. This is to reduce the
search to a manageable number of alternatives,
without overlooking entries which may well include the
one required.

ii) Different cultural groups classify and combine a person's name in a variety of radically different ways.

iii) Many specialist service departments seek to relate new findings with previous investigations for the same patient. They frequently maintain their own indexes and filing systems, multiplying the problems of inaccuracy and out-of-dateness.

iv) The scope and activities of specialist departments vary with time, and new departments are always forming. The pattern of health care is also changing rapidly, notably in the relationships between the basically independent groups for care through hospitals, general practitioners, dentists, community and social services.

v) There is no national U.K.policy as yet to define a standard for patient details, and there have been many diverse attempts to design index systems for specific application areas(FPC, hospital registration, laboratory records, etc.).

vi) Modern technology makes it simple to provide access to a centrally-maintained index of identified patients from a considerable number of specialised application areas. However, as soon as the "outstation" tries to add further patients or amend the details stored, complications can arise.

vii) "Outstations" usually want to file data from their own records against patient details. Complications arise when the reference copy of patient identification details is amended, especially Surname or Registration number.

viii) Many "outstations" in their records system need to include patients who are not on the reference index.

ix) "Outstations" require an absolutely reliable back-reference to the index on which they depend, if any sort of computer assistance is to be provided for their record-keeping.

There have been many studies into the most reliable items and combinations of items of information for establishing unique identity (e.g.Leguit); this paper instead concentrates on the principles and characteristics of an index suitable for use in a wide variety of specialist applications, considering particularly the evolving National Health Service.

3.   Advantages in using Computers

i)   The avoidance of mis-filing, which in a card file often results in entries being missed during a search. The card may have been placed in the wrong section of the file, or not returned to the file.

ii)   The ease with which changes to key items of information can be notified to specialist departments, to assist their own records management procedures.

iii) The possibilities for easy reproduction of the index for key users,for instance by producing microfiche copies or enabling remote computer terminals to interrogate the index directly. Real-time computer systems offer additional advantages, including the following.

iv)   Validation checks on the information as it is being submitted during the registration procedure. Registration can often take place when the patient is by the terminal operator, so queries can then be resolved immediately.

v)   The ability to enforce firmer control over the issue of fresh case-notes folders, in most cases avoiding duplicate registrations for the same patient and issue of the same record number to more than one patient.

vi)   The ability to update any peripheral files which contain copies of the key patient details(name, age, case-notes number, etc.) automatically, following authorised amendment of the patient index.

vii) The potential for completely reliable cross-references between the files for specialist departments and the central index, for functions such as the maintenance of cumulative laboratory reports.

4.   Particular Features of commonly used types of Patient Index

   4.1   Hospital Case Notes

      i)   A policy not to remove entries in the index, even after
            the death of a patient. Though the notes themselves may
            be culled and microfilmed after a period, the
            registration remains, and the notes may be reviewed from
            the archive. The only permitted deletion of entries on
            the index is when duplicate registrations or other
            errors are being corrected, by Medical Records staff.

     ii)   The typical size of index for a large teaching
            hospital is 1.2 million registrations growing at the
            rate of 35,000 per year (DHSS,1). A sizable pro-
            portion of patients (10% - 60%) may come from outside
            the Area which covers the local population.

    iii)   There are moves towards a pooled case-notes system
            within the Health District, where hospitals will use
            case-notes from other sites if the patient has
            previously been registered there, returning the notes
            to the place of registration on completion of the
            treatment episode.

            A combined hospitals index for the whole District will
            then be required, with provision for more than one
            registration for each patient.

            A complication is that case-notes numbers used in diff-
            erent hospitals sometimes overlap,so that the same number
            may refer to different patients, depending on the
            hospital of registration.

     iv)   Specialist service departments have traditionally used
            case-notes numbers as the key to their own records
            system. Such departments include Blood Tranfusion,
            Histopathology, Obstetrics, E.E.G.

            The possibilities for error within the department's own
            records system increase, as the service extends to cover
            more hospitals.

4.2   Specialist Medical Records

Numerous clinical specialties keep their own registers of patients, to aid functions such as the following:

a)   Re-call of patients to monitor treatment or check against recurrence of the condition

b)   To highlight the relevant features of the cumulative clinical record before subsequently examining the patient

c)   To facilitate the analysis of the records and the automated production of discharge summaries, statistics, etc.

Departments which act in this way include:

Diagnostic Radiology

Obstetrics

E.E.G

Intensive Therapy

Diabetic subsection of Metabolic Medicine

Bladder cancer

Cardiac (Pacemakers)

Features of such systems relevant to Patient Indexes include:

i)   Most or all patients are registered locally for case-notes, and so the specialist records can be filed according to case-notes number, avoiding the need for a separate patient index. If necessary, a supplementary file of records for unregistered patients, such as minor casualties for X-ray, is maintained alphabetically by patient.

ii)   Apart from Radiology, most such systems require files containing a few hundred to several thousand entries.

iii)   To give benefits to the people who record the information, the main emphasis of such systems is to aid the handling of the current live group of patients under treatment. Research and statistics are useless if the information is not accurate and reasonably complete, and this will only be so if the staff doing the data recording receive and acknowledge positive benefits from the procedure. This applies to accurate identification of the patient, as well as clinical data in the record.

4.3   Blood Transfusion Indexes

    i)   A local hospital index may be kept, with an entry for each patient who has had an Antibody Screen, and a note of any transfusion or cross-matching problems the laboratory becomes aware of. Features of this index are:

            a)   Only patients with a local set of case-notes are included, and case-notes number is used in conjunction with patient name to ensure 'identification' is correct at every stage. Laboratory staff often obtain blood specimens from patients themselves, in order to make absolutely sure that no mistakes are made.

            b)   Only current live patients are required on the index, as its primary function is to provide information when subsequent blood transfusion is being prepared for.

            c)   It is desirable to be able to highlight key items of information e.g. Haemophilia, on the normal Case-Notes Index.

    ii)   Local registers of patients with particular conditions requiring repeated transfusions of whole blood or blood products. These registers may be maintained by the Haematology Department, which is responsible for both the treatment of the patient and the running of the local Transfusion Laboratory. The registers are also used for tasks such as the management of stocks of specialist blood products. It is necessary for such patients to be suitably highlighted on the local laboratory index i above.

    iii)   Regional indexes of patients such as those in ii above.

    iv)   Regional indexes to donors which form the basis for such tasks as re-call for further donations.

     v)   Regional indexes to units of blood, noting their issue, re-use and any subsequent processing. There may be a call to link these records to donors and/or recipients of the units or subsequent blood products.

4.4   Pathology Indexes

i)   Most teaching laboratories will maintain an index to
        Histological sections exhibiting cancerous or other
        abnormalities. These indexes are usually held according
        patient name, so that previous slides may be re-examined
        during the subsequent investigations for a patient. To
        aid teaching and epidemilogical investigations, there is
        also a call to maintain a second index, based on a
        classification of the slide, such as the S.N.O.P.code.
        Because of the research uses, these indexes also are
        ever-growing, as they do not refer solely to the current
        population.

ii)   There are moves towards registers at Area or Regional level
        for Cytology. It would be medically desirable to combine
        such indexes with Histology ones, or at least make them
        readily accessible, as positive findings are very relevant
        to many cases. It is thought that Cytology indexes should
        be specific to the current live population, rather than a
        permanent, ever-growing file.

iii)   Many other types of laboratory also maintain indexes by
        patient name, to form the basis of cumulative records
        (Cavill).

iv)   A national cancer register is also being compiled.
        In many of these situations, there is a need to provide
        effective recall and remainder facilities, so that treatment
        can be monitored or recurrence of the condition looked for.
        One of the difficulties here is that the laboratory does
        not usually have direct contact with the patient; the
        identification details available are often just those
        written on a request form, and hence may be incomplete,
        or contain errors.

4.5   Family Practitioner Committee Indexes

i)   There is a central N.H.S. Register, used to manage the issue of N.H.S.numbers to the population nationally, and also to act as a clearing-house when members of the public transfer to a General Practitioner under a different Area Health Authority.

     Obviously this register is vastly larger than those of the size being considered in this paper. However, it would appear that a proportion of entries at the Area level (ii below) do not include N.H.S. number (Bussey, A.); this should be obtainable from the national register if it is requested.

ii)   At the Area Health Authority level a number of indexes and registers are maintained, covering the current, live population, so far as health-care is concerned. The two main indexes are the "Nominal Index", with an entry per live, registered member of the public, resident in the Area, or on the list of G.P in the Area, and a "Medical Register" which lists the patients registered under each General Practitioner who practices in the Area (DHSS,2).

     Some particular features of the Nominal Index are:-

a)   The size is between 0.5 and 2.0 million entries.

b)   Entries are deleted from the index if the person dies or moves from the Area, or comes under alternative medical care e.g on joining the Armed Forces.
It is quite possible that the entry for a person may be re-created, if they are subsequently re-registered with a GP in the Area. This has important implications for any case-notes or other cumulative records systems which may be linked with or based upon an Area Index.

c)   Each year about one third of the entries in the index are modified in some respect.(Addition, deletion, amendment)

d)   In many city areas there is a high immigrant population, causing extra doubts about the correctness of the identification.

e)   Although Dentists, Opticians and Pharmacists are also paid
       via the F.P.C., payment is on a "services provided" basis;
       the above registers are maintained specifically for
       General Practitioners, who receive a "capitation" fee.

A Plan for Progress in the use of Computer-based Indexes

5.1.   Where are we now?

Indexes based on patient names are currently operated to assist
in the following main types of situation.

   i)   National registers, which are beyond the scope of
          this paper.

   ii)   Specialist sub-groups of the <u>current live</u>
          population, including Blood donors, patients
          who happen to have investigations of a
          particular type, and patients under treatment
          by a specialist department.

   iii)   Reasonably comprehensive population registers,
          managed on an Area basis, for between 0.5 and 2.0
          million inhabitants. These are specifically for
          the <u>current live population</u>, and their total size
          is fairly static.

   iv)   Case-notes systems in hospitals, which currently
          grow continually and include a proportion of
          registrations for patients which do not and
          never have been resident in that Health Area.
          Such systems typically include between 0.3 and
          1.5 million registrations at present.

With many computer-based developments in the U.K. so far, the
starting point has been the existing hospital medical records
       procedures, particularly for laboratory and
       administrative systems(Wills). This is mainly because
       those records systems are local and tangible, and no
       satisfactory system of national unique personal
       identifier is in use, nor is one expected in the near
       future.

Operationally, these present systems provide considerable benefits
over their preceeding manual indexes, which start to become hard to
maintain when they grow to a million or more entries. Computer-based
hospital indexes provide particular benefits when various case-notes systems
in a health District are to be amalgamated, and this is part of the
reasoning behind current developments at the London Hospital.

At worst, computer assistance will gain a breathing space while the
National Health Service reviews its use of medical records, and hopefully
will re-consider the long-term storage of case-notes for deceased
patients. Until this is done, the chance of reconciling the conflicting
requirements for hospital versus population indexes is small. Meanwhile
the cost of storage,culling and microfilming case-notes must be enormous.

On the population register front, in the United Kingdom, prototype Area-
level Family Practitioner Committee indexes have been established, based
on batch computing facilities(Bussey). In Scandinavia, there are real-
time systems with firm restrictions, operating on a Regional basis, but
for numbers of residents equivalent to the larger health Areas in the
United Kingdom(Petersen).

5.2   Some of the first problems to be tackled

i)   Improving the identification of patients referred by
        General Practitioners for hospital treatment. Given
        the simplest of Area Population Indexes, it should be
        possible to supply hospital staff with a copy of the FPC
        patient identification details enabling them to identify
        an entry on their case-notes system, and record a
        suitable cross-reference on the hospital patient index.

ii)   Improving communication between the Hospital, General
        Practitioner, community and social services, when a
        patient is admitted and discharged from hospital. Again,
        access to a suitable cross-reference to the Area
        Population Index could provide a good basis for this.

iii)   To enable the Area Population Index to carry items of
        particular clinical significance, such as Blood Group,
        transfusion difficulties, drug allergies, entry on
        diabetic register, Australia Antigen positive; also to
        provide a reliable procedure to enable the appropriate

specialist departments to add such clinical details to
the Area Index.

Priority should be given to the development of real-time Area Population
Indexes using the lessons learnt already in Scandinavia and with the
batch FPC Index now working in three Area Health Authorities in the
United Kingdom. Real-time access to such an Index should be given to
acute-care hospitals to aid i) above, and so that the information
described in ii) above can be entered remotely.

5.3   Subsequent Developments

Given an effective Area Population index, with provision for storing a very
limited amount of important clinical information, opportunities exist for
developments such as the following:

> i)   Basing a number of separate specialist records systems
>   on the index, in a way that does not require modifica-
>   tions to the file structures of the index as the
>   applications are added (cf section 6).
>
> ii) Pursuing the integration of hospital case-notes
>   indexes with the Area population index. This can only
>   succeed if policies for medical records are revised
>   (see section 5.1).
>
> iii) Surveys of the Area index, to enable anomalies and
>   omissions relating to N.H.S.personal numbers to be
>   resolved.

The author does not see any significant advantages in providing a direct
linkage between national and Area indexes. "Upwards" access to view any
national index should be sufficient to resolve queries.

Similarly, given that acute hospitals and group practices could access the
Area index, and modify details over which they have been given control,
there is no great advantage in the Area authority being able to view
peripheral records systems based on the index. Indeed there are many
strong arguments against this being allowed, relying on the local
manager to supply a suitable digest of his records when requested.

6. <u>Important Design Features for any Real-time Computer Patient Index</u>

i)   The basic look-up file of patient details should contain
     only those details required for the construction of a list
     of possible matches. These would include flags to indicate
     registration, and perhaps status on all subordinate
     <u>indexes</u> or <u>major</u> record systems. Search procedures should
     allow for particular subsets to be specified, e.g
     patients currently under treatment at a particular
     hospital.

ii) The entries in the basic look-up file should be of
     variable length, so that new features can be added, and
     blank spaces in fields need not be stored.

iii) Requirements specific to Medical Records and FPC should
     be covered by <u>separate</u> associated files and indexes.
     Particularly, people additional to the current local
     population can then be added, e.g.N.H.S. personnel.

iv) A completely reliable, unique and permanent internal
     identification number must be given to each entry on the
     Index, which may be stored in any number of peripheral
     specialist records systems, without the need to maintain
     an associated forward reference to the peripheral file
     within the Index. Computer programs in the peripheral
     systems can then refer directly to the Index to obtain any
     details they require. It would then be impossible for such
     peripheral systems to have their privacy violated via
     record linkages through the central Index.

v)   It should be possible to amend, delete and merge
     registrations only from specified terminals and by
     authorised personnel. Note the interesting decisions and
     cross references that may need to be accommodated when
     two entries are to be merged! For instance, a
     subordinate index may already contain more than one entry
     referring to a single entry on the reference Index.

vi) There should be message-passing facilities between
     peripheral applications, quoting the unique Index entry
     identification number. Notification of changes to

centrally-managed entry details, which require
authorisation before the file can be modified,
could also be handled through such message-
passing facilities.

vii) Authorised changes to patient identification and
registration information should be logged, so that
relevant peripheral locations can be notified via
printed amendment lists, if they have crutial
manual files (e.g. X-ray films) organised according
to such details

viii) Index systems should be accessible to peripheral real-
time computer systems preferably by the systems
pretending to be a single terminal, or a cluster
of terminals. A visual display connected to a
hospital Medical Records or Admissions system could then
be used to search a centrally maintained Area Index,
copy details from a matching entry into the local
file, and lodge details of the local registrations in
the Area Index system.

7. Conclusion

Present plans to use computers to assist in the management of
patient indexes must take note of changes in the structure of the
Health Service. In the U.K, local indexes will be needed in
addition to Area and national indexes for a considerable time to
come. Local indexes and specialist records systems require local
control and privacy, but access to more comprehensive patient
identification systems would enable enormous advantages to be
achieved.

A series of design criteria for any such patient index system
has been presented. These features are not particular to any
computer hardware or database system. Without any adequately
planned approach to these problems, the prospects for major
improvements to patient administration and medical records are
slight. With a sound patient identification procedure, the many
advantages of better communication between health care units can
be achieved without many of the confidentiality problems feared
from fully integrated, over-centralised computer records systems.

REFERENCES

Association of Clinical Pathologists. "Data Processing in Clinical Pathology" 1968   J.Clin.Path 21(2)

Bussey, A. "The FPC - a possible Master Register ?" 1978 Seminar organised by the British Computer Society, Medical Specialist Group.

Cavill, I., Ricketts, C.,Jacobs, A. "Computers in Haematology" 1975 Computers in Medicine series.   Butterworths.

Department of Health and Social Security 1. "Computerisation of Hospital Patient Master Index" 1975   DHSS, Ray House, London

Department of Health and Social Security,2. "FPC Computer Study - Report of the steering Committee" 1978

Harding-Smith, R. "Experience of using an operational information system as the basis for a generalised package" 1977 Proc. Medcomp 77 Online Conferences Limited

Leguit, F., Mol, J. "Patient Identification in a real-time environment" 1977 Proc.Medcomp 77. Online Conferences Limited.

Petersen, H. "The Stockholm County Medical Information System" 1975 Computer Information Systems in Health Care - Sperry Univac

Wills, A. "A computer requesting and reporting system for a variety of clinical laboratories" 1977. Proc. Medcomp 77. Online Conferences Ltd.

Wadbrook D G	Royal Free Hospital	UK	545
Wieme R J	University of Gent	Belgium	339
Willems J L	University of Leuven	Belgium	1
Wills A R	London Hospital	UK	797
Wright P D	Royal Victoria Infirmary	UK	641
Ying Lie O	Institute of Nuclear Medicine	Netherlands	121
Zimmerman J	Washington University	USA	303
Zunzunegiu M V	Clínica Puerta de Hierro	Spain	189

SUBJECT INDEX